Resistance to airflow (Rrs) $\quad = \dfrac{Ppeak - Pplat}{FLOW}$

Pulmonary capillary content (Cc'_{O_2}) $= ([Hgb] \times 1.39) + P_{A_{O_2}} \times .0031$

Shunt fraction $(\dot{Q}s/\dot{Q}T)$ $\quad = \dfrac{Cc'_{O_2} - Ca_{O_2}}{Cc'_{O_2} - C\bar{v}_{O_2}}$

III. RESPIRATORY GAS TRANSPORT

Oxygen delivery $(\dot{O}_{O_2})$ $= \dot{Q}T \times Ca_{O_2}$

Aterial oxygen content (Ca_{O_2}) $= 1.39 \times Sa_{O_2} \times [Hgb] + .0031 \times Pa_{O_2}$

Mixed venous oxygen content $(C\bar{v}_{O_2})$ $= 1.39 \times S\bar{v}_{O_2} \times [Hgb] + .0031 \times P\bar{v}_{O_2}$

Arterio-venous oxygen content difference $= Ca_{O_2} - C\bar{v}_{O_2}$

Oxygen consumption $(\dot{V}_{O_2})$ $= \dot{Q}T\,(Ca_{O_2} - C\bar{v}_{O_2})$

Extraction fraction $\quad = \dfrac{Ca_{O_2} - C\bar{v}_{O_2}}{Ca_{O_2}}$

Respiratory quotient (RQ) $\quad = \dfrac{\dot{V}_{CO_2}}{\dot{V}_{O_2}}$

CO_2 production $(\dot{V}_{CO_2})$ $= f \cdot VT \cdot FE_{CO_2}$

O_2 consumption $(\dot{V}_{O_2})$ $= f \cdot VT \cdot (FI_{O_2} - FE_{O_2})$, when RQ = 1.0

PRINCIPLES
OF
CRITICAL
CARE

Companion
Handbook

NOTICE

Medicine is an ever-changing science. As new research and clinical experience broaden our knowledge, changes in treatment and drug therapy are required. The authors and the publisher of this work have checked with sources believed to be reliable in their efforts to provide information that is complete and generally in accord with the standards accepted at the time of publication. However, in view of the possibility of human error or changes in medical sciences, neither the editors nor the publisher nor any other party who has been involved in the preparation or publication of this work warrants that the information contained herein is in every respect accurate or complete, and they are not responsible for any errors or omissions or for the results obtained from use of such information. Readers are encouraged to confirm the information contained herein with other sources. For example and in particular, readers are advised to check the product information sheet included in the package of each drug they plan to administer to be certain that the information contained in this book is accurate and that changes have not been made in the recommended dose or in the contraindications for administration. This recommendation is of particular importance in connection with new or infrequently used drugs.

PRINCIPLES OF CRITICAL CARE

Companion Handbook

Jesse B. Hall, M.D.
Gregory A. Schmidt, M.D.
Lawrence D.H. Wood, M.D., Ph.D.

McGRAW-HILL, INC.
Health Professions Division

New York   St. Louis   San Francisco   Auckland   Bogotá
Caracas   Lisbon   London   Madrid   Mexico   Milan
Montreal   New Delhi   Paris   San Juan   Singapore
Sydney   Tokyo   Toronto

PRINCIPLES OF CRITICAL CARE
COMPANION HANDBOOK

1234567890   DOCDOC   987543

ISBN   0-07-025828-7

This book was set in Times Roman by Northeastern Graphic Services, Inc.
The editors were J. Dereck Jeffers and Peter McCurdy. Production
supervisor was Rick Ruzycka. R. R. Donnelly and Sons Company was
printer and binder.

Library of Congress Cataloging-in-Publication Data

Principles of critical care. Companion handbook / [edited by] Jesse B.
  Hall, Gregory A. Schmidt, Lawrence D. H. Wood.
    p.   cm.
    Includes index.
    ISBN 0-07-025828-7
    1. Critical care medicine.   I. Hall, Jesse B.   II. Schmidt,
  Gregory A.   III. Wood, Lawrence D. H.
    [DNLM: 1. Critical Care—handbooks. 2. Intensive Care Units—
  handbooks.   WX 218 P9573 1993 Suppl.]
  RC86.7.P752 1993 Suppl.
  616'.028—dc20
  DNLM/DLC
  for Library of Congress   93-48941
                                                                       CIP

To the many students
who have inspired
our teaching,

to our wives for their
limitless patience, and

to Cora Taylor, our secretary,
whose skill, efficiency, and spirit
earn our gratitude daily

CONTENTS

CONTRIBUTORS

This companion to *Principles of Critical Care* consists of brief summaries of chapters of that textbook, each reduced in length and complexity to be readily available as an introductory bedside guide. The original chapters and authors are listed at the end of each synopsis to guide the interested reader to more complete descriptions. The editors are indebted to the original authors for their most excellent and extensive reviews of these topics.

In the preparation of this companion text, the editors were assisted by a superb group of colleagues, each taking responsibility for summarizing a number of the original chapters. These individuals, all members of our training program in critical care, are:

Stephen Amesbury, MD
Shannon Carson, MD
Phillip Cozzi, MD
Phillip Factor, DO
Allan Garland, MD
Katrina Guest, MD
Manu Jain, MD

John Jordan, MD
Constantine Manthous, MD
Ted Naureckas, MD
Maurice Ndukwu, MD
Scott Neeley, MD
David Olson, MD
Kevin Simpson, MD

The editors thank these collaborators for their insights and efforts in the task of condensing such a large amount of information into the book you now hold.

PREFACE

Critical Care has evolved during the last four decades into a discipline combining the clinical scholarships of Anesthesia, Medicine, and Surgery. In editing the first edition of *Principles of Critical Care,* we encouraged our contributors to describe the differential diagnosis and management of each disease as the intensivist sees the critically ill patient. Written from this perspective, 189 chapters described the pathophysiology, diagnosis and management of critical illness and discussed the organization of critical care in 2432 pages. Because the bulk of this book makes it impractical to have available at all times, the editors, with the help of twelve senior critical care fellows, aimed to condense the clinical portions of PCC into this pocket-sized Companion Handbook, which practitioners of critical care can carry with them.

The Companion Handbook is meant to provide a brief introduction to, or reminder of, some aspect of critical care which intensivists may require when they cannot consult PCC. Users of the Companion Handbook should be warned that such a condensed, streamlined approach to critical illness can magnify several pitfalls intrinsic to critical care. By its very nature, critical care is exciting and attracts physicians having an inclination to action. Despite its obvious utility in urgent circumstances, this proclivity can replace effective clinical discipline with excessive, unfocused ICU procedures. We believe this common approach inverts the stable pyramid of bedside skills, placing most attention on the least informative source of data while losing the rational foundation for diagnosis and treatment. An associated problem is that ICU procedures become an end in themselves rather than a means to answer thoughtful clinical questions. Too often, these procedures are implemented to provide "monitoring," ignoring the fact that the only alarm resides in the intensivist's intellect. Students of critical care benefit from the dictum: "Don't just do something, stand there—take time to process the gathered data to formulate a working hypothesis concerning the mechanism(s) responsible for each patient's main problem(s) so that the next diagnostic or treatment intervention can best test that possibility." Without this exhortation to thoughtful clinical decision-making, students of critical care are swept away by the burgeoning tools of the ICU toward the unproductive subspecialty of Critical Care Technology. Furthermore, effective critical care is rarely based in brilliant, incisive, dramatic, and innovative interventions but most often derives from meticulously identifying and titrating each of the patient's multiple problems toward improvement at an urgent but continuous pace. This conservative approach breeds skepticism toward innovative strategies that are incompletely evaluated, and demands that the goals and adverse effects of traditional therapies be clarified so that the least amount of each intervention is employed to achieve its stated therapeutic goal, all in order to maximize one principle of patient care— "First, Do No Harm."

These several important principles of critical care necessarily get minimized in the Companion Handbook, which we consider to complement PCC as a single educational package. Accordingly, we recommend that relevant subjects in the standard textbook be consulted as soon as time permits. To facilitate this consultation, each of the critical illnesses and procedures discussed in the Companion Handbook refers to the relevant chapters in PCC. Used in this way, the companion handbook provides students, residents, fellows, and critical care physicians and nurses with quick access to essential information during the initial presentation or rapid evolution of critical illness in most ICU patients.

PRINCIPLES
OF
CRITICAL
CARE

Companion
Handbook

APACHE III and Assessment of Severity of Illness

Katrina A. Guest

SEVERITY OF ILLNESS AND RISK ASSESSMENT

Physicians admit patients with varied disease processes and degrees of physiologic impairment to intensive care units (ICUs). This decision is usually based on the perceived need for intensive treatment, expectant monitoring, or concentrated nursing care. Thresholds for using ICUs vary greatly and, in fact, no universal consensus on the appropriate use of intensive care resources exists. Quantitative tools that help specify severity of illness could assist in the determination of need for admission.

Beyond admission, prediction of outcome is the next and perhaps most important use of the measures of severity of illness (Table 1-1). The author of the APACHE, William A. Knaus, proposes four benefits derived from accurate predictive models:

1. They allow the physician to focus efforts on patients most likely to benefit.
2. They assist in the decision to limit or withdraw therapy.
3. They facilitate the comparison of performance between ICUs.
4. They facilitate the assessment of new technologies and allow for comparative analysis with standard therapy.

DEVELOPMENT OF PROGNOSTIC SCORING SYSTEMS

Historically, the first prognostic scoring systems were disease-specific prognostic indices, such as the Glasgow Coma Score for patients with acute neurologic injury, the Killip classification system for patients with acute myocardial infarction (Chap. 23), and the

TABLE 1-1 Outcomes of Critical Care of Clinical Importance

Mortality
Morbidity
  Nosocomial infection
  Reintubation
  Self-extubation
  Readmission to the ICU within 24 h
Length of survival following hospital discharge
Quality of survival
  Activities of daily living
  Satisfaction with quality of life achieved
  Return to work

Ranson criteria in acute pancreatitis (Chap. 62). While these systems achieve very reproducible results, they do not take into account comorbidities or underlying chronic disease.

Developed originally in 1981, APACHE sought to determine which clinical parameters best predicted outcome. The system consists of two parts: the Acute Physiology Score (APS), based on specified physiologic measures, and a preadmission health evaluation describing a patient's prior health status.

In 1985 the system was updated to APACHE II, in which several of the physiologic measures were deleted and the weights and thresholds of others were changed. The update also factored in chronic health problems and chronologic age.

The most current version, APACHE III, was published in 1991. It again revised the content and weight of the physiologic measures (Fig. 1-1). New to this revision are scores assigned to the bilirubin, albumin, glucose, urine output, and blood urea nitrogen (BUN) values. Clinical testing of APACHE versions has demonstrated that some physiologic measures were not independent predictors (e.g., urine output and creatinine, serum pH and P_{CO_2}, and respiratory rate with ventilator use were interrelated). Interestingly, serum potassium and serum bicarbonate were not related to outcome and so were deleted from the APS.

USING APACHE III

The total Apache III score is the sum of points from the 16 physiologic measures (Fig. 1-1), from the acid base abnormalities (Fig. 1-2), and from the neurologic assessment (Fig. 1-3), plus the points for chronological age and comorbid condition (Table 1-2). The worst observed abnormality in the first 24 hours of admission is used, and 0 is entered for any unknown values. If for example the patient's mental status was not assessed before sedation and paralysis was instituted, the neurologic score should be 0. This total APS score has a range of 0 to 254. The APS score alone when low (<20) or high (>140) has strong predictive value. In the middle range, a disease-specific coefficient is used to refine predictive value (Fig. 1-4).

Predicting Mortality

As alluded to above, the prediction of mortality requires the consideration of more than the APACHE III score alone. Dr. Knaus and his coinvestigators have determined the weighted coefficients for "reason for ICU care"; elective, emergent, or nonsurgical care; patient's most previous location; and the APACHE III score. Specific information on this weighting system has not been published, but can be obtained from Dr. Knaus, ICU Research Unit, Depart-

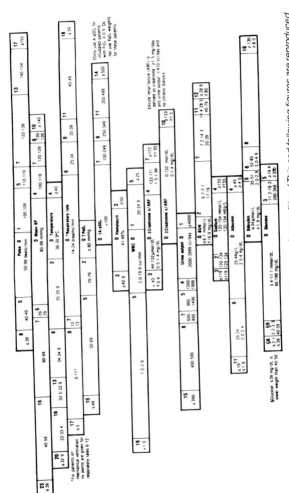

FIG. 1-1 APACHE III scoring for vital signs and laboratory abnormalities. (This and following figures are reproduced with permission from Knaus et al. APACHE III prognostic System. CHEST / 100 / 6 / DECEMBER 1991.)

pH \ pCO₂	<25	25-<30	30-<35	35-<40	40-<45	45-<50	50-<55	55-<60	≥60
<7.15				12				4	
7.15- <7.2									
7.20- <7.25		9		6		3		2	
7.25- <7.30									
7.30- <7.35		5		0				1	
7.35- <7.40									
7.40- <7.45			0		2			1	
7.45- <7.50									
7.50- <7.55			3				12		
7.55- <7.60									
7.60- <7.65	0								
≥7.65									

FIG. 1-2 APACHE III scoring for acid-base disturbances.

4

Eyes open spontaneously or to painful/verbal stimulation

verbal motor	oriented converses	confused conversation	inappropriate words and incomprehensible sounds	no response
obeys verbal command	0	3	10	15
localizes pain	3	8	13	15
flexion withdrawal/ decorticate rigidity	3	13	24	24
decerebrate rigidity/ no response	3	13	29	29

Eyes do not open spontaneously or to painful/verbal stimulation

verbal motor	oriented converses	confused conversation	inappropriate words and incomprehensible sounds	no response
obeys verbal command				16
localizes pain				16
flexion withdrawal/ decorticate rigidity			24	33
decerebrate rigidity/ no response			29	48

The shaded areas without scores represent unusual and unlikely clinical combinations. There were few or no cases in these cells. For the shaded areas with scores we had data that permit us to extrapolate values. Placing a patient in any of these cells should be done after careful confirmation of clinical findings.

FIG. 1-3 APACHE III scoring for neurologic abnormalities according to presence or absence of eye opening.

TABLE 1-2 APACHE III Points for Age and Chronic Health Evaluation

	Points
Age,yr	
≤44	0
45–55	5
60–64	11
65–69	13
70–74	16
75–84	17
≥85	24
Co-morbid condition*	
AIDS	23
Hepatic failure	16
Lymphoma	13
Metastatic cancer	11
Leukemia/multiple myeloma	10
Immunosuppression	10
Cirrhosis	4

*Excluded for elective surgery patients. Add only the highest score which applies.

APACHE III AND RISK OF DEATH: THE IMPORTANCE OF DISEASE

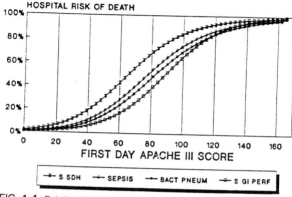

FIG. 1-4 Relationship between APACHE III score and predicted risk of hospital death for patients with postoperative subdural hematomas (S) (SDH), sepsis (other than urinary tract), bacterial pneumonia (BACT PNEUM), and postoperative gastrointestinal perforation (S GI PERF).

ment of Anesthesiology, George Washington University Medical Center, Washington, D.C.

Future Directions

Current research efforts are directed toward improving the accuracy and utility of prognostic scoring systems. The value of assessing severity of illness will become apparent to the clinician at the bedside when information is provided in real time to assist in individual patient decision making. Continued scoring over days of ICU stay is also likely to add predictive value to scoring systems and is the subject of ongoing research.

For further reading in *Principles of Critical Care*, see Chap 46 "Triage and Assessment of Severity of Illness" Carl A Sirio/ William A Knaus

2

Vascular Cannulation

Phillip Factor

PERIPHERAL VENOUS CANNULATION

The peripheral venous system refers to the veins found by palpation or observation in the subcutaneous tissues. These veins are the first choice for vascular access in hemodynamically stable patients. They are readily accessible in most patients and can often accommodate large bore catheters that may rival central lines in their fluid delivery rates. However, in the setting of hemodynamic compromise the time from fluid administration to arrival at the right atrium may be unpredictable.

Many factors affect periphal IV site selection, including adequacy of peripheral veins, required duration of cannulation, patient mobility and comfort, planned infusion rate, and catheter size. Infusion of hypertonic solutions and large bore catheters may prove inrritating to the endothelium, leading to discomfort, infusion phlebitis, and increased risk of catheter related infection. Central venous access may be preferable in these settings.

Complications of peripheral veinous cannulation include infection (cellulitis, septicemia), vasovagal responses, subcutaneous infiltration and skin necrosis, subcutaneous hematomas, and thrombophlebitis. Catheter care is an extensive subject, but based on a number of studies and the practices at our hospitals we recommend the following:

1. All peripheral catheters should be changed at intervals of 72 h or less.
2. Catheters inserted in emergency circumstances should be changed as soon as possible.
3. Dressing changes should be performed every 24 to 48 h, preferably by a dedicated IV team.

CENTRAL VENOUS CANNULATION

Central venous cannulation is preferred over peripheral access for the indications listed in Table 2-1. No absolute contraindication to central venous access can be identified. Other than coagulopathy and recent fibrinolytic therapy, contraindications are site specific (Table 2-2).

General Considerations

Regardless of the site or method chosen for central venous cannulation the patient must be well informed and appropriate consent

TABLE 2-1 Indications for Central Venous Access

Inadequate peripheral veins
Central venous pressure monitoring (CVP, PA catheters)
Administration of phlebitic medications (potassium, chemotherapy)
Extremely rapid fluid administration
Cardiopulmonary resuscitation
Intracardiac pacing
Frequent phlebotomies
Long term intravenous therapy (antibiotics, chemotherapy)
Hemodialysis
Hyperalimentation
Administration of vasoactive drugs

TABLE 2-2 Relative Contraindications to Central Venous Cannulation

General
Physician inexperience
Coagulopathy
Recent fibrinolytic therapy
Severe thrombocytopenia
Inability to identify pertinent landmarks
Infection or burn at planned catheter entry site
Uncooperative patient

Subclavian Vein
Upper thoracic trauma
Compromised pulmonary function (COPD)
High levels of PEEP
Coagulopathy
SVC Thrombosis

Internal Jugular Vein
Inability to identify landmarks
COPD, High levels of PEEP
Tracheostomy with excessive pulmonary secretions
SVC thrombosis

Femoral Vein
Absence of femoral pulse
Vena caval compromise: clot, extrinsic compression, IVC filter
Local infection at insertion site
Penetrating abdominal trauma
Cardiac arrest or low flow states
Requirements for patient mobility

obtained. All equipment should be at the bedside and the patient pre-positioned. In the absence of externalized cerebral ventricular drains or incipient respiratory failure, most patients can tolerate a few moments of reverse Trendelenburg positioning. Supplemental oxygen should be employed in patients at risk for arterial desaturation (e.g., lower lobe pneumonias or placement of sterile drapes over the face). Skin antisepsis should include an iodine based solution that should be allowed to air dry. Sterile technique is required with the placement of any central line. Inexperienced operators should be closely supervised. Selection of sedated, mechanically ventilated patients should be considered for physicians in training.

Critically ill patients who require central venous cannulation are frequently confused or uncooperative. Extreme caution must be exercised to prevent uncontrolled general anesthesia when parenteral sedation is used, especially in patients with compromised cardiopulmonary and neurologic function. Short acting parenteral benzodiazepines or sedating antihistamines are useful in this setting.

Following catheter placement adequacy of blood return should be reconfirmed. Post-procedure chest x-ray should be used to confirm catheter tip location (ideally 2 to 4 cm above the junction of the right atrium and superior vena cava) and to rule out pneumothorax.

Catheter Selection

Catheter-through-needle devices should be avoided. These cannulation devices require utilization of a larger than necessary needle and confer the additional risk of catheter emboli if the catheter is inadvertently withdrawn through the needle. Readily available catheter-over-needle devices and prepared guide wire kits make this method unnecessary, even in emergency situations.

Long arm catheters are placed via the antecubital veins and advanced into the central venous circulation. These devices are excellent choices for patients with coagulopathies. Advancement of these catheters into the thorax can be difficult. These catheters can occupy the entire lumen of an antecubital vein leading to venous stasis, endothelial injury, and thrombophlebitis.

The requirement for long term indwelling central venous catheters has been met with the development of barium impregnated silicone rubber (Silastic) catheters (i.e., Hickman, Gorshong, Quinton, Broviac) that can be tunneled beneath the skin prior to entry into a central vein. These "tunneled" catheters have a small Dacron cuff that is positioned subcutaneously to serve as a mechanical barrier to migration of bacteria along the catheter. These devices require a high level of care that includes frequent heparin flushes and dressing changes. Patients can be educated to care for their own catheters, allowing increased independence from health care facilities. Tunneled catheters are not without risk: Infection, central vein thrombosis, and thrombotic occlusion of the catheter are not uncommon problems. Slowed infusion rates or inability to withdraw blood may suggest catheter thrombosis. Administration of low dose streptokinase through the catheter may be useful in this setting.

Totally implantable catheter devices obviate some of the problems with tunneled catheters. These devices typically consist of a stainless steel or plastic portal with a self-sealing diaghragm connected to a central catheter. A Huber needle is inserted through the skin to access the device. The subcutaneous location eliminates the need for difficult dressing changes. Daily heparin flushes are not required. The reported infection rates are approximately one-third those of externalized, tunneled catheters. Mechanical problems such as occlusion and inability to withdraw blood occur frequently.

The high flows required for dialysis require the placement of large bore double lumen catheters into the central venous system. Stiff, large bore catheters limit patient mobility, are associated with venous perforation, and require frequent replacement. Utilization of flexible silicone rubber catheters with Dacron cuffs (e.g., Quinton Permacath) now allow these catheters to be left in place for several weeks pending creation and maturation of an AV graft or fistula.

Multiple lumen catheters have supplanted the need for multiple central venous lines. The use and development of these catheters has preceded adequate study of the risks, costs, and complications. Pending further study, several recommendations regarding their use can be made:

1. They should only be used when peripheral access is inadequate to support multiple lines;
2. The subclavian vein should be the preferred site of insertion;
3. These catheters should not be placed through catheter sheath introducers; and
4. a uniform, hospital-wide protocol describing catheter use and care (e.g., frequency of heparin flushes and dressing changes, specific port utilization) should be employed. No specific recommendations can be made regarding duration of cannulation. Routine catheter changes every 5 to 7 days may decrease the incidence of line related sepsis in some settings but are associated with an increased risk of insertion-related complications. In the absence of additional data at this time cannulation beyond 4 weeks can not be recommended.

Catheter sheath introducers are large bore catheters (8.5 F) that were developed to facilitate the placement of pulmonary artery catheters. The short, teflon coated catheters are also useful for rapid volume administration (see below). Several problems have been associated with these devices including vascular perforation, air embolism, and increased risk of air embolism. These catheters are not designed for long term use (i.e., > 72 h) and should not be left in place following restoration of intravascular volume or removal of a PA catheter.

Certain clinical settings require extremely rapid delivery of volume. Placement of a short, 8.5 F sheath introducer into a large central vein (internal jugular, subclavian or femoral vein) can allow for pressurized delivery rates of up to 1428 mL/min through the side port. Insertion of a 6-in. 14 gauge through the introducer's diaghragm can produce a venturi effect that will further increase delivery rates. Fluid administration rates in these ranges are most likely to be limited by the IV tubing. Use of blood infusion, large bore trauma, or urologic tubing will reduce this limitation.

COMPLICATIONS OF CENTRAL VENOUS CANNULATION

The complications of central venous cannulation are listed in Table 2-3. Pneumothoraces occurring from central venous cannulation do not always require tube thoracostomy. Chest tubes should be placed in patients with hemodynamic or respiratory compromise (e.g., tension pneumothorax) or nonresolving pneumothoraces. Uncomplicated pneumothoraces (i.e., no pleural fluid) can be treated with small diameter chest tubes attached to one-way valves (thoracic vents). Catheter embolism is typically associated with the use of catheter-through-needle devices. Removal of these

TABLE 2-3 Complications of Central Venous Cannulation

Pneumothorax
Catheter or guidewire embolism
Catheter knotting
Air embolism
Central vein thrombosis
Arrhythmias
Myocardial or central vein perforation
Cardiac tamponade
Infection (local or systemic)
Hydrothorax
Hematoma
Myocardial perforation
Phrenic nerve, brachial plexus damage
Subcutaneous emphysema or fluid infiltration
Arterial puncture and/or laceration
Catheter malposition
Thoracic duct laceration

emboli can present a difficult clinical challenge. Snares have been developed to facilitiate their removal. The sudden onset of mental status changes, hypotension, and rash (livido reticularis of the upper extremities) should suggest the diagnosis of air embolism. This complication can occur with any form of intravenous access. A churning, "cog-wheel" murmur may be heard. Patients should be placed in a left lateral decubitis position. Successful aspiration of air from the right ventricle has been reported using large bore central lines. Central vein thrombosis occurs in 20 to 70 percent of chronically cannulated patients. Most patients are asymptomatic. Diagnosis is based on clinical suspicion, reduced catheter flow rates, and signs of venous obstruction. Venography is the diagnostic procedure of choice. Doppler ultrasound and ^{125}I fibrinogen scanning are also diagnostically useful. Fibrinolytics can be useful in symptomatic patients; rarely is surgical thrombectomy required. Arrhythmias occur frequently with the passage of central lines into the right ventricle. Patients with pre-existing left bundle branch block may be at risk for complete heart block if the right bundle becomes injured during catheter placement. However, studies suggest that empiric pacemaker placement is not required; rather transcutaneous transvenous pacemakers should be readily available if required. Central venous and right ventricular perforations are unusual but not rare complications of central venous cannulation. Perforation typically occurs with the use of stiff catheters that are advanced too far into the central circulation. New pleural fluid collections or x-ray signs of a mediastinal hematoma should suggest the diagnosis if the perforation is above the pericardium. Right ventricular or SVC perforation is usually fatal and presents as cardiac tamponade. Cautious advancement of pliable catheters can prevent this problem. The distal portion of central catheters should be 2 cm or more above the junction of the right atrium and superior vena cava (SVC), and the catheter tip should lie parallel to the cannulated vessel, not under tension perpendicular to its wall.

In general, if catheter related infection is suspected, and the entry site appears clean, then the catheter can be changed over a guide wire pending the results of blood and quantitative catheter tip cultures. If the catheter tip culture yields more than 15 colony forming units (cfu) and the blood culture is positive for the same organism, then catheter related sepsis is likely. Positive catheter cultures (>15 cfu) and negative blood cultures indicate catheter infection. Catheter related sepsis requires that the line be removed and a new insertion site selected. Tunneled catheter related infections present a more challenging problem. Many cases of sepsis related to these lines can be treated with parenteral antibiotics. The catheter should be removed if signs of septicemia persist (>3–5 days) despite appropriate antibiotics, septic emboli appear, or if the catheter tunnel appears grossly infected. Successful treatment of fungal catheter infections is unlikely and should prompt removal of the catheter.

Following catheter removal, persistent bacteremia in the presence of documented central vein thrombosis suggests the diagnosis of catheter related septic central vein thrombosis (CR-SCVT). This condition can be treated medically with antibiotics and anticoagulation.

Routine changes of central lines over guidewires continue to be investigated and cannot be recommended at this time. Utilization of catheters designed for long term use, frequent inspection of the insertion site for signs of inflammation (every other day coupled with dressing changes), line and dressing care by a dedicated IV team, and limitation of central line manipulation can limit the incidence of line related sepsis. Catheters should be changed only in the presence of signs suggestive of line related sepsis (e.g., otherwise unexplained fever and leukocytosis). The routine changing of central lines at predetermined intervals is not recommended at this time.

ARTERIAL CATHETERIZATION

Arterial pressure monitoring has become commonplace in critical care settings because of improvements in the function and availability of bedside pressure monitoring devices and the increased use of arterial blood gases. Arterial lines can be used for infusion of fluids and nonvasoactive medications in emergency settings. Because of its peripheral and accessible location, the radial artery is the first choice for most patients. The axillary, dorsalis pedis, and femoral arteries are used less often, though when used in appropriately selected patients have similar overall complication rates as radial artery cannulation.

No absolute contraindication to radial artery cannulation can be offered other than absence of ulnar collateral flow. Patients with Raynaud's phenomenon, thromboangiitis obliterans, and other large vessel vasculitidies should be considered carefully prior to catheter placement. Fifteen to twenty percent of patients have inadequate collateral circulation to the hand. Allen's test should be performed in all patients prior to attempts at cannulation of the radial artery. Return of normal color to the fingers should occur within 7 s; longer than 14 s should definitely be considered abnormal. The limitations of this bedside maneuver are of note, thus ultrasonic flow analysis of the arterial supply should be employed whenever possible.

The overall complication rate of arterial catheterization is difficult to determine but appears to rise with underlying coagulopathy, hypotension, underlying peripheral vascular disease, duration of cannulation, placement by cutdown, wrist circumference, number of cannulation attempts, and catheter to artery diameter ratio. The three primary complications of note are bleeding, infection, and distal limb ischemia. Other less frequent complications are site related and peripheral nerve damage (especially the radial nerve), arteriovenous fistulas, pseudoaneurysm formation, air embolism, cerebral embolism, retroperitoneal hemorrhage, and peritoneal perforation.

ALTERNATIVES TO VENOUS CANNULATION

The extensive venous channels within the corpora cavernosa of the penis allow for its use as a short term venous access site. An 18 to 20 gauge needle can be inserted into one of the corpora. Drainage rates averaging 13.4 mL/s have been reported. Utilization of this route in emergency settings is untested.

Placement of a steel needle (16 to 20 gauge) into the marrow of the ribs or sternum in adults can allow for infusion rates in excess of 100 mL/h. Hypertonic and strongly alkaline solutions should be avoided. The theoretical risk of fat or cortical bone emboli has not been substantiated by clinical reports.

Subcutaneous infusions of small amounts of fluids and medications can be used when other routes are unavailable. Excessive delivery of fluids can result in impairment of blood supply to the skin with subsequent necrosis and sloughing. Subcutaneous administration of medications (e.g., epinephrine, terbutaline, insulin, heparin) is well documented to be safe. Absorption may be unreliable in patients with circulatory collapse.

Certain drugs can be administered via an endotracheal tube or directly into the peritoneum in emergency situations. Valium, atropine, lidocaine, isoproterenol, epinephrine, naloxone, and terbutaline have all been used endotracheally in the absence of intravascular access. Dosages require modification (e.g., double the usual epinephrine dose) to counterbalance reduced and delayed absorption.

INTRAVENOUS FLUIDS THERAPY

Table 2-4 lists currently available crystalloids and colloids. The selection of the appropriate fluid for intravenous therapy will vary with the clinical setting. Selection requires a thorough understanding of body fluid distribution and an ability to determine the type of deficit that a particular patient has. In general the decision must first be made if a patient is intravascularly depleted. If so then selection of an isotonic or hypertonic solution would be appropriate. Hypotonic solutions such as 5% dextrose are rapidly redistributed among both the intra- and extracellular compartments leaving

TABLE 2-4 Currently Available Intravenous Fluids

Crystalloids
  Dextrose (2.5%, 5%, 10%)
  Sodium chloride (0.45%, 0.9%, 3%, 5%)
  Ringers solutions (lactate, acetate, injection)
Colloids
  Albumin (5%, 25%)
  Starches (hetastarch, pentastarch)
  Dextran (40, 70)
  Gelatins
  Fresh frozen plasma
  Packed red blood cells
  Cryoprecipitate

only 8.5% of the administered volume in the vascular space. As such hypotonic solutions are principally used for treatment of electrolyte abnormalities such as hypernatremia. Twenty-five percent of a 0.9% NaCl solution will remain intravascular. In contrast, nearly 100% of administered colloids remain intravascular for hours to days. Crystalloid and colloid are both effective volume expanders when used for treatment of hypovolemic shock. When used in this setting less volume and times are required to volume resuscitate patients when colloid is used.

The complications associated with crystalloid use are those of inadequate (prerenal azotemia) and excessive volume resuscitation (pulmonary edema), electrolyte and acid base abnormalities (e.g. metabolic acidosis or alkalosis, hyperkalemia, hyponatremia), serum protein dilution and edema. In addition to their cost, colloids are not without their own complications which include; renal failure, coagulopathies, anaphylaxis, and electrolyte abnormalities.

For further reading in *Principles of Critical Care,* see Chap 24 "Vascular Cannulation" Phillip Factor/Jacob Iasha Sznajder

| **Blood Products and Plasmapheresis**

J. Edward Jordan

In this chapter, the types of individual blood products, indications for their use, and complications will be reviewed. Plasmapheresis, a method of exchanging existing blood components, will also be described.

Whole Blood

Whole blood is packaged and stored without removal of any components; however, blood stored for more than 24 h contains few active platelets or granulocytes. Factors V and VIII are present in greatly decreased amounts. Thus, whole blood transfusion does not render all of the biological activity of the original specimen. After transfusion with one unit of whole blood, 1.0 g/dL hemoglobin elevation will be noted in the absence of continued bleeding. The indications for transfusion with whole blood are limited but patients in hemorrhagic shock with coagulation factor abnormalities may benefit from its use.

Packed Red Blood Cells (PRBCs)

The red cell contents from a unit of whole blood are separated from the plasma and stored in glycerol. General indications for use include the replacement of hemoglobin for oxygen carrying capacity in patients with reduced hemoglobin, such as patients with major trauma and bleeding, shock secondary to acute blood loss, intraoperative blood loss >750 mL, and significant anemic states requiring intervention. Should the patient require, extra steps to remove platelets and leukocytes may be taken but are usually only performed to reduce the antigen load in patients who develop reactions to these products.

Complications from packed cell infusion are common. Acute hemolytic transfusion reactions are usually due to an antibody in the patient's plasma which reacts with donor red cells. The result can be intravascular or extravascular hemolysis. Intravascular hemolysis is often rapid, occurring with only a few milliliters of blood, and can lead to shock, acute renal failure, or bleeding due to disseminated intravascular coagulation (DIC) and hypofibrinogenemia. Symptoms include chills, fever, a burning sensation along the course of the vein, headache, oppressive chest pain, back pain, or facial flushing. The following steps should be taken in the event of such a reaction, or if incompatible PRBCs are being infused because of error:

1. Stop the infusion.
2. Quickly check the labels, forms, and patient identification.
3. Record and monitor urinary output.
4. Maintain urine output of at least 30 mL/h.
5. Measure the blood pressure and institute therapy for shock, if present.
6. Notify the blood bank and initiate transfusion reaction workup; send unused blood bag and freshly drawn blood samples to the blood bank with transfusion reaction workup request forms.
7. Perform baseline and follow-up lab studies including electrolytes, BUN, creatinine, PT, PTT, fibrinogen, platelet count, fibrin degradation products, D dimer, hemoglobin, urinalysis, serum evaluation for hemoglobinemia, and bilirubin with repeated bilirubin assays 5 to 7 h later.
8. The renal failure which may accompany hemolytic transfusion reactions is thought to be secondary to damage caused by hypotension and vasoconstriction following destruction of red cells with formation of red cell stroma-antibody complexes. In consultation with the renal and hematology services, consider whole blood or plasma exchange, dialysis, or heparin therapy, depending on the clinical condition of the patient and laboratory workup.

Extravascular hemolysis is usually not clinically severe but may present with chills, fever, or hyperbilirubinemia. Specific treatment for a purely extravascular hemolytic reaction is usually not necessary, although intravascular and extravascular reactions may occur together. In any event, the patient should be well hydrated and urine output and hematocrit monitored.

Massive Transfusion

Replacement of the patient's blood volume over a 24 h period defines massive transfusion and is associated with several potential complications. Platelets and coagulation factors may be diluted during massive transfusion. Aging red cell products also have potassium ions released from the red blood cells, and patients with shock, acidosis, and renal insufficiency may be at risk of iatrogenic hyperkalemia. Cold blood products may contribute to hypothermia. Transfusions also offer a significant volume challenge, and frequent assessment of patients receiving substantial blood products is required in order to detect volume overload.

Platelets

Transfusion of platelets is indicated for thrombocytopenia. Abnormalities in bleeding time (a measure of platelet function) usually do not appear until the platelet count drops below 50,000/mm^3. Prophylactic platelet therapy (to prevent spontaneous bleeding) is usually reserved for patients with platelet counts below 20,000/mm^3. Higher platelet counts are needed in patients with significant active bleeding in the setting of thrombocytopenia or thrombocytopathy. Adequate hemostasis can usually be achieved with platelet counts of 70,000 to 100,000/mm^3 for most surgical procedures. Replacement of platelets is generally not helpful in disease states where the platelets are destroyed or sequestered unless there is life threatening hemorrhage, and may not be effective in patients with hypersplenism, fever, sepsis, DIC, platelet antibodies, or alloimmunization to major histocompatibility antigens present on the donor platelets.

In a 70 kg adult, one platelet pack may be expected to increase the platelet count by 5,000 to 10,000/mm^3 1 h posttransfusion. After exposure to many platelet transfusions, sensitization may occur and the platelet count may fail to rise as predicted. Single donor platelet products are often used to limit the exposure of the patient to histocompatibility (HLA) antigens present on the platelets and reduce the likelihood of sensitization. Alloimmunized patients may show a rise in platelet count if they receive platelets from family members, especially siblings. If these platelets fail to raise the platelet count, several units of platelet concentrates can be administered at short intervals (4 units q 4–6 h) since transfusion of multiple units from different donors increases the chance of selecting histocompatible units.

Granulocytes

Granulocyte transfusions are reserved for febrile neutropenic patients (<500 neutrophils/mm^3) who have a good chance of bone marrow recovery and have bacterial or fungal infections unresponsive to antibiotic therapy. Granulocyte transfusions may also be considered for septic, pancytopenic neonates with decreased bone marrow reserve. Prior to granulocyte transfusion, non aspirin antipyretics, diphenhydramine, meperidine, and corticosteroids should be administered and concurrent use of amphotericin B avoided. Complications from these transfusions are common and include chills, fever, allergic reactions, and severe respiratory insufficiency. Febrile reactions can be distinguished from hemolytic reactions as outlined above. High fevers in this setting warrant blood cultures to rule out bacterial contamination. Some patients develop transient dyspnea due to noncardiogenic pulmonary edema in association with transfusion, which has been attributed to a reaction between leukoagglutinins and leukocytes. The transfusion should be stopped and intravenous corticosteroids are often given. Washed blood products may prevent further reactions.

Plasma Products

Plasma is indicated for patients with coagulation factor deficiency, hemolytic uremic syndrome, thrombotic thrombocytopenic purpura, and antithrombin III deficiency. Clotting factor concentrates may be indicated for certain factor deficiencies especially when the volume of plasma required would lead to excessive volume administration. It is not appropriate to administer plasma for volume expansion alone. Reactions to plasma are largely allergic in character. Asthma, glottal edema, urticaria, or other rashes may occur as a manifestation of an allergy to an antigen in the infusing plasma. These reactions are generally minor and an antihistamine may allow resumption of the infusion. Individuals who are IgA deficient may develop antibodies to transfused IgA, subsequently leading to an anaphylactic reaction which characteristically occurs after only a few milliliters of blood or plasma are infused. Further transfusions will require multiply washed red cells to eliminate IgA containing plasma.

Cryoprecipitate contains von Willebrand factor, factor VIII, fibrinogen, factor XIII, and fibronectin. It is used for therapy of von Willebrand's disease, hemophilia A, factor XIII deficiency, and fibrinogen deficiency. It must be ABO matched. Large amounts of cryoprecipitate have been associated with hyperfibrinogenemia, which may lead to bleeding.

Infusion of factor concentrates makes it possible to deliver large quantities of clotting factors in a minimal volume. Factor VIII concentrate is used for severe hemophilia A and in patients with significant factor VIII inhibitors. Overdose of factor VIII may also lead to hyperfibrinogenemia and bleeding. Factor IX concentrate is used to treat hemophilia B, deficiencies of factors II, VII, or X and factor VIII inhibitor. Side effects may include chills, fever, headache, nausea, flushing, thrombosis, and DIC.

Albumin and Plasma Protein Fraction

These products are derived from plasma, heat treated to prevent disease transmission, and indicated for patients who are hypovolemic *and* hypoproteinemic. Unlike plasma protein fraction, albumin may be given quickly, intra-arterially, and during cardiopulmonary bypass. A 5% concentration of either solution has osmotic and oncotic properties equivalent to plasma.

Disease Transmission

Donors with possible human immunodeficiency virus (HIV) infection are discouraged from contributing to the blood donor pool. In addition, all blood donations are submitted for enzyme-linked immunosorbent assay (ELISA), and, if positive, confirmatory Western blot, to insure that HIV infected blood does not freely enter the donor pool. It is important to recognize that there is a period during which the donor may be infected with HIV but has not yet formed the antibody which is discovered in the screening tests. Donated blood is now screened for hepatitis B and C, and it is hoped that the incidence of non A, non B hepatitis associated with transfusion therapy will fall with the ability to identify hepatitis C infected blood products. Bacteria are rarely present in blood products, causing septic reactions in the recipient. Most reactions are due to endotoxin produced by cold growing, gram negative species, including *Pseudomonas* species, *Citrobacter freundii, Escherichia coli,* and *Yersinia enterocolitica.* High fever, shock, hemoglobinuria, DIC, and renal failure have been reported. Cytomegalovirus and Epstein-Barr virus can be transmitted by leukocytes and can cause a post-perfusion syndrome at 21 to 42 days. Immunocompromised patients may develop fever, splenomegaly, liver dysfunction, and lymphocytosis.

Therapeutic Apheresis

Therapeutic apheresis is performed when it is desirable to remove a portion of a patient's blood that contains a pathologic component. Patients must be heparin anticoagulated and connected to specialized machines which exchange their plasma for an albumin-saline mixture. The heparin dose must be carefully monitored since the patients are predisposed to bleeding because of their underlying disease. In addition, citrate (which is used for plasma anticoagulation) may cause precipitous falls in serum calcium if infused rapidly. Diseases which are amenable to plasmapheresis include hyperviscosity syndromes, myasthenia gravis, rapidly progressive glomerulonephritis (idiopathic or secondary vasculitis), Goodpasture's syndrome, Refsum's disease, thrombotic thrombocytopenic purpura (TTP), thyroid storm, certain drug overdoses, severe acute polyradiculoneuropathy (Guillain-Barré syndrome), thrombocytosis, severe granulocytosis, lymphocytosis, and sickle cell disease.

For further reading in *Principles of Critical Care,* see Chap 35 "Blood Products and Plasmapheresis" Beverly W Baron/Joseph M Baron

---

4

Airway Management and Tracheostomy

Ikeadi Maurice Ndukwu

ENDOTRACHEAL INTUBATION

Translaryngeal endotracheal intubation (ETT) can dramatically stabilize a patient suffering from critical respiratory distress. Endotracheal intubation is generally performed to provide a reliable conduit for the delivery of inhalation or positive pressure therapy, to assure adequately low resistance pathway for pulmonary gas flow in patients who have severely impaired respiratory functions, and to protect the lungs from aspiration. The specific indications for ETT include airway support during cardiopulmonary arrest resuscitation, respiratory failure, frequent recurrent nonperfusing dysrhythmias, and hemodynamically compromising sepsis (Table 4-1).

The minimum required equipment for an ETT during cardiopulmonary arrest is a tube with a functioning cuff, stylet, laryngoscope, oxygen mask, suction, and a stethoscope. To enhance patient safety during the intubation process, the most experienced in ETT should perform the intubation. The patient should be evaluated for airway anatomy variance and neurologic status. Micrognathia, short neck,

TABLE 4-1 Indications for Intubation

Cardiopulmonary Arrest

Airway Support
  Mechanical airway obstruction (e.g., edema, pharyngeal mass)
  Pharyngeal instability (facial fractures)
  Depressed level of consciousness with absent gag reflex, absent cough, or inability to maintain airway with head in flexion.
  Bulbar or generalized motor weakness

Respiratory Failure
  Arterial blood gases with $PO_2 < 50$ torr or arterial hemoglobin saturation $< 85\%$ on $FlO_2 > .6$
  Severe respiratory acidosis or severe uncompensated metabolic acidosis without an obviously reversible etiology.
  Tachypnea > 35 breaths/min with accessory muscle recruitment and signs of patient distress (i.e., diaphoresis, tachy- or bradydysrhythmias, severe dyspnea, clammy cyanosis)

Miscellaneous
  Frequent recurrent non-perfusing dysrhythmias
  Hemodynamically compromising sepsis

(Reproduced with permission from Mitchell Keamy: Airway Management and Intubation, in Hall JB, Schmidt GA, Wood LDH: Principles of Critical Care, McGraw-Hill, New York, 1992.)

temporomandibular joint disease, or cervical spine immobility may make direct laryngoscopy problematic. Increased risk of aspiration should be expected. Adequate suction with a large bore rigid tip (Yankauer tip) should be available. Cricoid pressure (Sellick maneuver) prior to intubation provides relative protection against the risk of aspiration by physically occluding the esophagus. The pressure should be maintained until tube position is confirmed by auscultation of the lung fields and epigastrium.

Orotracheal intubation has the advantage of requiring minimal equipment and is the best technique in apneic patients. The necessity for suitable pharyngeal anatomy, risk of cervical spine injury, and need for sedation and paralysis to allow direct laryngoscopy, are some disadvantages of orotracheal intubation. Damage to patients' teeth, possible operator hand injury, and vision impairment by secretions, contribute to performance difficulties.

Nasotracheal intubation allows for favorable head and mandibular position during insertion, can be done blind, facilitates oral care, increases patient communication ability, and provides a stable taping position. The disadvantages to nasotracheal intubation include use of a smaller tube, hemorrhage secondary to burrowing under the nasal mucosa, risk of damage to turbinates and nares, and high incidence of purulent and serous otitis and sinusitis. Contraindications to nasal intubation include immunocompromise, acute facial or cerebral trauma, full therapeutic anticoagulation, platelet count below 80,000, and platelet dysfunction due to renal failure or drugs.

Cricothyrotomy performed at the level of the cricothyroid notch for insertion of a small tube (6.0) is reserved for true emergencies. It is indicated when the patient cannot be adequately ventilated and has sustained an unstable cervical spinal injury. Cricothyrotomy has the advantages of direct assess to the trachea. However, its disadvantage may be that a skilled physician may not be present.

Pharmacologic Aids

Pharmacologic aid to intubation has three goals: to establish sedation or paralysis; to provide patient comfort during the procedure; and to decrease hormonal, neurologic, and cardiovascular stress. The awake patient will benefit from some combination of amnesia, analgesia, hypnosis, muscle paralysis, and autonomic stabilization. Local anesthesia in the forms of topical oral anesthesia, transtracheal anesthesia, superior laryngeal nerve blocks, or 4% lidocaine nebulization not to exceed 4mg/kg, are excellent means to alleviate the pain and stress of intubation. Midazolam, a water soluble, potent anxiolytic, amnestic, and hypnotic, is most useful in the agitated, disoriented, combative, or uncooperative patient. A dose of 1 mg intravenously is an appropriate starting point. Demerol, alfentanil, and fentanyl are narcotics with rapid onset that blunt the pain of laryngoscopy and intubation. Succinylcholine (1.2 mg/kg) and vecuronium (0.1 mg/kg) are the most commonly administered paralytics for intubation.

Post-Intubation Care

Post-intubation care should include routine check of cuff pressure (maintain pressure < 25 cm H_2O); auscultation to evaluate patency, position, and leak; inspection of the tube's external fastening area for depth, skin integrity and minimal play; chest radiograph for assessment of tube position and barotrauma. Examination of the sinuses of nasally intubated patients should be part of the daily routine.

Complications of Intubation

Complications of intubation result from mechanical trauma and unrecognized prolonged malposition (Table 4-2). The most acute and potentially lethal complication of ETT is an obstructed tube. This can be caused by biting, kinking of the tube, or luminal obstruction with mucus, vomitus (which has leaked past the cuff and is coughed retrograde into the tube), or clot. An obstructed tube is an emergency situation. If the patient is aggressively bucking, has paroxysmal coughing, or is biting the tube, rapid paralysis will relieve the immediate obstruction and facilitate further assessment. If a suction catheter cannot be passed and no remediable kinking is obvious, the tube must be immediately replaced, or removed to allow bag-mask ventilation.

Dental trauma is common; dislodged teeth, if rapidly reimplanted, will usually maintain vitality. A protruding metal stylet may result in arytenoid dislocation, vocal cord tear, and esophageal or tracheal perforation. Mainstem intubation will result in hypoxemia due to pulmonary shunt, and, by exposing the ventilated lung to relatively large tidal volumes, may promote barotrauma.

Infections and localized trauma are the leading complications of chronic ETT. Pneumonia may result from aspiration of gastric contents or impaired mucociliary clearance system. Otitis and sinusitis are also common and can lead to fatal sepsis. Stridor may be secondary to posterior cricoarytenoid muscle edema and scarring, vocal cord synechiae, or tracheal stenosis. Tracheal necrosis leading to stenotic scar or perforation may occur because of excessive cuff pressure. A good outcome from ETT complications can be achieved with early recognition and proper management.

TABLE 4-2 Complications of Intubation

Peri-Intubation
  Right mainstem intubation
  Esophageal intubation
  Gastric aspiration
  Dental injury, tooth aspiration
  Tracheal or esophageal tear
  Hypertension/tachycardia with secondary cardiac or CNS injury
  Hypotension
  Temporomandibular joint dislocation
  Vocal cord tear or arytenoid dislocation
  Bronchospasm
  Epistaxis
  Nasopharyngeal mucosal tear
  Avulsed nasal turbinate
  Cardiac dysrhythmias
  Pain
Acute
  Obstructed ETT
  Right mainstem intubation
  Cuff leak
  Aspiration
Chronic
  Serous or purulent otitis
  Sinusitis, sepsis
  Nose or lip necrosis
  Tracheal mucosal injury
  Tracheomalacia
  Laryngeal stricture, secondary to:
    Posterior cricoarytenoid muscle edema, scarring
    Vocal cord synechiae
    Tracheal stenosis

(Reproduced with permission from Mitchell Keamy: Airway Management and Intubation, in Hall JB, Schmidt GA, Wood LDH: Principles of Critical Care, McGraw-Hill, New York, 1992.)

EXTUBATION

Extubation of the critically ill patient following more than 2 or 3 days of intubation should be approached cautiously. The patient should have adequate respiratory drive, level of consciousness and ability to generate sufficient pharyngeal muscle tone to support the upper airway. Prior to extubation, the patient should be suctioned, and the means for bag-mask ventilation and immediate intubation should be available. If intubation has been chronic (> 6 days), then passage of a small diameter fiberoptic bronchoscope to observe the tracheal anatomy and cord function as the tube is withdrawn past the glottis is prudent.

Patients with failed prior extubation and subsequent reintubation, those with facial burns or infections, or those with severe anatomic impediments to intubation benefit from a more deliberate approach to extubation. Delay extubation if tracheal or glottic edema is present as suggested by the absence of a leak past the tube into the pharynx when the tube cuff is deflated.

Inspiratory stridor or frank inspiratory obstruction is a rare complication of chronic intubation. Posterior commissure edema or retained secretions on the vocal cords commonly contribute. The initial management includes bag-mask ventilation, continuous positive airway pressure (CPAP) if available, and nebulized racemic epinephrine. Reintubate the patient if stridor, agitation, or blood gas derangement persists. The patient should be reintubated with a small tube (6.0 or 6.5) passed nasally to minimize the force applied to the posterior commissure. The patient should be treated with 4 mg dexamethasone every 6 h for 2 days, and a laryngologist should be consulted.

TRACHEOSTOMY

Indications for tracheostomy (tracheotomy) include overcoming upper airway obstruction, providing airway access for maintenance of tracheobronchial toilet or long-term assisted mechanical ventilation; and facilitating weaning from mechanical to spontaneous ventilation. The advantages of tracheostomy include a shorter and more direct route to the lower airways, accommodation of a large tube, increased comfort, improved ability to communicate, and increased stability, and better oral hygiene. Tracheostomy's few disadvantages include the remote possible hazards of the operation and a neck scar to remind the patient of the serious illness.

When to replace a tube with a tracheostomy is a topic of daily discussion in the ICU. There is agreement that for patients who are restless, moving about, swallowing and gagging frequently, with a fetid oral cavity, who have large amounts of tracheobronchial secretions that are difficult to clear, and who have an underlying condition that will not resolve in 7 to 10 days, an early tracheostomy is a reasonable course to take. Early tracheostomy should also be considered for patients with diabetes mellitus, purulent pneumonias, rheumatoid arthritis, ankylosing spondylitis, and in keloid formers because they are at risk for developing postextubation laryngeal complications. Stop gastric feeding at least 4 h before the procedure and aspirate the stomach. Tracheostomy should be postponed if the required fraction of inspired oxygen (FI_{O_2}) is greater than 0.6, if the positive end-expiratory pressure (PEEP) requirement exceeds 10 cmH_2O, or if the peak airway pressure is above 65 cmH_2O. Heparin infusions are stopped 6 h prior to surgery and resumed 12 h postoperatively. Thrombocytopenia below 50,000 and prothrombin time prolongation of greater than 20 percent beyond control are corrected with platelet, plasma or cryoprecipitate transfusions.

Complications

Early complications include hemorrhage, malpositioning or dislodgement of the tracheostomy tube, pneumothorax, and pneumomediastinum. Hemorrhage usually appears within a few hours of tracheostomy and is often due to improperly tied ligatures. Vessels commonly involved are the subcutaneous vessels, anterior neck veins, and thyroid vessels. Ventilator high pressure alarming or development of subcutaneous emphysema should be recognized as the signs of a malpositioned or dislodged tracheostomy tube. This complication will occur within a short time of tracheostomy and is potentially lethal if not corrected. No attempt should be made to reinsert a tube in a fresh tracheostomy without first regaining control of the airway by translaryngeal ETT. After ETT, the wound is re-explored to identify the tracheostomy tube over a catheter or fiberoptic bronchoscope. Pneumothorax occurring immediately after tracheostomy is usually due to inadvertent invasion of the pleural space by lateral and caudal dissection. Tube thoracostomy is the treatment of choice.

Late tracheostomy complications include hemorrhage, infection of the lower respiratory tract, tracheoesophageal fistula, and postdecannulation tracheal stenosis. Hemorrhage may be related to tube erosion into the innominate artery secondary to a low lying tracheostomy. Pulsatile hemorrhage or brief bright red "sentinel" bleeds are the signs of innominate artery erosion. Definitive management requires operative access with oversewing of the artery and repositioning of the tracheostomy tube higher in the neck.

Tracheal stenosis commonly occurs at the stomal site. The predisposing factors are female gender, duration of antecedent ETT, rheumatoid arthritis, diabetes mellitus, tendency to keloid formation, and suppurative pneumonia. Resection of the tracheal stomal stenotic area with primary reanastomosis is the procedure of choice.

UPPER AIRWAY OBSTRUCTION

Upper airway obstruction (UAO) may be caused by several conditions (Table 4-2): signs and symptoms include marked respiratory distress, aphonia or dysphonia, choking, cyanosis, inspiratory stridor or crowing, suprasternal and intercostal indrawing, facial swelling or prominence of neck veins, absent air movement with no air entry into the chest on auscultation, and tachycardia. Thoracoabdominal paradox is often prominent. As asphyxiation progresses, bradycardia, hypotension, and death occur.

Asthma is the leading differential diagnosis of UAO. Unlike asthma, UAO is associated with obstructive noises that are intensified on inspiration and are usually localizable to the upper airway. The pace at which assessment and diagnosis of the cause of UAO proceeds is dictated by the urgency of the patient's condition. The most important diagnostic procedure after a quick history taking and physical examination are the laryngoscope and the fiberoptic or rigid bronchoscope. These allow direct visualization of the oronasopharynx and larynx along with rapid translaryngeal intubation to secure patency of the airway. The patient with chronic UAO caused by goiter, thyroid malignancy, vascular arches, and mediastinal or paratracheal tumors may require a more deliberate diagnostic approach. Oropharyngeal and cervical plain radiograph, computed tomography, and flow volume loops may yield important diagnostic information. Patients suspected of having symptomatic chronic UAO should have diagnostic procedures performed under very close supervision. It is to be emphasized that since airway resistance varies inversely with the fourth power of the radius at the point of airway compromise, small advances in the underlying disease are likely to dramatically worsen the respiratory resistive load.

Securing and maintaining a patent airway is of paramount importance in the resuscitation of asphyxiating patients. The use of pharyngeal airways, endotracheal intubation, endoscopy with an open bronchoscope, helium-oxygen mixture, and various drugs may be necessary in the management of UAO.

Heliox, a helium-oxygen gas mixture, is effective in reducing the work of breathing by decreasing the resistive load by a decrease in the density-dependent pressure drop across the airway obstruction. The most effective helium-oxygen ratio is at least 70:30. Application of 21% heliox by mask with supplemental oxygen by nasal cannula titrated against pulse oximetery readings is an approach that avoids the time consuming adjustments of blenders used to achieve various helium-oxygen mixtures. Heliox is a temporizing measure that neither diagnoses nor corrects an obstructive lesion.

SPLIT-LUNG VENTILATION

Split-lung ventilation (SLV) or selective one-lung ventilation was developed to facilitate thoracic surgery. Indications for SLV in the intensive care unit (ICU) are evolving and so far include bronchopleural fistula, unilateral lung disease, bilateral lung dis-

ease, and airway hemorrhage. Bronchopleural fistula is a complication of acute lung disease, trauma, surgery, and positive-pressure
ventilation. If conventional ventilation fails, then SLV allows ventilation of the healthy lung while allowing the lung with the
bronchopleural fistula to rest.

Total unilateral atelectasis usually does not respond to conservative measures. When aggressive therapies (bronchoscopy, positive-
pressure ventilation) fail, SLV may be appropriate. Isolation of the
lungs allows for application of sufficient unilateral CPAP or PEEP
to reverse the atelectasis in the affected lung without causing barotrauma to the healthy lung.

Patients with bilateral lung disease (pneumonia, aspiration, pulmonary edema, and adult respiratory distress syndrome) have
shown improved gas exchange after institution of SLV. Selective
PEEP applied to the dependent lung with the patient in the lateral
decubitus position produces a significant reduction in venous admixture without the reduction in cardiac output usually seen in
conventional two lung ventilation with PEEP.

Immediate lung separation during acute airway hemorrhage may
be lifesaving. A bronchial blocker, double-lumen tube (DLT), or
an uncut endotracheal tube advanced into the main bronchus op-
posite the bleeding site are temporary measures used until the lesion
is identified and appropriate corrective treatment instituted.

Endobronchial blockade may be accomplished by intentionally
obstructing the bronchus of a lobe or whole lung with a gauze
tampon, cuffed rubber bronchial blockers, embolectomy balloons,
pulmonary artery or urinary catheters, or by specially designed
plastic tubes. Lung tissue distal to the obstruction collapses due
to continued absorption of alveolar gas (absorption atelectasis).
DLTs are the best bronchial blockers because they allow each
lung to be ventilated independently, collapsed and reexpanded or
examined at any time. Carlens and Robertshaw styles of DLTs
are available.

Malposition is the most common complication of DLTs. Common positioning problems are not passing the tube sufficiently far
into the bronchus, intubating the wrong bronchus, and passing the
tube too deep into the appropriate bronchus. Bronchoscopy immediately prior to intubation may be helpful.

Airway trauma, especially with some Carlens style DLTs, ranges
from ecchymosis of the mucous membranes to arytenoid dislocation and torn vocal cords. Pressure damage may occur because of
overdistension or uneven cuff distension. Airway damage may
present with air leak, subcutaneous emphysema, hemorrhage, or
cardiovascular instability from tension pneumothorax. Underinflation of the bronchial cuff can result in a cross-leak and ventilation
of the operated lung or contamination of the dependent lung. To

decrease the chances of injury, the bronchial cuff should be deflated before the patient is moved.

For further reading in *Principles of Critical Care,* see Chap 6, "Airway Management and Intubation" Mitchell Keamy, Chap 7 "Tracheostomy" EG King/SM Hamilton, Chap 10 "Split-Lung Ventilation" Jay B Brodsky/Frederick G Mihm, Chap 134 "Upper Airway Obstruction" EG King/GJ Sheehan/TJ McDonnell

---

5 | Resuscitation

Kevin Simpson

The American Heart Association (AHA) guidelines for resuscitation provide a rational general framework for resuscitation of patients in a wide variety of clinical circumstances. As such, these AHA protocols should form the basis of treatment of intensive care unit (ICU) patients in cardiopulmonary arrest. However, the AHA algorithms should not be viewed as all-encompassing or inflexible. Rather, an approach that creatively utilizes all the diagnostic and therapeutic modalities readily available in the ICU offers the greatest likelihood of successful resuscitation.

GENERAL PRINCIPLES

Cardiopulmonary arrest implies the state of profoundly inadequate tissue perfusion and oxygen delivery such that cell death is imminent. The absolute length of time that any given tissue bed can survive in this condition before irreversible damage results is controversial. Nonetheless, it is clear that unless resuscitated within a very few minutes, the patient who experiences cardiopulmonary arrest is very unlikely to survive to discharge. Hence, an organized approach to resuscitation that stresses the swift establishment of adequate circulation and ventilation is essential.

Control of the airway and provision of adequate ventilation are immediate objectives in all patients. The only circumstances which take precedence are initial attempts at defibrillation, the need to protect the patient from further injury, and compression of exsanguinating hemorrhage. This is not to say that every patient must be intubated, but rather that immediate assessment of airway and breathing coupled with measures to correct the deficiencies revealed are almost always the highest priorities.

Inadequate perfusion can certainly occur in the presence of a "normal" blood pressure. Therefore, assessment of circulation should include not only blood pressure and heart rate, but indicators of end-organ perfusion such as the temperature of the extremities, nailbed return, the quality of mentation and level of consciousness, and urine output as well. An adequate preload is essential and must be swiftly established through the rapid infusion of crystalloid, colloid, and/or red blood cells. Unlike many other clinical situations, volume resuscitation of the patient in cardiopulmonary arrest requires the ability to infuse liters of fluid within minutes. Hence, placement of short, large bore catheters is a high priority. Bradycardia and tachycardia likewise must be corrected expeditiously as discussed below. If a depressed inotropic state is suspected, empiric use of inotropic catecholamines is warranted. The primary indication for the use of a vasoconstrictor is the absence of appropriate vasoconstriction in the setting of hypotension. Use of these agents in other situations should be considered a temporizing measure only, until the underlying problem can be adequately addressed.

Ventricular Fibrillation/Pulseless Ventricular Tachycardia

Ventricular fibrillation is the most common cause of sudden death and the most amenable to treatment (Table 5-1). The absolute priority in any attempt at resuscitation from ventricular fibrillation or pulseless ventricular tachycardia is defibrillation. Neither cardiopulmonary resuscitation (CPR) nor attempts at intubation should be instituted until after the failure of the first three defibrillation attempts, assuming a defibrillator is immediately available. If initial attempts at defibrillation fail, attention should be turned towards optimizing myocardial responsiveness by improving oxygenation, acid-base status, and myocardial perfusion pressure. Correction of hypoxia and acidosis are best accomplished by securing control of the airway and assisting ventilation with 100% supplemental oxygen. A myocardial perfusion pressure (diastolic blood pressure minus right atrial pressure) of at least 15 mmHg appears to be critical for successful defibrillation. Hence, epinephrine is recommended in an attempt to raise mean arterial pressure. There is evidence, however, that the standard recommended dose of 0.5 to 1.0 mg IV push every 5 min may be grossly inadequate and consideration of much greater doses of epinephrine (up to 0.2 mg/kg) may be appropriate.

TABLE 5-1 Treatment of Ventricular Fibrillation/Pulseless Ventricular Tachycardia

Precordial thump if witnessed arrest
CPR only until defibrillator is available
Defibrillate at 200 J
Defibrillate at 200–300 J
Defibrillate at 360 J
Begin CPR, obtain IV access
Epinephrine, 0.5–1.0 mg IV push, every 5 min
Intubate
Defibrillate at 360 J
Bretylium, 5mg/kg IV push
(Consider bicarbonate)
Defibrillate at 360 J
Bretylium, 10 mg/kg IV push
Defibrillate at 360 J
Repeat Lidocaine or bretylium
Defibrillate at 360 J

Ventricular Tachycardia with a Pulse

The appropriate response to the patient experiencing ventricular tachycardia with a pulse depends upon how well the patient is tolerating the arrhythmia (see Table 5-2). Patients who are to be considered unstable, and therefore cardioverted at an early stage, include patients experiencing chest pain, dyspnea, congestive heart failure (CHF), hypotension, or other evidence of inadequate tissue perfusion. Even then, cardioversion should be attempted in a conscious patient only after sedation with a short-acting barbiturate or benzodiazepine.

Asystole/Bradycardia

Tables 5-3 and 5-4 detail the AHA algorithms for resuscitating the asystolic or bradycardic patient. There is some evidence that extreme vagal tone can lead to asystole and therefore a fully vagolytic dose of atropine (2.0 mg) may be considered as the initial dose rather than the traditional recommendation of 1.0 mg. In general, bradycardias require urgent treatment only when hemodynamically significant or when ventricular escape ectopy is apparent.

Electromechanical Dissociation (EMD)

The presence of a complex with a very weak or absent pulse should immediately generate a search for evidence of hypovolemia, hypoxia, pneumothorax, acidosis, pericardial tamponade, and pulmonary embolus. Swift correction of these conditions is essential for successful resuscitation from EMD. Institution of specific therapeutic interventions, however, may depend upon their availability, e.g.

TABLE 5-2 Ventricular Tachycardia with a Pulse

If Stable:
Oxygen, IV Access
Lidocaine, 1 mg/kg bolus
Lidocaine, 0.5 mg/kg every 8 min, until ventricular tachycardia resolved or total 3 mg/kg
Procainamide, 20 mg/min until ventricular tachycardia resolved or 1 g total
If Unstable (chest pain, dyspnea, CHF, hypotension, infarction): Oxygen, IV Access
Lidocaine, 1 mg/kg bolus
(Consider sedation)
Synchronized cardioversion at 50 J
Synchronized cardioversion at 100 J
Synchronized cardioversion at 200 J
Synchronized cardioversion at up to 360 J
If recurrent, lidocaine, procainamide, or bretylium
Repeat cardioversion at level previously successful

TABLE 5-3 Asystole

If possibly ventricular fibrillation, defibrillate
CPR, IV access
Epinephrine, 0.5–1.0 mg IV, every 5 min
Intubate when possible
Atropine, 1.0 mg IV, repeat X1 in 5 min
(consider bicarbonate)
Consider pacing

the immediate ability to perform pulmonary arterial embolectomy. In addition, as the goal of resuscitation is to prevent premature or unnecessary death but not to prolong the act of dying, reflexive institution of all heroic measures in every patient is probably not warranted.

Supraventricular Tachycardia

Patients who are hypotensive, experiencing chest pain, or are otherwise seriously threatened by the arrhythmia should be treated with synchronized cardioversion, using 50 to 360 J, whereas others less seriously threatened can be treated by vagotonic maneuvers and agents, overdrive pacing, and synchronized cardioversion if necessary. Not uncommonly it is unclear whether a tachycardia is supraventricular or ventricular in origin. The unstable patient should be promptly cardioverted in either case. In the stable patient, however, a trial of adenosine (6 mg injected quickly via central line followed by 12 mg if the tachycardia persists) may clarify the site of origin of the tachycardia.

Miscellaneous Issues

Bicarbonate is frequently administered to patients in cardiopulmonary arrest, often even in the absence of blood gas evidence of acidemia. Recently some have pointed out the lack of efficacy of sodium bicarbonate in cardiac resuscitation. Because of the ease with which carbon dioxide crosses cell membranes compared to the more polar bicarbonate ion, some investigators are concerned

TABLE 5-4 Bradycardia

If sinus, junctional, 1° AVB, or type I 2° AVB, treat only if signs or symptoms present. If type II 2° AVB or 3° AVB, treat even if asymptomatic:
Atropine, 0.5–1.0 mg IV
Repeat atropine every 5 min until total 2.0 mg
External pacemaker
or
Isoproterenol, 2–10 μg/min
Transvenous pacemaker

about the generation of a paradoxical intracellular acidosis. As such, routine administration of bicarbonate can not be recommended.

Calcium is an excellent inotrope in situations of decreased ionized calcium. Such conditions may exist in the patient coming off a bypass pump or who has received massive transfusions such as in the setting of liver transplantation. Additionally, calcium is effective in reversing the vasodilation produced by calcium entry blockers such as verapamil. However, there is no evidence that calcium administration improves survival rates during cardiopulmonary resuscitation. In addition, there is concern about the cytotoxic effects of calcium which could leak into ischemic cells.

Resuscitation in the intensive care unit may at times offer therapeutic modalities not often available on regular hospital wards. Fiberoptic bronchoscopy may be of use for clarifying appropriate endotracheal tube (ETT) placement and patency. Echocardiography allows rapid assessment of both left and right ventricular filling and function, as well as detection of pericardial effusions and assessment of their hemodynamic significance. End-tidal CO_2 monitoring may also allow assessment of ETT positioning as well as cardiac output. Hence, resuscitation in the ICU offers an opportunity for implementation of creative diagnostic and therapeutic approaches.

For further reading in *Principles of Critical Care,* see Chap 47 "Resuscitation and Stabilization" William F Rutherford/Edward A Panacek, Chap 114 "Shock" Keith R Walley/Lawrence DH Wood

---

6 | Mechanical Ventilation

Edward T. Naureckas

INDICATIONS FOR MECHANICAL VENTILATION

The application of mechanical ventilation allows the physician to temporarily reverse respiratory failure and sustain life. During the period of ventilator support, specific treatment is generally required to reverse the causes of respiratory failure and return the patient to his premorbid status.

While respiratory failure is commonly cited as an indication for ventilation, the term is imprecise and fails to convey any specific information about the underlying process for which mechanical ventilation is being initiated. One classification which overcomes this shortcoming groups disease processes into four categories:

1. Acute hypoxemic respiratory failure (AHRF); Those diseases such as adult respiratory distress syndrome (ARDS) and pulmonary edema in which shunt physiology predominates.
2. Those diseases such as obstructive airways disease or neuromuscular impairment which result in hypercapnia.
3. Post-operative atelectasis.
4. Acute medical and surgical cardiovascular syndromes, such as shock, where mechanical ventilation is used to decrease work of breathing.

GENERAL CLASSES OF VENTILATORS

Mechanical ventilators produce respiratory flows by generating positive pressures at the airway opening which are cycled with time. These ventilators can be of two subtypes, pressure cycled ventilators which deliver a preset pressure terminating the breath after a given time or flow rate, and volume cycled ventilators which deliver a preset volume. The tidal volume in a pressure cycled ventilator is determined by respiratory system mechanics. Hypoventilation may result if these change acutely. Until recently pressure cycled ventilation was used most commonly in the neonatal population, but has become more widely used in the adult ICU with the advent of pressure support and proportional assist ventilation. Volume cycled ventilation carries the potential risk of barotrauma from high airway pressures in cases of low lung compliance. In practice this is minimized by setting a pressure limit above which inspiration is terminated and by using physiologic tidal volumes (i.e., 5 to 8 cc/kg).

Negative pressure ventilators which include the "iron lung" and the more portable cuirass ventilator, produce cyclic pressure gradients across the chest wall by generating negative pressures at the chest wall surface. As in pressure cycled ventilation, tidal volumes are determined by the patient's respiratory system mechanics.

MODES OF VENTILATION

The pattern of machine-determined pressure or volume cycling used to drive gas flows during ventilation characterizes the mode of ventilator operation. It is important to note that while certain modes of ventilation exercise the respiratory muscles in a more physiologic pattern, no mode of respiration has been shown to significantly speed liberation from mechanical ventilation. The ability of patients to become independent of mechanical ventilation is more dependent on the resolution of the underlying respiratory pathology than on the mode of ventilation.

Assist-Control Mode Ventilation

In assist-control (AC) ventilation, a preset tidal volume is given to the patient every time an inspiratory effort is sensed as a fall in the pressure at the airway opening. A backup rate is also set to prevent hypoventilation in those patients who have a decrease spontaneous respiratory rate or are unable to generate sufficient negative pressure to trigger the ventilator. Exercise of the respiratory muscles can be accomplished by gradually increasing the magnitude of the negative pressure required to trigger the ventilator, thus increasing patient effort. (see Fig. 6-1.)

Theoretical disadvantages of this mode of ventilation include the potential for respiratory alkalosis in patients with increased respiratory drive related to factors other than hypercapnia or hypoxemia. This can be easily assessed by attention to blood gas parameters.

Synchronized Intermittent Mandatory Mode Ventilation

In synchronized intermittent mandatory ventilation (SIMV), the machine delivered breaths are triggered by the patient's inspiratory effort up to a preset rate. Any breaths over this preset rate will be unassisted. As in AC mode, a backup rate is provided if the patient's respiratory rate falls below the desired rate. (See Fig. 6-2.)

In order to provide exercise to the respiratory muscles on this mode, the rate of machine administered breaths or the tidal volume (Vt) are gradually reduced.

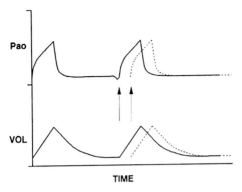

Pao

VOL

TIME

FIG. 6-1 Airway pressure (Pao) and lung volume during assist-control ventilation of a patient who is triggering the ventilator. The second breath was set to be delivered at the time marked by the dotted arrow; instead, the patient lowers the Pao, triggering the ventilator at the time marked by the solid arrow, thereby increasing the respiratory rate.

Pressure Support Ventilation

Pressure support ventilation may be used as a primary mode of ventilation, or as an adjunct to other modes of ventilation. In this mode, patients receive a preset pressure triggered by an inspiratory effort. The breath is terminated when the inspiratory flow, which is determined by the respiratory system mechanics, falls below a given level. The tidal volume is determined by the patient's respiratory system parameters such as lung compliance, chest wall compliance, the activity of the respiratory muscles, and to some extent, the airways resistance (R_{aw}). There is the potential for hypoventilation or hyperventilation if these parameters change. (See Fig. 6-3.)

Patient comfort has been shown to be increased on this mode of ventilation. Exercise in this mode is accomplished by initially setting the support pressure to that which provides full tidal volumes, then gradually decreasing the amount of pressure supplied with each breath.

Proportional Assist Mode Ventilation

Proportional assist ventilation (PAV) achieves greater patient comfort on the ventilator by scaling ventilator flow and volume to the patient's inspiratory effort allowing the patient greater control of

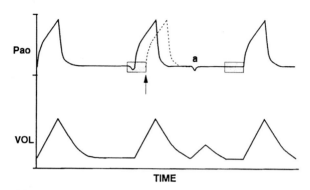

FIG. 6-2 Airway pressure (Pao) and lung volume (VOL) during SIMV. The first breath is a mandatory, nontriggered breath at the set tidal volume. The shaded rectangle near the second breath denotes the interval during which the ventilator will attempt to synchronize with the patient's inspiratory effort, delivering the mandatory breath slightly ahead of schedule. At the end of this time interval (arrow), a mandatory breath will be delivered (dotted tracing) if the patient has not triggered the ventilator. However, the patient does trigger the second breath within the window, and receives the same tidal volume as during a mandatory breath. The third breath is initiated before the synchronization interval (a), and is therefore not assisted. Tidal volume is totally determined by the patient. When the patient fails to trigger another breath within the next synchronization window, the fourth (mandatory) breath is delivered.

each machine delivered breath. This scaling is achieved by sensing the flow into the patient's lungs at a given pressure and using this information to determine the patients inspiratory effort. The results of these calculations are then used to adjust the ventilator pressure to deliver a flow and volume proportional to the patient's effort (as opposed to pressure support which delivers a fixed pressure regardless of patient effort).

The reputed benefits of this mode of ventilation include increased patient comfort, lower peak airway pressures (since pressure is applied in a profile parallel to the patient's inspiration). One potential of this system is that leaks in the ventilator circuit may be mistaken by the algorithm for patient effort and may cause over ventilation.

Respiratory muscle exercise may be accomplished in this mode by decreasing the scaling factor gradually so that a lesser amount of ventilatory assist is provided for a given effort.

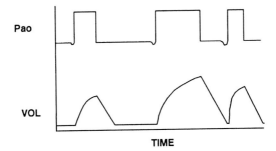

Pao

VOL

TIME

FIG. 6-3 Pressure-support ventilation. When a breath is triggered airway pressure (Pao) rises to the set level. Tidal volume depends on the Pao, respiratory system mechanics, and patient effort. The first breath shown represents a patient who triggers the ventilator, then remains fully passive. As long as there is no significant airflow obstruction, tidal nearly reaches the volume which would be predicted based on the compliance of the respiratory system times the increment in Pao. During the middle breath shown, the patient makes a small, but prolonged inspiratory effort. The Pao remains at the set inspiratory level as long as patient effort maintains flow, and a much longer tidal volume results. In the final breath, a much more powerful, but more brief inspiratory effort is made, generating a larger tidal volume than during the passive breath.

Inverse Ratio Ventilation

Inverse ratio ventilation (IRV) refers to mechanical ventilation in which the I:E ratio is set at greater than 1. This can be achieved by decreasing the inspiratory flow rate on a volume cycled ventilator such that the inspiration of a given volume requires a longer time (VC-IRV), by inserting a pause after inspiration at a normal flow rate (VC-IRV), or by applying a set pressure for a longer time on a pressure cycled ventilator (PC-IRV). The purported benefit of this mode of ventilation is that it may improve oxygenation in patients with AHRF who are unable to achieve adequate oxygen saturation with maximal positive end-expiratory pressure (PEEP) alone. There is some evidence to suggest that the effects of this mode of ventilation may be attributed to the presence of intrinsic PEEP (PEEPi), though some benefit may be attained by applying prolonged inflation to alveoli which require longer times to reopen (so called "long opening time constant" alveolar units). The disadvantage of this form of ventilation is that high levels of PEEPi (vide infra) can be seen in patients with increased airways resistance. This pattern of respiration is extremely uncomfortable for most patients, such that sedation and muscle relaxation are typically required. It is common with this mode of ventilation to start with an I:E ratio of 1:2 though ratios of as high as 1:4 have been used with careful monitoring for PEEPi.

Airway Pressure Release Ventilation

In this mode of ventilation, the pressure at the airway opening is held at a level to maintain lung volumes at greater than Functional Residual Capacity (FRC). Ventilation is then achieved by decreasing the pressure to a lower level, allowing expiration. The patient is able to take spontaneous breaths above the holding pressure. This mode of ventilation theoretically works in a fashion similar to pressure controlled inverse ratio ventilation by allowing the reopening of alveoli with longer time constants.

High Frequency Ventilation

High frequency ventilation is a nonconventional mode of mechanical ventilation which uses tidal volumes which are less than or equal to dead space volume. Three types of high frequency ventilation have been studied for clinical use, including high frequency positive pressure ventilation (HFPPV), high frequency oscillation (HFO) and high frequency jet ventilation (HFJV). HFPPV, one of the noisiest modes of ventilation, consists of an oscillating positive pressure wave applied at the airway opening by using a compressed gas source and a solenoid valve. Oxygen content is adjusted by entraining a stream of oxygen using a bias flow. HFO uses a piston pump that actively pulses gas both into and out of airways. HFJV uses a nozzle shaped jet centered at the endotracheal tube orifice with an angled side port for administering a bias flow and allowing for passive exhalation.

It was initially thought that the use of high frequency ventilation would decrease peak airway pressures and thus decrease barotrauma in patients with decreased lung compliance. These predictions have not been borne out in clinical trials of these modes of ventilation.

PEEP AND CPAP

PEEP and continuous positive airway pressure (CPAP) are not separate modes of ventilation but are used together with other modes of ventilation to improve oxygenation. PEEP specifically refers to the application of a fixed amount of positive pressure at the end of a mechanical ventilation cycle, whereas CPAP refers to the application of a fixed pressure throughout the respiratory cycle.

The benefits of applying positive airway pressure result from its potential ability to raise FRC and open closed alveolar units, which increases lung compliance and may reduce shunt. Used correctly, peak airway pressures may be significantly less than predicted simply from the sum of the peak airway pressure prior to PEEP plus the applied PEEP.

PEEP is initially applied in ARDS at a level of 5 to 10 cm of water. It is then increased in increments of 2.5 to 5 cm of water. Two of the potential complications associated with PEEP are barotrauma and altered hemodynamics. Hemodynamic monitoring may be helpful in managing PEEP.

MONITORING OF MECHANICAL VENTILATION

Assessment of Ventilation and Oxygenation

Oxygen delivery is proportional to hemoglobin concentration, hemoglobin oxygen saturation, and flow to a given tissue. During mechanical ventilation, saturation may be assessed in a number of ways. Most directly arterial blood samples may be drawn from a catheter inserted into the radial artery. This will also provide data regarding P_{CO_2} and acid base status (For a discussion of blood gas analysis, please see Chap. 57).

When a noninvasive approach is desired, pulse oximetry may be employed. This approach uses the absorption of light transmitted through a nailbed, earlobe, or other site to determine the hemoglobin saturation. These devices are accurate at high saturation but tend to overestimate the hemoglobin saturation at low oxygen tensions. They also tend not to work well in low perfusion states or other states with peripheral vasoconstriction.

Transcutaneous monitoring of P_{O_2} and P_{CO_2} relies on diffusion of gases from the vessels to the skin surface. Often the site is heated to dilate the capillaries and aid diffusion. This method is more applicable to pediatric populations and is rarely used in the adult setting.

Reflectance oximetry is often used to measure $S\bar{v}_{O_2}$ as an indication of oxygen delivery and extraction. The same information can be obtained from obtaining mixed venous blood gases from the distal port of a pulmonary artery catheter. In the setting of deranged oxygen extraction such as sepsis the $S\bar{v}_{O_2}$ may be normal despite inadequate tissue oxygenation.

Often it is useful to calculate the alveolar-arterial oxygen gradient to monitor the efficiency of oxygen exchange across the lung. The Pa_{O_2} can be obtained from blood gas analysis or calculated using pulse oximetry. The alveolar partial pressure of oxygen ($P_{A_{O_2}}$) is given by the following simplified formula:

$$P_{A_{O_2}} = P_{I_{O_2}} - P_{a_{CO_2}}/R$$

Where R is the respiratory exchange ratio, usually equal to approximately 0.8 with an average diet under normal conditions. $P_{I_{O_2}}$ is the partial pressure of inspired oxygen which is the $F_{I_{O_2}}$ multiplied by atmospheric pressure minus the water vapor pressure. The normal A-a gradient is less than ten but increases with increasing age and increasing $F_{I_{O_2}}$.

Monitoring Lung and Chest Wall Mechanics

Compliance measurements made during mechanical ventilation represent a summation of the effects of both the lung parenchyma and the chest wall. In order to calculate the compliance of the respiratory system (Crs) both a paused end inspiratory pressure at zero flow (Pplat) and the PEEP must be measured. Compliance can then be roughly calculated from the formula:

$$Crs = Vt/(Pplat-PEEP) \qquad (6-2)$$

The resistive component of the airway pressures can be calculated from the difference between the peak and pause pressures.

Intrinsic PEEP

When a tidal volume is given before the previous tidal volume can be completely exhaled, dynamic hyperinflation is present. This phenomenon is known as intrinsic PEEP (PEEPi) or "auto-PEEP." It is more likely to occur in settings of airflow obstruction especially with rapid rates or with inverse ratio ventilation. PEEPi can result in the same degree of barotrauma or hemodynamic compromise as PEEP set on the ventilator. It can be measured by pausing the ventilator at end expiration and closing the expiratory circuit to flow. If PEEPi is present it will be measurable at the airway opening with these maneuvers (see Chap. 32 for a description of the expiratory port occlusion technique).

Monitoring Strength

The most useful measure of respiratory muscle strength is the "maximal inspiratory pressure" (MIP), sometimes referred to as the "negative inspiratory force" (NIF). The MIP is determined by connecting the endotracheal tube to a pressure gauge manometer, then asking the patient to inspire with maximal effort. If the patient cannot cooperate, a brief period of airway occlusion will provoke attempts to maximally inspire. The most negative pressure achieved is the MIP. Although the MIP provides useful information regarding respiratory muscle strength, it gives no measure of endurance.

For further reading in *Principles of Critical Care,* see Chap 8 "Mechanical Ventilators" Edward P Ingenito/Jeffrey Drazen, Chap 9 "Current Controversies in Applying Specific Modes of Mechanical Ventilation" James K Stoller, Chap 14 "Monitoring the Respiratory System" John J. Marini/Jonathan Truwit

---

Conventional and Interventional Radiology in the ICU

Manu Jain

The increase in numbers of cardiac surgical procedures and transplant operations as well as more widespread use of assisted ventilation and hemodynamic monitoring has led to more bedside chest x-ray examinations. Unfortunately the technique of bedside radiography has remained largely unchanged for many years and inferior image quality is inevitable.

PORTABLE RADIOGRAPHS

General Considerations

Some important differences between portable chest radiographs and those obtained in the radiology department have important effects on interpretations (see Table 7-1). The most obvious differences are the increased cardiac magnification and wider mediastinum on portable radiographs. It is also important to interpret infiltrates in the context of pulmonary inflation and x-ray penetration. Thus it is helpful to view serial radiographs side-by-side to distinguish real interval change from artifactual changes. Various type of artifacts may overlie the lungs of ICU patients and can be mistaken for pathology. These include catheters, endotracheal tubes and electrocardiographic leads.

Abnormal Air Collections

Most abnormal air collections are iatrogenic and usually related to central venous access, thoracentesis or pulmonary barotrauma. In an erect patient without pleural adhesions a pneumothorax will accumulate at the apex. If adhesions are present, which is common in critically ill patients, atypical locations are more likely. Most atypical pneumothoraces are subpulmonic or anteromedial. If a pneumothorax is suspected an erect portable or a decubitus lateral radiograph may be necessary to confirm the diagnosis. It may be difficult at times to distinguish pneumothorax from a skin fold. Extension of shadow beyond the thorax, bilaterality, and vascular markings visible beyond a curved edge are all suggestions of skin folds. The most useful procedure is to repeat the radiograph.

Pneumomediastinum occurs spontaneously in asthmatics, in patients who are mechanically ventilated, and occasionally in patients with esophageal perforation or head and neck trauma. The most

TABLE 7-1 Differences Between Portable and Standard Chest X-Rays

Standard	Chest X-Ray	Portable Chest X-Ray	Comment
Position	Standing Posterior-anterior projection	Erect, sitting, semi-erect or supine Anterior-posterior projection	Increased cardiac magnification and limited pulmonary expansion on portable exam.
Beam Angle	Horizontal	Variable	Non-horizontal beam limits ability to detect free air, air-fluid levels, pleural effusions and pneumothorax.
Beam Energy	Kv:120 to 140 Exposure time < 1/10 s	Kv:80 to 100 Exposure time often > 1/10 s	Motion blurring more likely with portable technique.
X-ray Source	72"	40" to 72"	Shorter distances contribute to cardiac magnification.
Image Quality	Superior	Inferior	Mainly due to uncontrolled scattered radiation.

(From MacMahon H, Montner, SM, Chest Radiology In The ICU in Hall J, Schmidt G and Wood LDH, eds: Principles of Critical Care, McGraw-Hill 1992.)

45

important implication of a pneumomediastinum is that it may herald a pneumothorax. A pneumopericardium is virtually unknown in adults without trauma or surgery and usually is a pneumomediastinum in disguise.

Free intraperitoneal air usually indicates perforation of the gastrointestinal tract unless recent surgery has been performed. If a portable radiograph is unhelpful, a left-side-down lateral decubitus view of the upper abdomen is the most sensitive examination.

Pneumatoceles can be recognized by their relative spherical configuration and highly localized nature.

Pleural Effusions

Pleural effusions collect in the most dependent portions of the thorax. They are first seen as increased densities behind the domes of the hemidiaphragms on an erect film. As they enlarge one may see costophrenic angle blunting and separation of lung from the chest wall. On a supine x-ray only a hazy density is apparent over the affected lung.

Loculation of pleural fluid can take many forms. Subpulmonic effusions can be mistaken for an elevated hemidiaphragm, or fluid in a fissure can appear to be a cavity or a tumor. A lateral radiograph is helpful in such situations.

Adult Respiratory Distress Syndrome (ARDS)

The radiographic findings are not specific although there are suggestive features. Usually diffuse, patchy infiltrates develop which are indistinguishable from pulmonary edema of other causes. However, the heart does not enlarge and pleural effusions are not, typically, features of ARDS. One of the most suggestive findings is the stable appearance of the infiltrates over many days.

Aspiration

Aspiration refers to several different phenomena including aspiration of nasal-pharyngeal secretions or gastric contents. Radiographically the superior segments of the lower lobes are involved in patients who are supine whereas in patients who are more nearly erect the basilar segments of the lower lobes are more likely to be affected, especially on the right.

Atelectasis

Atelectasis is common in the ICU and is often multi-factorial in origin. Subsegmental atelectasis typically has a linear appearance and commonly occurs at the bases. On the other hand acute atelectasis of an entire lung is indicated by opacification of the hemithorax. This can be differentiated from a pleural effusion by noting that in atelectasis the mediastinum shifts toward the affected side, the ipsilateral ribs are approximated, and the ipsilateral hemidiaphragm is raised. Additionally one may see an apparent bronchial "cut-off" secondary to a mass or a mucous plug.

Pulmonary Edema

Because of pulmonary underinflation and cardiac magnification on portable radiographs, mild cardiomegaly and early interstitial edema may be difficult to detect. Additionally vascular redistribution, distention of the venous pedicle and indistinctness of pulmonary vessels are unreliable in patients who are not erect. Kerley B lines, however, are useful. Distinction between cardiogenic and noncardiogenic edema cannot be made reliably.

Pulmonary Infiltrates

Noninfectious infiltrates are common in ICU patients and the chest radiograph does not usually allow a specific diagnosis. In patients with pleural effusions, compression atelectasis can cause an infiltrate. Cardiac failure produces a large heart and interstitial edema, both of which can produce atelectasis, and give rise to air bronchograms at the basilar portions of the lungs. Pneumonia need not necessarily be considered unless pulmonary consolidation is disproportionately large.

When pneumonia is a consideration clinically, patients with normal immunity typically display focal or patchy infiltrates. Immunocompromised patients, on the other hand, commonly have diffuse, bilateral infiltrates which can resemble pulmonary edema.

Tubes, Lines and Catheters

Endotracheal and Tracheostomy Tubes

A chest radiograph is mandatory after placement of an endotracheal tube (ETT) to verify correct position and exclude complications. The tip of an ETT should be 5 to 7 cm above the carina with the head in a neutral position, while the ETT balloon must be below the vocal cords. In some patients the ETT will be as close as 2 cm from the carina in order to keep the balloon safely below the cords.

Although it is common to see small amounts of air in the subcutaneous tissue of the neck after tracheostomy tube placement, large amounts of air suggest a significant air leak. The tip of the tracheostomy tube should be one-half to two-thirds of the distance between the stoma and the carina. If the tip of the tube projects above the level of the clavicles, partial extubation should be suspected.

Venous Catheters

A chest x-ray should follow every successful or unsuccessful attempt at central venous access to verify location and exclude complications. The tip should lie in the innominate vein or superior vena cava but not the right atrium. If the course of a catheter is atypical, abnormal venous anatomy or entrance into a minor vessel should be suspected.

When evaluating the placement of a pulmonary artery catheter, one must assess its route and final location. The ideal resting position is in a central pulmonary artery. Common complications are formation of a loop within the heart and pulmonary infarction from an excessively distal location. Infarction most typically appears as a wedge-shaped, pleural based density.

Aortic counterpulsation balloon devices should be located in the descending aorta with the tip distal to the takeoff of the left subclavian artery.

Transvenous Pacemakers

Incorrect placement of a pacemaker can result in perforation of the right ventricle. This is suggested by an electrode that is located excessively far to the left and directed slightly cephalad. If a lead is directed superiorly and to the left in a more central location, cannulation of the coronary sinus should be suspected.

Thoracic Trauma

Blunt Trauma

Patients experiencing thoracic trauma are at risk for rib fractures, pneumothorax, hemothorax, pulmonary contusions or airway injury. Contusions appear as nonsegmental air-space infiltrates which appear shortly after the insult and usually disappear within 48 to 72 h. A pulmonary hematoma can appear as a multiloculated cavity with air-fluid levels or as a discrete nodule. Bronchial rupture is uncommon, but may be suggested by fracture of the upper three ribs, pneumothorax, pnemomediastinum or a collapsed malpositioned lung.

Rupture of the aorta or any of the great vessels causes mediastinal widening, although this finding is nonspecific. Other clues to vascular rupture include the loss of definition of the aortic knob, an abnormal density superior to the aortic knob extending to the left apex, a widened right paratracheal stripe and displacement of the left paraspinous line. If the chest film is inconclusive, either a CT scan or an angiogram may be diagnostic.

Penetrating Trauma

These injuries are usually caused by stabbing or gunshot wounds. In addition to the abnormalities seen in blunt trauma, one may see mediastinal air without evidence of lung injury. This suggests esophageal perforation which can be confirmed by ingestion of water-soluble contrast material and fluoroscopic examination.

ULTRASOUND AND COMPUTED TOMOGRAPHY (CT)

Ultrasound imaging is versatile in that it can be used at the bedside. It is useful in localizing fluid collections such as pleural effusions or ascites. Accurate determination of the location and size of a fluid collection can increase the yield of fluid aspiration. It is important, however, to scan the patient in the same position in which the procedure will be performed.

The advantage of CT is its ability to display anatomy in discrete axial planes with high resolution. It is more sensitive than plain X-rays for effusions, empyemas, abscesses, or loculated pneumothoraces. It is also useful in identifying malpositioned chest tubes and mediastinal disease. Because of the practical difficulties in transporting an ICU patient, additional conventional radiographic views or ultrasound should be considered before CT.

INTERVENTIONAL RADIOLOGY

Interventional radiology encompasses a variety of procedures having in common the placement of needles or catheters through the skin, usually under ultrasound, CT or fluoroscopic guidance. Since stabilization is not always possible, it is important that critically ill patients be appropriately monitored, have fluids and blood components available, and have a reliable airway. Since most interventional radiology procedures are performed in a special procedures suite, it is important that an ICU environment be reproduced as closely as possible. This means that in addition to basic electrocardiographic monitoring, noninvasive blood pressure and pulse oximetry devices, an ICU nurse should accompany the patient to radiology. In some circumstances an ICU physician may need to be present as well. Ultrasound, CT and fluoroscopy each have their advantages and disadvantages. Which modality to use for a particular procedure is best decided jointly in consultation between the interventional radiologist and intensivist.

Percutaneous Abscess Drainage (PAD)

In the last 10 to 15 years PAD has all but replaced surgical drainage as the treatment of choice for abscesses and other abnormal fluid collections. PAD is most successful when the fluid collection is well defined, unilocular and free flowing. In less optimal circumstances PAD may improve the patient's condition so that more definitive surgical drainage can be performed later. The only absolute contra-indication is lack of a safe access route, but this is rarely a problem with CT guidance.

In general, when placing a percutaneous catheter the shortest, straightest tract is best, always taking care to avoid bowel, pleura and major blood vessels. After placement, catheters are left to drain by gravity, although occasionally they may be connected to low suction. The catheter drainage should be monitored carefully. Only rarely is the material too viscous to drain. When necessary small 5 to 10 ml aliquots of sterile saline can be injected into the catheter and then allowed to drain. The catheter should be left in place as long as it continues to drain. If the patient remains febrile or the white blood cell count remains elevated, a follow-up CT should be obtained promptly and additional drainage catheters placed as needed. If drainage increases abruptly, a fistula may be the cause and should be looked for using contrast media with fluoroscopy. Complications from PAD include transient bacteremia, skin infection, bleeding, bowel perforation, and sepsis.

Percutaneous Cholecystostomy

Recently percutaneous cholecystostomy has emerged as an alternative to standard surgical therapy for patients too ill for cholecystectomy. Indications for this procedure are acute calculous or acalculous cholecystitis. Since acalculous cholecystitis is difficult to diagnose by conventional methods (i.e., ultrasound or hepatoiminodiacetic acid (HIDA) scans), percutaneous cholecystostomy can provide the diagnosis and definitive therapy. The procedure is performed at the bedside using ultrasound guidance and a pig-tailed catheter is left in the gallbladder and allowed to drain by gravity. When the patient's condition stabilizes, the cholecystostomy tube is injected under fluoroscopic guidance to evaluate for gallstones, and cystic and biliary duct patency. The cholecystostomy tube can be removed when a tract has formed, usually in 10 to 14 days. This procedure is successful in more than 95 percent of cases and complications are few.

Gastrointestinal Bleeding: Diagnosis and Treatment

Endoscopy and angiography are the two most helpful radiologic studies in localizing gastrointestinal (GI) bleeding. In upper GI bleeding, endoscopy should be performed before angiography. It can at least confirm active bleeding even if it can't localize it precisely.

Technetium labeled red blood cell studies are most useful in patients with bleeding distal to the ligament of Treitz. Because the agent is persistent in the bloodstream, extravasation of technetium can be monitored for 12 to 24 h after injection.

On the other hand, angiography requires active bleeding during the 10 s that the contrast material is injected into the artery. It is, however, the most accurate modality for anatomic localization of bleeding. In upper GI bleeding the celiac artery is the first vessel injected followed by the left gastric and gastroduodenal arteries. In lower GI bleeding both the superior and inferior mesenteric arteries must be studied. A bleeding rate of at least .5 mL/min is needed for angiographic visualization. If a site can be identified it can be controlled with either transcatheter embolization or selective vasoconstrictor infusion, usually with vasopressin. Vasopressin infusions generally begin at .1mL/min and can be increased to .4mL/min. The infusion should be continued for 12 to 24 h, then tapered over the next 24 to 48 h. Patients on vasopressin infusion should be monitored carefully for signs of gut, myocardial and peripheral ischemia. Other complications include arrhythmias, hyponatremia and thrombosis from prolonged placement of the intra-arterial catheter. Transcatheter embolization is accomplished using gelfoam surgical gelatin. Embolotherapy is most helpful in areas with rich collateral networks, such as the esophagus, duodenum, and rectum. Complications of embolotherapy are rare.

Foreign Body Retrieval

ICU patients have a multitude of intravascular catheters. Occasionally a catheter fragment may become dislodged into the vascular system. Major complications include vascular perforation, sepsis, arrhythmias or pulmonary embolism. Percutaneous retrieval of the intravenous foreign body is the procedure of choice. A snare made of very thin guidewire is the most common tool used, although baskets, graspers, or balloon catheters are occasionally used. Success rates range from 80 to 95 percent and complications are rare.

Percutaneous Vena Caval Interruption Devices

In patients with pulmonary embolism who cannot be anticoagulated or in whom anticoagulation has failed, mechanical devices can be used to prevent emboli from reaching the lungs. An inferior vena cavagram is performed before the device is inserted in order to facilitate placement directly below the renal veins. These devices are inserted through a small introducing sheath usually in the femoral vein, then expanded within the cava. A plain radiograph should be obtained 24 to 36 h after filter placement to serve as a baseline for detecting the filter. Complications of filter placement include bleeding, caval thrombosis, filter migration, and puncture site thrombosis.

Catheter-Directed Fibrinolytic Therapy

Catheter-directed fibrinolytic therapy can maximize fibrinolytic therapy at the site of vascular occlusion and minimize systemic side effects. This technique works best in acute thrombi or emboli. Urokinase is the agent of choice because it is not neutralized by circulating antibodies and is thought to have less bleeding complications. An adjunct to fibrinolytic therapy should be low-dose intravenous heparin to decrease the incidence of peri-catheter thrombosis and rebound thrombosis after discontinuation of fibrinolytic therapy. Additionally a fibrinogen level should be checked every 4 h and the infusion stopped if the level falls below 100 mg/dl. After successful lysis, underlying lesions should be dilated and the catheter removed. It is critical that care be delivered in conjunction with a vascular surgeon.

Complications are primarily related to bleeding, most often at arterial puncture sites. Significant bleeding is reported in 10 to 12 percent of patients. By limiting the length of infusion to 24 h or less and keeping the fibrinogen level greater 100 mg/dl, the risk of bleeding can be minimized. Occasionally patients may experience worsening of ischemic symptoms during fibrinolytic infusion. This is caused by distal embolization and usually responds to continued fibrinolytic therapy. However if clinical deterioration persists for longer than an hour, emergency surgery should be considered.

For further reading in *Principles of Critical Care,* see Chap 19 "Chest Radiology in the ICU" Heber MacMahon/Steven M Montner, Chap 20 "Interventional Radiology in the Intensive Care Unit Patient" Daniel Picus/Gregory A Schmidt

---

8 | Pulmonary Artery Catheterization and Interpretation

Scott P. Neeley

INTRODUCTION

The pulmonary artery (PA) catheter can yield information useful in a number of clinical situations at relatively small risk to the patient. Common applications of the PA catheter include determination of the etiology of pulmonary edema, hemodynamic management of patients with septic shock or adult respiratory distress syndrome (ARDS), and management of high risk cardiac and noncardiac surgery patients. Despite its usefulness, however, it is essential to recognize both the limitations of the PA catheter, as well as the potential negative impact of faulty data gathered from incorrect use of this device.

INDICATIONS

Table 8-1 lists clinical conditions for which placement of a PA catheter may provide useful clinical information, along with the commonly sought data point(s) for the given condition. Prior to PA catheter placement, it is important to consider conditions (such as coagulopathy) which may increase the risk of complication. The potential risks of empiric management (suboptimal gas exchange, decreased end-organ perfusion) must also be considered. A projected prolonged unstable course, along with high risks of empiric management would favor PA catheter placement. Finally, noninvasive options, such as echocardiography, should be considered in the diagnosis and management of conditions such as cardiac tamponade, valvular dysfunction, ventricular septal defect and acute right heart syndromes (see Chap. 9). In many of these circumstances, echocardiographic imaging provides information complementary to flow and pressure determinations by catheter technique.

POTENTIAL COMPLICATIONS

Potential complications consist of those related to obtaining vascular access (see Chap. 2), and those directly related to use of the PA catheter, discussed below.

Arrhythmia

Both atrial and ventricular arrhythmias occur during PA catheter placement, the most common being ventricular ectopy. Ventricular

TABLE 8-1 Clinical Uses of Bedside Pulmonary Artery Catheterization

Diagnostic Uses	
	Primary Data Sought
Pulmonary edema	Ppw
Shock	Q_T and SVR; Ppw; $S\bar{v}O_2$
Oliguric renal failure	Ppw, Q_T
Perplexing lactic acidemia	Q_T, $S\bar{v}O_2$
Pulmonary hypertension	Ppa, Ppad, Ppw
Cardiac disorders	
Acute mitral insufficiency	V wave
Ventricular septal defect	ΔO_2 saturation RA →PA
RV infarction	Pra, RVEDP, Ppw
Pericardial tamponade	Pra, RVEDP, Ppad, Ppw
Narrow complex tachyarrhythmia	RA waveform (flutter waves)
Wide complex tachyarrhythmia	RA waveform (cannon A waves)
Lymphatic carcinoma	Aspiration cytology
Microvascular thrombi (ARDS)	Angiography

Monitoring Uses
Assess adequacy of intravascular volume
Hypotension
Oliguria
High-risk surgical patient
Assess effect of change in Ppw on pulmonary edema
Assess therapy for shock
Cardiogenic (vasodilator, inotrope)
Septic (volume, vasopressor, inotrope)
Hypovolemic (volume)
Assess effects of PEEP on DO_2 in ARDS

Ppw, pulmonary wedge pressure; Q_T, cardiac output; SVR, systemic vascular resistance, $S\bar{v}O_2$, mixed venous oxygen saturation; Ppa, pulmonary artery pressure; Ppad, pulmonary artery diastolic pressure; Pra, right atrial pressure; RVEDP, right ventricular end-diastolic pressure; DO_2 oxygen delivery; RV, right ventricle; RA, right atrium.
(Reprinted with permission from Leatherman JW, Marini J: Clinical Use of the Pulmonary Artery Catheter, in Hall JB, Schmidt GA, Wood LDH: Principles of Critical Care, McGraw-Hill, New York, 1992.)

tachycardia (VT) is most often seen in the critically ill patient with risk factors such as myocardial ischemia, shock, hypoxemia, electrolyte disturbances, and exogenous or high endogenous catecholamine levels. Sustained VT requiring specific therapy is rare, as is ventricular fibrillation. Prophylactic lidocaine should be considered only after an initial attempt at PA catheter placement has failed and has induced VT. Emphasis should be placed on correcting arrhythmogenic conditions, use of a full 1.5 ml of air when inflating the catheter tip balloon, and minimization of procedure time.

Right bundle branch block (RBBB) occurs in 0.5 to 5 percent of PA catheter placements. This complication is usually of little con-

sequence, though it may be of concern in the patient with pre-existing left bundle branch block (LBBB). Fortunately, complete heart
block as a result of PA catheter placement is exceedingly rare, even
in the presence of LBBB. Thus, rather than routinely placing an
intravenous pacemaker prophylactically in patients with LBBB
undergoing PA catheter placement, it is acceptable to have external
pacing immediately available.

Thrombosis

Some degree of thrombosis at the catheter insertion site, within the
heart or within the pulmonary artery is common. These thrombi can
cause pulmonary emboli, though clinically significant events are
rare. The catheter itself can also cause pulmonary infarction, though
this is also unusual (0 to 1.4 percent). When infarction does occur,
it is often only apparent as a new radiographic abnormality.

Pulmonary Artery Rupture

This most serious of complications associated with PA catheter use
most frequently presents as brisk hemoptysis, from which 50 percent of patients will die. The incidence is less than 0.2 percent, with
risk factors being PA hypertension, cardiopulmonary bypass, and
anticoagulation.

Miscellaneous

Other complications of PA catheter use include sepsis, knotting,
endocarditis, pulmonic valve insufficiency, and balloon fragmenta-
tion and embolization.

PRESSURE MONITORING

The essential elements of the pressure monitoring system, including
the fluid filled catheter, connecting tubing, and a transducer to
convert the pressure wave to an electrical signal, are diagrammed
in Fig. 8-1. Appropriate damping of the system is important in
overcoming exaggeration of frequency components near the resonant frequency of the system. Overdamping, however, will smooth
tracings and eliminate important components of the waveform. The
most common causes of overdamping are air bubbles in the system,
fibrin or clot on the catheter, and kinking of the catheter. A simple
bedside test for appropriate damping is the "rapid flush test."
Opening the flush valve produces very high pressures in normally
patent systems. When the valve is closed, appropriately damped
systems will show a rapid fall in pressure with an overshoot and
prompt return to a crisp PA tracing (Fig. 8-2). Overdamped systems

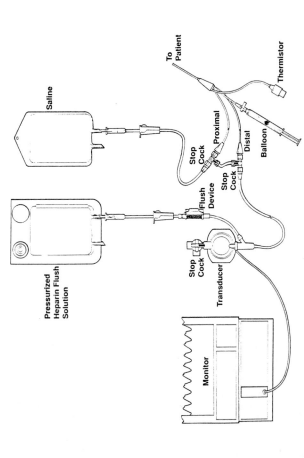

FIG. 8-1 Standard four-lumen PA catheter with pressure tubing, heparinized flush, transducer, and signal processing unit (monitor). PA or RA pressure can be displayed by stopcock adjustment. (Reprinted with permission from Leatherman JW, Marini JJ: Clinical Use of

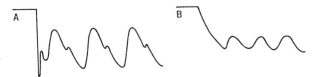

FIG. 8-2 Rapid-flush test. Appropriately damped system (*a*); overdamped system (*b*). *(Reprinted with permission from Leatherman JW, Marini J: Clinical Use of the Pulmonary Artery Catheter, in Hall JB, Schmidt GA, Wood LDH: Principles of Critical Care, McGraw-Hill, New York, 1992.)*

will show a gradual return to the baseline pressure without an overshoot.

Accurate measurement of pressures requires that the monitoring system be calibrated. First, the transducer is "zeroed" by isolating the catheter from the transducer with the stopcock, and then opening the transducer to atmosphere while it is at the level of the left atrium (LA, mid-axillary line at the fourth intercostal space). Once this is done, movement of the transducer above or below LA will result in over- or under-estimation of actual pressures. After zeroing, the amplification function of the transducer is calibrated. Most systems do this internally, though manual calibration can be performed by applying a known amount of pressure to the transducer by use of a fluid filled column of water or a three way stopcock, syringe and mercury manometer.

CATHETER INSERTION

The first step in PA catheter placement is selection of a vascular access site. The preferred sites are the internal jugular and subclavian veins because of ease of cannulation, easier advancement of the catheter across the tricuspid valve, and greater ease in catheter care. The left subclavian is often preferred over the right because of potential problems with catheter kinking with the right subclavian approach. Use of the femoral or antecubital veins introduces more frequent need for fluoroscopy and increased problems with catheter care. Nevertheless, these latter two approaches should be considered when coagulopathy or hyperinflation increase the risk for complications due to internal jugular or subclavian cannulation. Once the site is chosen, vascular access is obtained by insertion of an introducer with a side arm and safety seal feature. An 8.5 F introducer is adequate for passage of either a 7.0 or 7.5 F catheter.

Before insertion of the catheter care should be taken to:

1. Assemble and calibrate the pressure monitoring system and clear any air bubbles from the transducer and connecting tubing;

2. Check the integrity of the balloon by inflating with 1.5 ml of air;
3. Connect the appropriate pressure tubing to the distal catheter port and flush well;
4. Ensure the expected response to pressure changes on the monitoring system by jiggling the catheter tip; and
5. Position the sterile sheath over the PA catheter for later attachment to the introducer.

After the catheter is inserted 15 cm, the rapid flush test is performed to exclude an overdamped system. The balloon is then inflated with 1.5 ml of air, and the catheter gradually advanced into the right ventricle (RV). RV is usually reached 30 to 35 cm from the internal jugular or subclavian access sites. Once an RV tracing is obtained, it is usually not necessary to advance more than 15 cm to reach the PA. If a PA tracing is not obtained after advancing the catheter 15 cm from RV, the balloon should be deflated and the catheter pulled back to RV, as feeding excessive catheter promotes coiling and knotting in the RV. If difficulties persist in reaching PA, fluoroscopy is indicated. The PA tracing is recognized by a rise in diastolic pressure and by the appearance of a dicrotic notch due to pulmonic valve closing (Fig. 8-3). Once in the PA, the catheter is advanced until the balloon "wedges," recognized by transition to an atrial wave form and a fall in mean pressure. Once it is confirmed that balloon deflation is followed by transition back to a PA tracing, and that reinflation of the balloon yields a reliable PA occlusion (wedge) pressure (Ppw), the sterile sleeve can be attached to the introducer. Finally, a chest radiograph is obtained to confirm proper placement and assess for complications of the procedure.

The two most important criteria to confirm a Ppw tracing are an atrial pressure waveform and a fall in mean pressure relative to the pulmonary artery mean pressure Ppa. Damping of the PA tracing may appear atrial in nature but the mean pressure will not fall. Likewise, the "pseudowedge" tracing that sometimes appears as the

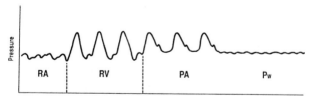

FIG. 8-3 Waveform transition as catheter is advanced from RA to wedge position. *(Reprinted with permission from Leatherman JW, Marini J: Clinical Use of the Pulmonary Artery Catheter, in Hall JB, Schmidt GA, Wood LDH: Principles of Critical Care, McGraw-Hill, New York, 1992.)*

catheter exits the RV usually has a pressure higher than RV mean pressure, and also appears before a convincing PA tracing is seen.

Several clinical conditions can cause difficulties in interpretation of PA waveforms. Hypovolemia can result in smaller than expected differences in transitions between waveforms. The transition from RV to PA may also be more difficult to appreciate when right ventricular end-diastolic pressure (RVEDP) approaches Ppad (pulmonary artery diastolic pressure) as a result of pericardial tamponade, RV infarction, or RV failure.

Catheter whip can exaggerate PA waveform excursions due to transmission of mechanical forces during ventricular contraction. For this reason it is important to measure Ppad at the plateau just before the systolic rise to avoid whip-induced undershoot of diastolic pressure.

Large V waves due to mitral regurgitation, a distended and noncompliant LA, or the presence of an acute VSD may cause the Ppw tracing to resemble the PA waveform. Furthermore, Ppw may approximate mean Ppa, making it appear as if the catheter has failed to wedge. In this situation, the transition from PA to Ppw is best judged by change in waveform, and by noting that the peak of the V wave occurs later in the cardiac cycle than the PA systolic wave.

Large swings in intrathoracic pressure may cause difficulty in recognizing the expected transition in waveforms during catheter insertion. If large respiratory fluctuations pose a problem during mechanical ventilation, sedation or temporary paralysis may aid in interpretation of waveforms and improve reliability of the measurements obtained.

PULMONARY ARTERY PRESSURE

PA pressure is a function of the right ventricular output, pulmonary vascular resistance, and downstream pressure. Normally, low pulmonary vascular resistance assures that Ppad approximates Ppw. Factors such as clot, hypoxia, fibrosis, sepsis, acidosis and drugs, which increase PVR, will cause Ppad to exceed Ppw. Indeed, a Ppad-Ppw gradient >5 mmHg is characteristic of ARDS, sepsis, excessive PEEP, and other conditions that increase PVR. In contrast, pulmonary HTN due to increased downstream (LA) pressure is characterized by normal Ppad-Ppw gradient (< 5 mmHg).

Increased cardiac output ($\dot{Q}_T$) alone will not cause pulmonary HTN. However, a modest increase in vascular resistance and a large increase in $\dot{Q}_T$ due to sepsis, cirrhosis or other factors may result in pulmonary HTN. The contribution of $\dot{Q}_T$ and PVR to pulmonary HTN can be assessed by measuring $\dot{Q}_T$ with thermodilution and calculating PVR [(mean Ppa − Ppw)/$\dot{Q}_T$]. This measurement can be confounded by the tendency of the pulmonary vascular bed to behave like a Starling resistor: resistance increases as flow (Q_T decreases. Thus, the calculated PVR must be interpreted with respect to the Q_T at the time the measurement is made.

PULMONARY CAPILLARY WEDGE PRESSURE

Intravascular pressure (Ppw) is obtained by inflating the catheter balloon with 1 to 1.5 ml of air, allowing the catheter to obstruct forward flow in a branch of the PA. The pressure recorded at the catheter tip is equivalent to the pressure in the occluded pulmonary vein where it intersects with flow from uninterrupted vessels (the j point). Ppw approximates LA pressure as long as there is not obstruction to flow downstream from the j point. Unfortunately, the use of Ppw as a basis for manipulations of intravascular volume and intravascular drugs is frequently complicated by a number of common errors in data acquisition and interpretation.

It should be recognized that while only Ppw is measured, it is the transmural pressure (intravascular-pleural, Ppw-Ppl) that is of interest, since for a given compliance of cardiac chambers, this determines ventricular volume and hence stroke volume. Thus, it is important to read Ppw from a strip recording (not the digital monitor) at end expiration. Assessment of Ppw at other points in the respiratory cycle will be influenced by the tidal variations in the intrathoracic pressure that surrounds the heart and pulmonary vasculature.

Ppw recorded at end expiration will overestimate transmural pressure (Ppw−Ppl) if intrathoracic pressure is positive at end expiration. This can be due to the presence of applied PEEP, auto-PEEP, or active exhalation. With relaxed respiratory muscles, the change in Ppl in response to PEEP is determined by the chest wall compliance (Cw) and change in lung volume; the lung volume change is in turn a function of PEEP and lung compliance (C_L). The formula $dPpl = PEEP \times C_L/(C_L + Cw)$ gives the pleural pressure change as a function of PEEP, C_L, and Cw. Under normal circumstances where C_L and Cw are roughly equal, this formula predicts that approximately 50 percent of a given PEEP is transmitted to the pleural space. A stiff chest wall enhances the fraction of PEEP transmitted to the pleural space, whereas stiff lungs (as in ARDS) result in decreased transmission of PEEP. While it is important to recognize these pressure relationships, practically speaking it is not possible to determine the actual juxtacardiac pressure at a given level of PEEP. Thus, in most types of clinical decision-making, use of the Ppw should not focus on the absolute number per se, but rather on changes in the Ppw with therapeutic interventions and their correlation with relevant end points (e.g., blood pressure, PaP_{O_2}, urine output).

An uncommon but serious problem in Ppw measurement occurs when Ppw actually reflects alveolar pressure. This occurs when the catheter is positioned in the lung such that Palv>Ppv (zone 1 and 2 lung) at end expiration. This situation will only occur when PEEP is present and PEEP exceeds Pla. Fortunately this condition seldom occurs in the absence of high levels of PEEP. It should be suspected, however, whenever there is a near 1:1 change in Ppw and PEEP on PEEP reduction or addition.

Auto-PEEP due to dynamic hyperinflation frequently leads to hemodynamic compromise as well as errors in PA catheter data interpretation. Auto-PEEP typically occurs in the setting of increased C_L (e.g., emphysema) and hyperinflation (due to airflow obstruction and high minute ventilation), resulting in a large component of Palv being transmitted to the juxtacardiac space with the potential for emergence of zone 2 lung conditions. Auto-PEEP can be estimated in the absence of respiratory muscle activity by measuring end-expiratory airway pressure with the airway occluded. Even in the presence of respiratory muscle activity, the hemodynamic significance of auto-PEEP can be assessed by observing changes in BP, Q_T, and Ppw during a brief interruption in positive-pressure ventilation. Finally, while auto-PEEP is most often suspected in airflow obstruction, it can occur in patients with ARDS when minute ventilation is high.

Large errors in Ppw measurement may occur when patients continue to actively expire at end exhalation. A respiration-related Ppw excursion of 10 to 15 mmHg suggests that end-expiratory Ppw overestimates the true transmural pressure. When this occurs, the use of sedation or paralysis in the mechanically ventilated patient may be necessary for reliable data aquisition.

Clinical Use of Ppw

In clinical practice, the Ppw is used primarily as an estimate of hydrostatic filtration pressure (Pcap) and as a measure of LV preload. Ppw is used as an estimate of Pcap in the diagnosis and management of pulmonary edema. However, an isolated Ppw reading does not reliably differentiate acute hydrostatic pulmonary edema from that due to altered permeability. Hydrostatic pulmonary edema may occur despite normal intravascular volume on the basis of diastolic dysfunction due to ischemia or accelerated hypertension. By the time a PA catheter is placed a previously elevated Ppw may have returned to normal. Thus, reliable assessment of the cause of pulmonary edema may require a period of observation. Normally, the expected Ppw threshold for hydrostatic pulmonary edema is 22 to 25 mmHg (this may be higher when Ppw is chronically elevated). Maintaining Ppw<18 should result in improvement in signs of hydrostatic pulmonary edema over 24 h if the situation is not complicated by intermittent elevation of Ppw due to myocardial ischemia, low plasma oncotic pressure, or altered pulmonary capillary permeability.

The use of Ppw to estimate Pcap is also useful in permeability pulmonary edema, where Pcap is a major determinant of lung water. Reducing Ppw by diuresis, ultrafiltration, or dialysis may markedly benefit gas exchange. There is no minimum value for Ppw below which removal of intravascular volume is contraindicated provided $\dot{Q}T$ is adequate.

The second major use of Ppw is as an indicator of the adequacy of LV preload. Ppw can be used to estimate LVEDP when there is neither mitral valve obstruction or very high filling pressures (>15 mmHg), where atrial systole will force LVEDP above mean Pla and Ppw. However, because the relationship between Ppw, LVEDP and $\dot{Q}T$ can be drastically affected by conditions such as ischemia, hypertrophy, shock and high doses of pressors, the optimal Ppw must be individually determined for each patient. Optimal Ppw can be defined as that above which further increase results in little rise in $\dot{Q}T$, stroke volume (SV) or LV stroke work (LVSW = SV × Pa − Ppw × 0.0136). In normal individuals LVSW usually plateaus at an LVEDP of 10 to 12 mmHg. In patients with septic shock the optimal Ppw usually lies between 10 and 14 mmHg. After acute myocardial infarction, or at high levels of PEEP, a Ppw of 18 mmHg may yield optimal $\dot{Q}T$. Similarly, after acute volume resuscitation of hypovolemic shock, a Ppw of 14 to 18 mmHg may actually represent relative hypovolemia because of reduced LV compliance. Thus the optimal Ppw should be defined for each individual patient if necessary by use of acute volume challenges followed by measurement of Ppw and $\dot{Q}T$ while holding PEEP and vasoactive drugs constant. Maintaining a Ppw higher than necessary to achieve optimal $\dot{Q}T$ may be detrimental in patients who have or are at high risk for ARDS. Conversely, in the individual whose primary problem is hypotension or shock, the Ppw should be increased with acute volume infusion until no further improvement in $\dot{Q}T$ can be achieved.

CARDIAC OUTPUT MEASUREMENT

The thermodilution technique for measuring cardiac output ($\dot{Q}Ttd$) is a method employing thermal depression as the indicator. Cold fluid is injected through the proximal lumen of the PA catheter into the RA and, after mixing in the RV with venous blood returning from the periphery, passes into the PA where a thermistor at the catheter tip senses dynamic changes in temperature. The Stewart-Hamilton formula relates $\dot{Q}T$ to temperature change over time:

$$\dot{Q}_T = V(TB - TI) \times K1 \times K2/\int TB(t)dt \qquad (8\text{-}1)$$

where V=injected volume; TB=blood temperature; TI=injectate temperature; TB(t)dt=change in blood temperature as a function of time; and K1 and K2 are constants.

Whether using iced or room temperature injectate, the $\dot{Q}_T$td compares favorably with output values obtained by Fick or dye dilution methods as long as careful technique is used. Errors may occur if the volume or recorded temperature of the injectate are incorrect or if the wrong computational constant for the catheter in use and injectate temperature is entered into the computer. Errors can also occur due to warming of the injectate due to delay or handling after the syringe is removed from the ice. Prolonged or uneven injections and thermistor contact with the vessel wall are other technical sources of measurement errors. Clinical conditions resulting in $\dot{Q}_T$td being an unreliable estimate of cardiac output include cardiac arrhythmias occuring during injection, left-to-right shunts (ASD, VSD), and significant tricuspid regurgitation. Finally, $\dot{Q}_T$td may vary based on the phase of the respiratory cycle at which the injection is begun. The average of multiple, randomly timed injections probably gives the most accurate assessment in this situation.

Measurement of $\dot{Q}_T$td allows calculation of vascular resistances: SVR=(meanBP−Pra)/$\dot{Q}_T$, PVR=(Ppa−Ppw)/$\dot{Q}_T$. The use of $\dot{Q}_T$ and SVR can be particularly helpful in management of septic shock, sepsis syndrome, and ARDS, where hypotension and hypoperfusion may be due to decreased cardiac output (myocardial dysfunction, increased venous capacitance, hypovolemia, pneumothorax, pulmonary emboli, increased PVR, change in PEEP or gas trapping) or low SVR due to vasodilation of sepsis.

MIXED VENOUS OXYGEN SATURATION

Measurement of mixed venous oxygen saturation ($S\bar{v}O_2$) allows an assessment of the relationship between O_2 delivery (DO_2, the product of $\dot{Q}_T$ and arterial O_2 content) and tissue O_2 consumption ($\dot{V}O_2$). Normally, $\dot{V}O_2$ is independent of DO_2, and is determined by metabolic activity of tissues. When DO_2 is insufficient to meet tissue requirements due to a reduction in $\dot{Q}_T$ or SaO_2, the result is a decrease in $S\bar{v}O_2$.

$S\bar{v}O_2$ should be assessed in PA blood after venous return from various organs has been thoroughly mixed in RA and RV. $S\bar{v}O_2$ obtained from a central venous catheter may not be reliable since normally $S\bar{v}O_2$ is lower in the SVC than in the IVC, whereas the reverse is usually true in shock. $S\bar{v}O_2$ can be assessed either by intermittent sampling of blood from the distal PA port or continuously with a fiberoptic PA catheter that measures O_2 saturation by reflectance oximetry. Intermittent sampling of $S\overline{v}O_2$ is accomplished by discarding the initial 3 mL of blood, then withdrawing a sample very slowly so as to avoid contamination with capillary blood. $S\overline{v}O_2$ should be measured directly by oximetry, since calculation of the $S\overline{v}O_2$ from measurement of $P\overline{v}O_2$, pH and temperature is often inaccurate due to the steep slope of the O_2 dissociation in the venous range. $S\overline{v}O_2$ measurement by reflectance oximetry using a fiberoptic PA catheter is a reliable method of $S\overline{v}O_2$ assessment providing the system is calibrated before insertion, an appropriate level of light intensity is used, and periodic comparison of displayed $S\overline{v}O_2$ with $S\overline{v}O_2$ measured on a sample of mixed venous blood is performed.

In the ICU, the primary use of $S\overline{v}O_2$ is in assessment of the adequacy of QT as it relates to tissue aerobic metabolism, or $\dot{V}O_2$. Normally the $SaO_2 - S\overline{v}O_2$ difference is 20 to 25 percent, yielding an $S\overline{v}O_2$ of 65 to 75 percent when arterial blood is well oxygenated. When DO_2 is insufficient to meet tissue requirements for aerobic metabolism due to hypovolemia, LV dysfunction or anemia, $S\overline{v}O_2$ will be decreased due to increased tissue extraction of O_2. This remains true as long as $\dot{V}O_2$ remains independent of DO_2. At a critically low level of $\dot{Q}T$, however, tissues are no longer able to meet their O_2 demands by increased extraction, and $\dot{V}O_2$ becomes flow dependent. At this point, $S\overline{v}O_2$ is no longer a reliable indicator of the adequacy of $\dot{Q}T$. Flow dependency is seen at levels of DO_2 that are at or above normal values in certain types of critical illness (see Chap. 57).

Other uses of the $S\overline{v}O_2$ include assessment of absolute level of $\dot{V}O_2$, use of $\dot{V}O_2$ to help guide nutritional support, and as an aid in the diagnosis of intra-cardiac left-to-right shunts.

MISCELLANEOUS APPLICATIONS OF THE PA CATHETER

Other diagnostic applications of the PA catheter that may on occasion prove useful in the ICU include bedside balloon occlusion pulmonary angiography, microvascular cytology, arrhythmia evaluation, and detection of intracardiac shunts.

For further reading in *Principles of Critical Care*, see Chap 25 "Clinical Use of the Pulmonary Artery Catheter" James W Leatherman/John Marini

Kevin Simpson

Doppler echocardiography is a relatively rapid, noninvasive, bedside imaging procedure that provides detailed structural and physiologic information about cardiac function. Serial examination is relatively inexpensive and poses no significant hazards to the patient, providing a means for monitoring and tracking a patient's condition and response to therapy. Clinical applications of echocardiography in the intensive care unit include the distinction of cardiac from noncardiac mechanisms of systemic hypoperfusion and hypotension, noninvasive assessment of volume status, determination of a source of systemic emboli, and early recognition of such processes as acute myocardial ischemia and pulmonary embolization of venous thrombi, tumor, or air.

ECHOCARDIOGRAPHY IN THE HYPOPERFUSED PATIENT

The first step in the evaluation of the hypotensive patient focuses on an assessment of volume status. Although chamber size is not exactly analogous to preload, certainly chamber size plays a large role in determining myocardial fiber length and ultimately cardiac output. Diastolic compliance of either ventricle can change acutely, rendering pressure measurements as a correlate of diastolic chamber size difficult to interpret and the lack of correlation of pulmonary capillary wedge pressure to left ventricular end-diastolic volume and stroke volume has been demonstrated. Echocardiography can potentially display a picture of any of the cardiac chambers directly, allowing immediate measurement of chamber dimensions. Hence, echocardiography offers an easy means of detecting hypovolemia and assessing the adequacy of volume resuscitation.

Direct assessment of myocardial fiber shortening and overall ventricular function can be achieved by quantitative echocardiographic analysis of end-diastolic and end-systolic dimensions. Indeed, it is possible to provide an immediate qualitative bedside description of global ventricular systolic function. In addition, the heterogeneity or regionality of segmental wall motion abnormalities, such as occurs following myocardial ischemia, can be judged by assessing whether individual myocardial segments thicken and move inward normally or not. Furthermore, Doppler techniques that measure flow velocity in the left ventricular outflow tract or aorta may be used to characterize left ventricular ejection and to measure cardiac output.

Dilated cardiomyopathies are characterized by a hypokinetic, enlarged left ventricle without significant increase in left ventricular wall thickness to radius ratio. In striking contrast, restrictive cardiomyopathies are typified by a normal to small left ventricle with preserved systolic function. If the restrictive process results from myocardial infiltration (e.g., amyloid), the myocardial walls will be increased in thickness relative to cavity size. Hypertrophic cardiomyopathies, whether acquired as a result of increased left ventricular afterload (e.g., systemic hypertension) or idiopathic, demonstrate normal to small left ventricular cavity size with marked increases in left ventricular wall thickness. The pattern of ventricular hypertrophy in idiopathic hypertrophic cardiomyopathy is usually nonuniform in contradistinction to the symmetric increase in left ventricular wall thickness observed in hypertensive heart disease. Until late in the disease left ventricular systolic function is normal if not hyperdynamic. In that unique subset of patients in whom the hypertrophic process is particularly marked in the left ventricular outflow tract, dynamic subvalvular left ventricular outflow tract obstruction may develop.

Doppler echocardiographic techniques are also useful for identifying mechanical complications of ischemic myocardial disease. Acute disruption of infarcting muscle resulting in left ventricular free wall rupture with pseudoaneurysm formation, ventricular septal perforation, or mitral regurgitation due to a flail mitral valve can all be diagnosed echocardiographically.

Pericardial Effusion and Tamponade

One of the earliest applications of echocardiography was the diagnosis of pericardial effusion detected as an abnormal relatively echo-free space surrounding the free walls of the heart. Early in the progression of hemodynamic deterioration, late diastolic and early systolic collapse of the right atrial free wall is noted. Subsequently, early diastolic collapse of the right ventricle is detected as cardiac output falls prior to the onset of systemic hypotension.

Right Ventricular Overload

Pure pressure overload of the right ventricle in patients free of left ventricular disease such as occurs in primary pulmonary hypertension, acute massive pulmonary embolism, chronic thromboembolic pulmonary disease, and pulmonary parenchymal diseases which secondarily compromise the pulmonary circulation results in right ventricular enlargement and secondary compression of the left ventricle by displacement of the interventricular septum. These alterations in left ventricular geometry profoundly influence left ventricular diastolic filling, resulting in a greater dependence on atrial systolic filling. Relief of right ventricular systolic hypertension results in reversal of left ventricular compression and improvement in early diastolic left ventricular filling. Right ventricular hypertrophy (RVH) is diagnosed by increased wall thickness, and signals chronic pulmonary hypertension (about 10 mmHg/mm RV wall thickness). The absence of RVH, as determined by echocardiography, in the setting of pulmonary hypertension suggests an acute elevation in pulmonary arterial pressure.

ADDITIONAL APPLICATIONS OF ECHOCARDIOGRAPHY

Two-dimensional and Doppler echocardiography have made their greatest impact on the diagnosis and characterization of valvular heart disease. Of particular interest to the intensivist is the characterization of valve-related masses which may explain systemic embolization, constitutional symptoms of endocarditis, sudden onset of valvular obstruction, or progressive valvular regurgitation.

Assessment of the great vessels in their proximal portions can be achieved by transthoracic echocardiography and, as such, echocardiography should be considered for use in the diagnosis of aortic dissection.

Contrast echocardiography is a technique in which intravenous echocardiographic contrast agents are used to improve the definition of endocardial borders, delineate intracavitary masses, detect bidirectional flow, and demonstrate intracardiac shunting.

Transesophageal Echocardiography

In the ICU, traditional transthoracic echocardiography is often unable to provide clear imaging of the heart due to interference from thoracic air which may be increased by positive-pressure ventilation, especially when end-expiratory pressure is applied. Furthermore, chest wall trauma, abdominal or thoracic surgery, burns, and dressings all may interfere with precordial imaging. Transesophageal echocardiography (TEE) is a technique that exploits the proximity of the esophagus to the heart to obtain anatomic and physiologic information that may not be possible with precordial imaging. This is of particular benefit when assessing the left atrium for the presence of intracardiac thrombi or masses. Not only does the proximal location of the probe to the left atrium allow visualization of this chamber, which is frequently impossible from the transthoracic approach, but, in addition, the superior resolution can permit distinction between tumor, thrombus, or vegetation in most cases. TEE is also the most sensitive technique for monitoring for intracardiac air or other embolic material.

Despite widespread use, few complications of TEE (e.g., esophageal perforation, aspiration, and arrhythmias) have been reported in the literature. TEE appears to be a safe modality even in the presence of anticoagulation, although esophageal pathology mandates that caution be used. Bacteremia can occur with pharyngeal and esophageal probe insertion and, therefore, most clinicians recommend antibiotic prophylaxis for patients at risk of endocarditis prior to undergoing TEE examinations.

For further reading in *Principles of Critical Care,* see Chap 21 "Doppler Echocardiography: Diagnostic Applications in the Intensive Care Unit" Eric K Louie/Steven N Konstadt, Chap 22 "Perioperative Transesophageal Echocardiography" Laurence Segil/Steven Konstadt

Bronchoscopy in the Critically Ill Patient

Katrina A. Guest

Fiberoptic bronchoscopy has a special role in the ICU setting. The indications, risks, and techniques are fundamentally different from routine diagnostic bronchoscopy.

INDICATIONS

Fiberoptic bronchoscopy is indicated in the ICU for:

1. Examining the placement site of the endotracheal tube (ETT);
2. Investigating the cause of lung collapse;
3. Extracting a foreign body;
4. Determining the site of bleeding in hemoptysis;
5. Obtaining reliable bacterial cultures using a protected brush;
6. Searching for possible tracheal or bronchial lacerations in trauma victims;
7. Examining the airways for stenosis or lesions;
8. Detecting the extent and severity of inhalational airways injury; and
9. Assisting in intubation or controlled extubation in patients at risk for airway complications.

PREBRONCHOSCOPY CONSIDERATIONS

As in elective diagnostic bronchoscopy, patient characteristics often contribute to the risk of the procedure. If intubated, the size of the ETT will dictate the size of the bronchoscope that can be used. In general an ETT of at least 8 mm internal lumen size is required. The stability or presence of neck fractures may determine the need for general anesthesia since the inevitable cough stimulated by the procedure may risk spinal cord injury. Posterior nosebleeds usually dictate use of a transoral route. Suspicion of epiglottitis requires the controlled atmosphere of the operating room.

The procedure required also dictates what type of bronchoscope should be used. Small scopes are adequate for children and for the purpose of viewing anatomic structures. The channel size in the smaller scopes is limiting for use of large forceps, baskets, or for suctioning. Therapeutic use of lasers also may require specific scope capabilities.

CONTRAINDICATIONS

Contraindications include: unstable angina or myocardial infarction (MI) in the past 6 weeks, ventricular tachycardia, oxygen saturations of less than 90 percent on 100 percent oxygen, and clotting abnormalities. If only airway inspection is performed, clotting variables need not be normal but nasal trauma should be avoided.

METHODS

In patients with a bleeding diathesis, attempts at correction are needed before biopsy or nasal intubation are attempted. In intubated patients routine consent and anxiolytic preparation is used but the pharynx need not be anesthetized. Biting of the ETT and consequent damage to the bronchoscope must be prevented with a bite block if the patient is orally intubated. The ETT is lubricated with 5 to 10 ml viscous lidocaine and the bronchoscope is then passed through an access elbow. At this point the bronchoscope allows for a leak of tidal volume, and causes incomplete obstruction of the airway. These may require adjustment in the ventilator such as increased $F_{I_{O_2}}$ (100 percent), increased tidal volume and altered inspiratory flow: expiratory flow (I:E) ratio. All patients should have continuous pulse oximetry in place. Airway anaesthesia is attained with small amounts (2 mL aliquots) of 1% lidocaine. The use of lidocaine is thought to decrease the yield of quantitative culture so its use should be minimized or eliminated if culture results are the primary goal.

Following general inspection of the airways, the first samples to be obtained should be those on a protected-lumen catheter for obtaining bacterial cultures. Following this, bronchoalveolar lavage and other procedures such as bronchial brushing for tumor cells, and biopsies can be done.

DIAGNOSTIC SAMPLING

Bronchoalveolar Lavage

This procedure is performed in the same way as in less ill patients with the expectation that the oxygenation will likely suffer for some hours after this procedure. A volume of 100 to 150 mL of saline solution is injected through the suction channel of a bronchoscope that has been wedged in a segmental bronchus. The saline and alveolar fluid is then aspirated through the bronchoscope into a collection trap. The resulting sample of bronchoalveolar lavage fluid contains a mixture of cells, microbes, surfactant, proteins, and debris. This information is best used to detect the presence of malignancy, tuberculosis, fungal infection, and *Pneumocystis carinii*. Viral pneumonia can be inferred from cellular abnormalities seen at cytology, direct florescent antibody stains, and culture of the virus. Bacterial infection is more difficult to discern since this fluid is uniformly contaminated with upper airway organisms. More than 10,000 colony-forming μ/mL of wash is suggestive of an etiology of pneumonia.

Bronchial Brushing

This technique is widely used for the diagnosis of endobronchial tumors and with a protected brush can be used for quantitative culture in the diagnosis of pneumonia. These cultures however require a labor intensive commitment from the bacteriology department. The criterion for pneumonia is the growth of more than 1000 colony-forming μ/mL of brush fluid, prepared by aseptically placing the brush, after its removal from the bronchoscope, in a volume of 1 mL nonbacteriostatic saline, and promptly delivering it to the microbiology laboratory. An unprotected brush sample is useful for the diagnosis of malignancy, tuberculosis, fungal organisms, or *P. carinii*.

Biopsies

Endobronchial biopsies are taken under direct vision from lesions within the airways. A transbronchial biopsy is taken by pushing the metal forceps through the wall of a small bronchus and sampling a piece of parenchymal lung tissue. This technique has a risk of pneumothorax which should be minimized for the critically ill patient by concomitant use of fluoroscopy. A judgment of whether or not a patient could withstand a unilateral pneumothorax should guide the decision to perform the test. Only one lung is biopsied to prevent the disastrous complication of bilateral pneumothorax. Patients requiring positive end-expiratory pressure (PEEP) have undergone transbronchial biopsy but their risk for pneumothorax is greater so open lung biopsy may be preferable. Transbronchial biopsy is particularly useful to diagnose miliary tuberculosis and coccioidomycosis, disseminated histoplasmosis, and certain noninfectious diseases such as alveolar proteinosis. In some cases, an untreatable diagnosis may be found, such as alveolar amyloid or lymphangitic cancer, but even these diagnoses have important implications for the patient's general prognosis. In every case, the benefits and risks of transbronchial biopsy must be weighed carefully because the danger of tension pneumothorax, air embolism, and bleeding is higher in critically ill patients.

UPPER AIRWAY OBSTRUCTION

Upper airway obstruction due to tumor or malignancy in the trachea, main carina, or mainstem bronchi can be treated either with endobronchial laser or radiation therapy. Laser bronchoscopy is a procedure done in the operating room in which a special bronchoscope with quartz fibers transmits laser energy capable of burning and evaporating tissue. Brachytherapy requires an endoscopically placed catheter for the administration of local radiation over a prescribed period of time. Either procedure achieves its end by increasing the diameter of the large airways and thereby relieving airway obstruction. This may be necessary either to relieve respiratory distress or obstruction resulting in pneumonia.

COMPLICATIONS

The complications of pneumothorax (simple or tension), hypoventilation, hypoxemia, and hemorrhage are made more ominous in the ICU by the patient's baseline poor physiologic state. Care must be taken in patient selection and execution of the procedure. The operator should take extra precautions to ensure adequate ventilation and oxygenation especially when the procedure significantly obstructs a small airway. Pneumothorax and hemorrhage can be minimized by using fluoroscopy for brush and transbronchial procedures and by careful attention to any coagulation abnormalities before the procedure is attempted.

For further reading in *Principles of Critical Care*, see Chap 17 "Bronchoscopy" Eugene F Geppert

11	**Control of Pain and Anxiety**
	Phillip Cozzi

In the intensive care unit setting, advances have been made in the control of pain and anxiety due to better drugs and improved methods of delivery.

DELETERIOUS EFFECTS OF PAIN AND ANXIETY

Pain and anxiety have harmful physiological and psychological effects. Abnormalities of mechanical pulmonary function and gas exchange consistently occur following major abdominal and thoracic surgery. Impairment in pulmonary function is worst following upper abdominal surgery, resulting in diminished cough, decreased vital capacity, inspiratory capacity, functional residual capacity, forced expiratory volume in 1 s (FEV_1), and forced vital capacity. These changes are most prominent in the elderly, obese, and those with cardiac disease.

Pain and anxiety contribute to the stress response, which is the pattern of biochemical changes following traumatic injury, sepsis, and surgery. These changes include alterations in the nervous system, humoral factors, coagulation and endocrinological milieu. A typical example of the stress response is the elevation of circulating catecholamines, contributing to hyperglycemia. The stress response also activates the sympathetic nervous system which increases heart rate, blood pressure, and myocardial oxygen consumption, predisposing to myocardial ischemia.

The ICU environment is particularly anxiety provoking. Patients being mechanically ventilated, for example, commonly sense agony, fright, and panic. Postoperative traumatic neurosis has been described in patients resulting from ICU experience. The beneficial effects of analgesia and sedation include reduction of acute emotional suffering, improvement in respiratory function and diminishment of diaphragmatic dysfunction.

ASSESSING PAIN AND SEDATION

Assessment of pain is invariably subjective. Rating scales are commonly used. One widely accepted instrument is the Visual Analog Scale (VAS), in which patients self-rate their pain by locating a point along a line with poles representing the extremes of "no pain" and "worst pain."

Assessment of sedation is likewise inexact. A commonly used six-point sedation scale incorporates identifiable clinical end-points (Table 11-1).

TABLE 11-1 Sedation Scoring for Critically Ill Patients

Level	Response
1	Anxious and agitated or restless or both
2	Cooperative, oriented, and tranquil
3	Responding to commands
4	Brisk response to stimulus[a]
5	Sluggish response to stimulus[a]
6	No response to stimulus[a]

[a]Light glabellar tap or loud auditory stimulus. *(Reproduced with permission from Drasner K, Katz JA, Schapera A: Control of Anxiety and Pain, in Hall JB, Schmidt GA and Wood LDH: Principles of Critical Care, McGraw-Hill, New York, 1992.)*

REGIONAL TECHNIQUES

Epidural Local Anesthesia

Epidural local anesthesia offers the easiest method for abdominal, thoracic and lower extremity analgesia. This technique provides profound analgesia while avoiding the risk of respiratory depression. Analgesia is best achieved using a catheter technique which permits intermittent or continuous infusions. Incorrect placement of the catheter can result in intrathecal injection (profound spinal blockade) or intravascular injection (CNS and cardiac toxicity). Distribution of analgesia depends on the concentration of the drug and the volume of delivery. Most anesthetists recommend using high volume and low concentration delivery of the drug, which results in better distribution and less profound motor blockade. Bupivacaine is the most widely used drug for epidural local anesthesia, because of its long duration of action and less motor blockade. Dosing begins with an initial bolus of 5 to 10 mg 0.25 to 0.5% bupivacaine, followed by continuous infusion of 0.125% solution at 8 to 20 ml/h depending on the location of pain. Side effects include motor blockade, sympathetic blockade resulting in hypotension, parasympathetic blockade resulting in urinary retention, catheter-related infections, and headache after accidental dural puncture. Contraindications to this technique include sepsis, coagulation defect, and local skin inflammation.

Spinal Narcotics

Selective spinal analgesia can be achieved using intrathecal opioid injection. This technique provides more profound analgesia compared to epidural injection, although it is associated with a higher incidence of side effects. The advantages of this technique are:

1. Selective effect for pain transmission,
2. No autonomic nor motor disturbance,

3. Sensation remains intact, unlike with systemic narcotics,
4. It provides analgesia to patients with tolerance to systemic opioids.

Morphine sulfate is administered by single injection (1 to 6 mg epidural or 0.1 to 1.0 mg intrathecal) or by continuous infusion of 0.2 to 1.5 mg/h. Epidural administration of fentanyl requires repeated bolusing or continuous infusion (2.5 to 10 μg per h). Side effects of spinal narcotics include respiratory depression (occasionally requiring naloxone reversal) nausea, vomiting, and pruritus. Combined epidural anesthetic and opioid can be used, typically including bupivacaine and morphine.

Intercostal Blockade

Intercostal blockade provides analgesia for somatic pain involving the thorax and upper abdomen. Bupivacaine (3 to 5 ml 0.5 percent with epinephrine 5μg per mL) is injected at the unilateral angle of the rib at the involved dermatome plus one intercostal space above and below. Rare side effects of this procedure include pneumothorax and systemic toxicity of the injected drug.

Intrapleural Anesthesia

Injection of anesthetic directly into the pleural space results in analgesia to unilateral dermatomes supplied by intercostal nerves. Intermittent injections of 20 ml 0.5% bupivacaine with epinephrine 5μg per mL provide excellent anesthesia. This technique also provides pain relief following cholecystectomy. Use following thoracotomy is limited by drug loss from the thoracostomy tube.

PARENTERAL NARCOTICS

Narcotics have threshold plasma concentrations at which they are effective. The goal in the use of narcotics is to provide adequate relief of pain with minimal side effects. Intramuscular administration of narcotics is inappropriate for most intensive care unit patients because of variable absorption and delay in efficacy. Intravenous administration provides more predictable drug levels and more rapid onset of action, but has increased side effects. Patient controlled analgesia is rarely useful in the intensive care unit because few critically ill patients are capable of using these devices.

Several narcotics are used in the intensive care unit, with varying pharmacokinetic characteristics (Table 11-2). Morphine is frequently used in the ICU and is inexpensive; however, it has slow onset of action, releases histamine, and morphine-6-glucuronide (a metabolite with four times the potency of morphine) accumulates

TABLE 11-2 Pharmacology of Intravenous Narcotics

| | Distribution Half-Life (min) | Elimination Half-Life (h) | Peak Effect (min) | Approximate Equinalgesic Dose | SUGGESTED INITIAL DOSE | | |
					Bolus	Continuous Infusion	PCA Bolus
Morphine	20	2–4	30	10	2–5 mg	2–10 mg/h	0.5–1.0
Meperidine	10	3–5	4	100	25–50 mg	Not recommended	5–10
Fentanyl	3	2–5	4	0.1	25–100 µg	25–100 µg/h	10–50
Sufentanil	1	2–3	8	0.01	2–10 µg	2.5–10 µg/h	2–5
Alfentanil	3	1–3	1	0.5	2–3 mg	0.5–3 mg/h	Not recommended

(Reproduced with permission from Drasner K, Katz JA, Schapera A: Control of Anxiety and Pain, in Hall JB, Schmidt GA and Wood LDH: Principles of Critical Care, McGraw-Hill, New York, 1992.)

in renal impairment. Meperidine has rapid onset of action and is a potent suppressor of shivering. Normeperidine, a major metabolite of meperidine, is a convulsant and accumulates in renal impairment. Fentanyl has rapid onset of action and pharmacokinetics which are not altered in hepatic cirrhosis and renal failure. Also, fentanyl may be useful for patients with significant reactive airway disease because it does not release histamine. Alfentanil has rapid onset of action, short duration of action, and no change in pharmacokinetics with renal disease, though hepatic disease prolongs elimination. Sufentanil is a highly potent narcotic, which may result in less tolerance. This drug, therefore, may be useful in patients requiring long-term administration of narcotic.

ANXIETY AND SEDATION

Heavy sedation is required with neuromuscular blockade. Otherwise, the patient should be sedated to the level of no distress. This strategy maintains some degree of spontaneous breathing and may shorten the period of immobility.

Administration of Sedation

Benzodiazepines are useful in the intensive care unit because of their anxiolytic, hypnotic, and amnestic properties. Although frequently used in the past, diazepam is less frequently used today because of its long elimination half life (24 to 40 h), prolonged elimination in liver and kidney disease, and associated thrombophlebitis and pain on injection. Midazolam has rapid onset of action and short elimination half life (1 to 4 h). Side effects include hypotension and respiratory depression; prolonged elimination is expected in hepatic disease. In ICU patients, sedation is initiated with 0.5 to 1.0 mg midazolam every one to three minutes until sedation is achieved; maintenance infusion rates range from 0.01 to 0.20 mg/kg/h. Flumazenil reverses benzodiazepine-related sedation and respiratory depression and may allow periodic assessment of neurologic status in patients requiring prolonged sedation. For the reversal of benzodiazepine overdose, the recommended initial dose is 0.2 mg flumazenil intravenously over 30 seconds, followed by 0.3 to 0.5 mg over 30 s at one-minute intervals up to a cumulative dose of 3.0 mg or the desired level of consciousness is reached. Seizures occurred in 1.3 percent of benzodiazepine overdose patients treated with flumazenil in U.S. trials. Since experience in the U.S. is limited, this drug should be used cautiously.

Phenothiazines, for example chlorpromazine, are infrequently used because of anticholinergic and α-adrenergic blocking properties. Butyrophenones, for example droperidol and haloperidol, are commonly used to control acute confusional states in the critically ill. Dosing of either droperidol or haloperidol is initiated with 2.5 to 5.0 mg by slow intravenous injection every thirty minutes until agitation ceases. Side effects include torsade de pointes and extrapyramidal reactions.

Propofol is a new intravenous anesthetic of the alkylphenol group. It is very short acting (elimination half life 1 to 3 h) and may, upon further investigation, have a role in sedation of critically ill patients, using subanesthetic doses.

Barbiturate use in the intensive care unit is limited by respiratory and cardiovascular depression, loss of thermoregulation, induction of hepatic microsomal enzymes, tolerance and withdrawal syndromes.

Ketamine is a phencyclidine compound and the only intravenous anesthetic that produces analgesia at subanesthetic doses. Side effects include systemic hypertension, increased intracranial pressure and hallucinations. Because of its short duration of action (8 to 10 min) it has been primarily used in the intensive care unit during short procedures such as wound debridement. Also, because of its sympathomimetic bronchodilatory effect, it may be useful for sedation of asthmatics requiring mechanical ventilation.

For further reading in *Principles of Critical Care,* see Chap 82 "Control of Pain and Anxiety" Kenneth Drasner/Jeffrey A Katz/Anthony Schapera, Chap 187E "Pain" Kathleen A Puntillo

---

12

Nutrition in the Intensive Care Unit

Constantine Manthous

Aggressive nutritional support must be considered routinely and early in the management of critical illness.

THE EFFECTS OF CRITICAL ILLNESS ON GUT PHYSIOLOGY

Critical illness often causes a hypersympathetic state in response to injury. Gut motility, especially of the stomach and small intestine, may decrease significantly. In addition, critically ill patients often receive narcotics for sedation, which may further inhibit normal peristalsis.

Absorption of drugs and nutrients may be erratic secondary to impaired motility and to abnormal function of villi when ischemia or necrosis has occurred. In these situations, integrity of the gut mucosal barrier function may also lead to increased translocation of bacteria and their toxins, which may suppress normal immune mechanisms and promote the activation of cytokine synthesis in the liver (see Chap. 15).

Total body metabolic demands often increase during critical illness. Overall energy expenditure increases by about 10 percent after elective surgery, 10 to 30 percent after trauma, 30 to 50 percent with sepsis and up to 100 percent with severe burns. Furthermore, the patterns of substrate utilization also change, probably as a result of increased catechols, glucagon and cortisol associated with the stressed state. Amino acids and fats become preferred to carbohydrates leading to increased nitrogen excretion, as well as glycerol and glucose concentrations. These patterns of utilization will vary from patient to patient and become important in formulating patient-specific diets, which must be modified as the acute injury gives way to healing.

COMPUTATION OF NUTRITIONAL REQUIREMENTS

Nutritional requirements may be determined by estimation, based on complex formulas which attempt to predict needs based on height, weight, and metabolic stress, or by measurement. As a rule, it is often difficult to predict caloric needs based on formulae because of the multi-factorial nature of critical illness, but these guidelines are useful for early management until direct measurement of nutritional requirements is accomplished. Table 12-1 suggests general guidelines for empiric nutrition in critically ill patients. 85 percent of ICU patients' caloric needs can be met by providing 2500 kcal/day, though more precise measurement is usually indicated.

TABLE 12-1 Nutritional Guidelines

1. Patients who are minimally injured and likely to resume eating in 3 days or less can be given dextrose-containing fluids alone.
2. Seriously injured or septic patients should receive 40 kcal/kg/day, with a ratio of 150 calories/g nitrogen. Carbohydrate should contribute 50–70% of nonprotein calories.
3. Malnourished patients who are not septic or seriously injured should receive 32.5 kcal/day with a ratio of 100 calories/g nitrogen. Carbohydrate should contribute 50–70% of nonprotein calories.
4. The enteral route should be used whenever possible, with a commercially available polymeric preparation.
5. The amount of CO_2 produced per calorie can be reduced by increasing the proportion of lipid. This may be appropriate in rare situations where a decrement in CO_2 production may facilitate successful spontaneous ventilation.

Caloric Requirements

The Harris Benedict formula has been the time-honored method of estimating caloric needs in patients (BEE = Basal Energy Expenditure in kcal/day).

$$BEE = 66 + (13.7)weight(kg) + (5)height(cm) - (6.8)age \text{ for males} \quad (12\text{-}1)$$

$$BEE = 655 + (9.6)weight(kg) + (1.8)height(cm) - (4.7)age \text{ for females} \quad (12\text{-}2)$$

These estimates of basal energy expenditure require modification for acute metabolic stresses. In the past, patients with burns, sepsis or other forms of severe metabolic stress, often received two to three times estimated BEE. More recently, researchers have found, using direct and indirect methods of calorimetry, that severe stresses usually require only 1.25 to 1.50 times normal BEE. Several studies have substantiated the inaccuracy of the Harris-Benedict formula for predicting actual caloric needs in critical illness, but it provides a caloric goal until measurements may be performed.

Indirect calorimetry measures the inspired and expired oxygen and carbon dioxide contents allowing calculation of caloric needs. Since

$$\dot{V}_{O_2} = (\dot{V}I \times FI_{O_2}) - (\dot{V}E \times FE_{O_2}) \quad (12\text{-}3)$$

and

$$\dot{V}_{CO_2} = (\dot{V}E \times FE_{CO_2}) - (\dot{V}I \times FI_{CO_2}) \quad (12\text{-}4)$$

where $\dot{V}_{O_2}$ is oxygen consumption, $\dot{V}_{CO_2}$ is CO_2 production, $\dot{V}I$ and $\dot{V}E$ are inspired and expired respiratory volumes, and FI and FE are the fractions of inspired and expired gases. FI_{CO_2} is very small so that steady state $\dot{V}_{CO_2}$ is simplified to:

$$\dot{V}_{CO_2} = \dot{V}E \times FE_{CO_2} \qquad (12\text{-}5)$$

These variables may be determined using a metabolic cart, both in ventilated and non-ventilated patients. Total energy expenditure may then be computed by:

$$EE \text{ (kcal)} = 3.6 \times \dot{V}_{O_2} + 1.4 \times \dot{V}_{CO_2}$$
$$- 1.2 \times \text{(nitrogen metabolism)} \qquad (12\text{-}6)$$

where the coefficients take into consideration differential energy yield for carbohydrate (4.4 kcal/g), protein (4.4 kcal/g), and fat (9.3 kcal/g), as well as differing amounts of O_2 and CO_2 liberated from the metabolism of each. Nitrogen metabolism varies over time, so that in catabolic, critically ill patients, it is estimated to be -21.5 kcal/day, so the final equation may be written:

$$EE \text{ (kcal)} = 3.586 \times V_{O_2}$$
$$+ 1.443 \times \dot{V}_{CO_2} - 21.5. \qquad (12\text{-}7)$$

These measurements can be made quickly and safely at the bedside in the intensive care unit. The main shortcoming of this approach is that metabolism may vary considerably, especially with fluctuations in body temperature, work of breathing, etc. Therefore, these limitations of this procedure must be noted and the measurements should be repeated as the clinical situation changes.

Indirect calorimetry also allows determination of appropriate fuel mixtures. A respiratory quotient below 0.7 suggests that the main fuel is fat, and when it is above 1.0 suggests lipogenesis. Since lipogenesis requires energy and liberates CO_2 (increasing the ventilatory demands of critically ill patients), it should be avoided.

The right heart catheter, used in many critically ill patients, can allow repeated safe determinations of oxygen consumption utilizing the modified Fick principle:

$$\dot{V}_{O_2} = \text{cardiac output}$$
$$\times \text{(arterio-venous oxygen content difference)} \qquad (12\text{-}8)$$

If one assumes a respiratory quotient ($\dot{V}_{CO_2}/\dot{V}_{O_2}$) of 0.85, each liter of oxygen consumed corresponds to the consumption of 4.9 kcal of nutrients. Therefore, the Fick equation may be modified to:

$$EE \text{ (kcal)} = \text{cardiac output} \times \text{Hgb}$$
$$\times \text{(arterial} - \text{venous O}_2 \text{ saturation)} \times 95 \qquad (12\text{-}9)$$

where cardiac output is expressed as L/min, hemoglobin as g/dL, and saturation as a fraction.

This measure has been correlated with indirect calorimetry, but varies as the respiratory quotient changes (as with varying the composition of feedings). As with indirect calorimetry, the Fick method only measures energy expenditure at a single point in time, but may be repeatedly determined to modify feedings.

Great care must be taken to avoid catabolism of constitutive proteins. Therefore, calculation of nitrogen balance is essential to providing an adequate amount of nitrogen-containing calories to prevent tissue catabolism. Positive nitrogen balance can be maintained by administering more nitrogen than is measured in the urine. A gram of urea nitrogen is liberated for each 6.25 grams of protein/amino acid. Since urinary urea nitrogen can be readily measured in a 24 h collection the following equation may be applied:

$$\text{Nitrogen balance} = \text{(grams of administered amino acid/6.25)}$$
$$- \text{([urine urea(g/l)} \times \text{urine volume(l)]}+4) \qquad (12\text{-}10)$$

where 4 is the estimated number of grams of nitrogen lost each day from feces and skin.

Two additional common situations which confound these measurements include gastrointestinal hemorrhage and proteinuria. In the former it is nearly impossible to estimate net protein loss in the stool (in the form of blood), but some attempts at quantification of blood loss may allow rough estimation of G.I. protein loss (concentration in mg/dl times number of dl estimated loss). Protein can be quantified in the urine as part of the 24 h collection and included in the computation of protein loss.

GENERAL NUTRITIONAL GUIDELINES

Nutritional support may be administered enterally or parenterally, through the use of hyperalimentation. As a general rule, the enteral route is always preferred when the gastrointestinal tract is functioning properly because it is safer, easier and less expensive than hyperalimentation. Furthermore, enteral feeding may prevent atrophy of gut villi, thus decreasing the possibility of bacterial translocation.

Enteral feedings. Access is obtained using a polyurethane feeding tube, although nasogastric tubes can be used for shorter term feeding. Some have advocated the placement of the feeding tube past the stomach into the duodenum, though no studies have shown clear mortality benefit from such a strategy. This can be accomplished by fluoroscopy or by rolling the patient into the right lateral decubitus position and advancing the tube when no resistance is felt. Tube placement should always be confirmed radiologically before any feedings are administered through the tube. When long-term feedings are anticipated in a patient who is unlikely to eat, gastrostomy or jejunostomy tubes are advisable.

The lack of bowel sounds should not prevent the use of enteral feedings as many patients without bowel sounds will tolerate enteral feeds. Feeds should begin at full strength, though some patients will develop diarrhea secondary to the hyperosmolarity of the solutions, requiring dilution and slow concentration to full strength. Feedings can occur continuously through a pump or every 3 to 6 hours. The head of the patient's bed should be kept at 30 to 45° and gastric residuals should be monitored to minimize the risk of aspiration.

Several complications can result from enteral feeds. When nasal tubes are used, there is a risk of sinusitis, especially when tubes remain in for long periods of time. Gastric residuals of more than 100 mL are often viewed as complications, leading to the cessation of tube feedings. Indeed, large gastric residuals (>200–300 mL) may increase the likelihood of aspiration. Still perseverance is indicated as maneuvers to increase gastric motility such as elevating the head of the bed, stopping narcotic sedation or adding a small dose of metaclopramide may improve motility. Diminishing the quantity of tube feeds or switching modes (continuous vs. bolus), should also be attempted before abandoning enteral feeding.

Diarrhea is also often cited as a reason to stop enteral feeds. Most commonly diarrhea is due to mucosal edema, villous atrophy or as a result of hyperosmolar feeds. If reduction of the osmolarity of the feeds and addition of stool bulking agents (fiber) is unsuccessful in decreasing the diarrhea, one ought to rule out infection (fecal leukocytes, etc.) and add immodium to the feeds (to decrease motility).

Lastly, special formulas have been developed for patients with specific organ failures. Although the data for such expensive products is not conclusive, they are commonly used in lieu of standard formulas to provide particular mixtures of components. Table 12-2 delineates the compositions of selected enteral formulations.

Indeed all attempts should be made to begin feeding to full caloric requirements within 24 to 48 h of entry into the ICU. Too often feeding is delayed or is inadequate for prolonged periods. Several studies have demonstrated improved nitrogen balance in burn patients who are enterally fed within the first 24 to 48 h of admission. When full calculated or measured needs cannot be delivered by gut, the difference should be delivered by hyperalimentation until such time as enteral feeds are fully tolerated.

TABLE 12-2 Some of the Polymeric, Semi-Elemental, and Elemental Formulas Available.

FORMULA	Caloric Density KCAL/ML	Protein G/L %KCAL	Fat G/L %KCAL	Carbohydrate G/L %KCAL	MOSM /kg
POLYMERIC:					
ISOCAL (Mead-Johnson)	1.06	34 13%	44 37%	132 50%	300
OSMOLITE HN (Ross)	1.06	42 14%	35 31%	134 55%	300
IMPACT* (Sandoz)	1.0	59 24%	28 25%	130 51%	<700
PULMOCARE (Ross)	1.5	63 17%	92 55%	102 28%	490
HEPATIC-AID (Kendall-McGaw)	1.1	44 15%	36 28%	169 57%	500
SEMI-ELEMENTAL:					
VITAL (Ross)	1.0	42 17%	11 9%	185 74%	460
CRITICARE HN (Mead-Johnson)	1.06	37 14%	3 3%	222 83%	650
ELEMENTAL:					
VIVONEX HN (Norwich-Eaton)	1.0	46 18%	1 1%	210 81%	810

*Only formula containing arginine, yeast RNA, and fish oil.

(Reprinted with permission from Singer P, Bursztein S, Askanazi J: Guidelines for Enteral and Parenteral Nutrition for Critically Ill Patients, in Hall JB, Schmidt GA, Wood LDH: Principles of Critical Care, McGraw-Hill, New York, 1992.)

Hyperalimentation. Two main forms of hyperalimentation may be used: peripheral and central. Peripheral hyperalimentation is delivered via a large-bore intravenous line, but this method has two main shortcomings. Full nutrition cannot be delivered by this route and the nutrients may irritate the peripheral vein. Hence peripheral hyperalimentation is ideal to provide the complement of calories to a patient who is unable to tolerate full enteral nutrition.

Central hyperalimentation may be used to deliver full caloric needs. Each day the hyperalimentation formula can be changed to modify its composition, or number of calories to meet the patients changing metabolic demands. In addition to the general guidelines for determining caloric and nitrogen needs, multi vitamins, electrolytes and trace elements should also be added to assure a full complement of nutritional requirements. When hyperglycemia is a problem, reversible causes should be treated, but insulin may be added to the formula, as needed, to prevent excessive hyperglycemia or ketogenesis.

Complications of hyperalimentation include line infections, hyperglycemia, hyperlipidemia, liver dysfunction (especially when excessive carbohydrates are being administered), and coagulation abnormalities. Electrolyte abnormalities as well as acid-base disturbances (especially metabolic alkalosis related to acetate in the formula) are also commonly encountered with hyperalimentation. The central line which delivers hyperalimentation should be placed under aseptic conditions and should not be used for any other purpose, as such use increases the likelihood of infection.

SPECIAL CONSIDERATIONS

Glutamine/Branched Chain Amino Acids (BCAAs)

Glutamine (and branched chain amino acids insofar as they give rise to glutamine) may be important nutrients in maintaining normal nitrogen balance, immune function and mucosal barrier function in critical illness. Numerous small studies have suggested that the addition of glutamine or branched chain amino acids to parenteral formulas may improve nitrogen balance and/or immune function in sepsis or surgical stress. However, it is not clear from these studies what groups of patients will benefit from BCAAs. The mixture of BCAAs and other calories also varied between studies. Therefore the role of BCAAs in supportive management of the stress state remains controversial.

Respiratory Failure

Since the elimination of carbon dioxide is a major metabolic function of the lungs, increased CO_2 production can greatly increase the work of breathing. In patients with respiratory muscle failure, all steps should be taken to minimize the work of breathing so as to prevent the need for, or aid in liberation from, mechanical ventilation. Since administration of excessive carbohydrate calories leads to lipogenesis, which increases CO_2 production, care should be taken to avoid overfeeding in patients with respiratory failure.

Renal Failure

Patients with renal failure may be very catabolic and in the setting of nephrotic or nephritic diseases may lose large amounts of protein in the urine. In this setting special care must be taken to meticulously determine nitrogen balance to avoid excess catabolism of muscle proteins that could otherwise be spared by the administration of adequate calories/protein in the diet.

Hepatic Failure

Many studies have examined the role of branched chain amino acids in the supportive care of hepatic failure. The rationale here is that these amino acids may be better metabolized by the failing liver and hence lead to less ammoniagenesis and release of other potential neurotoxins. This hypothesis has not been definitively proven, but several studies have suggested earlier recovery of hepatic encephalopathy especially when administered with hypertonic dextrose infusions.

For further reading in *Principles of Critical Care,* see Chap 5 "Gut Dysfunction and Nutrition" Gregory A Schmidt, Chap 90 "Fuel Utilization in Critical Illness" David H Elwyn/Jeffrey Askanazi, Chap 91 "Evaluation of Metabolic Requirements" Simon Bursztein/Jeffrey Askanazi, Chap 92 "Guidelines for Enteral and Parenteral Nutrition for Critically Ill Patients" Pierre Singer/Simon Bursztein/Jeffrey Askanazi, Chap 93 "The Role of Branched-Chain Amino Acids in Critical Illness" Björn Skeie/Eldar Söreide/Jeffrey Askanazi, Chap 94 "Nutrition and the Respiratory System" Simon Bursztein/Nicola P D'Attelis/Jeffrey Askanazi, Chap 95 "Choice and Care of Nutritional Access Site" Sylvie Anne Bursztein-de Myttenaere/Jeffrey Askanazi

| ## Complications of Critical Care

Shannon Carson

Survival from critical illness is often determined by the number and severity of complications related to life support and monitoring interventions. Daily rounds in the ICU should attempt to anticipate and prevent these adverse effects. This chapter describes many of the more common complications of critical care in an organ system review.

NEUROLOGIC COMPLICATIONS

Agitation in the Critically Ill

Episodes of abnormal behavior, perception, or cognition are estimated to occur in as many as 70 percent of adult patients admitted to an ICU. Physical and emotional stresses such as pain, sleep deprivation, loss of day-night cycles, and total invasion of privacy occur in conjunction with polypharmacy and neurologic consequences of underlying disease. *In making the diagnosis of 'ICU psychosis,' it should be emphasized that this is a diagnosis of exclusion and that other possibilities must be rigorously considered and sought.* Once abnormal behavior or perception has been observed or related to the physician, evaluation should be directed to a wide range of diagnostic possibilities (Table 13-1). Careful review of medication history is necessary, because critically ill patients receive numerous agents and toxicity is very common.

When organic processes have been excluded but behavior remains extremely inappropriate, the patient may require restraints and sedation until other measures have restored more normal function. In all but the most severe forms of abnormal behavior, major tranquilizers (haloperidol, thorazine, etc.) have little place since they do not facilitate communication with the patient and usually complicate already existing polypharmacy. It is usually preferable to institute a number of measures directed at the pre-

---

TABLE 13-1 Evaluation of the Critically Ill Patient with Abnormal Behavior

Perform neurologic examination to exclude a focal abnormality suggesting structural injury
Seek evidence of CNS infection
Exclude metabolic disturbances
Consider withdrawal state
Consider prior psychiatric disorder
Review medication history to exclude drug side effects
Consider 'ICU psychosis'

---

sumed causes of ICU psychosis. Efforts should be made to enhance quality of sleep. Constant attempts should be made by family, nurses and physicians to orient the confused or hallucinating patient. During the patient's more lucid intervals, attempts to interrupt the monotony of the ICU routine are often helpful. Finally, it is important to recognize underlying fears concerning death, desertion of family, or loss of control, and proper counselling should be initiated.

Stupor and Coma

Though many patients are admitted to the ICU with coma or stupor, it is equally common for a reduction in the level of consciousness to occur during their stay. As with abnormal behavior or hallucinations, assessment begins with a thorough neurologic examination. Focal abnormalities mandate brain imaging with computed tomography (CT) or nuclear magnetic resonance (NMR) scanning. Even for patients without focal findings, the threshold for imaging the brain should be low, unless another readily identifiable cause is present. Similarly, lumbar puncture should be considered early in this setting, once significant elevations of intracranial pressure have been excluded by brain imaging or careful fundoscopic examination. This procedure will identify infectious meningoencephalitis, carcinomatous meningitis, and subarachnoid hemorrhage (SAH).

Status epilepticus should be considered in all patients with profound reduction in level of consciousness. It is possible for intermittent seizure activity to produce coma without tonic-clonic motor activity. Clues to this etiology of coma include a prior history of seizures and an examination that varies significantly over short periods of time or between observers.

Certain encephalopathies are common in critically ill patients and must be excluded. Drug accumulations that are relatively common and should be considered include long-acting benzodiazepines given intermittently for sedation, particularly in the elderly; lidocaine in the elderly, in patients with hypoperfusion, or in patients with liver disease; prolonged (beyond 72 h) infusions or large doses of sodium nitroprusside, with consequent cyanide or thiocyanate accumulation; and the muscle relaxant pancuronium if given on a regular schedule in patients with renal dysfunction; the ensuing prolonged paralysis may mimic coma, although the patient may actually be conscious. Hypoxic and ischemic insult to the central nervous system (CNS) must be considered as well as electrolyte disturbances including marked hyponatremia, hypernatremia, and hypercalcemia. Sepsis frequently causes mild obtundation and on occasion coma, without direct involvement of the CNS. Hepatic failure may first manifest as coma or stupor. Finally, hypoglycemia must be excluded in all cases of coma and stupor.

PULMONARY COMPLICATIONS

Barotrauma

Barotrauma is defined as the presence of extraalveolar air in locations where it is not normally found in patients receiving mechanical ventilation. Clinical manifestations of barotrauma include pulmonary interstitial emphysema (PIE), pneumothorax, subcutaneous emphysema, pneumoperitoneum, tension lung cysts, hyperinflated left lower lobe, subpleural air cysts, and air embolization. Risk factors thought to predispose to barotrauma include high tidal volumes, high airway pressures, and positive end-expiratory pressure (PEEP). Barotrauma can also occur in patients with preexisting alveolar distention, i.e., in patients with primary diseases of high lung compliance (emphysema) and in patients with status asthmaticus. The clinician must rely on the proximal airway pressure, displayed on most ventilators breath to breath, to discover many of these risk factors. In general, the higher the peak airway pressure in patients with any given lung compliance, the greater the probability that barotrauma will occur.

Symptoms of barotrauma are unlikely to be specific in critically ill, ventilated patients unable to speak. Agitation, progressive hypoxemia, hypotension, or cardiovascular collapse may herald the appearance of pneumothorax, especially tension pneumothorax. Crepitation in the neck, face, chest, axillae, or abdomen by auscultation or palpation signifies subcutaneous emphysema. A "mediastinal crunch" is reported in 50 to 80 percent of patients with pneumomediastinum. Air embolization during mechanical ventilation may present with hypoxemia, CNS dysfunction, and livedo reticularis.

Radiographic evaluation is the usual method used to diagnose pulmonary barotrauma. Radiographic findings of PIE include small parenchymal cysts, linear streaks of air radiating toward the hilus, perivascular halos, intraseptal air collection, pneumatoceles, and large subpleural air collections. Critically ill patients are usually supine or semirecumbent at the time of radiologic examination, so locations of pneumothoraces include, in addition to the usual apicolateral location, anteromedial, subpulmonic, and posteromedial pleural recesses. Usual radiographic signs of tension pneumothorax include striking collapse of the lung, contralateral shift of the heart and mediastinum and inversion of the hemidiaphragm. Tension pneumothorax can also occur without these signs. Subtle signs of tension include slight flattening of the cardiac border and ipsilateral contour changes or depression of the diaphragm.

Standard methods to reduce the frequency of barotrauma include measures to decrease alveolar inflation and pressures, V_T, PEEP, and intrinsic PEEP (PEEPi). These measures include patient sedation and coordination with the ventilator, reduction in peak flow if it does not increase PEEPi, and perhaps adjustment of ventilator modes. Controlled hypoventilation to minimize peak airway pressures can reduce barotrauma in status asthmaticus and perhaps in other forms of respiratory failure as well. Pressure-assisted ventilation may also help reduce barotrauma compared to inverse ratio ventilation, since the latter may cause unduly large PEEPi.

Specific treatment modalities vary with the type of pulmonary barotrauma. Tube thoracostomy is appropriate therapy for pneumothorax or tension pneumothorax. Pulmonary interstitial emphysema is generally treated with nothing but the aforementioned methods to decrease lung distention. Pneumomediastinum and subcutaneous emphysema are generally thought to be benign but should heighten vigilance for further manifestations of barotrauma. The issue of "prophylactic chest tubes" in patients with pulmonary barotrauma but not pneumothorax is not resolved. We do not advocate routine tube thoracostomy unless pneumothorax has been identified or must be excluded.

Pulmonary Fibrosis

Diffuse interstitial fibrosis may follow lung injury of diverse causes, including acute respiratory distress syndrome (ARDS). When proliferative phase ARDS evolves rapidly in the patient still on the ventilator, a rather characteristic clinical pattern is often noted. The chest radiograph exhibits a "honeycomb" appearance, distinct from the typical pulmonary edema findings of the exudative phase. Lung compliance remains remarkably low, and the patient exhibits tachypnea and dyspnea. Shunt fraction often decreases relative to the acute phase of the illness, with lower PEEP and fraction inspired oxygen (FI_{O_2}) requirements. In contrast, dead space fraction rises dramatically in these patients, with minute ventilations of 20 to 30 L/min typical.

Specific therapies to prevent or reverse disordered healing and lung fibrosis have been entertained, but none demonstrated to be effective. Prevention of this entity centers on limiting exposure to toxic concentrations of oxygen and positive-pressure ventilation, the influences presumed to interact with the underlying lung injury to culminate in fibrosis. A reasonable goal for the clinician in the early phases of ARDS is the use of PEEP to achieve 90 percent saturation of arterial hemoglobin on a nontoxic FI_{O_2}. PEEP is usually well tolerated if used in conjunction with low V_T (6 to 7 mL/kg) to prevent barotrauma. Adjunctive therapies to maintain high oxygen delivery (maintain hematocrit >35, use of vasoactive drugs to augment cardiac output) and lower oxygen consumption (sedation and muscle relaxation, treatment of hyperthermia, modification of nutrition) may also be used to support the patient at the brink of gas exchange failure (see Chap. 30).

Complications Related to Airway Management

Complications are common during intubations performed in critically ill patients. If the intubation is prolonged, sequelae can include cardiac arrest, generalized seizure, gastric distention, and right mainstem intubation. Complications of endotracheal intubation result from injury to the hypopharynx, larynx and trachea, and are related to both the tube and cuff. Virtually all patients intubated for 2 or more days demonstrate laryngeal edema, ulceration, and hemorrhage. Less than 5 percent of these patients have clinical findings of stridor or upper airway obstruction upon extubation. Hoarseness occurs in three-fourths of patients but resolves within a month in the majority of patients. Paranasal sinusitis is found in as many as 25 percent of patients and can be the source of unexplained fever and sepsis.

Potential life-threatening complications of tracheostomy include tracheoinnominate fistula, tracheoesophageal fistula, and tracheal stenosis. Erosion into the innominate artery can produce sudden massive hemorrhage requiring immediate tamponade and surgery. Tracheal stenosis is a major complication occurring after tracheostomy in as many as 65 percent of patients, usually at the stomal site. Symptoms are rare unless there is a 75 percent reduction in tracheal lumen. Inspiratory and expiratory lateral soft tissue views of the neck together with fluoroscopy or tomography aid in the diagnosis.

Various factors have been implicated in laryngeal and tracheal injury, and daily management of the intubated platient is directed at minimizing the likelihood of complications. Measures outlined in Table 13-2 help minimize injury from ischemic or friction related mechanisms. Routine daily inspection of airway position with chest radiograph is advisable during the first week of critical illness. Appropriate endotracheal tube position is confirmed by chest radiograph when the tip is 3 to 5 cm above the carina. It is important to note that the tip will follow the direction of the patient's chin during neck flexion or extension and will move 2 to 4 cm from full extension to full flexion.

The duration of "safe" endotracheal intubation before reversion to tracheostomy is not known. We assess all patients carefully 7 to 10 days after intubation with a judgment as to whether extubation is likely within the next week; if it appears possible, we continue the translaryngeal intubation. If underlying disease has not been re-

TABLE 13-2 Daily Management of the Airway

Assure adequately sized tube with normal patency

Minimize cuff pressure by minimal leak or measured pressure < 25 mmHg

Minimize cuff movement and tube flexion or torsion

Confirm position by inspection, auscultation, palpation, and radiologic imaging

Assess duration of intubation

versed and the course is likely to continue over a prolonged period of time, tracheostomy is recommended.

All endotracheal tubes must be followed carefully on a daily basis for the development of obstruction. This is signaled by inability or difficulty in passing a catheter, rising peak airway pressures or failure to deliver an adequate V_T. On occasion the clinician will be required to evaluate the possibility of tube occlusion emergently. A concise and swift management plan is required. The patient should immediately be removed from the ventilator and hand-bagged with 100% oxygen. This eliminates ventilator malfunctions from consideration, and the clinician will be able to assess the resistance to inflation directly. If bagging is difficult and ventilation of the patient minimal, a catheter should be passed down the endotracheal tube. Failure to pass the catheter the full 25 to 35 cm to the trachea indicates tube obstruction. If immediately available, a fiberoptic bronchoscope is useful to determine tube patency and position. Preparation should be made for emergent reintubation. If the source of obstruction is clearly at the level of the teeth, a bite block may be applied or a paralyzing dose of succinylcholine may be given (see Chap. 11). If muscle relaxation does not immediately restore tube patency and ability to ventilate, the endotracheal tube should be removed, mask ventilation undertaken, and reintubation performed. In patients with obstruction below the level of the teeth, inability to pass a catheter, and complete inability to ventilate, cuff deflation should be performed to rule out cuff herniation over the endotracheal tube tip. Since most tube obstructions result from concretized secretions and mucous plugs, it is unlikely they can be removed once complete obstruction has occurred; reintubation should be performed quickly. If endotracheal tube obstruction has been ruled out as a cause of difficult ventilation, the patient should be immediately assessed for tension pneumothorax.

Approach to Arterial Hemoglobin Desaturation or Hypoventilation

Progression of primary causes of respiratory failure (ARDS, pneumonia, lung hemorrhage) or new lung insults (nosocomial pneumonia) may result in deterioration of gas exchange. These processes are usually readily identified by physical examination and chest radiograph. It is also common for desaturation to signal one of the less apparent complications of critical illness, and we therefore offer an approach to this observation. A recommended approach is given in Table 13-3. Hypoventilation will be signaled by the fall in Pa_{O_2} correlating to a rise in Pa_{CO_2} as dictated by the alveolar gas equation, and the $(A-a)_{O_2}$ will be unchanged. Ventilation/perfusion ($\dot{V}/\dot{Q}$) mismatching occurs with airway obstruction or with vasodilating drugs which increase blood flow to lung units with low ventilation. Increased ($\dot{V}/\dot{Q}$) variance is suggested by increased $(A-a)_{O_2}$ in the absence of increased shunt ($\dot{Q}s/\dot{Q}t$) or worsened hypoxemia on an $FI_{O_2} < 0.6$. The combination of worsened $\dot{V}/\dot{Q}$ matching and an increase in dead space should prompt consideration of pulmonary embolus. Development or worsening of intrapulmonary shunt is

---

TABLE 13-3 Causes of Worsening Hypoxemia in the Critically Ill

1. Artifact
2. Alterations in FI_{O_2}
3. Hypoventilation (A–a gradient unchanged)
   a. Diminished patient effort (fatigue, depressed drive)
   b. Ventilator malfunction or inadvertent change in settings
   c. Gas leak
   d. Alterations in physiologic dead space
      Hypovolemia
      PEEPi
      Increased alveolar pressures in restrictive lung disease
4. Ventilation-perfusion mismatch
   a. Airway
      Bronchospasm
      Secretions
      Mucous plugging
      Endotracheal tube suctioning
   b. Vasculature
      Use of vasoactive drugs
      (Inhaled or intravenous)
5. Shunt
   a. Atelectasis
   b. Pulmonary edema
   c. Pulmonary hemorrhage
   d. Positional change in nonhomogeneous disease
   e. Lobar collapse (acutely)
   f. Pneumonia
   g. Cardiac shunt
6. Mixed Venous Hypoxemia
   Low O_2 delivery due to reduced flow, hematocrit or saturation, or to increased $\dot{V}O_2 \rightarrow$ low mixed venous saturation $\rightarrow$ arterial hypoxemia in shunt or lung disease with large number of low $\dot{V}/\dot{Q}$ units.
7. Miscellaneous
   a. Dialysis
   b. Pulmonary embolus

suggested by severe hypoxemia refractory to oxygen therapy. A number of processes will increase intrapulmonary shunt, the common feature of which is filling or collapse of alveolar spaces. Thus, the chest radiograph will identify most such processes, with the exception of diffuse microatelectasis. As with $\dot{V}/\dot{Q}$ mismatch, vasoactive drugs like nitroprusside, dopamine, dobutamine, and other pulmonary vasodilators increase shunt. Right-to-left shunt in the heart should be considered when $\dot{Q}s/\dot{Q}t$ is out of proportion to the air space filling on the chest radiograph. It is useful to follow the mixed venous oxygen saturation as well as parameters of perfusion (heart rate, blood pressure, cardiac output, urine output) when evaluating hypoxemia to rule out circulatory disturbances as a cause.

Atelectasis and Lobar Collapse

Increasing age, obesity, volume overload, supine positioning, and smoking history are risk factors for substantial atelectasis. In addition, patients undergoing intubation and mechanical ventilation are at risk for lobar collapse, particularly if airway secretions are tenacious, the artificial airway is malpositioned, or there is underlying neuromuscular weakness. Atelectasis or lobar collapse is usually identified by abnormalities in gas exchange, physical examination, or chest radiograph.

To prevent the development of atelectasis, three-point turning, early mobilization to a chair, incentive spirometry, and the upright position should be applied to patients at the earliest possible time. Mechanically ventilated patients often require ventilator adjustments to prevent atelectasis, and it is our clinical impression that sighs and low levels of PEEP (3 to 7 cmH$_2$O) are helpful in this regard.

Once lobar collapse has occured, reexpansion can often be accomplished by gradually increasing the V_T at the bedside. When recruitment of the lobe is accomplished, the airway pressure will be seen to no longer rise with the increased V_T and may actually fall, corresponding to the recruitment of collapsed lung. If a collapsed lobe cannot be recruited before airway pressures of 50 to 55 cmH$_2$O are reached, chest physiotherapy, vigorous airway suctioning, and PEEP should be used for 12 to 24 h to achieve lobe expansion. If this is unsuccessful in reexpanding the lobe, fiberoptic bronchoscopy should be performed to confirm or establish airway patency.

CARDIOVASCULAR COMPLICATIONS

Pulmonary Emboli

The source of pulmonary emboli in critically ill patients has been thought to be due primarily to deep venous thrombosis (DVT), especially of the lower extremity. DVT has been found to occur in 13 to 29 percent of patients in an ICU. Another source of pulmonary emboli in critically ill patients can be thrombus associated with intravenous catheters. The diagnosis of pulmonary emboli must be considered whenever acute unexplained dyspnea, hypoxemia, pulmonary hypertension, or hypotension develops in the critically ill patient. Definite diagnosis can be made with lung scanning in the appropriate setting, but this test loses value and can actually confound diagnosis in patients with radiographic infiltrates or clinical evidence of airway disease (see Chap. 24). Thus in many instances, pulmonary angiography is necessary, although difficult to arrange due to the many impediments to transporting and investigating critically ill patients.

Prevention of pulmonary emboli in populations at risk is centered on prophylaxis of DVT or in the use of devices which prevent the migration of intravenous clot to the pulmonary circulation. For most patients, we prefer the use of subcutaneous heparin at a dose of 5000 U every 8 to 12 h. If the patient does not have contraindications to anticoagulants but cannot tolerate heparin (i.e., heparin-induced thrombocytopenia), warfarin is an acceptable alternative. Patients with absolute contraindications to low dose heparin therapy should have intermittent venous compression pneumatic devices applied to the lower extremities. Multiple trauma patients present a particular challenge for DVT prophylaxis. The incidence of this complication is high in this group, but lower extremity injury may preclude compression device use, and active bleeding may make anticoagulation unwise. A Greenfield filter may be placed in the inferior vena cava to prevent pulmonary embolization in these patients, but this approach has not been evaluated prospectively.

Complications Associated With Pulmonary Artery Catheters

Major complications of pulmonary artery catheter insertion include pneumothorax, air embolism, arrhythmias, phrenic or brachial nerve injury, carotid or sublcavian injury, hemothorax, cardiac perforation with tamponade, and intrapleural or intramediastinal infusion of fluid. In our view, the most commonly overlooked complication is misinterpretation of the hemodynamic data obtained and the consequent erroneous titration of patient care.

Arrhythmias, especially ventricular arrhythmias, are frequent. In general, premature ventricular contractions are self-limited and resolve with forward movement of the catheter. Risk factors for sustained ventricular tachycardia include myocardial infarction (MI) or ischemia, hypoxemia, and acidosis. Prolonged catheterization is another risk factor. Bundle branch block occurs much less frequently; right bundle branch block is usually transient with resolution in 10 to 24 h. Complete heart block is very infrequent. Treatment of ventricular tachyarrhythmia is standard. Prophylactic lidocaine may be helpful in high risk patients with prolonged (>20 min) catherization time. Transvenous pacemakers are not suggested in patients with chronic left bundle branch block but are recommended in patients with acute MI and left bundle branch block. Pulmonary artery catheters with a pacemaker channel may be useful in this setting, as may external cardiac pacemakers.

Major complications seen after placement include pulmonary artery rupture, infection, and thrombosis. Pulmonary artery rupture is infrequent but often fatal. Risk factors include pulmonary hypertension, age >60 years, and improper location and inflation of the balloon. Arterial trauma can also result in dissection of the pulmonary artery. It often presents with hemoptysis, and a well-developed mass or nodule adjacent to the pulmonary artery catheter position can be seen radiographically. Diagnosis requires pulmonary angiography, and ablation of the aneurysm can be accomplished with steel coil transcatheter embolization. Thrombosis as a complication of the pulmonary artery catheter occurs in several ways. Persistent wedging in small pulmonary arteries causes thrombosis at the catheter tip with resultant infarction. However, this is an infrequent complication. A fibrous sheath or sleeve clot is the most common form of catheter-associated clot. It originates at the point of intimal injury where the catheter enters the vein. The clinical significance of fibrin sheath formation is uncertain. Mural thrombus can form where the catheter is in contact with the venous, endocardial, or pulmonary arterial wall. Clinical symptoms can result from occlusion of the vessel by the mural thrombus or embolization of thrombus into the pulmonary arteries. Effective measures to prevent catheter-associated thrombus have not been determined.

Ischemia

Myocardial ischemia is likely common during critical illness, although it is difficult to detect because of impaired patient perception and communication and atypical presentation. Although ischemia may be signalled by typical chest pain, other presentations are common and are listed in Table 13-4. When these phenomena are noted, further evaluation with ECG and serum enzyme analysis is recommended. Echocardiography may be useful here, with transient segmental wall-motion abnormalities suggesting regional ischemia.

TABLE 13-4 Presentations of Myocardial Ischemia in the Critically Ill

Typical chest pain
Agitation with heart rate abnormalities
Sudden pulmonary edema
Sudden elevation of pulmonary capillary wedge pressure
Electrocardiographic or echocardiographic abnormalities noted during "routine" monitoring

Arrhythmias

Both bradyarrhythmias and tachyarrhythmias are extremely common in the course of critical illness, and the clinician must be familiar with the principles of specific diagnosis (see Chap. 25). Many are complications of therapy and should be recognized as such, obviating unnecessary diagnostics. As noted above, atrial and ventricular tachyarrhythmias as well as heart block are common during right heart catheterization or with routine central venous catheters during guidewire placement. Metabolic disturbances associated with arrhythmias include electrolyte disturbances (particularly hypokalemia and hyperkalemia, hypocalcemia, and hypomagnesemia) and hypoxia.

Drug effects must be considered as a cause of observed atrial and ventricular arrhythmias in the critically ill. Catecholamine infusions frequently result in (worsened) sinus tachycardia and ventricular extrasystoles or ventricular tachycardia. Inhaled catecholamines rarely cause symptomatic arrhythmias in ambulatory patients. In critically ill asthmatic patients, however, these drugs are often used in sufficiently high doses to result in dysrhythmias. It is advisable to infuse theophylline through peripheral catheters to avoid high local concentrations in cardiac conduction tissue, and theophylline levels should be determined frequently.

Severe lung disease and pulmonary hypertension are associated with atrial arrhythmias such as multifocal atrial tachycardia (MAT) and paroxysmal atrial tachycardia (PAT). These often respond to verapamil, but this agent can result in significant hypotension. More recently, adenosine infusion has been suggested in this setting, because its MAT-terminating effect is comparable and associated hypotension less.

GASTROINTESTINAL COMPLICATIONS

Alterations in gastrointestinal motility occur in up to 50 percent of patients with acute respiratory failure, especially those who are mechanically ventilated. Early aggressive correction of electrolyte abnormalities, reduction of morphine and other drugs which reduce motility, discontinuation of enteral feedings, and suction from above and below will decrease the morbidity from progressive bowel dilation. Diarrhea also occurs frequently in ICU patients, and causes include enteral alimentation, medications such as antacids or cimetidine, infection, hypoalbuminemia, and dietary lipids. Definitive treatment of diarrhea requires modifying known causes of diarrhea.

Complications of rectal tube use are frequent and include discomfort, local ulceration and necrosis, secondary infection, and perforation with extraperitoneal migration and contamination. It is recommended that rectal tubes be used only for clear indications and that these indications be reviewed on a daily basis so that the device does not become a nursing and physician "convenience." In addition, it is advisable to deflate the tube at least twice daily to inspect for related injuries.

Gastrointestinal Hemorrhage

Critically ill patients with multisystem disease who present with nongastroenterologic disease such as acute respiratory failure can develop gastrointestinal hemorrhage later in their ICU course as a complication of critical illness (see also Chap. 60). In these instances, hemorrhage is most commonly caused by, but not limited to, acute gastric ulceration. Acid and pepsin are generally thought to be required for the development of stress ulceration, but the primary mechanisms of ulceration are tissue acidosis or ischemia which result in impaired mucosal handling of hydrogen ion already present.

The clinical diagnosis of gastrointestinal hemorrhage is made by the appearance of hematemesis, melena, bright red blood per nasogastric tube, or signs of hypovolemic shock. Hematest-positive nasogastric aspirate in the absence of other signs of acute blood loss is a less reliable sign of significant gastrointestinal hemorrhage. It should be emphasized that nasogastric suction itself frequently causes multiple small mucosal erosions. Severe or massive gastrointestinal bleeding occurs in about 5 percent of medical ICU patients. Risk factors for the development of gastrointestinal hemorrhage include major trauma, shock from any cause, sepsis, renal failure, jaundice, and acute respiratory failure. Bleeding occurs more frequently in ARDS than in other causes of acute respiratory failure. Also, patients who are ventilated have a higher incidence of bleeding than nonventilated patients with lung disease, and risk of bleeding increases with prolonged (>5 days) mechanical ventilation. Coagulopathy also increases bleeding.

Therapy of stress ulceration should correct conditions favoring its development. Correction of hypoperfusion and acidosis are prime considerations. Prophylactic measures have centered on neutralizing gastric acidity with antacids or decreasing gastric acid secretion with histamine-receptor blockade such as cimetidine or ranitidine. Sucralfate appears to provide stress ulcer protection without reducing levels of gastric acid. Antacids require large nursing time commitment to administer these agents every 1 to 2 h with intragastric pH measurement. Both antacids and H_2 blockers are associated with gastric colonization caused by alkalinization of gastric pH. Resultant transmission of gastric organisms into the airways with the development of nosocomial pneumonia is a possibility. Sucralfate may lessen this complication. Nutrition may also be a useful prophylaxis against stress ulceration. Gastric colonization with resultant nosocomial pneumonia can also occur with enteral feeding.

Nutritional Complications

Nutritional complications in critical illness include the adverse effects of malnutrition on the cardiopulmonary system as well as complications associated with the administration of either parenteral or enteral nutrition. Malnutrition reduces diaphragmatic strength with an impairment in respiratory muscle function. Malnutrition also reduces ventilatory response to hypoxemia and adversely affects cell-mediated immunity. Clinical sequelae of altered respiratory muscle strength, ventilatory drive, and immune mechanisms could include precipitation of hypercapnic respiratory failure, difficulty in weaning from mechanical ventilation, and infection, particularly nosocomial lung infection.

Complications associated with enteral nutrition can be classified into mechanical, gastrointestinal, and metabolic categories. Mechanical complications include inadvertent nasotracheal passage, clogging, obstruction of the tube and aspiration of enteral feeding. Pleuropulmonary complications include pneumothorax, pneumomediastinum, subcutaneous emphysema, and death. A common finding in these cases is the use of a wire stylet to assist passage of the flexible feeding tube. Radiologic confirmation of placement is essential.

Prevention of gastric content aspiration should be directed at minimizing the mechanical factors contributing to regurgitation such as patient elevation and improper tube placement. Gastric residual should be checked frequently, especially in patients at risk for slowed gastric emptying.

Gastrointestinal complications of enteral feeding include vomiting, abdominal distention, and diarrhea. Metabolic complications of enteral nutrition include electrolyte abnormalities, especially hyperglycemia and hypophosphatemia.

Complications related to total parenteral nutrition (TPN) are also multiple and are classified into mechanical, infectious, or metabolic categories. Mechanical complications include those of catheter placement including pneumothorax and line sepsis.

Major metabolic complications include hyperchloremic acidosis, hyperglycemia, and hypophosphatemia. Hepatic abnormalities are frequent in patients receiving TPN. Histologic findings of fatty liver, cholestasis, and triaditis develop after short term TPN. The cause of liver function abnormalities remains obscure. Current recommendations to diminish hepatic injury include avoidance of excessive quantities of carbohydrates and protein with 10 to 30 percent of nonprotein calories supplied as lipid. Serum enzyme studies should be performed weekly.

Worsening hypercapnia can occur in patients receiving either enteral or parenteral nutrition and is often associated with excess carbohydrate calorie administration. This problem can be avoided by identifying patients at risk (chronic obstructive pulmonary disease [COPD], the "difficult to wean" patient), avoiding excessive calorie administration, and providing a high percentage (40 to 50 percent) of calories as lipids in the appropriate patient population.

INFECTIOUS COMPLICATIONS

When clinical evidence suggests the presence of infection in the critically ill patient, an early search for the infectious source is indicated. Beyond the initial surveillance cultures of blood, sputum or endotracheal secretions and urine, most such critically ill patients benefit from an aggressive systematic top-to-bottom search for additional sites of infection: meningitis, sinusitis, septic thrombophlebitis, line sepsis, endocarditis, nosocomial pneumonia, empyema, pericarditis/pleuritis, abdominal or pelvic abscess, rectal abscess, peritonitis, acalculous cholecystitis, decubitus ulceration, and arthritis.

Nosocomial Pneumonia

Nosocomial pneumonia is a frequent complication of critical illness with multiple adverse sequelae. It occurs in 20 percent of mechanically ventilated patients in a medical ICU and as many as 68 percent of patients with ARDS. Gram-negative bacilli represent over half the organisms responsible for infection. Sources for potential nosocomial pathogens are multiple and include invasive monitoring devices, respiratory therapy equipment, medical personnel, and sites in the ICU such as food or sinks. Despite these exogenous sources for nosocomial pathogens, however, most infections appear to result from endogenous sources.

The primary pathogenetic mechanism of nosocomial lung infection relates to oropharyngeal colonization with subsequent tracheobronchial colonization by gram-negative organisms. Although microorganisms can reach the airway by inhalation, inoculation from contiguous sites of infection, or hematogenous spread, aspiration of colonized oropharyngeal contents is generally thought to be responsible for most cases of tracheobronchial colonization and pneumonia. In addition, however, gastric colonization with subsequent tracheal appearance of gastric organisms has been found in patients undergoing gastric pH manipulation with antacids or cimetidine. Enteral nutrition, in the absence of antacids or H_2 blockers may also result in gastric colonization.

The diagnosis of nosocomial pneumonia is very difficult, particularly in patients with radiographic infiltrates already present. These patients may also have other causes of fever, leukocytosis, and positive sputum cultures, the traditional diagnostic guidelines of pneumonia. Thus, the distinction between tracheobronchial colonization and pneumonia is difficult if not impossible. Because diagnosis is difficult, new techniques and technologies have been introduced to improve diagnostic sensitivity and specificity of nosocomial pneumonia. Most interest has centered around the use of the protected specimen brush (PSB) or BAL with bronchoscopy. The PSB attempts to bypass upper airway contamination by using a telescoping cannula brush to obtain lower airway secretions. Quantitative PSB cultures have been shown to be highly accurate in diagnosis of nosocomial pneumonia. Quantitative BAL cultures may also have utility in the diagnosis of nosocomial pneumonia.

General strategies aimed at the prevention of nosocomial pneumonia include efforts to improve host defense mechanisms as well as measures directed at decreasing airway colonization and bacterial inoculation into the lower airway. In the setting of clinically suspected nosocomial pneumonia in mechanically ventilated patients, empirical antibiotics are often administered either before or in lieu of culture data. Studies indicate even adequate or appropriate antibiotic therapy is not beneficial. Antibiotics may not only be ineffective but may also increase the rates of serious gram-negative or difficult to treat gram-positive pneumonia, so routine antibiotic prophylaxis cannot be recommended at this time.

Bacteremia and Sepsis

Bacteremia is defined classically as the presence of bacteria in the bloodstream as determined by blood cultures. Clinical sepsis or the sepsis syndrome occurs when fever, hypotension, tachycardia, alterations in mental status, or leukocytosis occur with or without positive blood cultures. Sources of secondary bacteremia are those secondary to a known infection. Primary bacteremia originates most frequently from intravascular devices. Other components of the system besides the catheter itself can cause bacteremia. Stopcocks, pressure transducers, and flush solutions can become colonized and release organisms into the circulation. Line sepsis is best prevented by meticulous attention to detail in line maintenance and early discontinuation, generally within 48 to 72 h, for catheters placed in the ICU. When assessing the patient for possible line sepsis, culturing through the suspect catheter and from peripheral sites is helpful. Persistently positive cultures obtained through the catheter, with negative cultures at other sites, strongly suggests at least colonization of the catheter.

ACUTE RENAL FAILURE

The development of renal failure in patients with critical illness, particularly acute respiratory failure, is an ominous prognostic sign. An early response to oliguria or new increases in blood urea nitrogen (BUN) and creatinine levels should occur immediately. Common causes of acute renal failure in the ICU include hypoperfusion with prerenal azotemia, acute tubular necrosis (ATN) caused by decreased renal perfusion, and tubular dysfunction following nephrotoxic drug administration. Despite its relative rarity, the index of suspicion for obstructive uropathy must be high, since therapeutic approach will be different from other etiologies of renal dysfunction. Renal ultrasound is an excellent screening test for this possibility. Every patient with renal dysfunction in the ICU should have a careful review of medication history. Therapy of acute renal failure should be directed at its apparent cause.

Alterations in renal hemodynamics and tubular function are common in critically ill patients as a result of hypoxemia, acidosis, mechanical ventilation, PEEP, and postoperative changes in water balance. Adverse consequences include positive water balance, edema, hyponatremia, and possible increased mortality. Weight changes, serum sodium concentration, and fluid intake and output should be monitored daily and compared with previous days' records.

HEMATOLOGIC COMPLICATIONS

Hematocrit drops of more than two to three percent in 24 h should prompt consideration of excessive blood loss, underproduction, or both. Traumatized, anticoagulated, or instrumented patients may have loss at relatively occult sites such the retroperitoneum. CT scanning can be of help in such settings. Not uncommonly, evidence of hemolysis is sought or reported late in the critically ill patient. The significant amount of blood removed for laboratory testing or flushing and clearing of right heart and arterial catheters is a frequent contributor to the anemia observed in the course of critical illness.

Thrombocytopenia can be caused by both increased consumption and decreased thrombopoiesis in acute respiratory failure. Other causes of increased platelet consumption include disseminated intravascular coagulation (DIC) and intravascular pressure monitoring devices. Observation of significant thrombocytopenia should prompt careful medication review. Most drug-related thrombocytopenia results from diminished production. By contrast, heparin can induce antiplatelet antibody formation in approximately five percent of patients receiving this drug. These antibodies cause platelet aggregation with resulting thrombotic and hemorrhagic complications.

ENDOCRINOLOGIC COMPLICATIONS

Thyroid function tests are frequently abnormal in acutely ill patients with nonthyroidal disease. The term "euthyroid sick syndrome" is used to describe these patients. Thyroxin (T_4) levels are low, while free T_4 and thyrotropin (TSH) values are within normal limits. Thyroid function studies should not be routinely ordered in critically ill patients unless a clinical suspicion of hypothyroidism or hyperthyroidism exists.

Glucose intolerance is extremely common as well, particularly during sepsis or the hypermetabolic phase of multisystem organ failure (MSOF). Euglycemia may be achieved only with great effort, and it is unclear what benefit is conferred on the previously nondiabetic patient to have blood sugar levels dropped from the 150 to 200 mg/dL range to normal by insulin infusion.

De novo adrenal insufficiency is uncommon in critical illness, but can result from shock (hemorrhagic and septic) and has been associated with certain drug use, in particular ketoconazole and rifampin. More common is the circumstance of iatrogenic adrenal insufficiency preceding or accompanying acute illness. When adrenal insufficiency is suspected and the patient is hemodynamically unstable, stress doses of dexamethasone should be administered while a cortisol level is obtained before and after an adrenocorticotropic hormone (ACTH) stimulation test is performed (see Chap. 64).

For further reading in *Principles of Critical Care,* see Chap 52 "Prevention and Early Detection of Complications of Critical Care" Susan K Pingleton/Jesse Hall

---

14 | Oxygen Delivery and Pathological Supply Dependence of Oxygen Utilization

Allan Garland

The normal functioning of every organ and cell in the body is dependent upon an adequate supply and normal utilization of oxygen. There are pathologic states, such as shock, in which delivery of oxygen is clearly inadequate, with subsequent organ system dysfunction. However, interpreting the oxygen delivery in many critical care situations is often more challenging. Some evidence suggests that states such as sepsis and adult respiratory distress syndrome (ARDS) may alter the normal relationship between tissue oxygen delivery and oxygen uptake. *Pathologic supply dependence of oxygen utilization* refers to an impaired ability of tissues to extract oxygen from the blood even at levels of oxygen supply which would normally be sufficient to ensure adequate oxygenation. If such pathologic supply dependence of oxygen utilization does occur, then tissue oxygen availability can be impaired even when total body oxygen delivery is normal, or even elevated. In this chapter we will briefly examine the normal physiology of oxygen delivery and uptake, and discuss the possible existence and clinical significance of pathologic supply dependence of oxygen utilization.

NORMAL PHYSIOLOGY OF OXYGEN DELIVERY AND UPTAKE

Total body oxygen delivery ($\dot{Q}_{O_2}$) is the product of the O_2 content of arterial blood (C_aO_2) and the rate of delivery of blood to body tissues, i.e. the cardiac output ($\dot{Q}_T$). The total oxygen content of arterial blood is comprised of that which is bound to hemoglobin, and a normally much smaller amount (about 2% of the total) which is dissolved in the plasma; the precise relationship is given by: $\dot{Q}_{O_2} = \dot{Q}_T \times C_aO_2 = \dot{Q}_T \times [(1.39 \times Hb \times S_aO_2) + (0.0031 \times P_aO_2)]$, where Hb is the blood hemoglobin level in mg/dl, S_aO_2 is the fractional oxygen saturation of arterial blood, and P_aO_2 is the partial pressure of dissolved O_2 in arterial blood. Total body oxygen uptake ($\dot{V}_{O_2}$) is the difference between the arterial O_2 delivery, and the amount of O_2 that returns in the mixed venous blood, and is given by $\dot{V}_{O_2} = \dot{Q}_T \times (C_aO_2 - C_vO_2)$.

Under normal resting conditions, tissues are able to obtain as much oxygen as they require to meet their functional requirements, and thus they operate aerobically. With a normal $\dot{Q}_{O_2}$ Of 16 ml/kg/min, and a normal $\dot{V}_{O_2}$ of 4 ml/kg/min, the usual total body *oxygen extraction fraction* (OEF=$\dot{V}_{O_2}/\dot{Q}_{O_2}$) is about 25%. As $\dot{Q}_{O_2}$

rises (as a result for example of raising cardiac output with dobutamine), $\dot{V}O_2$ remains essentially unchanged (because it is determined by cellular oxygen demand) and consequently OEF declines. As $\dot{Q}O_2$ is progressively reduced, $\dot{V}O_2$ remains stable and OEF rises, until a point is reached when the tissues are unable to extract a great enough fraction of oxygen from the blood to meet their metabolic and functional needs. This *critical point* occurs at a mean OEF of about 70 percent; as $\dot{Q}O_2$ falls further below this point the tissues no longer are able to maintain the $\dot{V}O_2$ that they desire—$\dot{V}O_2$ falls and they become anaerobic. Fig. 14-1 shows this normal relationship wherein $\dot{V}O_2$ is nearly independent of $\dot{Q}O_2$ (the flat portion of the curve), until $\dot{Q}O_2$ falls below the critical point, after which oxygen uptake becomes delivery-dependent (i.e., the sloped portion of the curve to the left of the critical point).

At the organ system level, studies in animals have demonstrated that different organs possess different patterns of oxygen delivery-oxygen uptake relations. Thus, skeletal muscle and the intestinal tract have $\dot{Q}O_2$–$\dot{V}O_2$ curves like that of the whole body. On the other hand, because of their unique physiologies, the $\dot{V}O_2$ of the heart and kidneys is dependent upon their $\dot{Q}O_2$ at all values of $\dot{Q}O_2$. The liver is intermediate; it has a critical point above which there remains a

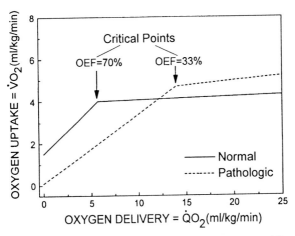

FIG. 14-1 Idealization of the normal relationship between oxygen delivery and oxygen uptake, and with pathologic supply dependence. In the latter, baseline oxygen demand is increased, while the critical point at which uptake becomes supply-limited occurs at a higher oxygen delivery, and lower oxygen extraction fraction (OEF).

significant (though lesser) dependence of $\dot{V}o_2$ upon $\dot{Q}o_2$. At the cellular level, the rate determining step of O_2 utilization is within the mitochondria. The functioning of these organelles does not become limited by O_2 supply until the local Po_2 falls below 1 to 2 mmHg.

Organisms respond to limitations in oxygen delivery at many levels. At the behavioral level, injured animals become lethargic, thermally insulate themselves, and conserve energy to the best of their abilities. As peripheral tissues are challenged by limitations in O_2 delivery, sympathetic and hormonal regulation of regional vasomotor tone acts to preferentially protect the heart and brain from hypoxia, and to optimize O_2 delivery to other tissues so that one organ will not be overperfused while another is underperfused. Within tissues, local metabolic control acts to increase the number of perfused capillaries by opening pre-capillary sphincters, and thus attempts to insulate cells from the effects of underperfusion by decreasing the mean distance that oxygen must diffuse to get from capillary to cell.

As tissue oxygen supply falls, cells may exhibit protective reductions in their individual oxygen demands. Cells have many avenues of energy consumption and loss that could conceivably be suppressed in times of threatened O_2 supply. While such mechanisms have been hypothesized in animal models, to date there has been little investigation of these mechanisms in humans.

PATHOLOGIC SUPPLY DEPENDENCE OF OXYGEN UTILIZATION

Conflicting data has emerged over the past 20 years about whether the normal relationship between oxygen delivery and oxygen utilization is altered in critical illness.

Some studies in animal models of ARDS and of sepsis have found altered $\dot{Q}o_2-\dot{V}o_2$ relationships for both the whole animal and for individual organ systems. These changes consist of defective extraction of oxygen, and an increased peak oxygen uptake. The maximal fraction of delivered oxygen which tissues are able to extract (OEF) falls considerably below its usual value (to as low as 30 percent), resulting in a shift of the critical point up and to the right; this corresponds to an O_2 uptake which is dependent upon the level of O_2 delivery at supranormal values of $\dot{Q}o_2$ (Fig. 14-1). However, the validity of these findings has been brought into question by the existence of some well-done studies which have failed to find such changes, as well as by a spirited debate concerning experimental methods.

In humans, investigations have been carried out in groups of patients with ARDS, sepsis and end-stage cardiogenic shock; these have been plagued by the same methodologic questions that arise in the animal experiments, as well as by the limitations necessarily imposed on data collection in clinical studies of critically ill patients. The results have been conflicting. Pathologic dependence of $\dot{V}_{O_2}$ upon $\dot{Q}_{O_2}$ has been found in some studies, but not in others; some investigators who did see an oxygen extraction defect found a plateau phase at high $\dot{Q}_{O_2}$, while others have not. To compound the difficulty in interpreting this data is the fact that almost none of this work has been done using techniques sufficiently sensitive to be able to detect changes of the magnitude observed in the animal experiments.

If it exists, pathologic supply dependence might result from any mechanism which either: **1.** alters the normal homeostasic regulation of blood flow distribution between or within tissues, or **2.** impairs the ability of cells to take up and/or utilize oxygen. Numerous normal and abnormal substances (e.g., cytokines, tumor necrosis factor, bacterial endotoxin) having effects on virtually every cell type circulate in states such as sepsis and ARDS, and are putative mediators of such abnormalities in vascular and cellular function.

RELEVANCE OF ALTERED OXYGEN UPTAKE AND UTILIZATION

Pathologic supply dependence of oxygen utilization represents tissue hypoxia, and thus may be an important contributor to the multi-system organ failure frequently seen in the ICU. Because this tissue hypoxia begins at a level of total body $\dot{Q}_{O_2}$ which would normally be sufficient to ensure adequate oxygenation, it may go unrecognized. Indeed, all available clinical indices of tissue perfusion and oxygenation (see below) are merely indirect measures and in the critically ill patient can be difficult to interpret, and even misleading. For example, such a patient may well have a normal blood pressure and even a supranormal cardiac output.

The ongoing debate over the available data should not overshadow the recognition that these issues might be of considerable consequence even if the shape of the $\dot{V}_{O_2}$–$\dot{Q}_{O_2}$ curves for each organ is unaltered by the pathologic state. Even if the whole body $\dot{Q}_{O_2}$ is normal, maldistribution of blood flow amongst tissues could still create a situation whereby some tissues are operating below their critical point, and thus are ischemic.

MANAGEMENT

Principles

The approach to correction of an imbalance between oxygen utilization and delivery begins with treating the underlying cause, e.g., sepsis. Beyond that, physiologic principles suggest that in selected cases it could be beneficial to use interventions which: **1.** decrease total O_2 demand, **2.** increase total body O_2 supply, and **3.** improve the regional and local distribution of oxygen delivery.

Selective improvement of maldistributed blood flow is an intriguing concept, but at present there are no such selective therapies available.

Oxygen demand may be lowered by treatment of fever and anxiety, avoidance of overfeeding, and judicious use of sedation, muscle paralysis and mechanical ventilation.

Elevation of total body $\dot{Q}O_2$ can be accomplished by raising (either individually, or together) the patient's hemoglobin concentration, arterial oxygen saturation, and cardiac output.

The oxygen carrying capacity of blood can be raised with red blood cell transfusions; a rise in hemoglobin from 9 to 12 mg/dL raises oxygen delivery by 33 percent if nothing else changes. Because of concern about elevated hemoglobin levels causing increased blood viscosity, and thus decreasing microvascular flow, our recommedation for anemic patients in the ICU with documented or suspected tissue hypoxia is to correct their hemoglobin up to 12 to 13 mg/dL.

In hypoxemic patients, oxygen delivery can be raised by increasing the oxygenation of arterial blood. In patients with ARDS, use of supplemental oxygen, PEEP and other ventilator manipulations will usually succeed in achieving a minimal goal of maintaining greater than 90 percent saturation on a nontoxic level of inspired oxygen (i.e., < 50 to 60 percent).

Elevation of the cardiac output may be effected by augmenting preload with intravascular volume infusion, decreasing afterload with vasodilators (which is often impractical in an already hypotensive patient), and increasing the inotropic state of the heart with drugs such as dobutamine.

Practical Considerations

The parameters commonly utilized to assess the adequacy of tissue perfusion and oxygenation are: a clinical assessment of organ system functioning (e.g., normal renal function and mentation), blood pressure, cardiac output, arterial pH and oxygen saturation, serum bicarbonate and lactate concentrations, mixed venous oxygen saturation, and the calculated $\dot{V}O_2$. However, in critically ill patients the interpretation of these parameters is often challenging. In addition to the uncertainties in knowing what value of blood pressure or cardiac output (or any other numerical parameter) is "adequate" for a given patient, critically ill patients often have complex pathologic states which can make interpretation of these parameters difficult; for example, rather than indicating tissue hypoxia, an elevated serum lactate level could reflect hepatic dysfunction, or the catabolic state which frequently accompanies severe illness. It is not rare to be faced with a body of seemingly inconsistent data. In those situations, practitioners must use knowledge of the clinical setting to accurately interpret, prioritize and integrate the various parameters into a coherent impression of the status of tissue oxygenation. Because these patients are almost always unstable, and because the best clinical evaluation of total body oxygen delivery and uptake requires measurement of mixed venous blood gases and thermodilution cardiac outputs, these patients should generally have pulmonary artery catheters placed for use in management.

Beyond interventions to correct a pathologically elevated oxygen demand (which, like treatment of fever, are often implemented for independent reasons in these patients), the intensivist is often faced with the question of whether to use potentially dangerous interventions (particularly inotropic drugs) to increase the cardiac output of patients who, despite a value of $\dot{Q}_T$ within or above the "normal range," have clinical or laboratory findings which suggest tissue hypoxia. This decision is usually clouded by the uncertainties present in evaluating the presence of an oxygen extraction defect, along with the difficulty in knowing what level of $\dot{Q}_{O_2}$ is adequate for a given patient. Our approach in the patient in whom an oxygen extraction defect is suspected despite a total body oxygen delivery which is seemingly adequate, or even supranormal, is a therapeutic trial of interventions aiming to further increase the cardiac output; if subsequent re-evaluation fails to suggest improved tissue oxygenation, then the interventions are withdrawn. A typical example is a septic, hypotensive patient with elevations of serum lactate and of the pulmonary artery wedge pressure, along with Hb=12 mg/dL, P_{aO_2}=85 mmHg, and $\dot{Q}_T$=9 L/min. In this situation it would be reasonable to perform a therapeutic trial of dobutamine to raise the Q_T to >11 L/min, using the parameters discussed in the previous paragraph to evaluate the success of such an intervention.

For further reading in *Principles of Critical Care*, see Chap 57 "Pathologic Supply Dependence of Oxygen Utilization" Richard W Samsel/Paul T Schumacker

15

Multiple Systems Organ Failure

Constantine A. Manthous

Multiple systems organ failure (MSOF) is a common phenomenon, occurring in up to 15 percent of patients admitted to the intensive care unit. MSOF refers to the severe, acquired dysfunction of at least two organ systems lasting for more than 24 h. Table 15-1 summarizes the defining criteria for this diagnosis. Many diseases can lead to MSOF, likely through common or similar biologic and molecular mechanisms. Therefore, a thorough understanding of the pathogenesis may allow the clinician to prevent or treat this process, as therapies directed against the mechanisms of MSOF are developed.

TABLE 15-1 Modified Apache II Criteria for Organ System Failure

If the patient had one or more of the following during a 24 h period (regardless of other values), organ system failure (OSF) existed on that day.

Cardiovascular Failure (presence of one or more of the following):
   Heart rate $\leq$54/min
   Mean arterial blood pressure $\leq$49 mmHg (systolic blood pressure $\leq$60 mmHg)
   Occurrence of ventricular tachycardia and/or ventricular fibrillation
   Serum pH $\leq$7.24 with a $Paco_2$ of $\leq$40 mmHg
Respiratory Failure (presence of one or more of the following):
   Respiratory rate $\leq$5/min or >49/min
   $Paco_2 \geq$50 mmHg
   $Aado_2 \geq$350 mmHg $Aado_2 = 713 \, FIO_2 - Paco_2 - Pao_2$
   Dependent on ventilator or CPAP on the second day of OSF (i.e. not applicable for the initial 24 h of OSF).
Renal Failure (presence of one or more of the following):*
   Urine output $\leq$479 ml/24 h or $\leq$159 ml/8 h
   Serum BUN $\geq$100mgm/100 mL (*>36 micromoles/L*)
   Serum creatinine $\geq$3.5 mgm/100 mL (*>310 micromoles/L*)
Hematologic Failure (presence of one or more of the following):
   WBC$\leq$1,000 μL
   Platelets $\leq$20,000 μL
   Hematocrit $\leq$20 %
Neurologic Failure
   Glasgow Coma Score $\leq$6 (in absence of sedation)
   Glasgow Coma Score: Sum of best eye opening, best verbal, and best motor responses.

Scoring of responses as follows (points):

Eye   Open: spontaneously (4); to verbal command (3); to pain (2); no response (1).

TABLE 15-1 Modified Apache II Criteria for Organ System Failure *(continued)*

Motor	Obeys verbal command (6); response to painful stimuli-localized pain (5); flexion-withdrawal (4); decorticate rigidity (3); decerebrate rigidity (2); no response (1); movement without any control (4).
Verbal	Oriented and converses (5); disoriented and converses (4); inappropriate words (3); incomprehensible sounds (2); no response (1). If intubated, use clinical judgment for verbal responses as follows: patient generally unresponsive (1); patient's ability to converse in question (3), patient appears able to converse (5).

Hepatic Failure (presence of both of the following):
Serum bilirubin >6 mg %
Prothrombin time >4 s over control (in the absence of systemic anticoagulation)

min=minutes; mmHg=millimeter of mercury; mgm/100 mL=micrograms per 100 milliliters µL=cubic millimeter; WBC=White blood count; BUN=Blood urea nitrogen; $Paco_2$=Partial arterial pressure of carbon dioxide; $Aado_2$=Arterial-alveolar difference in oxygen tension; Flo_2=Fraction of inspired oxygen; Pao_2=Partial arterial pressure of oxygen; CPAP=Continuous positive airway pressure.
*Excluding patients on chronic dialysis prior to hospital admission.
Modified from Knaus et al. (14)
(Reprinted with permission from Matuschak GM: Multiple Systems Organ Failure: Clinical Expression, Pathogenesis, and Therapy, in Hall JB, Schmidt GA, Wood LDH: Principles of Critical Care, McGraw-Hill, New York, 1992.)

COMMON ORGAN FAILURES

The lung is the most common organ to fail in MSOF. Acute respiratory distress syndrome (ARDS), detailed in Chap. 30, is the most typical lesion. Numerous precipitants of ARDS, including aspiration, pneumonia and sepsis contribute to the inflammatory events underlying its pathogenesis. Mortality from ARDS alone is 50 percent or more, and the brisk inflammatory response (to be described later) may secondarily involve other organs. ARDS, by itself may lead to MSOF.

Acute renal failure, secondary to acute tubular necrosis (ATN), is the renal lesion commonly seen with MSOF. This usually occurs after an episode of shock. Renal failure has also been noted in MSOF in the absence of well-defined episodes of hypoperfusion. The complex hemodynamic alterations that typify sepsis, in which renal blood flow is often preserved, but with increased metabolic demand, may explain how ATN occurs in the absence of overt shock. The superimposition of nephrotoxins such as antibiotics, etc., may also contribute to the renal failure of MSOF.

Encephalopathy, similar to septic encephalopathy, mild cardiac depression, bone marrow insufficiency and liver synthetic dysfunction also occur in MSOF, though less commonly than ARDS and ATN. The clear etiology of all of these organ failures seems intertwined insofar as a fundamental dysregulation of host inflammatory mechanisms appears to run amuck, leading to organ failure rather than organ protection.

PATHOGENESIS

The most common etiology for MSOF is shock; most often septic shock. Yet many other disease processes including pancreatitis, thermal injuries, trauma, connective tissue diseases and liver failure can lead to MSOF. It has been proposed that each of these processes activates the host's defense responses leading to a common final pathway of humorally-mediated end organ damage and, finally, failure. These responses generally protect the host from external insults, such as microbes and other foreign bodies. But these very same inflammatory/wound responses, normally an adaptive advantage to the host, may become deleterious if over-activated. This is the presumed mechanism whereby a large variety of different insults can activate the same set of defenses—eventuating in a form of self-perpetuating inflammation unto organ damage. This damage, in turn, incites activation of more mediators which propagates the hemodynamic and humorally-mediated organ failure which define MSOF. Hence the initial precipitating event may be treated, but the humoral cascade may autoactivate in self-perpetuating intravascular inflammation. Figure 15-1 summarizes the mechanisms that are thought to lead to this disruption of normal host homeostasis.

A Model for MSOF

The most widely accepted model for MSOF suggests that the gut may play a pivotal role as the so-called "engine" of MSOF. This model holds that the numerous disease processes mentioned earlier—shock, infection, pancreatitis, burns etc.—upregulate gut metabolism and thus oxygen demand ($\dot{V}O_2$) and/or transiently limit oxygen supply ($\dot{Q}O_2$) leading to gut ischemia. The villi, which normally prevent large amounts of luminal bacteria-derived endotoxin from entering the portal circulating, fail, leading to portal endotoxaemia. In the liver, endotoxin is readily taken up by Kupffer cells which then produce tumor necrosis factor and numerous other cytokines which then activate the humoral cascade (see Fig. 15-2). These mediators, in turn, may cause further increases in gut $\dot{V}O_2$ in the face of insufficient $\dot{Q}O_2$ leading to the translocation of more endotoxin. When the capacity of the liver to clear endotoxin is exceeded, it enters the hepatopulmonary axis. Lung macrophages likely act as the second line of defense against circulating endotoxin. Endotoxin is a known experimental precipitant of ARDS, and endotoxaemia may explain some cases of ARDS in MSOF. Meanwhile, the inflammatory mediators are also causing end organ damage which itself may contribute to cascade autoactivation. Other factors which promote the translocation of endotoxin include total parenteral nutrition and disruption of the balance of endogenous bowel flora, which are common in such critically ill patients.

PROGNOSIS

Table 15-2 summarizes data compiled by Knaus et al., examining prognosis in patients who satisfied the criteria for MSOF. Quite simply, prognosis relates to the number and duration of organ failures. Though the pooled data regarding prognosis cannot be applied directly to a particular patient, it may be used as a rough guideline to determine when therapy or support should be withdrawn. As a general guideline, if 3 or more organ systems are failed for more than 3 days, the patient is very unlikely to live, and withdrawal of therapy is often justified, especially if no improvement has been noted.

TREATMEMT

Table 15-3 presents potential interventions to improve morbidity and mortality in MSOF. There is no proven efficacious treatment for multiple systems organ failure per se, but some recent work suggests future avenues of management. If the gut is the engine of sepsis one would hypothesize that antiendotoxin therapy might be useful. Though the studies utilizing antiendotoxin antibodies for the treatment of sepsis were not designed to address the role of such therapy for MSOF, many of the patients in the studies satisfied criteria of MSOF. One study demonstrated a 15 percent reduction in mortality among gram negative bacteremic patients treated with HA-1A, a monoclonal antiendotoxin antibody. These results cannot be readily extrapolated to MSOF patients without gram negative infection. In fact, this therapy had no proven efficacy for septic patients with other etiologies of infection, suggesting that MSOF and death in these patients may not have related to endotoxaemia. Therefore further studies to examine the role of antiendotoxin therapy for MSOF are needed before any conclusions can be drawn.

Steroids have been examined for both ARDS and sepsis syndrome. Numerous large prospective studies have failed to show any benefit from the use of steroids in these patients, many of whom had MSOF. Therefore steroids are unlikely to be of use in MSOF.

Small studies in humans using nonsteroidal anti-inflammatory

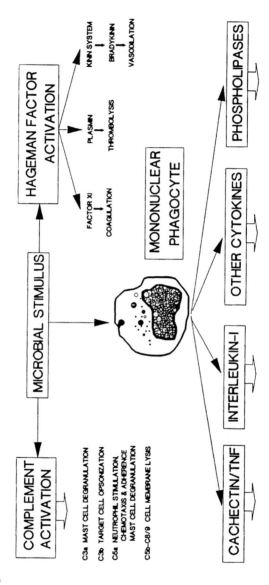

FEVER

LIPOPROTEIN LIPASE
SUPPRESSION
→ HYPERTRIGLYCERIDEMIA

↑ VASCULAR PERMEABILITY
INTRACELLULAR FLUID SEQUESTRATION
→ ↓ BLOOD VOLUME
→ HEMOCONCENTRATION

ENDOTHELIAL CELL DAMAGE
ENDOVASCULAR COAGULATION
→ ISCHEMIC TISSUE DAMAGE
→ CONSUMPTIVE COAGULOPATHY

NEUTROPHIL ACTIVATION

FEVER

↑ ACUTE PHASE PROTEIN
SYNTHESIS
↓ ALBUMEN SYNTHESIS

SKELETAL MUSCLE
PROTEIN BREAK-DOWN
→ AMINO ACID RELEASE

B&T LYMPHOCYTE ACTIVATION

NEUTROPHILIA &
NEUTROPHIL ACTIVATION

CYTOTOXIC LYMPHOCYTE
ACTIVATION

B CELL ACTIVATION
→ ANTIBODY PRODUCTION

BONE MARROW
CELLULAR PROLIFERATION

MACROPHAGE & NEUTROPHIL
ACTIVATION

↑ FREE FATTY ACID AVAILABLE
FOR PROSTAGLANDIN & LEUKOTRIENE
SYNTHESIS & RELEASE
MEDIATORS OF:
VASODILATION/VASOCONSTRICTION
PLATELET AGGREGATION
VASCULAR PERMEABILITY
MACROPHAGE CHEMOTAXIS
CACHECTIN & IL-I EFFECTS

FIG. 15-1 *A humoral-cellular model for the pathogenesis of MSOF. (Reprinted with permission from Light RB: Sepsis Syndrome, in Hall JB, Schmidt GA, Wood LDH:* Principles of Critical Care, *McGraw-Hill, New York, 1992.)*

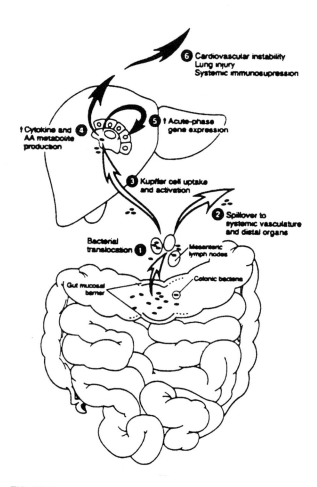

FIG. 15-2 Sequence of events in the gut-liver axis involved in bacterial translocation. *(Reprinted with permission from Matuschak GM: Multiple Systems Organ Failure: Clinical Expression, Pathogenesis, and Therapy, in Hall JB, Schmidt GA, Wood LDH:* Principles of Critical Care, *McGraw-Hill, New York, 1992.)*

TABLE 15-2 Mortality Statistics in a Large Cohort of Patients with MSOF.

Number of Organ System Failures	Day of Failure						
	1st	2nd	3rd	4th	5th	6th	7th
1	440/2297 19% / 37% 488/1323	294/1291 23% / 41% 347/842	248/1036 24% / 46% 309/672	221/846 26% / 47% 264/561	198/729 27% / 48% 235/491	170/615 28% / 50% 222/441	145/542 27% / 51% 179/353
2	313/718 44% / 64% 267/419	262/561 47% / 73% 221/302	219/415 53% / 71% 153/214	185/350 53% / 73% 139/191	160/311 51% / 72% 128/178	146/270 54% / 80% 111/138	126/217 58% / 83% 87/105
≥3	404/491 82%	302/322 94%	208/223 93%	152/159 95%	127/131 97%	103/105 98%	103/105 98%

Legend (1 and 2 OSFs):
Deaths/patients
% mortality <65 age / % mortality age >65
Deaths/patients

Legend (≥3 OSF):
Deaths/patients
% mortality all ages

(Knaus et.al., Critical Care Clinics, 1989) *(Reprinted with permission from Knaus W: Multiple Systems Organ Failure: Epidemiology and Prognosis, in Pinsky MR, Matuschak GM: Critical Care Clinics, Saunders WB, Philadelphia, 1989.)*

TABLE 15-3 Mechanism-Oriented Prophylactic and Therapeutic Options for Sepsis-Induced MSOF

Active immunization, passive protection by antisera/purified immunoglobulins against *Enterobacteriaceae, Pseudomonas sp.*, endotoxin

Reduction in frequency/duration of deficits in global O_2 delivery by maintenance of intravascular blood volume

Therapeutic goals for O_2 delivery based on values from survivors

Source control of infection
  Antibiotics
  Drainage of purulent collections

Prevention of mesenteric/hepatic ischemia during vasoactive drug infusions
  Selective mesenteric dopaminergic receptor stimulation (e.g., dopamine 1–3 µg/kg/min)

Inhibition of xanthine oxidase-mediated generation of O_2 free radicals during resuscitation for circulatory shock
  Allopurinol, other agents

Administration of opsonic plasma fibronectin during states of consumptive hypo-opsonemia

Extracorporeal filtration to dampen malignant intravascular inflammation
  Plasma exchange
  Specific absorption (e.g., polymyxin B for endotoxin)

Administration of monoclonal Abs directed against TNF-α

Pharmacologic modulation of intracellular cyclic AMP in inflammatory cells by therapy
  Pentoxifylline
  PGE$_2$
  Dibutyryl cAMP

Pharmacologic modulation of cytokine gene expression or tissue effects
  Corticosteroids

PAF synthesis inhibitors or PAF receptor blockade

Cyclooxygenase pathway inhibition (e.g., ibuprofen)

Lipoxygenase pathway inhibition or leukotriene receptor blockade, especially with preexisting liver damage

Preservation of gastric acidity to decrease incidence of nosocomial pneumonia

Meticulous management of intravascular lines

(Reprinted with permission from Matuschak GM: Multiple Systems Organ Failure: Clinical Expression, Pathogenesis, and Therapy, in Hall JB, Schmidt GA, Wood LDH: Principles of Critical Care, McGraw-Hill, New York, 1992.)

agents, mainly ibuprofen, have suggested minor benefits in patients with sepsis, but have not been tested in MSOF. Insofar as ongoing prospective clinical trials of anti-inflammatory drugs, including anti-TNF antibodies and interleukin-1 receptor antagonists, will address the role of such therapies in sepsis, some conclusions regarding interruption of MSOF may also be possible. No studies have addressed the role of such anti-inflammatory therapies for MSOF, in the absence of detectable infection. Such studies would require large numbers of patients and extended life-support, and are, thus, unlikely to be performed.

Therefore prevention of MSOF is essential; shock should be treated aggressively so as to avoid tissue ischemia and end-organ failure (see Chaps. 22 and 37). Organ-specific supportive therapy such as mechanical ventilation, renal dialysis and nutritional support are indicated while reversible precipitants of MSOF are treated. Some have hypothesized that adequate nutrition, particularly if delivered enterally, may better maintain mucosal barrier function of the gut thus preventing or attenuating MSOF. This hypothesis has not been proven.

For further reading in *Principles of Critical Care,* see Chap 53 "Multiple Systems Organ Failure: Clinical Expression, Pathogenesis, and Therapy" George M Matuschak, Chap 67 "Prevention and Management of Multiple Systems Organ Failure Following Trauma" James R Macho

---

| **Intensive Care Management of Trauma**

J. Edward Jordan

Care for the trauma patient may be categorized as either pertaining to acute resuscitation or management of complications due to the original injury. Priorities must be set early and the intensivist must be aware of the life threatening implications of specific injuries. Control of the airway and ventilation must be secured first. Neck manipulation during airway management is a critical issue as the trauma patient may have sustained a cervical spine injury. All seven cervical vertebrae must be visualized on lateral neck films before ruling out these injuries and removing the cervical collar. If there are any clinical signs of a cervical spine injury the cervical collar should remain in place. Many techniques to establish an artificial airway put the cervical spine at risk of further injury resulting in permanent neurological deficits, paraplegia, or death. The neck should not be turned, extended, or flexed in patients suspected of having a cervical spine fracture. Nasotracheal intubation should be considered for conscious and breathing patients, however apneic patients should be orally intubated. With the head in the neutral position, midline traction should be maintained while an airway is placed. If these techniques are unsuccessful, the patient may require cricothyroidotomy to establish an artificial airway.

Once the airway is in place and ventilation assured, shock must be corrected. The patient should be examined early for thready pulse, pallor, poor capillary refill, tachycardia and cool extremities, all of which are highly suggestive of hypoperfusion. Hypoperfusion in the trauma patient is most commonly a consequence of hemorrhage and is not always signaled by hypotension. Other causes of shock include tension pneumothorax, cardiac tamponade, myocardial contusion, open pneumothorax, and flail chest.

The cause of hypoperfusion must be quickly located and reversed. Direct pressure on bleeding sites and aggressive volume replacement with several large bore IV catheters is preferred. It is best not to place IV catheters in limbs with significant soft tissue injuries. If peripheral access is difficult to obtain, central access should be rapidly secured. If the source of hemorrhage cannot be determined by chest x-ray and physical exam, consideration must be given to abdominal or thoracic sources which peritoneal lavage or computed tomographic (CT) scans may quickly identify. The pelvic girdle and extremities may conceal profound bleeding.

If volume infusion is not adequate to maintain blood pressure with a pneumatic antishock garment deflated, the patient should be taken to the operating room where the garment can be deflated and the search for the source of hemorrhage immediately undertaken. If it is impossible to deflate the garment because of persistent hypotension, thoracotomy and temporary clamping of the aorta above the diaphragm may be necessary before deflating the garment and proceeding to exploratory laparotomy. The garment should not be inflated for prolonged periods of time (> 4 h) because of possible complications, such as a compartment syndrome or ischemia of an extremity requiring amputation.

A vagally mediated bradycardia may result from massive blood loss and must not be mistaken for adequate volume resuscitation. Blood should be substituted for crystalloid when 50 mL/kg has been administered in emergent conditions, and blood products should be warmed in cases of massive blood transfusion. Hypothermia impedes clotting; therefore, core temperature monitoring should be added to electrocardiogram (ECG) and blood pressure monitoring in severe cases of trauma. When the trauma patient fails to respond to massive volume infusion, thoracotomy allows for rapid identification of intrathoracic emergencies such as cardiac tamponade, hemorrhage, and allows for the initiation of cardiac massage, cross clamping of the aorta, and relief of tension pneumothorax. Inotropic agents may also be employed for the stabilization of the hypotensive patient in this setting, but should never take the place of adequate volume repletion.

When the respiratory and hemodynamic states have been stabilized, neurologic assessment should follow. Central nervous system injury is implied when the patient has a change in the level of consciousness after trauma. Initial assessment should include an appraisal of appropriateness to commands and type of stimulus required to elicit a response. If the exam is abnormal, the cause should be quickly identified. One of the commonest causes of a depressed level of consciousness in the multiple-injured patient is uncorrected hypovolemia resulting in hypoperfusion and cerebral hypoxia. There is also a high incidence of intracranial bleeding which must be addressed urgently. Fractures usually do not present an immediate threat to life unless they are associated with massive hemorrhage; however, unstable fractures may cause arterial spasm or arterial injury leading to ischemia of a limb or compartment syndrome. An assessment should be made of neurovascular integrity and if questions remain, arteriography should be performed to insure an adequate blood supply.

When the issues above have been addressed, a thorough and systematic assessment of the patient should follow before transfer to the intensive care unit. This includes a detailed examination of the unclothed patient from head to toe, careful inventory of subtle injuries and injuries to the back, rectal examination for gastrointes-

122 PRINCIPLES OF CRITICAL CARE COMPANION HANDBOOK

tinal bleeding and pelvic injury, and tetanus immunization. All patients with severe traumatic injuries should have a nasogastric tube placed (if there are no posterior pharyngeal injuries), and a Foley catheter inserted. A complete history of the mechanism of injury and episodes of loss of consciousness should be recorded. Consultants from the appropriate surgical services should be called when injuries are noted. Ideally, vital signs should be completely stabilized and urine output monitored. A complete review of all laboratory data, radiographs, and ECG should occur before the patient is transferred to the intensive care unit. If immediate surgical intervention is not needed, repeat clinical examinations and close observation should ensue.

ACUTE HEAD INJURIES

Evidence of an intracranial hematoma is present in 25 to 50% of patients with coma due to acute head injury. Prophylactic antibiotics (cloxicillin 4 to 6 g/day and chloramphenicol 4 g/day) should be administered prior to surgery. After surgical evacuation of an intracranial hematoma, intracranial pressure monitoring should be used to follow the course of intracerebral swelling. A cerebrospinal fluid (CSF) leak sometimes first presents in the intensive care unit after a basal skull fracture. CSF otorrhea usually stops spontaneously without further therapy. CSF rhinorrhea usually requires elective surgical repair.

A neurologic examination should be performed hourly. Neuromuscular blocking agents should be withheld every 12 to 24 hours to allow for a more complete examination when the neurological status is in question. Arterial pressure monitoring, intake and output assessments, and pulmonary artery wedge pressures (especially during mannitol use) are employed to insure stable hemodynamics. Intracranial pressure (ICP) monitoring is useful since many pathogenic processes are reflected by increasing intracranial pressure. Increased ICP is correlated with poor patient outcome. The degree of slowing as revealed by the electroencephalogram (EEG) is correlated with depth of coma and evidence of increasing frequencies over the first week is associated with improved survival. Evoked potentials are very useful in predicting outcome after acute head injury. Deterioration in serial-evoked potentials with secondary injury to the brain correlates with poor patient outcome. Other parameters which predict poor outcome include a low score on the Glasgow Coma Scale, advanced age, intracranial hematoma, and significant systemic injury.

The medical management of acute head injury involves control of ICP, prompt treatment of seizures, infusion of fluids and electrolytes, and provision of nutrition. Normal ICP is 10 torr and treatment to reduce ICP is indicated for persistent elevation to 20 to 25 torr. In preoperative cases of cerebral contusion, an increased ICP may reflect a need for surgical removal of contused brain. In all cases of increased ICP, impeded venous return should be ruled out. If there is no surgically treatable cause for an elevated ICP, hyperventilation and pharmacotherapy may be used to control the ICP. By intubating and hyperventilating the patient to a P_{CO_2} of 30 to 34 torr (if necessary as low as 25 torr), ICP may fall due to decreased blood flow to the brain. Morphine (or analog) should be used for sedation during forced hyperventilation. If the ICP remains unacceptably elevated, paralysis should be induced with pancuronium. Febrile patients should have their core temperature reduced to 37°. If these maneuvers fail to sufficiently reduce the ICP, cerebrospinal fluid should be removed by an interventricular drain on an hourly basis as necessary. Mannitol should also be considered for the reduction of ICP. Mannitol is given 0.5 to 1.0 g/kg IV as a 20% solution. The effect usually lasts two to six hours and the drug may be given repeatedly. Serum osmolarity should be monitored and mannitol should be withheld when the serum osmolarity is greater than 320 mosm/L. Excess urine loss should be replaced to maintain a normal pulmonary capillary wedge pressure, serum osmolarity less than 300, and normal serum electrolytes. When mannitol fails to lower ICP, pentobarbital can be used as either a bolus or constant infusion. The endpoint of pentobarbital use is either a satisfactory reduction in ICP or hypotension. The hypotension induced by pentobarbital may be responsive to IV dopamine.

Seizures should be treated prophylactically. Patients at risk for seizures include those with severe injuries or an intracranial hematoma. Phenytoin is typically used and is continued for 6 to 12 months. The nutritional requirements of a patient with a severe head injury are similar to those of patients with a 20 to 40 percent area burn. The syndrome of inappropriate antidiuretic hormone (SIADH) often complicates the care of patients with head injury and usually responds to fluid restriction to 1 L per day. Diabetes insipidus may also occur and control is best obtained with desmopressin acetate (DDAVP). The dosage is 1 to 2 µg IV two to four times a day to control excessive urine output. The patient should be evaluated for rehabilitation soon after admission to the ICU.

SPINAL INJURIES

Complete radiographic characterization of spinal injuries and neurosurgical consultation should occur prior to admission to the ICU. Spine injuries must be considered in all patients with significant head or facial injuries. Patients with abnormal spinal anatomy may also suffer significant spinal injury after trivial insults. A history should be taken of present and past neurologic injuries, motor deficits, and changes in bladder function. Abrasions, contusions, paradoxical breathing patterns, and priapism should be noted on the initial physical examination. A detailed neurologic exam and flow sheet will allow a continuous assessment of neurologic function. All suspected spinal injuries must be immobilized until stabilized or radiographically cleared. The Po_2 should be maintained over 100 and systolic blood pressure greater than 100 mmHg in order to provide adequate O_2 supply to areas of spinal injury at risk for ischemia. Patients with spinal injuries should have secure IV access, a nasogastric tube placed, and a Foley catheter.

Complications following spinal cord injury should be anticipated. Neurologic shock following spinal cord injury is best treated by correction of any preexisting hypovolemia, and vasoactive drugs if necessary. Bradycardia responds to atropine. Occult sources of bleeding should always be sought. Hypothermia, autonomic dysreflexia, and myositis ossificans ("swollen limb") may complicate the management of spinal injury. Patients with high cervical spine injuries are at risk of phrenic nerve paralysis. Substantially increased left ventricular afterload may follow spinal injury and cause pulmonary edema. Spinal injury may also cause an otherwise unexplained ileus. Patients with spinal injuries should have close attention to pulmonary embolism prophylaxis, nutrition, and skin care after arrival in the ICU.

Two principles which guide therapy of spinal injuries are to decompress the cord and provide an adequate perfusion pressure with well oxygenated blood. Surgical intervention is indicated for **1.** progressive neurologic loss after spinal injury, **2.** failure to improve with nonoperative decompression, and **3.** incomplete cord or cauda equina lesions with residual compression. Surgical intervention is not indicated for complete spinal cord lesions without spinal shock or progressive neurologic loss secondary to cord ischemia in the absence of a compressive lesion. Adjunctive measures to reduce spinal cord compression include corticosteroids (methylprednisolone 30 mg/kg IV within 8 h of the injury followed by 5.4 mg/kg/h for 23 h) and nimodipine plus epinephrine which may increase blood flow to areas of the cord with poor perfusion.

NONSPINAL NECK INJURIES

Penetrating neck wounds which violate the platysma may result in vascular or airway injury and thus should almost always be surgically explored in the operating room. Airway compromise may result from direct laryngotracheal injury, compression and edema secondary to an expanding hematoma, or massive intraoral bleeding leading to suffocation. Neck structures may also be injured as a result of therapeutic and diagnostic maneuvers. Perforation of the cervical esophagus may follow endotracheal intubation, placement of a nasogastric tube, or endoscopy. Subcutaneous emphysema may be an important clue to the discovery of this complication. The diagnosis is confirmed by gastrograffin (preferable) or barium swallow. Attempts to secure venous access in the neck may result in pneumothorax or arterial puncture. A chest radiograph should be obtained after all attempts to place a central line in the neck to detect a possible pneumothorax. Arterial punctures during the placement of a central line require direct pressure over the puncture site for several minutes to stop the bleeding and usually no further therapy is required.

Orotracheal intubation is the method of choice in the management of the patient with an upper airway injury, although emergency cricothyroidotomy may be necessary. Indications for surgical intervention in cases of upper airway injury include airway obstruction, shock, uncontrolled bleeding, and a rapidly expanding hematoma. Questions concerning the integrity of vascular structures in the neck should be answered by angiography if time permits.

TORSO TRAUMA

Thoracic Injuries

Open pneumothorax, massive hemothorax, flail chest, and aortic rupture require stabilization and characterization prior to admission to the ICU. The following traumatic injuries are more likely to require diagnosis and management in the ICU.

A *tension pneumothorax* is caused by an intrathoracic leak of air into the pleural space and is suspected when there is hyper-resonant percussion, tracheal shift, dyspnea, and hypotension. The trapped air can be immediately released by inserting a large needle into the second intercostal space at the midclavicular line. A chest tube should be placed under water seal since the underlying disorder will usually take days to resolve.

Cardiac tamponade follows when the pericardial sac fills with enough fluid to inhibit proper ventricular filling, thus reducing stroke volume and cardiac output. Tamponade may follow blunt or penetrating trauma and should be suspected when there is evidence of an elevated central venous pressure, hypotension, and muffled heart sounds. Cases of hemodynamically significant tamponade may demonstrate a pulsus paradoxus greater than 10 mmHg. Urgent pericardiocentesis is indicated in cases of life threatening tamponade. A long (6 in.) 16 or 18 gauge needle is attached to an empty 50 mL syringe and inserted below the xiphoid process at a 45° angle aimed cephalad toward the tip of the left scapula. An electrocardiographic lead is attached to the hub end of the needle and monitored for electrocardiographic evidence of myocardial injury. If the syringe is filled with clotting blood and the patient fails to improve hemodynamically, the myocardium may have been punctured which could require operative repair. When tamponade is not immediately life threatening, the pericardium should be drained with a pericardiostomy tube in the operating room.

Lung contusion results from direct injury to the lung parenchyma. Many patients require no specific therapy while others may develop respiratory failure requiring mechanical ventilation. *Myocardial contusion* occurs during blunt trauma to the chest when the sternum impacts the heart. Whenever the sternum is fractured, myocardial contusion should be assumed. The diagnosis is suggested by an elevated CPK (MB), nonspecific ECG abnormalities, and abnormal echocardiographic findings. Electrocardiography may show persistent tachycardia, premature ventricular contractions, dysrhythmias, bundle branch block, and ST segment changes (which may appear ischemic). These patients should be monitored in an ICU because of the risk of life threatening dysrhythmias. Therapy should include effective analgesia, supplemental oxygen, and other supportive care as indicated. Patients with *flail chest* are mechanically ventilated only if the defect is too large for the patient to effectively sustain respiration. A chest tube should be placed on the side of the flail and adequate analgesia should be given to control discomfort. A *diaphragmatic rupture* may be mistaken for an elevated left hemidiaphragm on a chest radiograph. Since the degree of symptomatology is highly variable, surgical repair is not usually an emergency.

Abdominal Injuries

Patients with intra-abdominal injuries should be evaluated and stabilized prior to admission to the ICU. A detailed discussion of the diagnosis and therapy of the traumatized abdomen is outside the scope of this text, however several principles apply. With the exceptions of cardiac tamponade and traumatic air embolism, unstable patients with torso trauma and functioning chest tubes demonstrating no free blood or continued major air leak must be considered to have an intra-abdominal source of bleeding. Such patients should generally have urgent exploratory laparotomy. When the abdominal examination is compromised by obstruction, cord injury, or drugs, peritoneal lavage may be useful to determine the need for laparotomy. Abdominal CT scanning is also useful in the evaluation of abdominal trauma, although CT scans of the abdomen may fail to reveal some life threatening intra-abdominal injuries.

PELVIC TRAUMA

Pelvic injuries may be a source of major hemorrhage, as well as neurological, vascular, and visceral injury. It is therefore important to determine the stability of the pelvic ring in cases of severe traumatic injury. Palpation and manipulation of the pelvis will readily determine whether instability secondary to pelvic ring fracture is present. Routine anteroposterior radiographs of the inlet view of the pelvis may clearly reveal areas of pelvic fracture. A CT scan of the pelvis is the single best tool to define pelvic injury as the sacroiliac complex is visualized well. Complete instability of the pelvic ring is associated with ten percent mortality and requires immediate resuscitation and surgical stabilization.

ICU management of pelvic injuries is troubled with complications of multiple systems organ failure, sepsis, and fat emboli. These patients are placed at significant risk of pulmonary thromboemboli and must receive prophylactic therapy until they are adequately mobilized. Pelvic injury predisposes to nocosomial pneumonia, thus these patients benefit from rotational beds and chest physiotherapy.

INJURIES TO EXTREMITIES

Compartment Syndrome

Compartment syndromes should be anticipated after complicated trauma. The syndrome is defined as an elevation of the interstitial pressure in a closed osseofascial compartment resulting in microvascular compromise and may occur in the forearm, leg, hand, foot, or thigh. It may be the result of prolonged external pressure, direct trauma (with or without underlying fracture), or reperfusion of an ischemic limb. Other risk factors include multiple trauma, history of hypotension, use of antishock trousers, coagulopathy, and crushing injury. The diagnosis is suggested when pain is disproportionate to the apparent injury, or there is swelling, tenderness, hypesthesia, severe weakness, or pain on passive stretch of the involved muscle. In unresponsive patients the diagnosis is difficult. Intercompartmental pressure monitoring may be helpful, but the diagnosis is largely clinical. Treatment consists of fasciotomy performed within eight hours and generally results in good functional recovery. Prior to fasciotomy, the extremity may be raised to the level of the heart which may reduce the neurovascular compromise. If this maneuver is going to be effective, it will work within one hour.

Peripheral Nerve Injury

Peripheral nerve injury is common in cases of significant trauma. Management of these injuries includes detailed and serial examinations of limbs with known injury, with special attention to innervation of distal sensory areas and muscle groups which have the least cross innervation and whose function is not inhibited by pain. If the nerve is not lacerated, regeneration which has not already occurred in 3 to 6 weeks will proceed at a rate of 1 mm/day plus 1 month delay. A positive Tinel's sign is suggestive of nerve regeneration. If recovery does not follow the above schedule, a primary (within 7 days) or secondary nerve repair is indicated.

Vascular Injuries

Vascular injuries may be due either to penetrating or blunt insults. Penetrating vascular injuries are usually obvious before admission to the emergency room and require operative repair prior to ICU admission. Blunt vascular injury, however, may not become apparent until the patient is followed serially in the ICU. Pain, pallor, paresthesia, paralysis, and pulselessness are clinical features of blunt vascular injury. Further evaluation is aided by Doppler ultrasonography (in the setting of stable hemodynamics) to detect flow in peripheral arteries. If concern remains, arteriography of the vessel in question is indicated. In the setting of possible arterial occlusion, early consultation with a vascular surgeon is recommended. The therapeutic aim is to restore blood flow to ischemic areas within 6 h. When the patient's medical condition permits, arterial reconstruction should begin.

Fractures and Joint Injuries

The principles of definitive management of fractures are reduction, maintenance, and rehabilitation. Early operative intervention to stabilize fractures with early mobilization of the patient results in a significantly decreased incidence of pulmonary complications. Compound fractures with disruption of the integument are frequently contaminated with *Staphylococcus aureus* although, depending on the circumstances of the injury, gram negative or clostridial organisms may also be present. The initial antibiotic of choice is cefazolin (Ancef) with a loading lose of 2 g IV followed by 1 g every 8 h. If gram negative contamination is likely (including high velocity injuries with severe crushing and the presence of skin flaps), an aminoglycoside should be added. Penicillin G should be added in cases where wounds are possibly contaminated by clostridium.

Fat Embolism

Fat embolism syndrome occurs in 2 to 5 percent of patients with long bone fractures and 5 to 10 percent of victims of multiple trauma. The full syndrome typically occurs 48 to 72 h after the initial injury. Clinical features include respiratory insufficiency, cerebral involvement, and petechial rash. Subtle features include pyrexia, tachycardia, anemia, thrombocytopenia, and lipiduria. Chest x-ray may show a diffuse alveolar infiltrate. ECG may show evidence of right ventricular strain. Hypoxemia may be severe. Early definitive fracture splinting is probably the most effective method of circumventing this syndrome and avoidance of hypotension may help to lessen its severity. Aggressive supportive care and early stabilization of long bone fractures are the most reliable treatment modalities. Corticosteroid use in this setting is controversial.

ELECTRICAL TRAUMA

Patients who encounter electrical trauma may suffer a wide variety of sequelae. Electrical trauma victims should always be regarded as victims of blunt trauma and treated as such. Of note, these patients require aggressive fluid resuscitation which is usually grossly underestimated. Isotonic solutions should be administered to provide a urine output of 0.5 to 1.0 mL/kg/h. The presence of myoglobinuria and hemoglobinuria requires an increased urine output for preservation of renal function, thus urine output should approach 2 mL/kg/h. It may be useful to employ mannitol in conjunction with vigorous fluid administration to insure proper renal clearance. Intravenous bicarbonate has also been used to prevent the precipitation of myoglobin in the renal tubules and may be administered by adding one ampule per liter of isotonic solution until urinary myoglobin has cleared. Acetazolamide should be used to reverse systemic alkalosis. Loop diuretics should not be used to improve urine output.

When mental status is abnormal, traumatic causes should be eliminated first. Patients with electrical trauma often manifest a variety of ECG changes suggestive of cardiac ischemia, and routine diagnostic evaluation is not helpful in eliminating the diagnosis. However, since it is unusual for victims of electrical injury to suffer myocardial infarction, needed surgical procedures should not be delayed. Potentially fatal arrhythmias are unusual once the patient is stabilized. The pulmonary sequelae of electrical injury are not specific. When the electrical path passes through the pharynx, local edema may cause upper airway obstruction. All patients at risk of upper airway obstruction should have serial endoscopic examinations and early intubation is hypopharyngeal edema if found. Abdominal complications of electrical injury are infrequent although gastric atony and adynamic ileus are sometimes seen.

Any aspect of neurologic function may be affected by electrical injury with transient or permanent sequelae. Immediate deficits occur in forty percent of patients. Spinal cord injuries can present as complete motor and sensory loss which may resolve over the course of days. Delayed symptoms are more ominous and less likely to resolve. Peripheral nerve injury is common and may require surgical release from compression. Compartment syndromes are common and should be anticipated.

For further reading in *Principles of Critical Care,* see Chap 59 "Priorities in Multisystem Trauma" J Ali, Chap 60 "Closed and Open Head Injury" Richard J Moulton, Chap 61 "Spine Injuries" GE Johnson, Chap 62 "Other Neck Injuries" D Ian Soutter, Chap 63 "Torso Trauma" J Ali, Chap 64 "Pelvic Trauma" Marvin Tile, Chap 65 "Extremity Injuries" GE Johnson/AR Downs, Chap 66 "Electrical Trauma" Lawrence Gottlieb/Jonathan Saunders/Raphael Lee

---

| **Burns**

Scott P. Neeley

The burn patient presents particularly complex, and rapidly evolving management problems. The optimal environment for such a patient is a burn center, but if not available, an ICU modified for the special needs of the burn patient can be adequate. Burn patients require increased room temperature and strict adherence to infection control principles. Vascular access problems may necessitate increased reliance on noninvasive measure of fluid status and cardiopulmonary function.

Many of the problems unique to burn patients are predictable and must be prevented rather than treated as they develop. Discussion of these burn-related issues will therefore be divided into three time periods: the initial resuscitation period (0 to 36 h), the early postresuscitation period (2 to 6 days), and the inflammation-infection period (day 7 to wound closure).

RESUSCITATION PHASE (0 TO 36 h)

This period is characterized by life-threatening airway and breathing problems and hypovolemia due to loss of plasma volume into burn tissue. The burn itself is of less immediate concern. It is essential to remember that the burn patient is a trauma patient and the standard approach to trauma resuscitation must be followed (see Chap. 16).

Airway and Pulmonary Abnormalities

Pulmonary insufficiency caused by inhalation of heat and smoke accounts for over 50 percent of fire-related deaths. These injuries are due in large part to inhalation of superheated or toxic fumes, and are comprised of three distinct pathophysiologic processes: carbon monoxide (and cyanide) toxicity, upper airway obstruction, and chemical burn to the lung. Lung changes associated with skin burn and impaired chest wall compliance also contribute to burn-related morbidity and mortality.

Carbon Monoxide and Cyanide Toxicity

Carbon monoxide (CO) toxicity usually occurs when carboxyhemoglobin concentration exceeds 15 percent, and is characterized by symptoms of decreased tissue oxygenation, metabolic acidosis and neurologic manifestations (see Chaps. 66 and 68). Cyanide toxicity presents similarly with severe metabolic acidosis and obtundation. While cyanide levels are not always available or reliable, normal levels are <0.1 mg/L, with levels of near 1.0 mg/L being lethal. Intoxication and head trauma should also be considered in the differential for a burn patient with neurologic dysfunction.

The diagnosis of CO or cyanide toxicity is suggested by persistent metabolic acidosis despite adequate volume resuscitation and cardiac output. Arterial PO_2 may be normal in CO toxicity since the amount of oxygen (O_2) dissolved in arterial plasma is not affected. However, measured hemoglobin saturation (SO_2) will be decreased relative to PO_2. Once a high carboxyhemoglobin or cyanide level is found, a significant smoke exposure is confirmed, and a chemical burn to the airways should be suspected

Upper Airway Obstruction from Airway Edema

Inhalation of air heated to 150° C (318° F) or higher results in immediate injury to the face and the mucosa of the oropharynx and upper airway. Although this injury is immediate, clinically significant physiologic changes may not be apparent for 12 to 18 h. The presence of a body burn increases the severity of airway edema in proportion to the size and depth of the burn, in part due to fluid resuscitation. Face or neck burns complicate the management of airway edema because of anatomic distortion and external compression of the airway.

Clinical symptoms of airway obstruction cannot be relied upon, since stridor and dyspnea do not develop until critical airway narrowing is present. Inspection of the oropharynx for soot or evidence of heat injury should be routine. Spirometry detects early airway obstruction but requires a cooperative patient without severe facial burns. Both fiberoptic bronchoscopy and laryngoscopy will demonstrate the presence of mucosal injury at or above the cords and provide information about the need for intubation. These studies must be performed serially to be maximally effective. The absence of upper airway injury almost always means absence of lower airway injury.

If severe facial or neck burns are present, or if initial evaluation reveals potential for development of airway problems, it is best to proceed with intubation. Progressive edema, especially when combined with anatomic distortion from face or neck burns, may make delayed intubation difficult and dangerous. A large oral endotracheal tube (at least 7 mm internal diameter) should be used in order to allow for adequate clearance of thick secretions. Patients not intubated need to be placed with head elevated, receive careful fluid resuscitation to minimize edema formation, and be monitored by experienced ICU personnel ready to intervene if necessary.

Chemical Burn to Upper and Lower Airways

Toxic gases contained in smoke as well as carbon particles coated with aldehydes and organic acids can injure both upper and lower airways. In the conscious patient, breath-holding and laryngospasm protect against excessive exposure to gases. A history of loss of consciousness or confinement in a closed space should raise suspicion for this type of injury.

Symptoms may be absent on admission, only becoming apparent after 24 to 48 h. Early symptoms consist of wheezing and bronchorrhea. Soot in the lung secretions is evidence of smoke exposure but is not a necessary finding. Physical findings on admission suggestive of smoke exposure include facial burn, soot in the sputum, dyspnea, coughing, wheezing, and bronchorrhea.

Treatment consists of upper airway maintenance and careful fluid resuscitation, combined with aggressive efforts to maintain small airway patency and remove soot and mucopurulent secretions. Endotracheal intubation and positive end-expiratory pressure (PEEP) may decrease early pulmonary deaths after severe burns and smoke inhalation. Bronchospasm should be treated with parenteral or inhaled bronchodilators. Elevation of the patient's head and chest 20 to 30° may help control airway edema. Corticosteroids increase burn-related mortality and should be avoided, as should prophylactic antibiotics. Close monitoring of adequacy of gas exchange with an indwelling arterial line or pulse oximeter is required.

Impaired Chest Wall Compliance

Chest wall burns can markedly impair respiratory excursion. The loss of elasticity of the chest wall increases the work of breathing. Reduced functional residual capacity, in conjunction with elevated closing volume causes airway closure with ventilation perfusion ($\dot{V}/\dot{Q}$) mismatching and atelectasis. Increased work of breathing can lead to hypoventilation and respiratory failure, particularly when hypoxia, hypovolemia, pain, or sedation accentuate lung dysfunction.

Symptoms may not be evident until edema formation peaks. The first evidence of chest wall restriction is often labored breathing, often rapidly followed by respiratory failure. Clearance of secretions may be impaired, due to inability to generate hyperinflation. The increased intrathoracic pressure required to expand the chest wall may impede venous return, complicating concomitant hypovolemia.

Treatment consists of measures to reduce edema, possibly with surgical decompression of the chest wall. The head of the bed should be elevated 30° when possible, and fluid resuscitation should be well controlled. If chest wall restriction develops with a third degree burn, escharotomy is required. Escharotomies are usually not required in a second-degree burn unless the burn is very deep or edema is massive.

Restoration and Maintenance of Hemodynamic Stability

Pathophysiology of Burn Shock

After a major burn, massive intravascular volume loss into burn tissue occurs as a result of increases in vascular permeability and in burn tissue osmotic pressure. The markedly abnormal vascular permeability in burn tissue leads to a loss of the gradient between plasma and interstitial protein contents, even for very large molecules. However, the rate of initial fluid loss from the microcirculation into interstitium of burn tissue is greater than can be explained by increased vascular permeability alone. It has been hypothesized that an increase in burn tissue osmotic pressure due to sodium binding to injured collagen explains the rapid rate of fluid loss. Increased vascular permeability in burn tissue also results in substantial protein losses from plasma into the interstitium of burn tissue and subsequent hypoproteinemia. Fluid and protein losses are greatest in the first 6 to 8 h because of the combined effect of increased permeability and increased interstitial osmotic pressure.

The interstitial edema fluid appears to form a gel after about 12 h, probably due to leakage of clotting proteins and fibrin deposition. This causes obstruction of local lymphatics, and impairs edema clearance. Tissue oxygenation also decreases as edema fluid increases the distance between viable cells and the closest capillaries. Resolution of edema depends on restoration of lymphatic patency, which may take a number of days to weeks.

Generalized edema also occurs in nonburned tissues in patients with burns exceeding 30 percent of total body surface area (TBS). This process appears to be due to alterations in microvascular interstitium due to low protein content, changes in cell membrane potential and cellular swelling associated with shock, and plasma hypoalbuminemia. Vascular permeability is only transiently altered in nonburned tissues.

Hemodynamic changes associated with the early stages of burn shock are primarily those of hypovolemia. Cardiac output (CO) is usually low due to intravascular volume loss—actual depression in myocardial contractility may be seen with very severe burns due either to myocardial edema or a circulating myocardial depressant factor. Systemic vascular resistance (SVR) is increased due to circulating vasoactive mediators such as catecholamines. Tachycardia is typically present, and helps to restore CO toward normal even before normal plasma volume is restored.

Treatment

Intravenous access should be obtained via peripheral vein catheter through nonburn tissue when possible. Central vein or pulmonary artery catheters are required for monitoring resuscitation primarily in the elderly patient, or in those with severe cardiac or renal disease. Very high rates of infectious and embolic complications of central catheters have been reported in burn patients, and thus such devices should be removed as soon as they are no longer needed. Central line sites (when not dedicated to total parenteral nutrition) should be rotated every 3 days to minimize the risks of catheter sepsis.

No single perfusion parameter is a completely reliable indicator of tissue oxygenation in the burn patient. Therefore, several parameters and laboratory tests should be monitored. *Baseline body weight* helps in estimation of fluid infusion rate, assessment of nutrition needs and drug dosages. *Tachycardia* is inevitable with the exception of elderly patients and those with underlying heart disease. As a rule, a pulse of 120 usually indicates adequate volume, while a pulse >130 indicates that more fluid is needed. *Urine output* (UOP) is a useful reflection of renal perfusion in the absence of factors such as renal insufficiency, osmotic agents, or inappropriate sodium and water retention. UOP of 0.5 to 1.0 mL/kg/h normally reflects adequate renal blood flow. A value of <0.5 mL/kg/h indicates renal hypoperfusion, while a value >1.0 mL/kg/h usually means that too much fluid is being given. *Arterial pH* is an extremely useful measure of tissue oxygenation. Acidosis during this phase usually reflects impaired tissue oxygenation due to hypoperfusion, or carbon monoxide or cyanide toxicity. *Temperature* should be monitored closely and maintained at 37 to 37.5° C (98.6 to 99.9° F) during this period. Burn patients are prone to hypothermia during early resuscitation. *The central venous pressure* (CVP) is usually low (0 to 5 mmHg) during this period, as is *pulmonary capillary wedge pressure* (Ppw) (6 to 10 mmHg), even with adequate fluid resuscitation. Thus, use of arbitrary endpoints for CVP or Ppw may risk increased edema formation due to excessive fluid resuscitation. *Cardiac output or cardiac index* may not be predictive of adequate tissue oxygen delivery in the burn patient due to increased tissue demands, though the *mixed venous* P_{O_2} can greatly assist in this determination.

In general, crystalloid fluids containing at least as much salt as is contained in plasma are appropriate for use in resuscitation: restoration of sodium lost into the burn is essential. Fluids should be free of glucose (except in small children) since glucose intolerance is common. Isotonic solutions such as Lactated Ringers or normal saline are acceptable. A common practice is to use a solution with a sodium content of approximately 240 meq/L by adding 2 ampules sodium lactate to each liter normal saline. The serum sodium level should not be allowed to exceed 160 meq/L. A more isotonic solution should be instituted once a hyperosmolar state develops. Colloid infusion beginning at about 8 to 12 h may be appropriate if edema in noninjured tissue and fluid requirements are to be minimized. The use of fresh frozen plasma should be reserved for correction of documented clotting abnormalities. A 6% albumin infusion can be used to replace albumin losses. A rate of between 0.5 and 1 mL/kg/% burn may be used as an arbitrary guideline for albumin infusion during the first 24 h. Nonprotein colloids, such as Hetastarch, are less expensive than albumin and may be equally effective in maintaining early hemodynamic stability.

The rate of fluid administration is that necessary to maintain adequate perfusion. An initial rate can be estimated using the size of the burn relative to weight:

$$24 \text{ h volume} = 4 \text{ mL} \times \% \text{ burn} \times \text{weight (kg)} \qquad (17\text{-}1)$$

Any formula is only an initial guide. If shock is present, a bolus of fluid should be administered. After perfusion is restored, fluid should be infused at a relatively constant rate, making small changes to maintain perfusion. Boluses are disadvantageous since they may transiently increase microvascular pressure, increasing rate of fluid loss into the burn. Approximately half of the first 24 h requirements should be given in the first 8 h. Beginning at 8 to 10 h, an attempt should be made to gradually decrease the rate to the lowest needed to maintain perfusion.

Inotropic support is indicated if adequate perfusion cannot be maintained without excessive fluid administration. This problem is most frequently encountered in elderly patients, those with underlying heart disease, or in patients requiring positive pressure ventilation. Dobutamine is most often the agent of first choice.

Management of the Burn Wound

Assessment of the Burn Wound

Traditionally, burn depth has been classified in degrees of injury based on the amount of epidermis and dermis injured. A *first-degree burn* involves only the thin outer epidermis, and is characterized by erythema and mild discomfort. Tissue damage is minimal, and complete healing takes place uneventfully. *Second-degree burns* are those in which the entire epidermis and variable portions of the dermis are destroyed. *Superficial second-degree burns* involve heat injury to the upper third of the dermis and are characterized by blister formation. Despite loss of the entire basal layer of the epidermis, burns of this degree will heal with minimal scarring in 7 to 14 days. *Deep dermal (or deep second-degree) burns* extend deep into the dermal layer, leaving few viable epithelial cells. Blister formation is unusual, and the wound surface is usually red with white areas in deeper parts. Dense scarring usually occurs if the wound is not excised and skin grafted. *Full thickness or third-degree burns* involve destruction of the entire epidermis and dermis. The wound is usually a waxy white color. If the burn extends into fat or there is prolonged contact with flame, it will have a black or brown charred appearance. The wound will not re-epithelialize, and the area not closed by wound contraction will require skin grafting. Nerve endings are destroyed in third-degree burns, leading to a lack of painful sensation. This characteristic can be used to distinguish second-degree from third-degree burns.

The size of the burn is defined in terms of total body surface area (TBS). A useful initial guide is the "rule of nines" where the body is divided into areas each with 9 percent of TBS: the head and each arm are considered 9 percent of TBS, while the chest and abdomen, the back and each lower extremity are considered to be 18 percent of TBS. The Lund and Browder chart is more accurate and should be used for more precise calculation.

Treatment

The major objectives in initial management of the burn wound are to decrease the potential for further local damage and to decrease the systemic abnormalities produced by the loss of the skin barrier function. In severely injured patients, adequate control of the airway, gas exchange, and restoration of fluid loss should precede attempts to clean and debride the wound.

The first step in management is neutralizing the source of burn injury. Rapid removal of burned clothing is essential. Cooling of the burn is recommended for initial heat neutralization and to control pain in superficial second-degree burns <15% TBS. Cooling should be avoided in more severe burns as it increases the rate of heat loss, increases oxygen and glycogen consumption by causing shivering, and decreases blood flow to the skin.

Heat loss from the burn wound should be controlled by placing dry dressings over the wound and by placing the patient in a warmed external environment. Wound debridement and washing should not be initiated on a large burn until the external temperature is controlled. The optimum environment for cleaning of the major burn is one where temperature control and aseptic technique can be observed. Intravenous narcotics are indicated for pain control.

Tetanus prophylaxis is necessary. Prophylactic systemic antibiotics are contraindicated with the exception of low dose penicillin for protection against β-hemolytic streptococcus in patients at high risk for this organism (known carrier or recent exposure). Topical antibiotics (e.g., Silvadene) are indicated for dirty superficial second-degree burns and for all deeper burns.

Edema formation can increase tissue pressure to a point which impedes arterial blood flow, particularly in the circumferential burn. Perfusion of the distal extremity must, therefore, be closely monitored. A warm extremity indicates adequate perfusion, though a cool extremity may indicate hypovolemia and shock as well as hypoperfusion due to burn constriction. Monitoring of the distal pulse by palpation or Doppler flowmeter is the most practical manner of assessment. Tissue pressure measurements using a small needle can be obtained, but introduce increased risk of infection. Tissue pressure exceeding 25 to 30 mmHg indicates the need for escharotomy. Decreasing distal flow with a proximal deep burn is also an indication for escharotomy.

POSTRESUSCITATION PHASE (DAY 2 TO DAY 6)

The early postresuscitation phase is a period of transition from the shock characteristic of early severe burn injuries to the hypermetabolic state seen in later stages of severe burn injuries. The patient's cardiovascular condition can deteriorate rapidly with the onset of hypermetabolism and sepsis. The early wound excision and grafting approach is initiated during this period, as increased wound blood flow and infection have not yet peaked. The exceptions to this rule are patients with severe lung injury, and patients who are hemodynamically unstable.

Pulmonary Abnormalities

Upper Airway Obstruction

Continued airway maintenance with an endotracheal tube may be required during this period as facial and airway edema slowly resolve. Elevation of the patient's head to 30 to 45° will allow faster resolution of edema. Optimal timing of extubation can be difficult to determine since no single measure adequately assesses airway patency. Laryngoscopy to determine the presence of cord edema can be helpful, as is deflation of the endotracheal tube cuff to determine if air moves around the tube. Persistent edema of the false cords and supraglottic tissue, or external compression from a neck burn may compromise the airway after extubation however, even if cord edema has sufficiently resolved. Therefore, the patient should be closely monitored during this period in case reintubation is needed.

Decreased Chest Wall Compliance

Even after escharotomy, significant impairment in chest wall compliance may persist for days due to loss of elasticity in burn tissue and persistent edema. This impairment results in decreased FRC and vital capacity, and increased work of breathing and energy requirements. Potential therapeutic measures include measures to minimize edema, and mechanical ventilation, to maintain FRC, and minimize atelectasis and oxygen demands. Early excision of the full-thickness wound can improve chest wall motion by removing both edema and noncompliant tissue.

Tracheobronchitis from Inhalation Injury

Persistent cough, bronchorrhea and mucus production are characteristic of even mild to moderate inhalation injury. After severe injury, damaged mucosa becomes necrotic 3 to 4 days after injury and begins to slough. Increased secretions can lead to airway obstruction, atelectasis, and a high risk for pneumonia.

Clinical findings of respiratory compromise, such as dyspnea, tachypnea, wheezing and rhonchi precede radiographic findings. Common X-ray findings include diffuse atelectasis, pulmonary edema or focal infiltrates. Repeated blood gas analysis and changes in sputum characteristics should be noted.

Treatment includes vigorous efforts to clear soot, purulent exudate and sloughing mucosa. Endotracheal intubation and mechanical ventilation may be necessary. Aerosolized bronchodilators, frequent postural changes, and chest physiotherapy are very helpful. A continuously rotating bed to promote postural drainage is ideal for the patient with an inhalation injury and a large body burn in whom movement is limited by pain and stiffness. Infection surveillance is crucial to detect bacterial bronchitis. Bacterial colonization is inevitable, and can lead to a diffuse tracheobronchitis with subsequent severe diffuse pneumonia. Sputum smears are useful as initial guides, though are fair at best in predicting infection and the organisms involved. Systemic antibiotics should not be given prophylactically, but should be initiated when a bacterial tracheobronchitis becomes evident.

Pulmonary Edema

The most common causes of pulmonary edema during this phase are volume overload due to mobilization of edema and excess infusion of fluid in the presence of myocardial dysfunction, and non-cardiogenic pulmonary edema due to progression of a smoke inhalation injury. In the setting of severe burn or smoke inhalation injury, these etiologies may be difficult to distinguish by clinical assessment. Pulmonary artery catheterization and/or echocardiography may contribute to decision making in these circumstances. Therapy may include reduction in fluid infusion rates, use of low-dose dopamine, and judicious use of diuretics and vasoactive agents (e.g., dobutamine).

Maintaining Hemodynamic and Metabolic Stability

Pathophysiologic Changes in the Postresuscitation Period

Intravascular volume loss due to edema formation is maximal in the first 30 h after burn injury. After this time, evaporation from the surface of the burn becomes a major source of water loss that persists until the wound is closed. A reasonable estimate of loss can be obtained from the following formula:

$$\text{Evaporative water loss (mL/h)} = (25 + \%\text{burn}) \times (\text{m}^2 \text{ body surface area}) \qquad (17\text{-}2)$$

Despite these losses, continued caution in fluid administration is necessary to prevent further increases in edema and the development of volume overload.

Despite evaporative losses, intravascular fluid may increase during the postresuscitation period due to mobilization of edema. The actual rate of edema resorption is highly variable. Loss of lymphatics in full thickness burns, fibrin deposition in burn edema, and high central venous pressures all retard edema resorption. Edema resorption is much more rapid in superficial burns, and is also improved by increased muscle activity. For these reasons, the magnitude of tissue edema is a poor reflection of intravascular volume and should not be used to determine fluid replacement.

Hepatic albumin synthesis is markedly diminished in favor of acute-phase protein synthesis. Resulting hypoalbuminemia may contribute to persistent edema in burn and non-burn tissues, and may contribute to abnormal pharmacokinetics due to loss of normal protein binding.

Red blood cell mass decreases markedly during this period because of an increased rate of red blood cell breakdown and decreased production. Typically the hematocrit falls to between 30 and 35, or lower, several days postburn. Losses from escharotomies, wound debridement and phlebotomy may further contribute to anemia.

The restoration of blood flow to the burn tissue results in the resorption of a large load of osmotically active solutes from disrupted cells and proteins. This results in an obligate solute diuresis manifested by a high-specific gravity urine. The increase in urine output may be mistaken for fluid resorption and hypervolemia unless the specific gravity is followed carefully.

After initial stability in the early postresuscitation phase, the onset of a hypermetabolic state often manifests beginning at day 5 or 6. The metabolic rate gradually increases from a normal level of 35 to 40 cal/m^2 per h (25 cal/kg per day) to levels ranging from 2 to 2.5 times normal at about day 10. The magnitude of increase is related to burn size, and is typically greater in younger patients. The hypermetabolic state is characterized by increased oxygen consumption, hyperglycemia, and increased protein catabolism. Body temperature increases to between 100 and 101° F (38 to 38.5°C), making the diagnosis of infection more difficult. Cardiac output usually begins to increase and to exceed normal values as a hyperdynamic state evolves, and tachycardia (100 to 120 beats per minute) is common. SVR begins to decrease, with the increased vascular space causing increased requirements for fluids, colloid and red cells.

Hemodynamic Management

Assessment of the adequacy of perfusion, tissue oxygenation, and fluid and electrolyte needs can be difficult during this period. Many of the same parameters are monitored as before. However, interpretation of some of the physiologic values differs from that during initial resuscitation. UOP usually exceeds 0.5 mL/kg per h as edema fluid and solute load are mobilized, but may not reflect adequacy of perfusion due to the obligatory solute diuresis. Intake usually exceeds UOP during this period, though the major output, evaporative loss, is not directly quantitated. The absolute body weight cannot be used to reflect blood volume during this transition period, though if weight is increasing, excess fluid (and salt) is probably being given. Arterial blood pressure and pulse rate are difficult to interpret due to the effects of pain, elevated temperature, narcotics and increasing metabolic rate.

CVP greater than 15 mmHg usually indicates hypervolemia or impaired venous return (e.g. from PEEP). Ppw greater than 15 suggests the possibility of heart failure, hypervolemia or increased intrathoracic pressure (e.g. PEEP). VO$_2$ typically increases 50 to 100 percent with the development of hypermetabolism. Cardiac output increases with O$_2$ demand and typically doubles with burns greater than 30 percent of TBS.

Isotonic or hypertonic crystalloid fluid is generally no longer needed during this period, and may contribute to hypernatremia and volume overload. A 5 percent glucose containing fluid with a low sodium content is the fluid of choice for replacement of evaporative and urinary losses. The addition of 20 to 30 meq of potassium per L is usually indicated to replace urinary potassium losses. If plasma albumin cannot be sustained at a level of 2.5 g/dL with nutritional support alone, it may be reasonable to continue albumin infusion during this period. Finally, it is frequently necessary to administer red blood cells. The hematocrit should be maintained at least in the low 30's to optimize oxygen delivery.

Nutritional Support

Nutritional support should be started early in the post-resuscitation period. The enteral route is preferred because of lower rates of infectious complications and cost. However, ileus is common in patients with large burns, frequently necessitating the use of parenteral nutrition. In order to provide necessary support for energy needs, energy expenditure needs to be determined for each patient. Energy expenditure is determined by the basal metabolic rate (BMR), muscle activity, and stress-induced energy needs. The BMR is the energy requirement necessary to maintain cell integrity in the resting state, and is dependent on body surface area, age and sex (see Chap. 12). Muscle activity is usually minimal in the critically ill burn patient and is typically estimated at 25% of BMR, though excessive work of breathing or agitation may markedly increase energy expenditure. Stress-induced energy needs are those related to the hypermetabolism induced by the burn. The stress factor is a multiple of the BMR, and is primarily related to the size of the burn (see Table 17-1). An estimation of caloric needs is based on the following formula:

$$\text{Energy requirement} = \text{BMR} \times 1.25 \text{ (Activity)} \times \text{stress factor} \quad (17\text{-}3)$$

This formula may be used as a guideline in many patients. However, more precise estimation of caloric needs with indirect calorimetry (see Chap. 12) may be indicated in patients with rapidly changing metabolic requirements.

TABLE 1

Burn Size (%TBS)	Stress Factor
10	1.25
20	1.5
30	1.7
40	1.85
50	2.0
60-100	2.1

(Reprinted with permission from Demling R: Burns: Inflammation-Infection Phase (Day 7 to Wound Closure), in Hall JB, Schmidt GA, Wood LDH: Principles of Critical Care, McGraw-Hill, New York, 1992.)

Approximately 60 percent of estimated nonprotein caloric requirements should be given as glucose. Fat can be used for the remaining 40 percent of nonprotein calories. Triglyceride values should be monitored 4 h after cessation of lipid infusion and should not exceed 250 mg/dL. A standard estimate of protein requirements of 1.5 to 2.0 g of protein per kg body weight per day can be used for all major burns. A more specific quantitative estimate may be made based on the calorie nitrogen ratio (see Chap. 12). Vitamin A should be given in a daily dose of 10,000 to 50,000 units, and vitamin C in a daily dose of 1 g. Zinc should be replaced with 220 mg $ZnSO_4$ twice daily orally, or 45 mg daily parenterally. Vitamin B complex needs are 5 to 10 times the RDA in burn patients. Other specific trace element requirements are less well defined.

Care of the Burn Wound

Pathophysiologic Changes in the Burn Wound

The burn wound, relatively inert at 24 h, becomes a focus of intense inflammation at about 7 to 10 days in full-thickness burns, and several days sooner in partial thickness burns. This change is related to increased vascularity in the wound, with increased release of inflammatory mediators. The eschar of a deep burn becomes more prominent during this period, and may be indistinguishable from the yellow to white appearance initially seen with a full-thickness injury. The subeschar tissue changes dramatically, first with neutrophil infiltration (2 to 3 days), followed by intense macrophage infiltration during peak inflammation (7 to 10 days). Bacterial colonization is usually evident at 2 to 3 days, though invasive wound infection is not common in the first week unless gross wound contamination occurred initially.

Wound conversion, the process by which marginally viable tissue is converted to nonviable tissue, occurs during this period. This occurs most often in deep second degree wounds, and is accentuated by wound infection. Spontaneous surface sloughing of the eschar occurs towards the end of this period due to inflammatory liquefaction of the eschar and subeschar tissue.

Management of Burn Wound Infection

Loss of skin barrier, the presence of dead tissue, impaired blood flow, and systemic immunosuppression all contribute to the development of burn wound infection. Movement of organisms by hand contact, from area to area on the patient, or between patients is the major factor leading to bacterial contamination of the wound. This problem can be attenuated with enforced hand washing.

Diagnosis of wound infection may be difficult since colonization is inevitable. Fever, leukocytosis, tachycardia and fever are characteristically seen with or without infection. Wound purulence is a reliable indicator of infection only if the purulence is in the subeschar space. Surface cultures of the wound should be taken after the exudate has been removed. Such cultures are not diagnostic of infection, but may assist in identifying the type of bacteria present. *Staphylococcus aureus* is the most common organism in wound cultures in the first week, though β-*hemolytic streptococci* are also seen early. Gram-negative organisms become more common after the first week. Enterococci and *Candida albicans* are being seen with increasing frequency. The most reliable method for diagnosing a burn wound infection is analysis of a wound biopsy. A small, full-thickness portion of eschar along with some underlying viable subcutaneous tissue is removed by punch biopsy instrument or scalpel. 10^5 organism per g of tissue is the bacterial load that is preinvasive. Even more reliable is histologic inspection of biopsy tissue. Bacterial invasion of viable tissue indicates true infection and the need for systemic antibiotics. Routine biopsies every 3 to 4 days provide continuing information on microbiologic changes in the wound.

Early Wound Excision and Grafting

Early excision and grafting should be considered for all burns that will not heal within 3 weeks. Full-thickness burns require grafting unless they are smaller than 3 to 4 cm. The more rapidly the wound is closed the better. Burns covering less than 30 percent of TBS can often be rapidly closed as adequate donor sites are available. The key issue is to balance risks of surgery against the potential benefits of early wound closure.

INFLAMMATION-INFECTION PHASE (DAY 7 TO WOUND CLOSURE)

Pulmonary complications and sepsis are the most common causes of mortality during this period. Nosocomial pneumonia is particularly common in mechanically ventilated patients and those with smoke inhalation injury. The development of the adult respiratory distress syndrome (ARDS) or multisystem organ failure (MSOF) due to sepsis, lung injury or persistent severe wound inflammation may be particularly difficult to reverse in the burn patient (see Chaps. 15 and 30). Manipulation of the burn wound should be limited during this period because of infection and hypervascularity. Continued attention to adequate nutritional support and pain management is of utmost importance.

Pulmonary Abnormalities

Nosocomial Tracheobronchitis and Pneumonia

The development of bacterial tracheobronchitis after smoke inhalation injury is a major risk factor for the development of bacterial pneumonitis. Other factors contributing to the development of pneumonia in burn patients include colonization due to carriage of resistant and/or virulent bacterial strains by ICU personnel and equipment; aspiration potentiated by sedation, impaired cough, NG tube placement and endotracheal tube placement; and impaired mucociliary clearance. The usual criteria for diagnosis of pneumonia (fever, leukocytosis, purulent sputum, radiographic findings, sputum smears and cultures) are unreliable in critically ill burn patients. Quantitative cultures of protected brush or BAL specimens obtained by bronchoscopy may be of use in diagnosis and therapy (see Chap. 41). In addition to appropriate antimicrobial therapy, efforts should focus on maintaining adequate oxygenation, tissue perfusion, nutrition, and pulmonary toilet.

Hypermetabolism-Induced Respiratory Muscle Fatigue

The increase of O_2 consumption and CO_2 production during this period imposes increased demand on the respiratory system. Multiple causes of increased ventilatory load and decreased neuromuscular competence commonly present in critically ill burn patients can lead to frank respiratory failure during this period. In addition to controlling edema and infection, maintaining nutrition, and providing adequate rest and exercise, efforts should be made to control CO_2 production by avoiding excess carbohydrate calories and controlling hyperthermia.

Infection and Sepsis

Pathophysiology

The sepsis syndrome is clinically similar to the postburn hypermetaboic state; it is characterized initially by fever, leukocytosis, tachycardia, and a hyperdynamic state reflected by increased cardiac output, decreased SVR, and increased O_2 consumption. Evidence of impaired tissue oxygenation is present, however, as is lactic acidosis and hypotension. These signs are unusual with hypermetabolism alone. The most common sources of infection in the burn patient are the lungs, the burn wound, and vascular access catheters. Septic thrombophlebitis should be suspected in the presence of repeatedly positive blood cultures and appropriate physical findings. Intraabdominal processes, such as acalculous cholecystitis and pancreatitis are less common, but well recognized sources of sepsis. The high risk of intravascular lines can not be over-emphasized. Lack of a positive blood culture does not rule out an infected line, and a high index of suspicion must be maintained. Sometimes the only proof is resolution of the septic episode after removal of the catheter.

Treatment

Empiric antibiotics should be begun promptly when infection is suspected. Combined therapy with a cephalosporin or extended spectrum penicillin plus an aminoglycoside is usually appropriate initial management. Suspicion for line sepsis may be an indication for the use of vancomycin. The antibiotic regimen should be altered appropriately when culture data and diagnostic studies become available. Careful attention should be given to dosing: burn patients may require larger total antibiotic doses due to hypermetabolism and loss of antibiotics from the wound. On the other hand, renal impairment may mandate lower doses. Monitoring of aminoglycoside levels should be routine.

As with any form of sepsis, the removal or control of the septic focus is of primary importance. Mafenide cream is the agent of choice for topical management of wound infection. Debridement should be performed gently to unroof pockets of infection and allow for better local wound care. Large incisions are often poorly tolerated because of dissemination of infection and blood loss. Tender or inflamed peripheral veins should be inspected via a cutdown and surgically removed if there is any question of purulence. Careful physical examination should be performed to look for evidence of line-related infection or soft tissue abscess. In the absence of other sources of infection, abdominal etiologies should be considered and appropriately investigated (see Chap. 36).

For further reading in *Principles of Critical Care,* see Chap 68 "Burns: Resuscitation Phase (0 to 36H)" Robert H Demling, Chap 69 "Burns: Postresuscitation Phase (Day 2 to Day 6)" Robert H Demling, Chap 70 "Burns: Inflammation-Infection Phase (Day 7 to Wound Closure)" Robert H. Demling

---

18

Organ Procurement and Management of the Multiorgan Donor

Kevin Simpson

Although transplantation has developed into an important treatment for both acute and chronic organ failure, donor organ shortage is the rate-limiting factor in most types of transplantation. Through the early recognition of potential organ donors, accurate and efficient declaration of brain death, and skillful donor management prior to procurement, it will be possible to increase the number of beneficiaries of organ transplantation.

ORGAN PROCUREMENT

Recognition of a Potential Organ Donor

There are both general and organ-specific exclusion criteria for organ donation. General absolute exclusion criteria include age greater than 70; malignancy (primary cerebral malignancy, skin cancer, and lip cancer are usually not regarded as exclusions); documentation of hepatitis, human immunodeficiency virus (HIV) infection or active tuberculosis; systemic infection; and current intravenous drug abuse.

In addition to general exclusion criteria, there are organ-specific issues. Kidneys usually are not procured if there is evidence of long-standing severe hypertension or diabetes, or evidence of chronic renal disease. Specific exclusionary criteria for the pancreas include a history of diabetes and compelling evidence of pancreatitis. Livers are not obtained from donors who have histories of chronic alcoholism or show other evidence of liver disease. Livers from donors with elevated serum glutane-pyruvic transaminase (SGPT) and/or bilirubin levels may be accepted if the trend is downward on serial testing. Potential lung, heart, and heart-lung donors are usually less than 45 years of age and there must be no history of pre-existing cardiac or pulmonary disease. In the case of lung donation, sputum cultures must confirm no evidence of ongoing infection and bronchoscopy is performed to exclude anatomic lesions and aspiration of either gastric contents or foreign bodies. Furthermore, the PaO_2: FIO_2 ratio should be at least 250 mmHg and peak airway pressures should be less than 30 cmH_2O when ventilated with a tidal volume of 15 mL/kg and a positive end-expiratory pressure (PEEP) of 5 cmH_2O. In the case of heart and heart-lung transplantation, the ability to maintain a systolic blood pressure of 90 mmHg or above on moderate doses of dopamine is considered to be evidence of adequate cardiac function. Pulmonary or cardiology consultation is mandatory. Finally, it is important to remember that exclusionary criteria for organ donation vary from transplant center to transplant center and that the regional transplant team should be contacted before a possible organ donor is rejected.

Obtaining Permission for Organ Donation

At the time of brain death in a patient who meets the criteria for organ or tissue donation, the designated hospital representative, or the local organ procurement coordinator, should approach the legal next of kin to offer the family of the deceased the option of organ or tissue donation. A professional who is knowledgeable and comfortable with brain death and organ transplantation is best able to interact with the next of kin in an objective, yet compassionate, way. Acceptance of death is an absolute prerequisite to familial consent for organ donation; therefore, brain death must be explained thoroughly and succinctly.

Brain Death

Brain death is a medically and legally definable state synonymous with death of a human being (see Chap. 46). Brain death is defined as the total lack of function of the whole brain, including the brain stem and is recognized when **1.** cerebral functions are absent, and **2.** brain stem functions are absent. Irreversibility is recognized when **1.** the cause of coma is established and is sufficient to account for the loss of brain functions, **2.** the possibility of recovery of any brain functions is excluded, and **3.** the cessation of cerebral and brain stem function persists for an appropriate period. The determination of brain death can be complicated by drug intoxication, neuromuscular blockade, metabolic derangement, and hypothermia. Hence these conditions must be excluded or reversed in order for the clinical determination of brain death to be reliable.

Once the criteria for brain death have been satisfied, an apnea test should be performed in which the patient is ventilated for ten minutes with 100% O_2 and the minute volume adjusted to allow the arterial P_{CO_2} to rise above 40 mmHg. Minute ventilation is then reduced to allow the P_{CO_2} to rise above 60 mmHg, while pulse oximetry guarantees adequate arterial saturation. The absence of respiratory efforts confirms the state of apnea.

The diagnosis of brain death should be clearly documented in the chart by a physician not directly associated with organ transplantation.

MANAGEMENT OF MULTIORGAN DONORS AND COMPLICATIONS ENCOUNTERED AFTER BRAIN DEATH

The primary goals of routine donor care are to maintain organ perfusion and tissue oxygenation, reduce the risk of infection, and monitor for complications. Routine management including regular nursing care directed towards skin care, catheter and dressing changes, charting of vital signs, and culturing of potentially infected sites is essential.

Cardiovascular instability is very common in brain-dead patients and a central venous catheter, arterial line, and Foley catheter are necessary to monitor the adequacy of perfusion and tissue oxygenation. The best signs of an acceptable cardiac output are adequate systolic blood pressure and good urine output (at least 0.5 to 1 mL/kg per h). The most crucial aspect of maintaining organ viability is obtaining adequate systemic perfusion and a systolic pressure of 100 mmHg is a reasonable goal. The most common cause of hypotension is inadequate volume resuscitation; thus, if hypotension develops, the central venous pressure should first be increased to 8 to 10 cmH$_2$O by boluses of colloid, crystalloid, or blood, and the hematocrit should be kept in the range of 25 to 35 percent. If the blood pressure is still low after adequate hydration, vasoactive drugs may be necessary. Dopamine is added first in low doses (2 to 3 µg/kg per min). When an inotrope is needed in addition, dobutamine or a higher dosage of dopamine is used. Epinephrine, norepinephrine and dopamine at doses higher than 10 µg/kg per min can adversely affect the kidney and liver and should be avoided if possible. Because of the risk of infection, use of right heart catheters should be avoided except when adequate systemic perfusion cannot be maintained without resorting to high doses of vasoactive drugs.

Bradyarrhythmia and systemic hypertension (Cushing's reflex) may be seen at the time of brain herniation. Unless these are associated with instability, treatment is unnecessary. Bradyarrhythmias are not responsive to atropine and treatment entails a catecholamine, such as isoproterenol, or electrical pacing. There may also arise tachyarrhythmias related to the release of catecholamines; these often respond to β-blockers.

Cardiac arrest by itself does not exclude the use of an organ donor. Treatment should be undertaken in the same manner as for patients who are not brain-dead, with two exceptions; **1.** atropine is ineffective; and **2.** organ viability is the most important limiting factor, so the tolerances acceptable to the transplant team should be known.

Ventilatory management of the organ donor includes routine suctioning, turning and manual lung expansion to help prevent atelectasis and pneumonia. Up to 5 cmH$_2$O of PEEP may also be helpful in this regard, although higher levels may impair venous return or selectively reduce hepatic perfusion. In patients who are not suitable for heart-lung donation, it is preferable to use a high FI$_{O_2}$, rather than a high level of PEEP, to maintain oxygenation when necessary. In a lung donor, the endotracheal tube should be placed high in the trachea to avoid injury at potential suture lines. Treatment of pulmonary edema focuses on reducing filling pressures to the lowest level consistent with an adequate cardiac output and using PEEP to recruit alveoli.

Diabetes insipidus is common in brain-dead organ donors and is treated with desmopressin acetate (DDAVP), a synthetic analogue of arginine vasopressin, titrated to keep urine output greater than 100 mL/h and less than 250 mL/h. Coagulopathy and disseminated intravascular coagulation (DIC) are seen in a high percentage of head-injured patients. Appropriate therapy may include warming the patient (for hypothermia), platelet transfusion, or component therapy; ε-aminocaproic acid should not be used, however, because of the risk of inducing microvascular thrombosis with resulting ischemic organ damage. Hypothermia may cause coagulation defects, cardiovascular arrhythmias, decreased cardiac output, and other adverse effects; it can usually be prevented or managed by heating blankets, warmers for blood and fluid infusions, and warming (to 40°C) of the humidified gas supplied through the mechanical ventilator. Finally, at the first sign of infection, cultures of urine, blood, wound and endotracheal secretions should again be collected. Since the recipient of the donor organ will be immunosuppressed, transplantation of infected organs can have disastrous consequences.

19

Immunotherapy and Organ Transplantation

Edward T. Naureckas

Improvements in immunosuppression have led to a dramatic increase in organ transplants. This has led to an increase in the number of transplant recipients in the general public and has been paralleled by an increase in the number of centers doing organ transplants.

ALLOGRAFT REJECTION

There are three types of allograft rejection. Hyperacute rejection presents almost immediately after revascularization of the grafted organ. At present there is no treatment for this form of rejection.

Chronic rejection is characterized by progressive vasculitis leading to graft ischemia, fibrosis, and loss of function. This form of rejection tends to be refractory to immunotherapy and is the most frequent cause of late graft failure.

The greatest gains in transplantation therapy have come from the prevention of acute rejection. This form of rejection is initiated by T lymphocytes responding to foreign MHC antigens from the allograft.

IMMUNOSUPPRESSIVE AGENTS

Immunosuppressive agents, while effective in decreasing the incidence of acute rejection, have many side effects and predispose patients to infection. In order to avoid the toxicities of particular agents, immunosuppressive regimens are often modified. A number of immunosuppressive agents and their toxicities are listed in Table 19-1.

Cyclosporin

Cyclosporin is thought to act by inhibiting the production of IL-2 by T-lymphocytes. It is currently used in combination with prednisone as the mainstay of maintenance therapy. Its administration is generally begun near the time of transplantation at approximately 8 to 10 mg/kg/day divided into two daily oral doses. When it is necessary to give the drug by intravenous route one-third the oral dose is given. As the drug undergoes enterohepatic circulation, increased doses may be required in liver transplants with external bile drainage. Cyclosporin levels, while available, do not reliably indicate the presence of toxicity nor the adequacy of immuno-

TABLE 19-1 Non-Infectious Complications of Immunosuppressive Drugs

Side Effects of Cyclosporine	Nephrotoxicity Hypertension Tremor Psychosis	Seizures Hypertrichosis Hyperkalemia Hepatotoxicity
Side Effects of Corticosteroids	Hyperglycemia Muscle wasting Impaired wound healing Gastritis Cataracts	Masking of infections Adrenal suppression Bone demineralization Cushingoid facies
Side Effects of Azathioprine	Neutropenia Hepatotoxicity	Squamous and basal cell skin cancer
Side Effects of ALG	Fever Chills Thombocytopenia	Hypertension Pruritis Serum sickness
Side Effects of OKT3	Fever Bronchospasm Seizures Tachycardia Hypertension Headache	Pulmonary edema Rigors Formation of anti-OKT3 antibodies Nausea and vomiting Diarrhea

(Reproduced with permission from Bruce D, Thistelthwaite: Immunotherapy in the Transplant Patient, in Hall J, Schmidt G and Wood C, eds: Principles of Critical Care, McGraw-Hill, New York, 1992.)

suppression. Many drugs may interact with cyclosporin to raise or lower its serum level.

The most significant toxicity of cyclosporin is nephrotoxicity. Special regimens reduce the dose of cyclosporin, or substitute other drugs, until the post-transplant acute tubular necrosis (vide infra) has resolved in order to minimize the impact of cyclosporin nephrotoxicity.

Corticosteroids

Corticosteroids were one of the original immunosuppressive agents used in transplants. Among their many effects, these drugs cause lymphopenia with redistribution of lymphocytes to lymphoid tissues and inhibit IL-2 production.

Corticosteroids are used in large doses for the induction of immunosuppression and treatment of episodes of acute rejection. Much smaller doses are used in multi-drug regimens for the maintenance of immunosuppression.

The numerous side effects of corticosteroid use are well known and many are listed in Table 19-1. The most serious effect of corticosteroid therapy is its nonspecific suppression of host immune defenses leaving the patient susceptible to a number of infections. Corticosteroids can also mask the signs and symptoms of acute infection such as peritonitis and meningitis.

Azathioprine

Azathioprine interferes with DNA and RNA synthesis by competitively inhibiting purine metabolism. As it affects primarily rapidly proliferating cells, it blocks the clonal expansion of T and B lymphocytes and their development into effector cells. Its role in immunotherapy has been reduced somewhat by the introduction of cyclosporin and it is now used in combination with cyclosporin and corticosteroids to reduce the doses of those drugs.

Antilymphocyte Antibodies

The first antilymphocyte antibody preparation used in transplantation therapy was polyclonal antilymphocyte globulin (ALG). A monoclonal antibody, OKT3, which binds to CD3 positive cells is now also available. Both of these agents are used either for induction of immunosuppression or for treatment of acute rejection. They are given as a 7 to 14 day course at a dose of 5mg/day for OKT3 and 1000 to 1500 mg/day for ALG. Their long term use is precluded by the formation of antibodies to them and their substantial toxicities. These toxicities include fever, chills, and hypotention and are attributed to an initial non-specific activation of lymphocytes leading to the release of IL-2, IL-6, and tumor necrosis factor.

INFECTIOUS COMPLICATIONS OF IMMUNOSUPPRESSION

Bacterial Infections

Defense against bacterial infections is mediated primarily by neutrophils, macrophages and the humoral immune system. Thus, cyclosporin and OKT3, which mainly affect T cell function, do not greatly impair resistance to bacterial infections. Many more bacterial infectious complications are seen with corticosteroids and azathioprine. These infections are usually seen within the first month of transplantation and reflect the flora of the transplantation site. For example, gram negative aerobes and enterococci are the most common pathogens following liver transplantation. Other common sites of bacterial infection in transplant patients are the urinary tract, the respiratory tree, and indwelling devices such as central venous catheters. It is important to note that immunosuppression may mask the signs and symptoms of infections such as peritonitis and meningitis and a high degree of suspicion for such infections needs to be maintained.

Fungal Infections

Fungal infections usually occur within 1 to 2 months of transplantation and are more common with high dose corticosteroid use. Repeated courses of broad spectrum antibiotics, multiple reoperations and prolonged ICU course also predispose patients to fungal infections. *Candida* is the most frequent organism. Infections range from minor infections such as oral or bladder involvement which can be treated with oral nystatin or amphotericin bladder irrigation, to invasive pneumonitis, fungemia, and intraabdominal infection. The more serious infections need to be treated with a full course of intravenous amphotericin B therapy. Other fungi, such as *Aspergillus* and *Cryptococcus*, do not respond well to therapy and carry a high mortality.

Viral Infections

As most immunosuppressive therapies are targeted at T cells, and defense against viral disease is primarily T lymphocyte mediated, viral infections are a major problem in transplantation. Cytomegalovirus (CMV) is the most important pathogen. These infections can be due to reactivation of CMV in a previously infected recipient or to the transplantation of CMV infected organs or blood products into a patient with no prior exposure to CMV. Reactivation occurs within 1 to 4 months of transplantation and is usually more mild than primary infection.

CMV may cause several different clinical syndromes including pneumonitis, hepatitis, nephritis, and gastrointestinal ulceration. The most common presentation, however, is fever and leukopenia, often presenting together with thrombocytopenia and atypical lymphocytes. Diagnosis is confirmed by tissue invasion with nuclear inclusions seen on liver or lung biopsies.

The therapy of CMV infections depends on the severity of the disease. Many infections resolve with no treatment or with reduction of immunosuppression. For more severe infections the use of gancyclovir and CMV immune globulin are currently under investigation.

Many other types of herpes viruses are commonly seen in transplant recipients including herpes simplex virus, and varicella zoster (shingles). These infections are troublesome but are generally not life threatening.

Parasitic Infections

Pneumocystis carinii pneumonia is the most common parasitic infection in the transplant recipient. This typically occurs several months after transplantation and should be suspected in any transplant patient presenting with a pulmonary infiltrate. Diagnosis can often be made with bronchoscopy with bronchoalveolar lavage. Intravenous trimethoprim/sulfmethoxazole (TMP/SMX) is the agent of first choice in treatment, but pentamidine may be used in case of allergy or other adverse reaction to TMP/SMX.

Approach to Patients with Pulmonary Infiltrates

The most common serious infection occurring more than one month following transplantation is pneumonia. As pneumonia may progress rapidly in the immunocompromised host, pulmonary infiltrates need to be rapidly diagnosed and treated. Infiltrates in these patients are usually diffuse and bilateral and sputums are often nondiagnostic. In this case, presumptive coverage should be broadened by adding TMP/SMX to cover pneumocystis, and bronchoscopy with broncho-alveolar lavage should be performed. A non-diagnostic bronchoscopy should be followed by open lung biopsy.

MODIFICATION OF IMMUNOSUPPRESSION IN INFECTION

Immunosuppression must often be reduced or withheld in the presence of severe infection. This may present a dilemma in heart or liver transplant recipients where life depends on the continued function of these grafts. It should be noted that the discontinuation of immunosuppression does not always lead to rejection in critically ill patients.

Immunosuppression Related Neoplasms

Prior to the introduction of cyclosporin, CNS lymphomas and skin cancers were the malignancies most often associated with transplantation. Cyclosporin appears to be more closely associated with B cell lymphomas occurring outside of the CNS, possibly due to reactivation of Epstein-Barr virus. This condition usually responds to a reduction in the level of immunosuppression. If immunosuppression is not reduced a malignant B cell lymphoma can develop.

DIAGNOSIS AND TREATMENT OF ACUTE REJECTION

Most rejection episodes occur within the first year after transplantation. In general rejection episodes present with fever or symptoms or laboratory values suggesting inflammation or dysfunction of the graft. Biopsies should be used following the initial evaluation of graft function to diagnose rejection.

Initial therapy is usually high dose corticosteroids followed by OKT3 or ALG therapy if the presence of rejection is confirmed.

ORGAN SPECIFIC ISSUES

Renal Transplant

As the post-transplant period is usually marked by transient acute tubular necrosis (ATN) in the transplanted kidney, therapies with reduced nephrotoxicity are often chosen in renal transplantation. Specifically, ALG or OKT3 are often substituted for cyclosporin in the induction of immunosuppression. Alternatively, a reduced dose of cyclosporin is used.

Rejection is rarely the cause of immediate post-transplant graft dysfunction and is usually due to ATN, vascular occlusion, or obstruction of the urinary collecting system.

Liver Transplant

Liver transplant is now the standard therapy for end-stage liver disease. As the decision to transplant is often prompted by acute complications of liver failure such as esophageal bleeding, critical care is often required in the pretransplant setting as well as in the perioperative period and in the management of acute complications of transplantation.

Liver transplantation is a difficult and lengthy surgical procedure. Operative blood loss can be used as a means to quantify the magnitude of the surgical injury and also correlates both with preoperative risk factors and postoperative prognosis. Postoperative therapy should be aimed at the rapid withdrawal of invasive therapy in order to minimize iatrogenic complications. Postoperative complications include infection, encephalopathy, high cardiac output hypotension, pulmonary edema (both cardiogenic and non-cardiogenic), and hepatorenal syndrome. Postoperative recovery results in the gradual restoration of multisystem physiology deranged by liver failure and cirrhosis. This may require days to months depending on the duration and severity of preoperative disease.

Following discharge from the ICU the patient remains at high risk for vascular complications and cardiopulmonary decompensation. The risk for life threatening infections persists despite full apparent recovery following transplantation.

Lung Transplant

The main indication for single lung transplantation is end stage fibrotic lung disease. Double lung transplantation is almost exclusively used for end stage septic lung disease where a remaining diseased lung would infect the newly transplanted lung.

In selecting donor lungs the following criteria apply: Donor lungs must be normal by chest x-ray and must be capable of maintaining the donor's PaO_2 above 300 mmHg with a FIO_2 of 1.0 and a PEEP of 5.

As corticosteroids have been implicated in non-healing at the anastomotic site, they are often used at low dose or are omitted from induction immunosuppression in lung transplantation until healing has occurred. While it is advisable to have a fully primed bypass machine available during the actual transplantation, cardiovascular bypass is required in only about 20 percent of single lung transplants. Double lung transplant has usually always required bypass but with the use of sequential single lung transplants, bypass can sometimes be avoided.

In the first 24 h following transplantation, cardiovascular instability is often seen with high cardiac output hypotension. Pulmonary edema, both cardiogenic and from capillary leak is also seen. Following this initial rocky course, an average of 2 episodes of acute rejection are seen during the first 3 weeks after transplantation. While common in heart-lung transplantation, bronchiolitis obliterans occurs rarely in single and double lung transplants. Infections, on the other hand, represent the greatest threat to long term survival. Late airway stenosis, while common, can usually be managed by repeated dilations and the use of endoluminal silicone stents.

Heart-Lung Transplantation

Heart-lung transplantation is usually reserved for patients with combined end stage respiratory and cardiac disease. The survival rate for this procedure has been increased markedly by improvements in procuring and preserving donor organs. In addition the management of these patients has been aided by the early use of transbronchial biopsy to diagnose acute rejection or opportunistic infection allowing for rapid and specific intervention.

As with other organs, rejection is often indicated by dysfunction of the transplanted organ. This can be monitored by the recipient by means of a portable spirometer. A sustained fall in function should prompt evaluation by the managing physician including transbronchial biopsy. One of the major long term complications of heart-lung transplant is obliterative brochiolitis. This complication may be prevented by early detection and treatment of acute rejection.

For further reading in *Principles of Critical Care,* see Chap 77 "Immunotherapy in the Transplant Patient" David S Bruce/J Richard Thistelthwaite, Chap 78 "Lung Transplantation" E Vallieres/TR Todd, Chap 79 "Critical Care of the Recipients of Heart and Heart-Lung Transplants" Chris Dennis/John Wallwork/Tim Higenbottam, Chap 80 "Critical Care of Liver Transplant Patients" Jean C Emond

Phillip Cozzi

The risk of postoperative complications can be modified by pre-, intra-, and postoperative medical intervention. This chapter focuses on risk assessment for cardiac and pulmonary postoperative complications, as well as the management of critically ill patients requiring surgery.

There is no single test which can predict morbidity and mortality associated with surgery. Each test lacks sensitivity, specificity, or both and, therefore, its value for predicting outcome is limited. The sensitivity and specificity are stable properties of a test which do not change depending on the population being tested. The clinically relevant characteristics of a test include the positive and negative predictive values. These properties depend on the prevalence (pretest likelihood) of a condition in a specific population. When the prevalence of a condition placing the patient at risk is 40 to 60 percent, decision making is facilitated by use of the test. If the pretest likelihood is very high or very low, the test provides little additional information.

CARDIAC RISK

Risk assessment. Perioperative cardiac complications occur in approximately 10 percent of patients undergoing major abdominal or thoracic surgery. Specifically, cardiac complications include myocardial infarction, arrhythmia, cardiac failure and cardiac death.

Since no single clinical parameter is both sensitive and specific in predicting postoperative complication, multifactorial symptoms for risk assessment have been developed, including the American Society of Anesthesiologists Classification of Physical Status and the cardiac risk index (CRI). In computing the CRI, points ascribed to various clinical parameters are summed (Table 20-1). The total point score is used in classifying the patient into one of four groups, in which risk of postoperative complication has been retrospectively analyzed (Table 20-2). Exercise stress testing is sensitive though variably specific in predicting postoperative cardiac complications. The inability to exercise is a significant predictor of perioperative cardiac morbidity, although the reason remains unclear. Preoperative Holter monitoring is predictive of postoperative unstable angina, pulmonary edema, and myocardial infarction. Coronary artery angiography is not of value in predicting outcome. Ventriculography may be better, as it more accurately reflects the physiologic reserve of the heart.

TABLE 20-1 Computation of the CRI

Criteria	Points
1. *History*	
a. Age >70 year	5
b. MI within previous 6 months	10
2. *Physical examination*	
a. S_3 gallop or JVD	11
b. Important valvular aortic stenosis	3
3. *ECG*	
a. Rhythm other than sinus or PACs on last preop ECG	7
b. >5 PVCs/min documented at any time before operation	7
4. *General status*	3
$Po_2 < 60$ or $Pco_2 > 50$ mmHg, K < 3.0 or	
$HCO_3 < 20$ meq/L,	
BUN > 50 or Cr > 3.0 mg/dL,	
abnormal SGOT, chronic liver disease, or	
bedridden from noncardiac causes	
5. *Operation*	
a. Intraperitoneal, intrathoracic, or aortic operation	3
b. Emergency operation	4
Total possible	53

JVD, jugular vein distention; PAC, premature atrial contraction; PVC, premature ventricular contraction.
Reprinted by permission of the New England Journal of Medicine (297:848, 1977.)

Dipyridamole-thallium scanning (DTS) has been used to quantify cardiac reserve in patients who cannot exercise. In patients with known ischemic heart disease, this test is both sensitive and specific and has a good positive predictive value. As a screening procedure for the general population, however, this test is less useful. DTS should be performed preoperatively in vascular surgery patients who have one to two clinical risk factors for postoperative cardiac

TABLE 20-2 CRI

Class	Point Total	No or Only Minor Complication (N = 943)	Life-Threatening Complication[a] (N = 39)	Cardiac Deaths (N = 19)
I(N = 537)	0–5	532 (99)[b]	4 (0.7)	1 (0.2)
II(N = 316)	6–12	295 (93)	16 (5)	5 (2)
III(N = 130)	13–25	112 (86)	15 (11)	3 (2)
IV(N = 18)	≥26	4 (22)	4 (22)	10 (56).

[a]Documented intraoperative or postoperative MI, pulmonary edema, or ventricular tachycardia without progression to cardiac death.
[b]Figures in parentheses denote percentage.
Reprinted with permission from the New England Journal of Medicine (297:848, 1977).

complications. These clinical risk factors include age over 70, arrhythmias requiring treatment, Q-waves on ECG, a history of angina, and diabetes mellitus. In the absence of clinical risk factors, the risk of postoperative cardiac event is less than 3 percent. In the presence of more than two risk factors, the risk of postoperative cardiac event exceeds 50 percent, and DTS does not improve risk prediction in this high risk group.

In multivariate analyses, congestive heart failure has been shown to be independently associated with perioperative cardiac event. Recent myocardial infarction (MI) (less than 6 months) is associated with increased risk of perioperative reinfarction. It remains controversial as to whether age and diabetes are major risk factors for perioperative cardiac event independent of the patient's overall health.

Risk modification. Coronary artery bypass grafting (CABG) has been used prophylactically to reduce cardiac risk. Those patients who survive cardiac surgery are at no greater risk of perioperative cardiac event than those patients without known cardiac disease. Controversy remains, however, as to whether prior bypass grafting improves overall survival or simply selects for lower risk patients (those who survive cardiac surgery). In addition, randomized prospective studies are needed to elucidate the role of coronary angioplasty in modifying perioperative cardiac risk.

Intensive perioperative management may modify many of the cardiac risk factors such as congestive heart failure, MI, and arrhythmia. Preoperative ICU admission for pulmonary artery catherization is performed in some centers, although the value of this approach remains uncertain. For patients within 6 months of MI, the use of pulmonary artery catheterization is reasonable, because aggressive perioperative control of hemodynamics in this population significantly reduces reinfarction rate. ICU monitoring of all patients postoperatively is not a possibility because of financial limitations. Recent studies suggest that over 75 percent of postoperative ischemic events occur within 26 h postoperatively, suggesting a short period of monitoring may be sufficient.

The choice of anesthetic technique may alter outcome of various procedures. For ophthalmalogic surgery and transurethral prostectomy, regional anesthesia offers improved outcome in morbidity and mortality compared to general anesthesia.

PULMONARY RISK

Risk assessment. Pulmonary complications are common following surgery, particularly abdominal procedures. Cough, sputum production, dyspnea, chest pain, fever, or radiographic changes occur in approximately half of such patients, with respiratory failure necessitating mechanical ventilation occurring in 0 to 21 percent.

The value of spirometry in predicting pulmonary complications is unproven. A better indicator of risk may be the inability to improve abnormal spirometry preoperatively. In a prospective study, preoperative chest physiotherapy, bronchodilators, intermittent positive pressure breathing, and cessation of smoking were utilized to improve spirometric values; those without response had an increased incidence of respiratory failure.

Malnutrition is a major risk factor for perioperative pneumonia and other pulmonary complications. Other clinical factors which have been identified inconsistently as risk factors for pulmonary complications include age and smoking. There are no proven multifactorial risk indices for predicting pulmonary complications; however, nutritional status, obesity, smoking history, age and severity of underlying lung disease should be considered in assessing risk.

Risk modification. Patients at high risk for perioperative pulmonary complications show improved outcome when treated pre-operatively with bronchodilating drugs, inhalation of humidified air, smoking cessation, chest physiotherapy, and delay of surgery, if necessary. Less severe pulmonary complications and shorter hospitalization result. Improvement in lung function occurs with cessation of smoking over a period of 1 to 12 months. For CABG patients, a period of 8 weeks is needed to cause significant reduction in complications. Deep breathing exercises, intermittent positive pressure breathing, and incentive spirometry reduce postoperative pulmonary complications to 30 percent of non-treated controls. Intermittent positive pressure breathing is not recommended because of expense and poor tolerance by patients. Incentive spirometry and deep breathing exercises may be equally efficacious.

The type of surgical incision may significantly modify pulmonary function and risk of pulmonary complication. Upper abdominal incision, for example, results in 50 to 60 percent reduction in vital and functional residual capacities, as well as a 20 percent reduction in tidal volume. A subcostal incision for cholecystectomy results in less reduction in vital capacity and pulmonary complications than midline incision. Reduction in vital capacity and functional residual capacity are important factors in the development of pulmonary complications.

Postoperative pain control is important in limiting risk of postoperative atelectasis. Standard narcotic analgesia as well as all forms of regional anesthesia (epidural narcotics, epidural local anesthetics, intercostal nerve blocks, and intrapleural local anesthetics) can produce beneficial changes in pulmonary function postoperatively.

SURGICAL RISK IN THE ICU PATIENT

Because of the complexity of care of the ICU patient, general preoperative management begins with good communication between all physicians involved. Since transportation of the patient to the operating room is often complicated, support systems of the ICU environment must be transported with the patient. ECG monitoring with defibrillation capability, oxygen, portable infusion pumps, and skilled personnel including an ICU nurse and an ICU physician or anesthesiologist should accompany the patient. Similar attention should be given to the return trip from the recovery room. Oxygen delivery to the periphery and cardiac output should be maintained at all times, utilizing inotropes if necessary. Because of the increased frequency of renal and hepatic dysfunction in the ICU patient, derangements in drug clearance should be kept in mind. Since this population is at risk for developing ARDS, the left atrial pressure should be kept as low as possible to limit transcapillary fluid flux; intraoperative fluid management should be conservative.

For further reading in *Principles of Critical Care,* see Chap 81 "Preoperative Assessment of the High-Risk Surgical Patient" John D Haigh

---

Phillip Factor, D.O.

More than 300,000 surgical cases involving cardiopulmonary bypass (CPB) are performed each year and all of these patients require postoperative intensive care. Coronary artery bypass grafting (CABG) constitutes the majority of these procedures. Percutaneous transluminal coronary angioplasty is increasingly used to treat low risk patients. Consequently CABG patients tend to be older and sicker and have more complications of critical illness than in the past. Large prospective trials have demonstrated that the risk of operative mortality increases with advanced age, emergency operation, evidence of left ventricular dysfunction, renal dysfunction and repeat operation. An awareness of these issues and the details of open heart surgery and CPB are crucial prerequisites to the management of these critically ill patients.

INTRAOPERATIVE MANAGEMENT

The Prebypass Period

The sequence for placement of intravascular access lines and monitors varies between institutions. Large bore intravenous access (central and peripheral), direct intraarterial pressure monitoring, and continuous electrocardiogram (ECG) monitoring are typically established. Pulmonary artery catheters are also typically used despite clear evidence of their efficacy in this setting. In some centers transesophageal echocardiography (TEE) is used adjunctively to provide assessment of cardiac function and ventricular volumes, and to signal the presence of acute myocardial ischemia (usually by detecting wall motion defects). Hemodynamic goals during this period are determined by the underlying cardiac pathophysiology. A balance must be struck between intravascular volume, anesthetic medications, and vasoactive drugs that allows maintenance of tissue perfusion and myocardial function until the surgical procedure is finished.

Occult myocardial ischemia is a common problem in CABG patients that is associated with a high incidence of perioperative myocardial infarction (MI). While most of these MI's are silent, hemodynamic disturbances can occur. Intraoperative management for CABG patients should focus on limitation of myocardial oxygen consumption and avoidance of tachycardia. High dose narcotics (fentanyl, sufentanil) are commonly used to blunt the catecholamine response to the stimulation of intubation and surgery. Valvular surgery presents additional problems that depend on the degree of cardiac hypertrophy or dysfunction present. Patients with left ventricular (LV) hypertrophy due to aortic stenosis are intolerant of reductions in preload or myocardial depression. They are also more prone to myocardial ischemia due to the limited subendocardial coronary blood flow attendant to high intraventricular pressures. The dilated LV seen in patients with aortic insufficiency requires that afterload be reduced and diastolic filling time be increased (by avoidance of tachycardia). Both mitral stenosis and insufficiency can produce pulmonary hypertension and cor pulmonale. Optimization of RV function and avoidance of stimuli that increase pulmonary artery pressures (hypoxemia, acidosis, vasoconstrictors) are essential in these patients. Like aortic insufficiency, mitral regurgitation patients can be optimized by reductions in LV afterload.

Management of Cardiopulmonary Bypass

The effects of cardiopulmonary bypass (CPB) are responsible for many of the critical care issues that arise in the postoperative period. Complement activation, elevated catecholamines, release of bradykinin, loss of platelet number and function, hemolysis, intrapulmonary neutrophil sequestration, loss of T lymphocytes, renal dysfunction, and cerebral capillary closure are among the phenomena associated with CPB. Most of the common complications of cardiac surgery (Table 21-1) have been shown to increase with CPB times over 150 to 180 minutes. In most cases CPB is achieved by placement of right atrial and aortic root cannulas. While on CPB patients are systemically anticoagulated with heparin (300 to 400 u/kg to produce activated coagulation times of >400 to 480 s). After initiation of CPB the patient is cooled, and following fibrillation of the heart, the aortic root is cross clamped. Myocardial protection during this time is achieved with topical and systemic hypothermia and hyperkalemic blood or crystalloids.

TABLE 21-1 Postoperative Morbidity Associated with Prolonged CPB

Cardiac Dysfunction	*Infection*
Low output syndrome	Mediastinitis
Right heart failure	Sternal wound
IABP requirement	Pneumonia
Neurologic Dysfunction	*Metabolic*
Global	Catecholamine release
Focal	Bradykinin levels
Delirium	Complement activation
Respiratory Problems	*Renal Failure*
Delayed extubation	*Gastrointestinal Complications*
ARDS	Hepatic dysfunction
Coagulopathy	Pancreatitis
Platelet dysfunction	Gastrointestinal bleeding
Fibrinolysis	
Dilutional coagulopathy	

The longer the cross clamp time, the greater the incidence of myocardial dysfunction after discontinuation of CPB. The likelihood for needing postoperative pharmacologic or mechanical support also depends on the baseline cardiac function, surgical technique and effectiveness of myocardial preservation but increases with cross clamp times in excess of 120 min. Occasional procedures such as the repair of aortic arch aneurysms require interruption of CPB. Profound hypothermia (20° C) can allow safe circulatory arrest times of up to 45 min in some patients.

Separation from CPB is attempted only after rewarming, correction of electrolyte and hematologic abnormalities and reinstitution of assisted ventilation. Defibrillation usually occurs with reperfusion and the washing out of the cardioplegic solution from the myocardium. Complete heart block is not uncommon in these patients, thus some institutions routinely place epicardial pacing wires. Inotropic support is frequently required at this time. Calcium is also used for its positive inotropic effect and its ability to counter the residual effects of hyperkalemic cardioplegia on the conducting system. As cardiac function returns the venous drainage to the pump is gradually occluded and blood remaining in the pump is returned to the patient via the aortic line.

Intra-aortic balloon counterpulsation (IABP) should be considered in patients who require high doses of inotropes, show signs of persistent ischemia, or have refractory ventricular dysrhythmia. A small group of patients may not respond to this type of mechanical and pharmacologic support. For these individuals left or right ventricular assist devices can be utilized. Transient ischemia may develop shortly before or after separation from CPB, especially in the territory of the right coronary artery. This is thought to be due to embolization of small air bubbles to the right coronary artery. Treatment includes nitroglycerin, augmentation of coronary perfusion pressure and occasionally reinstitution of CPB. Persistent ischemia may suggest graft occlusion or spasm and may require topical papaverine or sublingual nifedipine.

Right ventricular dysfunction is common, particularly in the setting of pre-existing pulmonary hypertension or RV dysfunction. Inotropic support, pulmonary vasodilation, prevention of RV overdistention, and maintenance of coronary perfusion pressure are useful therapeutic aims. Selective infusion of norepinephrine via left atrial lines, right atrial infusion of amrinone and prostaglandin E_2 have been tried. Other therapeutic alternatives include IABP and right ventricular assist devices.

Following separation from CPB heparinization is reversed (initially with protamine). Desmopressin has also been used to augment platelet function and increase serum factor VIII levels. Epsilon-amino caproic acid (EACA) has been advocated to ameliorate fibrinolysis initiated by CPB. Finally, blood products may be required depending on the extent of anemia and thrombocytopenia induced during CPB.

POSTOPERATIVE MANAGEMENT

Initial postoperative care focuses on restoration of normal body temperature and monitoring of hemodynamic, respiratory, electrolyte and fluid status and blood loss from mediastinal and pleural drains. Cardiac tamponade or excessive bleeding may require emergent reoperation. The presence of mediastinal blood loss of more than 300 ml in the first h, 250 mL in the second h, or 150 mL/h thereafter has been correlated with surgically correctable bleeding. Early return to the operating room may prevent catastrophic hemodynamic collapse, excessive transfusion requirements, and decrease the incidence of wound infection. Patients with excessive bleeding should be evaluated for residual thrombostatic defects. In addition to routine coagulation parameters, thromboelastography may be helpful in defining common problems such as heparin rebound, platelet defects, or fibrinolysis. For patients with persistent bleeding, empiric protamine sulfate (50 to 100 mg) can be tried. Desmopressin and EACA are also used in some centers. Platelet transfusion should also be considered as platelet defects are common following CPB. Administration of red blood cells, fresh frozen plasma, cryoprecipitate, and other blood products should be based on appropriate laboratory values. Positive end-expiratory pressure (PEEP) can also be employed to compress small mediastinal and chest wall bleeding sites. It should be carefully titrated to effect to prevent untoward hemodynamic effects.

Ideal anesthetic management should be tailored such that the patient awakens in the ICU only after they are completely rewarmed, hemodynamically stable, and blood loss has ceased. This is most often achieved with high dose narcotics as mentioned above. Delayed emergence and prolonged respiratory depression may occur with these agents. Residual narcotics have been reported to cause late truncal rigidity, decreased chest wall compliance and hypoventilation. These complications are especially common following early extubation in the presence of hypothermia. Naloxone can be used, but overzealous utilization can be complicated by severe hypertension that can precipitate hemorrhage, ventricular failure, pulmonary vasoconstriction, or arrhythmias. In many situations reintubation may be preferable over the use of naloxone. The early period after CPB is characterized by a progressive temperature drop that occurs as blood from poorly perfused tissues returns to the central circulation. Once core temperature begins to increase, it does so quickly, although peak temperatures may not be reached until 8 h after ICU admission. Postoperative shivering is common with resultant increased CO_2 production which increases minute ventilation, myocardial work and O_2 consumption. Extubation should be delayed until rewarming is complete. Treatment, in addition to active and passive rewarming, can include meperidine if the patient is responsive and hemodynamically stable. If severe, or when there is hemodynamic instability, sedation and paralysis should be utilized.

COMPLICATIONS OF CARDIAC SURGERY

Cardiovascular

Postoperative arrhythmias are common and may be due to electrolyte shifts, myocardial ischemia, acid-base abnormalities, hypothermia, catecholamine overload, conduction abnormalities, and surgical trauma. Consideration of each of these etiologies is required for appropriate management of these patients. Supraventricular arrhythmias are common during the first postoperative week. Beta blockers (e.g., esmolol) and calcium channel blockers (e.g., verapamil) are effective if myocardial depression can be tolerated. Magnesium is useful for treatment of ventricular dysrhythmias.

Tamponade

The signs of cardiac tamponade in the postoperative period may be atypical as the pericardial sac is typically left open after cardiac surgery. Even echocardiography may be difficult due to bandages, edema and positive pressure ventilation. The possibility of isolated left or right atrial tamponade further clouds the diagnosis of this problem. The diagnosis of tamponade must be entertained with any hemodynamic deterioration. Equalization of end diastolic pressures or abrupt reductions in chest tube output should suggest the diagnosis. Cardiac compression is usually due to excessive blood and clot in the mediastinum. Pericardiocentesis is rarely useful as clot typically can not be aspirated through a needle. These patients should be taken to the operating room and their chests reopened utilizing minimal anesthesia. Additional anesthesia can be administered following restoration of hemodynamic stability. In the presence of complete circulatory collapse opening of the chest should not be delayed pending transfer to the operating room.

Low Output Syndrome

Low output syndrome, defined as a cardiac index of <2.2 l/min/m², is associated with a high incidence of postoperative respiratory, renal, hepatic and central nervous system (CNS) failure, gastrointestinal bleeding, disseminated intravascular coagulation (DIC), and death. Inotropic support should be initiated only after correction of preload deficits. Specific etiologic considerations in these patients include the effects of vasoactive drugs on the coronary circulation, the type of bypass grafts used (internal mammary artery [IMA] vs. saphenous vein [SV], treatment of tachyarrhythmias with β-agonists, the possibility of adrenergic receptor down regulation from previous catecholamine therapy, and RV failure. IMA (as opposed to saphenous) grafts remain innervated and can be anticipated to behave as would any other artery in the face of catecholamine therapy. Whenever possible, the mean arterial pressure should be maintained above 70 mmHg to maintain flow through IMA grafts; β-agonists can be used to achieve this goal once preload and inotropic intervention have been exhausted. Ischemic electrocardiographic changes may be nonspecific in the presence of ventricular dysfunction or arrhythmias and may warrant TEE or emergent coronary angiography to further define the problem. Valve replacement patients (especially mitral insufficiency), in general, are more at risk for low output syndrome than are CABG patients. Acute changes in afterload are problematic in patients with decompensated, dilated ventricles. These patients often require significant inotropic support and meticulous attention to preload and afterload. After valve surgery, cardiac pacing may be required for treatment of transient or permanent heart block. An IABP is occasionally required for management of intractable cardiac failure following CPB. IABP induced improvements of cardiac index, the presence of good urine output, and high-normal SVR and PCWP suggest a favorable prognosis.

Postoperative Hypertension

Significant hypertension develops in up to 40 percent of patients. It is typically due to increased circulating catecholamine levels associated with hypoxemia, hypercapnia, ventilatory difficulties, pain, shivering, or manipulation of the great vessels. Treatment is directed at eliminating the primary cause. Pharmacologic therapy typically includes sodium nitroprusside, but other vasodilators (hydralazine, prazosin) and antihypertensives (clonidine, captopril, nifedipine, labetalol) can be used. If the cardiac index is adequate, β blockers (labetalol, esmolol) are attractive antihypertensive agents due to their negative chronotropic effects.

Neurologic

Potential neurologic problems following CABG include focal cerebral lesions, severe global encephalopathy, peripheral neuropathies, spinal cord ischemia and subtle neuropsychiatric disorders.

Risk factors for CNS injury include emergency operation, severe LV dysfunction, advanced age, carotid bruits, peripheral vascular disease, IABP support, prolonged bypass time (>142 min), and associated valvular procedures or ventriculotomy. Air or particulate emboli originating within the heart or at the cannulation site appear to be major causes of postoperative cerebral dysfunction. Patients who fail to awaken on the first postoperative day should have all sedatives and muscle relaxants discontinued. Computed tomography should be obtained to rule out structural problems and cerebral edema and an electroencephalogram (EEG) should be obtained to rule out subclinical status epilepticus. Prevention of CNS injuries remains the principal therapeutic modality as little can be done once the insult has been discovered. Transient postoperative delirium is common within the first postoperative week. Reassurance and orientation of the patient, relief of mechanical problems (full bladder), and treatment of pain or anxiety usually eliminate the problem. Intravenous haloperidol can be useful if necessary.

Respiratory Care

Maintenance of oxygenation and ventilation and protection of the airway while preserving hemodynamic stability are the major goals of postoperative respiratory care. Weaning and extubation can be accomplished when the patient is alert, warm, hemodynamically stable, chest output is minimal and oxygenation is acceptable. Common respiratory problems following CPB that can impede extubation include atelectasis, pleural effusions, pulmonary edema, loss of lung volume and phrenic nerve injury.

Following median sternotomy and CPB, vital capacity (VC) is significantly reduced (by up to 50 percent), reaching its nadir on the second and third postoperative days. Reductions in functional residual capacity also occur and can persist through the seventh postoperative day. Atelectasis is an almost universal problem especially of the left lower lobe. This occurs due to lack of lung inflation during CPB, general anesthesia, surgical compression, diaphragmatic dysfunction, pleural effusion or blood, pain, and decreased surfactant production following hypothermia. IMA grafts are associated with more impairment of pulmonary function than are SV grafts. Upon arrival to the ICU patients should be ventilated according to their clinical situation. High concentrations of O_2 (60%) are typically used to protect against possible hypoxemia during hemodynamic instability or shivering. PEEP is used to recruit lung volume but must be used cautiously in hypovolemic patients. Before extubation the patient should be awake, cooperative, hemodynamically stable and without acutely evolving problems.

Table 21-2 lists risk factors predisposing patients to prolonged postoperative ventilation. Weaning these patients can be difficult and a planned approach that includes attention to respiratory muscle training, nutrition, reversal of correctable abnormalities (infection, electrolyte disorders), appropriate diuresis, and patient education should be successful (see Chaps. 29 and 31). The role of tracheostomy in these patients is similar to that of other clinical situations complicated by prolonged respiratory failure. The proximity of the mediastinal wound to the tracheostomy must be considered. Once the mediastinal wound is healed and the potential for mediastinitis is considered low tracheostomy can be entertained.

The reported incidence of phrenic nerve injury varies. It can be injured both transiently and permanently at a number of points as it traverses the thoracic cavity. The nerve may be thermally injured when cold cardioplegics are placed in the pericardial sac, or mechanically injured during IMA dissection or reoperation. Intercostal nerves can also be injured as a result of chest retraction. Injury to these nerves may contribute to ventilator dependence, especially in patients with borderline preoperative pulmonary function. Tachypnea with paradoxical abdominal respiratory motion, lower than expected VC, elevation of the diaphragm on x-ray, reduced negative inspiratory force and reduced VC when supine should suggest the diagnosis of phrenic nerve impairment. Fluoroscopy and ultrasound can be used to suggest the diagnosis but are not diagnostic in many cases. Diaphragmatic paralysis is uncommon and tends to spontaneously resolve, usually within several weeks. Diaphragmatic paralysis should not prevent weaning.

TABLE 21-2 Factors Predisposing to Prolonged Ventilation after Open Heart Surgery

Stormy postoperative course (IABP)
Reexploration for bleeding or tamponade
Emergency procedure
Valve operation
LV dysfunction
Renal failure
Fluid overload
Infection (sepsis, mediastinitis, pneumonia)
Malnutrition
Bronchospasm
Phrenic nerve injury
Pulmonary hypertension
MSOF
Advanced age
Neurologic injury (stroke, encephalopathy)

Renal Failure

Renal failure after open heart surgery is a serious problem. Preoperative renal dysfunction (serum creatinine >1.7 mg/dL) increases the risk of further creatinine elevation, anuria, need for dialysis, and mortality. Risk factors for the development of postoperative renal failure include low cardiac output at the end of CPB, age, preoperative elevation of creatinine, preoperative cardiac failure, need for postoperative circulatory support, blood transfusion, and bypass time. No known therapeutic measures can definitively prevent renal failure. Close attention to urine output is essential. Mannitol is frequently used, as is low dose dopamine to promote a diuresis during the perioperative period.

When renal failure does occur, it follows one of three patterns. Abbreviated acute renal failure occurs after an isolated insult at the time of surgery, results in the creatinine peaking during the fourth postoperative day, and is followed by a prompt recovery. In overt renal failure the acute insult is followed by prolonged circulatory failure and runs a longer course with recovery occurring during the second or third postoperative week. A second insult (sepsis, hypotension) occurring during recovery from overt failure can result in the third pattern, protracted acute renal failure which may result in lifelong dependency on dialysis. This third pattern is typically accompanied by the development of adult respiratory distress syndrome (ARDS) or multiple system organ failure (MSOF).

The development of postoperative oliguria should be met with appropriate diagnostic measures such as fluid challenge, augmentation of cardiac output, and bladder catheterization. If hemoglobinuria or myoglobinuria are present alkalinization of the urine may be of benefit. Obstructive etiologies are rare but should be evaluated with appropriate studies.

Infectious

Pneumonia, sepsis, wound infections, mediastinitis, and urinary tract infections are frequent complications after open heart surgery. Current prevailing opinion is that a single dose of cefazolin or vancomycin should suffice for prosthetic valve and other open heart surgery. Cefamandole and cefuroxime are reportedly associated with fewer wound infections than cefazolin. Infections occurring after prophylaxis are frequently due to resistant organisms (*Pseudomonas* sp., *Klebsiella, Serratia, Providentia*). Treatment of these infections should include a penicillinase resistant penicillin and an aminoglycoside. Use of broad spectrum antibiotics can lead to infection with more unusual organisms that include yeast.

Sternal wound infections occur in 1 percent of median sternotomies. Predisposing factors include diabetes mellitus, low cardiac output, use of bilateral IMA grafts, and reoperation for excessive mediastinal bleeding. Mediastinal infection may manifest as unexplained fever, inability to wean, or an unstable sternum. Risk factors for suppurative mediastinitis include chronic obstructive pulmonary disease, repeat operation (including reexploration), pyuria, low ejection fraction, high left ventricular end diastolic pressure, valve or aortic aneurysm repair, prolonged bypass time or return to bypass, cardiopulmonary resuscitation, and mechanical ventilation for >48 h.

Gastrointestinal

Gastrointestinal (GI) problems are uncommon but are associated with a high postoperative mortality. Postoperative ileus and upper GI bleeding are the most commonly encountered problems, although pancreatitis, cholecystitis, hyperbilirubinemia, bowel perforations, and infarctions are also encountered, especially in high risk patients. Risk factors include prolonged bypass time, concurrent renal failure, and prolonged ventilatory support. Jaundice occurs in 20 percent of CPB patients and is a risk for subsequent mortality. Jaundice is associated with multiple valve replacement, higher transfusion requirements, and longer bypass times. It also occurs following otherwise uncomplicated procedures where it may be due to a defect in hepatic bilirubin excretion. Acute pancreatitis is uncommon but conveys a poor prognosis. It is often seen in the setting of MSOF. Severe fulminant pancreatitis leading to death, less severe pancreatitis with abscess formation, or mild chemical pancreatitis without clinical sequelae are noted in these patients.

Mesenteric ischemia due to low flow or atheroembolic phenomena are rarely seen. The gastroepiploic artery is sometimes used in bypass grafting. These patients are prone to postoperative ileus. Nasogastric suction should be used until bowel activity is assured in these patients.

RISK FACTORS PREDICTING MORBIDITY AND MORTALITY

Factors commonly cited as risks for operative mortality following CABG include advanced age, female gender, congestive heart failure, LV dysfunction, left main coronary disease, emergency operation and reoperation. Factors predisposing to risk following valve surgery include advanced age, endocarditis, female gender, impaired LV function, concurrent ischemic disease, mitral regurgitant lesions, the need for tricuspid annuloplasty, previous operation, diabetes mellitus, and ascites. At present there is no prospectively tested scheme that takes into account the relative importance of each of these factors in predicting patient outcome following open heart surgery.

VASCULAR SURGERY

Patients with significant arteriosclerotic vascular disease frequently have concomitant illnesses such as hypertensive or ischemic cardiovascular disease, chronic obstructive pulmonary disease, diabetes mellitus or chronic renal insufficiency. Identification of patients at greatest risk for perioperative morbidity and mortality must be accomplished preoperatively. Close monitoring, including pre- and postoperative intensive care may limit perioperative complications in some patients. Cardiovascular complications (perioperative myocardial infarction, arrhythmias, heart failure) account for 50 percent of the perioperative mortality in these patients (2 to 6 percent for elective vascular reconstructive procedures). Utilization of invasive cardiopulmonary monitoring in tandem with large bore venous access should be employed, especially when major reconstructive procedures are planned or if the patient presents as a high risk for perioperative complications. Transesophageal echocardiography is also useful for detection of acute myocardial ischemia intraoperatively.

AORTIC SURGERY

Surgical outcome in patients undergoing aortic surgery can be linked to the extent of operative dissection and blood loss. Techniques such as aneurysmorrhaphy (as opposed to aneurysmectomy) and retroperitoneal vs. transabdominal approaches can limit these problems.

The clamping and unclamping of the aorta remain crucial events during aortic surgery. Acute elevations of myocardial preload and afterload can occur with aortic cross clamping. Nitroprusside and/or nitroglycerin may be required to treat associated myocardial ischemia. Reduction of renal cortical blood flow during cross clamping requires that ischemic time be kept to an absolute minimum. Utilization of low dose dopamine (3 to 5 μg/kg/min) or mannitol (25g) prior to cross clamping may help maintain renal function. The acute reduction in afterload that follows unclamping of the aorta ("declamping shock") is the result of the sudden release of vasoactive products from reperfused ischemic tissues. Cautious volume infusion, discontinuation of negative inotropes and vasodilators, and gradual declamping may limit this problem. If acidosis or hypotension persist, some authors recommend utilization of $NaHCO_3$ and $CaCl_2$.

Inadequate hemostasis at suture lines, heparinization, dilution coagulopathy, hypothermia and unexpected venous injury are a few of the causes of significant bleeding during aortic surgery. Preoperative planning (cell savers, autotransfusions) can limit the blood bank requirements of these patients.

CEREBROVASCULAR SURGERY

Carotid endarterectomy is among the most commonly performed vascular procedures. Combined morbidity and mortality rates of <5 percent and permanent neurologic deficit rates of <2 percent can be anticipated when attention is paid to preoperative evaluation, anesthetic management and the technical aspects of the operation. Anesthetic approaches include general anesthesia with continuous EEG monitoring, local anesthesia with parenteral sedation, or regional nerve blocks. The last two approaches permit awake evaluation of cerebral function.

Maintenance of cerebral blood flow during this procedure is often difficult. Patients with cerebrovascular disease may have disordered vascular autoregulation and as such may be sensitive to swings in blood pressure. Hypoxemia and hypercapnia should be avoided as reductions in cerebral blood flow may occur.

MESENTERIC AND RENAL RECONSTRUCTION

Endarterectomy and aortomesenteric bypass have been employed as operative treatments for patients with intestinal ischemia due to celiac or superior mesenteric artery atherosclerotic disease. These procedures require extensive exposure and manipulation of the bowel leading to sequestration of fluid in the bowel wall. Cautious pre- and intraoperative volume restoration should be employed to prevent the hemodynamic consequences of volume shifts.

Hydration and glucagon (0.06 mg/kg/h) should be utilized in patients with abdominal angina and intestinal viability. Glucagon reduces splanchnic vascular resistance and should be continued for 36 to 48 h postoperatively. Mannitol is also frequently used to promote diuresis postoperatively.

A high cardiac output, low SVR state may develop due to mechanisms related to reperfusion. Broad spectrum antibiotics and volume expansion are the principal modes of therapy. Vasoconstrictors may compromise splanchnic blood flow in this setting, further compromising ischemic tisues.

INFRAINGUINAL VASCULAR SURGERY

Patients requiring infrainguinal vascular reconstruction typically have diffuse multilevel atherosclerotic disease that often requires a combination of procedures. Aorto–femoral bypass, femoral–femoral bypass and percutaneous transluminal angioplasty may be used prior to reconstruction of distal vessels. Patients with distal disease tend to have multiple medical problems and reduced life expectancy as compared to patients with aortoiliac disease. Despite this, functional limb salvage can be obtained in 85 percent of patients with a procedural mortality of 3 percent.

POSTOPERATIVE MANAGEMENT OF THE VASCULAR SURGERY PATIENT

Most life-threatening complications in vascular surgery occur in the early postoperative period, thus major reconstructive procedures warrant ICU monitoring.

Of particular importance is frequent assessment of the reperfused vascular bed (e.g., cerebral function, renal function). Following peripheral vascular reconstruction, distal pulses can be used to assess vessel patency. In the absence of palpable pulses bedside Doppler devices should be employed to obtain hourly ankle-brachial pressure indices. Absent or monophasic signals indicate a failing graft or distal thromboembolism and require immediate evaluation.

Leg edema is a common consequence of limb reperfusion and typically resolves with leg elevation alone. Other etiologies such as deep venous thrombosis, compartment syndromes, and tense wound hematomas must always be considered.

Other postoperative issues for these patients include delivery of adequate analgesia, stress ulcer prophylaxis, and prevention or treatment of hypothermia.

Vascular surgery patients are frequently malnourished at presentation due to the presence of other underlying disease processes. As with all critically ill patients, nutritional therapy appropriate to the situation should be considered.

MANAGEMENT OF THE CARDIOPULMONARY SYSTEM

Cardiopulmonary complications are the chief causes of morbidity and mortality in vascular surgery patients. Anticipation of cardiopulmonary instability should be among the principal aims of perioperative management. When appropriately used, invasive hemodynamic monitoring (e.g., arterial and pulmonary artery catheters) may facilitate optimization of cardiovascular function and limitation of myocardial ischemia.

Postoperative hypertension is a frequent occurrence following vascular surgery (e.g., aortic and extracranial carotid surgeries). Treatment should include pain control, optimization of intravascular volume status, and antihypertensive pharmaceuticals. Labetalol, nifedipine, nitroprusside and nitroglycerin are useful when tailored to the clinical setting.

Blood pressure instability postoperatively often occurs following carotid endarterectomy due to stretching of the carotid bulb. Hypertension followed by hypotension is probably due to disturbances of the carotid body baroreceptor reflex. Hypotension can be supported with ephedrine until reflex hyperactivity subsides. Hypertension can be treated as described above. Pharmacologic treatment should employ short acting agents.

Tachycardia is common to all postoperative patients. Treatment should emphasize control of pain, correction of volume status, anemia, hypoxemia, and evaluation for cardiac ischemia and pulmonary embolism. If no cause can be found then treatment may be indicated to limit myocardial oxygen consumption. Esmolol (20 mg IV push test dose, then 10 to 30 μg/kg/min), a short acting selective β blocker can be useful. Persistent tachycardia can be treated with metoprolol (50mg po). Relative contraindications to β-blocker therapy include obstructive lung disease and cardiac failure.

RENAL FUNCTION

Postoperative renal failure in vascular patients portends a poor prognosis (50 to 75 percent mortality). Therapeutic efforts should be aimed at maintaining renal blood blow and urine output. Adequate intravascular volume must be assured. Osmotic diuresis due to hyperglycemia or preoperative contrast studies is a common cause of hypovolemia in these patients. Beyond volume expansion, low dose dopamine, diuretics and mannitol may be useful in producing diuresis (1 to 1.5 ml/kg/h). In patients with evidence of rhabdomyolysis following tissue reperfusion, alkalinization of the urine may be useful.

If oliguric or anuric renal failure occurs, early continuous arteriovenous hemofiltration should be instituted to prevent additional morbidity associated with volume overload.

INFECTION

First generation cephalosporins are typically used prophylactically and should be continued through the postoperative period until the threat of wound and graft infection no longer exists. Early postoperative wound infections can be life and limb threatening and are most commonly caused by *Staphylococcus* species (*S. aureus* or *S. epidermidis*). Antibiotic selection should be directed toward these organisms. Fresh prosthetic grafts are particularly susceptible to bacterial seeding, thus close attention should be paid to all indwelling devices used in these patients.

Persistent signs suggestive of occult sepsis are uncommon in these patients. MSOF can develop and is usually preceded by a period of hypoperfusion. Common sites for infection should be investigated. In their absence, ischemic pancreatitis, acalculous cholecystitis, ischemic colitis and small bowel ischemia should be considered and treated as dictated by the clinical setting.

CRITICAL ILLNESS AND VASCULAR DISEASE-SPECIAL CONSIDERATIONS

Symptomatic, synchronous disease of the carotid and coronaries is not uncommon. Treatment priorities should be based on the most threatening problem. Combined procedures have not been shown to be of benefit to patients undergoing CABG. Carotid endarterectomy is usually well tolerated in patients with mild to moderate coronary artery disease. Situations remain where both carotid and coronary disease is severe and symptomatic and though a slightly higher risk of stroke has been reported, combined surgery is warranted.

THORACOABDOMINAL ANEURYSM REPAIR

Thoracoabdominal aneurysm (TAA) repair is a formidable procedure that is associated with a high rate of morbidity and mortality. Most TAA repairs require reimplantation of visceral arteries and prolonged periods of ischemia to the organs these vessels supply. The usual surgical approach for this procedure is a left thoracoabdominal incision with transection of the left hemidiaphragm. Postoperative care requires careful attention to pain control and pulmonary toilet.

Paraplegia is an unpredictable complication of this procedure. It can occur immediately postoperatively or days later. Despite improved techniques, complete prevention of neurologic deficits is virtually impossible.

VASCULAR EMERGENCIES ARISING IN THE ICU

Acute limb ischemia in the ICU can be due to thromboembolism, thrombosis during low flow states, overzealous use of vasoconstrictors, and thrombosis related to intra-arterial catheters. Detection of limb ischemia can be difficult in patients with hypothermia, cyanosis, or those receiving vasoconstrictors. All patients admitted to the ICU must have initial and routine documentation of their peripheral vascular examination.

Treatment of these problems should focus on the primary etiology whenever possible. Thrombotic events should be treated with anticoagulation. Intravascular catheters should be removed if they are in the threatened extremity.

For further reading in *Principles of Critical Care,* see Chap 86 "Management of the Critically Ill Vascular Surgery Patient" Giancarlo Piano/John Alverdy/Christopher Zarins, Chap 87, "Cardiac Surgery" Joseph P Coyle/Thomas L Higgins

22

Shock

Constantine A. Manthous

DEFINITIONS

Shock is the underperfusion of multiple organ systems. Since body tissues depend upon the cardiovascular and respiratory systems to supply adequate oxygen and fuel for metabolic function, this definition may be further refined as: substrate supply ($\dot{Q}_{O_2}$) inadequate to meet demand ($\dot{V}_{O_2}$). Clinical signs of hypoperfusion include tachycardia, diminished mean blood pressure, altered mental status, and decreased urine output. Lactic acidosis may also be a marker of shock although it does not necessarily reflect anaerobic metabolism (see Chap. 37). Hypotension, defined as a systolic blood pressure less than 90 mmHg or a mean pressure less than 60 mmHg, often occurs with shock states, but is not always present. Indeed, eclampsia and hypertensive emergency are shock states with elevated blood pressures.

PRIMARY SURVEY

Since morbidity and mortality are determined by the rapidity of diagnosis and treatment, a simple bedside algorithm for assessing the patient is presented. The two determinants of systemic pressure are cardiac output (CO) and systemic vascular resistance (SVR). Quite simply, hypotension is due to inadequate CO (most commonly hypovolemic or cardiogenic shock) or an abnormally low SVR (typically septic shock). Right heart catheterization allows measurement of chamber pressures and flows, which may assist in the diagnosis and management of shock. However, a right heart catheter should be placed to test a clinical hypothesis (e.g., is the patient hypovolemic?) which cannot be answered less invasively, rather than as a routine part of care. The following algorithm aids prompt delineation of these major categories (see Table 22-1).

1. Is this high or low output shock? The patient with high output shock is warm, well-perfused, with brisk capillary refill, bounding pulses, widened pulse pressure, reduced diastolic (more than systolic) blood pressure with a strong apical cardiac impulse. The great majority of patients with this form of shock are septic. If the patient is cool, poorly perfused, with poor capillary refill, thready pulses, reduced pulse pressure, and weak apical cardiac impulse, then the patient is most likely in hypovolemic or cardiogenic shock.

2. Is the heart too full? The patient with hypovolemic shock, usually due to hemorrhage, has reduced jugular venous pressure, normal lung and heart examination (save tachycardia and tachypnea), normal chest radiograph and electrocardiogram (ECG), and, often, overt evidence of bleeding (e.g., hematemesis, hematochezia, melena, expanding abdomen, hemothorax or a tense lower extremity). The patient with cardiogenic shock is also poorly perfused, but instead has increased jugular venous pressure, an S3, crackles on auscultation of the chest, peripheral edema, a large heart and pulmonary edema pattern on chest radiograph, and often ECG abnormalities.

3. What doesn't fit? When the bedside examination yields unclear or conflicting information, one must consider the possibility of a mixed shock picture, such as sepsis complicated by myocardial infarction. In these situations more information in the form of echocardiography or right heart catheterization may be required to sort out the precise etiology of the shock state, but it does not change the approach to early management—the prompt restitution of an adequate intravascular volume with fluids or blood. Table 22-2 presents recommendations for urgent resuscitation.

INITIAL MANAGEMENT

The mainstays of shock therapy are to **1.** improve oxygen delivery (by raising hemoglobin concentration, cardiac output, or arterial saturation); **2.** reduce oxygen consumption, and **3.** identify and treat the precipitants of hypoperfusion. It takes no more than a few minutes to perform the clinical assessment outlined above and to formulate a hypothesis as to the type of shock. At the same time the ABCs (airway, breathing, and circulation) are evaluated.

Improving Oxygen Delivery

Airway and breathing. As depressed mentation is common in patients with shock, tracheal intubation is often indicated to protect the lungs from aspiration of oropharyngeal or gastric contents. Acute hypoxemic respiratory failure often complicates shock, in which case mechanical ventilation serves to improve oxygenation through the delivery of increased inspired oxygen and positive end-expiratory pressure (PEEP). Lastly, metabolic (lactic) acidosis prompts increased respiratory drive, causing a dramatic elevation in respiratory muscle oxygen demand at the same time that oxygen delivery is impaired. In order to prevent respiratory arrest, patients in shock should be intubated electively, especially when there is distress, tachypnea, or use of accessory muscles of respiration.

TABLE 22-1 Early Formulation of a Working Diagnosis of the Etiology of Shock

Shock Features	Septic	Cardiogenic	Hypovolemic
Blood pressure	↓	↓	↓
Heart rate	↑	↑	↑
Respiratory rate	↑	↑	↑
Mentation	↓	↓	↓
Urine output	↓	↓	↓
Arterial pH	↓	↓	↓
Is Cardiac Output Reduced?	No	Yes	Yes
Pulse pressure	↑	↓	↓
Diastolic pressure	↓↓	↓	↓
Extremities/digits	Warm	Cool	Cool
Nailbed return	Rapid	Slow	Slow
Heart sounds	Crisp	Muffled	Muffled
Temperature	↑ or ↓	↕ ↓	↕ ↓
White cell count	↑ or ↓	−	−
Site of infection	++	−	−

Is the Heart Too Full?	No	Yes	No
Symptoms/clinical context	Sepsis/liver failure	Angina/ECG	Hemorrhage/dehydration
Jugular venous pressure	↓	↑	↓
S_3, S_4, gallop rhythm	–	+++	–
Respiratory crepitations	–	+++	–
Chest radiograph	Normal	Large heart ↑ upper lobe flow Pulmonary edema	Normal

What Does Not Fit?
Overlapping etiologies (septic + cardiogenic, septic + hypovolemic, cardiogenic + hypovolemic)

Short list of other etiologies	*High output hypotension*	*High right atrial pressure hypotension*	*Nonresponsive hypovolemia*
	Thyroid storm	Cardiac tamponade	Adrenal insufficiency
	Arteriovenous fistula	Right ventricular infarction	Anaphylaxis
	Paget's disease	Pulmonary hypertension	Spinal shock

Get more information — Echocardiography, right heart catheterization

(Reprinted with permission from Walley KR, Wood LDH: Shock, in Hall JB, Schmidt GA, Wood LD: Principles of Critical Care. McGraw-Hill, New York, 1992.)

TABLE 22-2 Urgent Resuscitation of the Patient with Shock; Intravenous Volume and Vasoactive Drug Therapy

Hemorrhagic Shock including Trauma, Ruptured Aneurysms	Nonhemorrhagic Hypovolemia including Septic Shock	Cardiogenic Shock due to Myocardial Ischemia
	Volume therapy	
Elevate legs, MAST	Elevate legs	When heart is "too full," ↓ blood volume (rotating tourniquets, phlebotomy, nitroglycerin, morphine, diuretics).
Access/infuse emergency blood	3 L/20 min warmed saline	
Group/match/administer warmed blood/ components	Group/match packed RBCs and plasma re dilutional anemia	
> 3 L/20 min warmed saline	Continue aggressive volume infusion until blood pressure normal or heart "too full"	If the heart is not "too full," or blood pressure ↓ with above interventions, NS 250 ml/20 min
Equal volumes of colloid or substitutes (albumin, dextran, hetastarch)		
Continue aggressive volume infusion until blood pressure normal	Detect and treat tamponade with pericardiocentesis, thoracostomy, peritoneal drainage, or reduced PEEP	Repeat if blood pressure ↑ until heart too full
Consider early surgical hemostasis		

Vasoactive drug therapy

Awaiting adequate volume repletion, institute multipurpose agent (*dopamine* or *epinephrine*) and increase dose from 1 toward 10 (μg/kg/min for dopamine; μg/min for epinephrine) as needed to maintain blood pressure. If higher doses are needed, add *norepinephrine* (2–20 μg/min). Discontinue these drugs as urgently as volume repletion and hemostasis allow (see second column).	Avoid vasoactive drugs until heart "too full." Except *dopamine* (2–5 μg/kg/min) for renal perfusion early. Nitroglycerin and nitroprusside are contraindicated. Vasoconstrictors delay adequate volume repletion (see left column). In right heart overload with shock *norepinephrine* (2–20 μg/min) may help by maintaining RV perfusion; in septic shock, vasoconstrictors may help when adequate volume replacement provides inadequate perfusion pressure (see text).	*Dobutamine* (5–15 μg/kg/min) to enhance contractility without excess tachycardia, arrhythmia, or vasoconstriction; higher doses dilate skeletal vascular bed. *Dopamine* (2–5 μg/kg/min) to preserve renal cortical blood flow; at higher dose (4–12 μg/kg/min), increases heart rate, contractility, venous tone, and preload, like *epinephrine*. *Nitroglycerin* (5–250 μg/min) for venodilation with minimal arterial dilation except for the coronary circulation. *Sodium nitroprusside* (0.1–10 μg/kg/min) for arterial dilation to reduce afterload and allow greater ejection from a depressed left ventricle or regurgitant aortic/mitral valve.

(*Reprinted with permission from Walley KR, Wood LDH: Shock, in Principles of Critical Care, McGraw-Hill, New York, 1992.*)

185

Circulation. Early assessment must rule out the possibility of shock secondary to tension pneumothorax or arrhythmias since these are rapidly treated by tube thoracostomy or electrical cardioversion (see Chap. 5). Thereafter, the therapeutic approach to the circulation in nearly all forms of shock is aggressive volume resuscitation to decisively assure an adequately filled cardiovascular system. Warmed blood or crystalloid administered "wide open" through at least two large caliber intravenous lines should begin immediately until the cardiovascular system is filled. Indices of "full" include resolution of hypoperfusion or elevation of central venous or other intravascular pressures. Too often vasoactive agents are administered before adequate intravascular volume is assured, compromising subsequent delivery of fluid. The exceptions to aggressive volume resuscitation are in patients with right heart syndromes (vide infra) or ischemic heart disease, when more modest volume challenges (e.g., 500mL) are indicated. Nevertheless, many patients with acute myocardial infarction are hypovolemic and improve with judicious fluid resuscitation.

Since blood offers both oxygen carrying capacity and effective intravascular replacement, it should be used first, up to a hematocrit of around 40. Maximizing the hematocrit is especially useful when shock is complicated by acute hypoxemic respiratory failure. Steps to maximize hemoglobin saturation include the addition of high concentrations of inspired oxygen and PEEP. The temporary use of 100% inspired oxygen, until initial resuscitation has succeeded, is therefore advisable. PEEP has the potential to improve oxygen delivery (by reducing shunt in diffuse lung lesions) or worsen it (by compromising cardiac output).

Vasoactive drugs. Vasoactive agents often treat the blood pressure but not the patient. Tables 22-3 and 22-4 outline these drugs and their useful dose. Vasoconstrictors such as dopamine, norepinephrine, phenylephrine and pseudoephedrine, increase the systemic vascular resistance while constricting the venous capacitance vessels, thus increasing venous return: an autotransfusion. This is a poor substitute for adequate volume resuscitation. Furthermore, these agents may reduce blood flow to vital tissues (through vasoconstriction), which is antithetical to the objective of treatment. Military anti-shock trousers (MAST) have long been used for similar effect in hemorrhagic shock. If used properly, they may cause a similar auto-transfusion effect without reducing vital organ flow while vigorous volume replacement is undertaken. Positive inotropes such as dobutamine and dopamine (in the 5 to 10 mcg/kg/min range) are useful for the acute management of most forms of cardiogenic (and sometimes septic) shock. These drugs should be given and adjusted based on physiologically relevant

TABLE 22-3 Drugs to Increase Cardiac Contractility

Drug Name	IV Dose Range	Oral Dose Range
Dobutamine	2–15 µg/kg/min	NA
Dopamine	0.5–10 µg/kg/min	NA
Isoproterenol	1–8 µg/kg/min	NA
Digoxin	0.25–1.0-mg loading dose, followed by 0.125–0.25 mg/day	Same as IV or slightly higher due to decreased bioavailability
Amrinone	0.75 mg/kg loading dose, then 5–10 µg/kg/min	NA
Milrinone	50 µg/kg over 10 min, then 0.375–0.75 µg/kg/min	7.5–10 mg q.i.d. or q 4 h

(Reprinted with permission from Elliot WJ: Vasoactive Drugs, in Hall JB, Schmidt GA, Wood LDH: Principles of Critical Care, McGraw-Hill, New York, 1992.)

TABLE 22-4 Drugs to Increase Systemic Vascular Resistance

Drug Name	IV Starting Dose	Maintenance Dose
Dopamine	1–2 µg/kg/min	0.5–50+[a] µg/kg/min
Norepinephrine	2 µg/min	2–20 µg/min
Epinephrine	0.1–0.25-mg bolus, but may be given by constant infusion (0.01–0.3 mg/min)	0.5–1 mg q 5 min (during CPR)
Metaraminol	0.5 mg over 2–3 min	0.5–5 mg slow IV push over 2–3 min
Phenylephrine	0.5 mg over 2–3 min	0.5–5 mg slow IV push over 2–3 min

[a]At the higher doses of infused dopamine, α-agonism becomes the overwhelming pharmacologic effect. Higher doses are often necessary in patients with congestive heart failure or acidosis. For some physicians, norepinephrine is the α-agonist preferred over dopamine at the higher doses (exceeding 20–50 µg/kg/min).

(Reprinted with permission from Elliot WJ: Vasoactive Drugs, in Hall JB, Schmidt GA, Wood LDH: Principles of Critical Care, McGraw-Hill, New York, 1992.)

endpoints, such as adequacy of perfusion, rather than titrated to arbitrary levels of blood pressure. Dopamine, at 2 to 3 mcg/kg/min, is frequently administered in the management of shock to improve renal and mesenteric blood flow, though its efficacy has not been demonstrated.

Reducing Oxygen Consumption

Mechanical ventilation reduces, but does not usually eliminate, the work of breathing. Additional steps to sedate, and often to relax muscles, may be necessary. Since fever increases oxygen demand by about 10 percent per degree centigrade above 37°C, antipyretics should be given early in the acute management of hyperthermic (usually septic) shock. Cooling blankets should be restricted to paralyzed, sedated patients since they cause shivering which can increase oxygen consumption.

SPECIFIC THERAPY FOR SHOCK

Though the urgent resuscitation of shock is not based on the specific etiology, subsequent management depends upon the specific underlying disease.

Septic Shock

Septic shock is examined in great detail in Chap. 37. Briefly, broad spectrum antibiotics which target suspected pathogens, must be initiated immediately upon recognition of the high output shock. Once gram stain results of relevant body fluids are known, broad coverage can be instituted for the first 24 to 48 h until culture data allows narrowing of the antibiotic spectrum. Early management also includes drainage of collections such as intra-abdominal, intrapelvic, bony, or soft tissue abscesses since antibiotics alone will not eradicate the infection. Antiendotoxin antibodies, antitumor necrosis factor antibodies, interleukin-1 receptor antagonist, and nonsteroidal anti-inflammatory drugs remain investigational. Corticosteroids are not efficacious.

Myocardial Infarction

The most common cause of cardiogenic shock is acute myocardial infarction. Therapy is focussed on improving coronary blood flow, while reducing myocardial work (detailed in Chap. 23). The former is addressed with aspirin, nitrates, heparin, thrombolysis, balloon counterpulsation, coronary angioplasty, and coronary artery bypass. Myocardial work is decreased by the careful use of sedation, analgesia, nitrates, and afterload reduction. Routine management of myocardial infarction utilizes β-blockers, which are contraindicated in the setting of acute myocardial infarction with shock. Dobutamine augments myocardial performance while afterload reducing the heart, thus improving performance at minimal energetic cost. Dopamine is often positively chronotropic in 5 to 10 mcg/kg/min doses and thus may augment cardiac output but at a higher energy cost. In general, vasoconstricting drugs should not be used in acute myocardial infarction since they increase afterload and reduce perfusion. Afterload reduction, as with nitroprusside, can reduce cardiac work. Very careful titration of dose while monitoring with a right heart catheter is essential since hypotension can worsen ischemia. Acute valvular dysfunction and ventricular septal defect may be amenable to surgical repair and so should be excluded early.

Acute Hemorrhage

Trauma and gastrointestinal bleeding are the most common causes of hypovolemic shock. The initial urgent management includes the placement of at least two large bore, short-length intravenous catheters with the rapid administration of warmed blood and crystalloid until the circulation has been restored. Trauma is discussed in Chap. 5 but several points bear emphasis. The site of bleeding must be recognized early to direct lifesaving surgical intervention. Occult sites of blood loss include the abdomen, retroperitoneum, thorax, and thighs. Clues may come from serial physical examinations, plain radiographs of the chest, computed tomography, or peritoneal lavage.

Likewise, gastrointestinal bleeding (reviewed in Chap. 60) requires early diagnosis (sampling of nasogastric and fecal material for blood) and aggressive management. This often mandates emergent upper endoscopy to examine for esophageal, gastric, or duodenal bleeding. Endoscopy may also be therapeutic when electrocoagulation or sclerotherapy is available. Diagnosis of lower gastrointestinal bleeding may require angiography, a radio-labelled bleeding scan, or direct visualization of the bleeding site. Therapies include endoscopic laser cautery, embolization, local infusion of vasoactive agents, sclerotherapy, or surgical extirpation of bleeding segments.

OTHER SHOCKS: THE LONGER LIST

Table 22-5 offers a more extensive list of the less common etiologies of shock. In those cases in which no infection, acute hemorrhage or myocardial infarction is found, other diseases must be considered.

Non-Septic High Output Hypotension

In the absence of an infection, very few diseases cause high output hypotension. These include advanced liver disease, the hypermetabolic stage of a thermal injury, severe pancreatitis, thyrotoxicosis, wet beri beri, adrenal insufficiency, and severe salicylate poisoning. The first three may be related to endotoxemia. Fulminant hepatic failure, most commonly secondary to viral or toxic hepatitis, is treated with supportive management and liver transplantation (Chap. 61). (See Chap. 17 for burns and Chap. 62 for pancreatitis).

TABLE 22-5 Causes of and Contributors to Shock

Decreased Pump Function of the Heart—Cardiogenic Shock

Left Ventricular Failure
  Systolic dysfunction—Decreased contractility
    myocardial infarction
    ischemia and global hypoxemia
    cardiomyopathy
    depressant drugs: β-blockers, calcium channel
      blockers, antiarrhythmics,
    myocardial contusion
    respiratory acidosis
    metabolic derangements: acidosis,
      hypophosphatemia, hypocalcemia
  Diastolic dysfunction—Increased myocardial diastolic stiffness
    ischemia
    ventricular hypertrophy
    restrictive cardiomyopathy
    consequence of prolonged hypovolemic or septic shock.
    ventricular Interdependance
    external compression (see cardiac tamponade below)
  Greatly increased afterload
    aortic stenosis
    hypertrophic cardiomyopathy
    dynamic outflow tract obstruction
    coarctation of the aorta
    malignant hypertension
  Valve and structural abnormality
    mitral stenosis, endocarditis, mitral/aortic regurgitation
    obstruction due to atrial myxoma or thrombus
    papillary muscle dysfunction or rupture
    ruptured septum or free wall
  Arrhythmias
Right Ventricular Failure
  Decreased contractility
    right ventricular infarction, ischemia, hypoxia, acidosis
  Greatly increased afterload
    pulmonary embolism
    pulmonary vascular disease
    hypoxic pulmonary vasoconstriction, PEEP, high alveolar pressure
    acidosis
    ARDS, pulmonary fibrosis, sleep disordered breathing, COPD
  Valve and structural abnormality
    obstruction due to atrial myxoma, thrombus, endocarditis
  Arrhythmias

**Decreased Venous Return With Normal Pumping
Function—Hypovolemic Shock.**

Cardiac Tamponade (increased right atrial pressure—central
  hypovolemia)
  Pericardial fluid collection
    blood
    renal failure

TABLE 22-5 Causes of and Contributors to Shock *(continued)*

Decreased Venous Return with Normal Pumping Function—Hypovolemic Shock.

    pericarditis with effusion
  Constrictive pericarditis
  High intrathoracic pressure
    tension pneumothorax
    massive pleural effusion
    positive pressure ventilation
  High intraabdominal pressure
    ascites
    massive obesity
    post extensive intra-abdominal surgery
Intravascular Hypovolemia (reduced Pms)
  Hemorrhage
    gastrointestinal
    trauma
    aortic dissection and other internal sources
  Renal losses
    diuretics
    osmotic diuresis
    diabetes insipidus
  Gastrointestinal losses
    vomiting
    diarrhea
    gastric suctioning
    loss via surgical stomas
  Redistribution to extra vascular space
    burns
    trauma
    post surgical
    sepsis
Decreased Venous Tone (reduced Pms)
  Drugs
    sedatives
    narcotics
    diuretics
  Anaphylactic shock
  Neurogenic shock
Increased Resistance to Venous Return (RVR)
  Tumor compression or invasion
  Venous thrombosis with obstruction
  PEEP
  Pregnancy

High Cardiac Output Hypotension

  Septic Shock
  Sterile Endotoxemia with Hepatic Failure
  Arteriovenous Shunts
    dialysis
    Paget's disease

TABLE 22-5 Causes of and Contributors to Shock *(continued)*

Other Causes of Shock with Unique Etiologies

Thyroid Storm
Myxedema Coma
Adrenal Insufficiency
Hemoglobin and Mitochondrial Poisons
  cyanide
  carbon monoxide
  iron intoxication

(Reprinted with permission from Walley KR, Wood LDH: Shock, in Principles of Critical Care, *McGraw-Hill, New York, 1992.)*

Miscellaneous Causes of Cardiogenic Shock

Though ischemic heart disease is the most common form of cardiogenic shock, other forms must also be considered since appropriate definitive management depends upon prompt recognition. A few of the more common forms of cardiogenic shock in the absence of infarction are discussed below.

Acute valvular disease. The acute failure of an aortic or mitral valve may lead to acute cardiogenic shock. This most often occurs in the setting of infective endocarditis (Chap. 42) or as a complication of myocardial infarction. The sudden onset of symptoms and signs of pulmonary edema with a new murmur should prompt consideration of sudden valvular failure. Initial diagnosis is obtained with a bedside echocardiogram, followed by left heart catheterization if necessary. Management includes reduction of left ventricular afterload using a drug such as nitroprusside. Surgical management is typically required to re-establish hemodynamic stability in particularly severe cases.

Acute right heart syndrome. Acute pulmonary embolism (PE) is discussed in Chapter 24. In the setting of shock, a definitive diagnosis is essential in order to guide specific, often risky, therapy. The diagnosis may be suspected based on the history, electrocardiogram, chest radiograph, or echocardiogram, but a high probability ventilation perfusion lung scan or positive angiogram provide a more firm foundation to guide management. Thrombolytic therapy may be useful for shock due to PE. In addition to anticoagulation, patients in shock should also have a vena caval interrupting device placed to eliminate the risk of recurrent embolization.

Shock due to PE is due to acute right heart failure. These patients are often intravascularly overfilled and fluid administration may dilate the right ventricle, further compromising forward flow. Hemodynamic support includes dobutamine to augment right ventricular output. In hypotensive patients, vasoconstrictors, such as norepinephrine, may relieve right ventricular ischemia and improve cardiac output. Such drugs should only be given when they improve cardiac output, not to raise blood pressure.

Another relatively common right heart syndrome is the superimposition of any disease state which requires an acute increase in cardiac output on chronic pulmonary hypertension. The most common causes for chronic pulmonary hypertension include chronic obstructive pulmonary disease, chronic pulmonary embolism, and sleep apnea. When metabolic demand increases or systemic vasodilation occurs as with sepsis, cardiac output must increase. Right-sided pressures rise and the patient exhibits signs of right heart failure–peripheral edema, elevated neck veins, ascites, and hepatic congestion. As with pulmonary embolism, dobutamine and norepinephrine may be useful in improving right heart output until the precipitating stress is corrected.

Cardiac tamponade (see Chap. 26). Patients with tamponade are generally short of breath without pulmonary edema but have signs of elevated filling pressures, including jugular venous distension, peripheral edema and hepatojugular reflux. A pulsus paradox is often present and a friction rub may be heard on auscultation of the heart. The cardiac silhouette is often enlarged, sometimes in the classic "water bottle" configuration. The electrocardiogram may reveal low voltage, diffuse ST elevation (when pericarditis is present), or electrical alternans. The echocardiogram is the diagnostic test of choice. Effusions can be readily identified and the signs of tamponade including right atrial and ventricular collapse during diastole, may be seen. Right heart catheterization can be used to confirm the diagnosis (equalization of pressures during diastole) but urgent relief of tamponade by pericardiocentesis or surgical pericardiostomy is indicated. While awaiting surgical therapy, great care must be taken to avoid hypovolemia. Vasoactive agents should be avoided.

Nonhemorrhagic Hypovolemic Shock

Although hemorrhage is the most common form of hypovolemic shock, anaphylaxis and adrenal insufficiency occur with enough regularity to warrant consideration in patients with hypovolemic shock and no readily identifiable source of hemorrhage.

Hypersensitivity reactions. Anaphylaxis must be considered in the differential diagnosis of hypovolemic shock, especially in the appropriate clinical context. The clinical history often includes exposure to a new drug or food, or an insect sting. Symptoms may include rhinorrhea, shortness of breath, cough, chest tightness, dizziness, general skin itchiness, and a feeling of impending doom. Signs on examination include wheezing, stridor, cyanosis, nonpitting edema, urticaria and hypotension. In the setting of shock with this constellation of signs and symptoms urgent resuscitation is carried out as above, but definitive therapy includes epinephrine, 0.05 to 0.1 mg intravenously every 1 to 5 min, as needed in conjunction with fluids. Since laryngeal edema often accompanies anaphylaxis, early intubation is indicated if any stridor is noted. Additionally, care must be taken to assure that the offending agent has been removed, if this is possible. Antihistamines and steroids may also be beneficial as adjuncts to primary therapy.

Adrenal insufficiency (see Chap. 64). Adrenal crisis occurs most commonly in patients who are suddenly withdrawn from chronic steroid therapy, or who develop critical illness while receiving small, but suppressive doses of corticosteroids. Less commonly there is adrenal infarction or infection. Although eosinophilia, hyponatremia and hyperkalemia may be present these findings are not necessary to make the diagnosis. Often the hypotension of adrenal crisis is refractory to fluid management even though the patient is hypovolemic by exam. In these cases, 4 mg of intravenous dexamethasone should be administered immediately and a rapid adrenocorticotropic hormone (ACTH) stimulation test performed as soon as possible. Dexamethasone does not affect the results of the ACTH stimulation test. Following the test, hydrocortisone, 100mg intravenously every 6 h, should be substituted.

For further reading in *Principles of Critical Care,* see Chap 2 "The Cardiovascular System" LDH Wood, Chap 114 "Shock" Keith R Walley/Lawrence DH Wood, Chap 125 "Vasoactive Drugs" William J Elliott/Daniel D Gretler

---

23

Ischemic Heart Disease and Thrombolytic Therapy

Stephen R. Amesbury

In patients with noncardiac critical illness, the common manifestations of myocardial ischemia and infarction may be subtle or absent. The critical care physician must maintain a high index of suspicion for myocardial ischemia in the hemodynamically unstable patient in the ICU setting. This chapter will review the diagnosis and management of myocardial ischemia and acute myocardial infarction.

MYOCARDIAL ISCHEMIA

Diagnosis of Myocardial Ischemia

Myocardial ischemia is most commonly manifested as constant substernal chest tightness or pressure which is typically left-sided and may radiate to the throat, jaw or left arm. It may be accompanied by dyspnea and diaphoresis. Pericarditis, pleuritis, dissecting aortic aneurysm, pulmonary embolism, musculoskeletal pain, costochondritis, and pain of gastrointestinal origin may mimic myocardial ischemia. Examination of the precordium may demonstrate the presence of a fourth heart sound, the emergence of a mitral regurgitant murmur, a third heart sound, an elevated jugular venous pressure, or pulmonary crackles.

The electrocardiogram (ECG) abnormalities in myocardial ischemia are widely variable. T wave changes in the leads reflecting the anatomic area of myocardium in jeopardy are the first ECG changes. If the occlusion of the coronary vessel is complete, the T wave is peaked. Previously flattened or inverted T waves may revert, masking ischemic changes—the so-called pseudonormalization of T waves. Hyperacute ST segment elevation is indicative of transmural ischemia.

Conduction disturbances such as first degree atrioventricular (AV) block, sinus or junctional bradycardia, or complete heart block with a narrow QRS complex are associated with occlusion of the right coronary artery. Occlusion of the left anterior descending coronary artery may lead to right bundle branch block (RBBB), left bundle branch block (LBBB), or bifasicular block. Ventricular ectopic beats and ventricular arrhythmias are common during ischemic episodes. Supraventricular arrhythmias can also occur in ischemic syndromes. Atrial fibrillation accompanies acute myocardial infarction (MI) approximately 10 to 15 percent of the time.

The most useful and reliable enzyme determination for MI is creatine kinase (CK). CK released from the myocardium begins to appear in the plasma within 4 to 8 h after onset of infarction, peaks at 12 to 24 h, and returns to base line at 2 to 4 days. To be diagnostic for MI, total plasma CK must be above the upper limit of normal and must be at least 3.0 percent MB fraction. Therapeutic interventions should not be delayed pending assay results. Some of the causes of false-positive elevations of CK-MB include myocarditis, pericarditis, myocardial trauma, hyperthermia, hypothermia, renal failure, hypothyroidism, subarachnoid hemorrhage, rhabdomyolysis, abdominal surgery, and tumors. Serum lactic dehydrogenase (LDH) is of utility in diagnosing infarction when the normal pattern of LDH isoenzyme 2 > LDH isoenzyme 1 is inverted ("flip" to $LDH_1 > LDH_2$).

An echocardiogram can detect discrete segmental wall motion abnormalities of the left ventricle suggesting ischemia, mitral regurgitation secondary to papillary muscle dysfunction, and can rule out other diagnoses, such as aortic dissection, cardiac tamponade, and pericarditis.

Treatment of Unstable Angina

When angina is of recent onset, or occurs at rest, there is a moderately high probability of the development of a MI within the next few days. This is unstable angina.

Nitrates are a mainstay of therapy for unstable angina because of their efficacy and rapid onset of action. Nitroglycerin decreases preload, at higher doses decreases afterload, and dilates epicardial coronary arteries, including arteries with stenoses. Sublingual doses of 0.4 mg may be administered every 5 to 10 min to a total of three doses, if required to control pain. Frequent blood pressure checks are required. Should hypotension develop, place the patient in the Trendelenburg position and give intravenous saline boluses. Topical nitroglycerin ointment, 0.5 to 2 in. every 6 to 8 h may be applied after angina has resolved with sublingual doses. If pain persists, intravenous nitroglycerin may be initiated at 10 to 20 μgm/min and titrated upward at 10 to 20 μgm/min increments every 5 to 10 min until pain resolves or the systemic systolic pressure is 95 to 110 mmHg. An upper limit of 400 μgm/min is usually accepted as maximal.

Narcotics can be given as the dose of nitroglycerin is being titrated upward. Morphine is the initial agent used, and because it decreases left ventricular preload, it is especially beneficial when pulmonary edema is present. Morphine can increase vagal tone which, in the setting of inferior wall MI, can lead to bradycardia. Hydromorphone (1 to 3 mg) is more potent than morphine and less vagotonic.

β-blockade is important, especially in the setting of angina with tachycardia and hypertension. β-blockers are relatively contraindicated in patients with marginal blood pressure, bradycardia, AV conduction disturbances, and left ventricular failure. Short-acting esmolol is useful in patients with the potential for hemodynamic instability. Otherwise, metoprolol at a dose of 15 mg intravenously over 15 to 20 min until the heart rate is between 60 and 70 beats/min, provided the systolic blood pressure does not fall below 95 mmHg, is preferred. Thereafter, 50 mg every 6 h is given orally.

Calcium channel blockers may relieve the component of epicardial coronary artery occlusion due to vasospasm by direct dilation of vascular smooth muscle. Nifedipine is preferred for vasospasm and when angina persists despite nitrates and narcotics because it has the least cardiodepressant action (along with nicardipine). A rapid fall in blood pressure can occur with nifedipine, so hypotension should be anticipated. The illicit use of cocaine causes coronary vasospasm and angina, and responds well to treatment with calcium channel blockers.

Aspirin for patients presenting with unstable angina reduces the incidence of refractory angina, MI, and cardiac death. It should be used routinely in all patients with unstable angina. A single tablet of 164 or 325 mg, taken immediately and daily thereafter is sufficient to effectively inhibit platelet activity.

Heparin is as effective as aspirin for both treating patients with unstable angina and in preventing MI. Patients with unstable angina treated with aspirin who continue to have ischemic episodes should receive heparin. A bolus of 5000 to 10,000 U followed by 1000 U/h to maintain the activated partial thromboplastin time (PTT) at one and a half to two times the control is the usual therapy.

Thrombolytic therapy for unstable angina has not demonstrated added benefit over treatment with aspirin alone. Because of the significant risk of bleeding with thrombolytic agents, their routine use in unstable angina cannot be recommended at this time.

Coronary angiography should be reserved for unstable patients in whom a possible revascularization procedure is anticipated in the near future. Angiography is of little tangible value if coronary artery bypass graft (CABG) surgery or angioplasty are not viable options. In cases in which the patient stabilizes readily with pharmacologic agents and aspirin/heparin, there is no need for early angiography.

An intra-aortic balloon pump (IABP) is indicated in unstable angina when the angina and attendant ECG abnormalities are persistent and refractory to maximal pharmacologic therapy. It is particularly indicated in this situation when coronary angiography or possible revascularization cannot be performed within a reasonably short time or as a method to control progressive unstable angina to allow coronary angiography to be performed safely.

Potential complications of IABP include aortic dissection, femoral artery laceration, hematomas, femoral neuropathies, renal failure from renal artery occlusion, arterial thrombi and emboli, limb ischemia, and line sepsis. Once inserted, the patient should be placed on full doses of heparin by constant infusion. Prophylactic administration of antibiotics, such as oxacillin or a cephalosporin, is usually instituted.

ACUTE MYOCARDIAL INFARCTION

Symptoms suggestive of MI are usually similar to those of ordinary angina, but the intensity and duration of symptoms are greater. The initial treatment with oxygen, nitrates, and narcotics to relieve pain are similar as well.

Therapeutic Approach

β-blockers have been shown to be beneficial in q wave infarctions, but not in non–q wave infarctions. Administration of 15 mg metoprolol intravenously over 15 to 20 min and then 50 mg orally every 6 h thereafter has been shown to reduce mortality and to preserve myocardial function postinfarction. Contraindications include overt cardiac failure, second degree AV block, hypotension, sinus bradycardia, and of course, cardiogenic shock. A history of bronchospastic pulmonary disease is a relative contraindication.

Thrombolytic therapy is beneficial if it is initiated within 4 to 6 h of symptom onset. The two principal thrombolytic agents in use today are streptokinase (SK) and tissue plasminogen activator (TPA). Another less commonly used thrombolytic agent is acylated plasminogen streptokinase activator complex (APSAC). There is no clear benefit of SK over TPA in terms of mortality reduction or preservation of left ventricular function. Absolute contraindications include any active or recent bleeding other than menstruation, intracranial neoplasm, AV malformation or aneurysm, stroke or neurosurgery within the past 6 months, or head trauma within 14 days. Relative contraindications include major thoracic or abdominal surgery within 10 days, diabetic retinopathy, pregnancy, coagulation disorders, bacterial endocarditis, uncontrolled hypertension (above 200/110 mmHg), and prolonged or traumatic cardiopulmonary resuscitation. Thrombolytic agents should be used only if angina is excluded, and there is firm ECG evidence for infarction: at least 1 to 2 mm ST elevation in at least two contiguous leads. When the diagnosis of MI is in doubt, emergent echocardiography may be helpful.

Tissue plasminogen activator is given as a 10 mg bolus intravenously followed by 50 mg over the next hour by constant infusion. Then, 20 mg is administered in the second hour, and an additional

20 mg over the third hour, to a total of 100 mg over 3 h. *Streptokinase* is administered over 1 h to a total of 1,500,000 U by constant infusion. Since SK is derived from bacteria and is potentially antigenic, its administration may result in anaphylactic reactions. For this reason, 100 mg hydrocortisone is commonly administered immediately prior to intravenous SK. APSAC is given as a 30 mg bolus over 2 to 4 min, and like SK, is antigenic and generates a profound systemic lytic state, leading some to feel it offers no advantage over SK. Aspirin 325 mg should be started concomitantly with thrombolytic therapy, and continued as 325 mg orally daily thereafter. Heparin is started as a bolus of 5000 to 10,000 U, followed by 1000 U/h by constant infusion to achieve an activated PTT of one and a half to two times control. It is continued for 3 to 7 days or until coronary angiography is performed. Beta blockers should be initiated in concert with thrombolytic therapy according to the protocol previously given.

Angioplasty in acute MI is reserved for patients with hemodynamic instability during or after thrombolytic therapy, or in patients with refractory chest pain despite therapy. Patients presenting with *cardiogenic shock* are best managed with emergency percutaneous transluminal coronary angioplasty (PTCA). The risk of untoward complications in such patients, who ordinarily require multiple lines, is high if a thrombolytic agent is administered.

EVOLVING MYOCARDIAL INFARCTION

After these interventions in the first 6 h, the goals of treatment of acute MI are to monitor and prevent lethal ventricular arrhythmias and to treat hemodynamic instability.

Patients are placed on intravenous nitroglycerin infusion as described for unstable angina patients. Calcium channel blockers may be continued or increased if angina recurs. Nifedipine and nicardipine have the most vasodilating effect and least cardiodepressant effect. Diltiazem and verapamil slow conduction in the AV node and therefore should be used cautiously in combination with beta blockers and in inferior wall MIs. Diltiazem has been proven to have benefit in patients with non-q wave MIs, who do not have evidence of congestive heart failure. It is given at a dose of 30 to 60 mg every 6 to 8 h.

Left ventricular thrombus develops in approximately 30 to 40 percent of anterior wall MIs, and 10 to 15 percent of these embolize. Therefore, in patients with no contraindications to heparin therapy, we recommend routine anticoagulation.

The incidence of sustained ventricular tachycardia or fibrillation is highest within the first 3 to 4 h, but may occur at any time. The prophylactic use of lidocaine is controversial, but we recommend its use, especially in the first 6 h after MI. A loading dose of 50 to 100 mg should be administered, followed by a drip of 1 to 2 mg/min. If complex ectopy persists, additional boluses may be given to a total of 220 mg, with adjustment in the drip, to a total of 4 mg/min. If frequent ectopy persists, or if salvos of nonsustained ventricular tachycardia persist, procainamide is added at a loading dose of 1000 mg at a rate of 20 to 50 mg/min followed by a drip of 1 to 4 mg/min. Procainamide is the initial drug of choice if there is coexisting ventricular tachycardia and sustained supraventricular tachycardia. Breakthrough ventricular tachycardia/fibrillation resistant to these drugs should be treated with bretylium, started at a 500 mg loading dose over 30 min followed by a 1 to 4 mg/min drip. We also recommend lidocaine administration prophylactically when an accelerated idioventricular rhythm is present.

Ectopy may be caused by acidosis, hypoxemia, and hypokalemia. Magnesium depletion is also an important cause of persistent ectopy. Even normal serum magnesium levels may not reflect myocardial concentrations. Therefore we administer 2 to 4 g $MgSO_4$ in divided doses over 24 h when ectopy persists, provided renal failure is not present.

Hemodynamic monitoring with a pulmonary artery catheter is indicated whenever hemodynamic instability is present that does not improve relatively quickly with simple therapeutic maneuvers (e.g., saline bolus, intravenous loop diuretics, nitroglycerin). A PA catheter is indicated when pulmonary edema is suspected, when intravenous inotropes or vasodilators are used, and when the cardiac versus pulmonary origin of hypoxemia and infiltrates on chest x-ray cannot be differentiated clinically. PA catheters are not indicated in uncomplicated MIs or when minor pulmonary edema can be managed with small doses of diuretics and nitrates. Since many patients with acute MI are candidates for thrombolytic and anticoagulant therapy, it is prudent to use insertion sites for a PA catheter which are easily compressible should significant bleeding occur.

Pharmacologic Support for the Failing Left Ventricle

Overall treatment of the failing ventricle emphasizes reducing preload, decreasing afterload, and increasing cardiac contractility. Decreasing resistance to outflow is particularly beneficial in mitral regurgitation and ventricular septal defects.

Intravenous nitroglycerin is an ideal agent to use for both preload and afterload reduction. It is administered according to the protocol previously described. The other intravenous vasodilator preparation is nitroprusside, which is more potent than nitroglycerin.

Nitroprusside may cause diversion of blood flow from ischemic to nonischemic zones because of its very potent vasodilating properties ("coronary steal" phenomenon). Nitroprusside is metabolized to thiocyanate, a metabolic poison that can accumulate after 48 h of infusion (sooner in the face of renal dysfunction). If nitroglycerin at reasonably high doses (300 to 600 µgm/min) does not adequately reduce systemic vascular resistance (SVR), nitroprusside is started at 0.5 µgm/kg/min and gradually increased. Serum thiocyanate levels should be determined after 24 h and if found to exceed 10 mg/dL, nitroprusside should be discontinued.

Diuretics are used to treat pulmonary edema resulting from an elevated pulmonary capillary wedge pressure. When furosemide or bumetanide at high doses (40 to 80 mg every 6 to 8 h for furosemide and 1 to 2 mg every 6 to 8 h for bumetanide) do not produce adequate diuresis, oral doses of metolazone (5 to 10 mg daily) may be added. Serum potassium and magnesium levels must be closely monitored.

Dobutamine is an intravenous inotrope which may be needed to augment cardiac output. It is initiated at 5 µgm/kg/min and may be increased to 10 to 20 µgm/kg/min. Since it is an adrenergic agonist, dobutamine can be arrhythmogenic. Dopamine may be beneficial in low doses (2 to 5 µgm/kg/min) to augment renal blood flow and urine output.

Amrinone is an alternate inotropic agent which also acts as a vasodilator and decreases SVR. It is started with a loading dose of 0.75 mg/kg over 15 to 30 min, followed by constant infusion at 5 to 15 µgm/kg/min. Ventricular arrhythmias, elevation of liver transaminase levels, and thrombocytopenia are potential complications.

Digoxin therapy for congestive heart failure complicating acute MI is controversial, but its use to control ventricular rate in atrial fibrillation is unequivocally beneficial. Digoxin may be loaded with 0.25 mg to 0.5 mg intravenously initially, followed by an additional 0.5 mg to 0.75 mg in divided doses in the next 24 h. Subsequent doses should be adjusted if there is renal failure.

Hypotension in the setting of acute MI, unresponsive to dobutamine and cessation of nitrates, should be treated with high dose dopamine starting at 10 µgm/kg/min; it may be titrated to as high as 20 µgm/kg/min as needed to achieve a systolic blood pressure of 90 to 100 mmHg, so that perfusion to the coronary and systemic vascular beds is maintained. Hypotension refractory to dopamine is treated with norepinephrine starting at 2 to 4 µgm/min and titrating upward as needed. If high doses of pressors are needed to support blood pressure, serious consideration must be given for placement of an IABP in an effort to increase cardiac output and reduce myocardial oxygen requirements.

CARDIOGENIC SHOCK

Hemodynamic instability may not be present initially in some MI patients who ultimately slip into shock several hours to days after onset of infarction. Emergency angiography followed by either PTCA or emergency CABG surgery should be performed in such patients to reperfuse the myocardium as quickly as possible. If there is a delay in mobilizing the appropriate staff, an IABP should be inserted to stabilize the patient and facilitate catheterization. Where catheterization and PTCA or CABG surgery are not available, thrombolytic therapy should be instituted, perhaps even in patients who are at high risk for bleeding complications, since the alternative to no reperfusion is bleak. Other causes of shock should be excluded in such cases (tamponade, free wall rupture, ventricular septal defect, or rupture of a papillary muscle) prior to administering thrombolytic therapy.

RIGHT VENTRICULAR INFARCTION

The right ventricle is involved to varying extents in inferior-posterior wall MI in about 30 percent of cases. Because the left heart filling pressures are low, there is ordinarily absence of pulmonary edema, despite jugular venous distention. Administration of even small doses of nitroglycerin to these patients may further decrease preload, possibly resulting in hypotension. Marginal hypotension in right ventricular infarct usually responds to augmentation of preload with boluses of saline solution. Nitroglycerin may be administered to control recurrent episodes of ischemia, but it should be administered in concert with fluid. Dobutamine is necessary to augment both right and left ventricular forward flow when hypotension is present that is unresponsive to fluid boluses. When transvenous pacing is required for a conduction disturbance, dual chamber AV sequential pacing affords better right ventricular contraction than does single chamber pacing.

INDICATIONS FOR TEMPORARY PACING IN ACUTE MI

Disturbances of conduction distal to the AV node and His bundle, as occurs in complete heart block with a ventricular escape rhythm, are worrisome, even if they are tolerated well hemodynamically. Ventricular foci are unstable and their discharge rate may vary widely, with abrupt acceleration to ventricular tachycardia or deceleration to asystole. Any bradyarrhythmia unresponsive to atropine that results in hemodynamic compromise requires pacing. Pacing for LBBB remains controversial. Other indications include third degree AV block in the presence of anterior-lateral MI, alternating LBBB and RBBB, new bifasicular block, new RBBB, new first degree AV block and LBBB or RBBB, new first degree AV block and pre-existing bifasicular block, and type II second degree AV block with wide complex QRS. Another indication considered controversial is third degree AV block or type II second degree AV block with narrow QRS escape in inferior wall MI that is tolerated well hemodynamically.

For further reading in *Principles of Critical Care,* see Chap 116 "Myocardial Ischemia" John T Barron/Joseph E Parrillo, Chap 119 "Anticoagulants and Thrombolytic Agents" Gregory A Schmidt

J. Edward Jordan

Approximately 630,000 cases of pulmonary embolism (PE) occur each year resulting in nearly 200,000 deaths. Present estimates suggest pulmonary emboli are undiagnosed at death in 70 percent of patients. The mortality in correctly diagnosed and treated cases is 8 percent but may be as high as 30 percent in untreated cases. Barriers to the assessment of history and physical exam in the setting of organ failure, pulmonary infiltrates, and cardiovascular dysfunction complicate diagnosis in critically ill patients. Accurate diagnosis is required due to the 10% risk of significant bleeding with systemic anticoagulation.

PATHOPHYSIOLOGY

Clinical manifestations of thrombus embolization are due to occlusion of the pulmonary vessels with subsequent hemodynamic and gas exchange abnormalities. Occlusion of the pulmonary vasculature creates areas of lung which are ventilated but not perfused (dead space). Patients will typically increase minute ventilation ($\dot{V}_E$) in order to maintain a constant or reduced $Paco_2$. Mechanically ventilated patients who cannot increase $\dot{V}_E$ will experience a rise in $Paco_2$, a fall in end tidal CO_2, ($ETCO_2$), and an increasing disparity between the two. Patients who hyperventilate will usually not show a precipitous fall in PaO_2, however, the alveolar-arterial O_2 gradient ($[A–a])O_2$) will widen. Since many patients with pulmonary emboli will not demonstrate hypoxemia, a normal PaO_2 should not be used to exclude the diagnosis of PE. Severe pulmonary outflow tract obstruction may reduce cardiac output ($\dot{Q}_T$), lowering mixed venous oxygen saturation (S_VO_2). If the increase in right sided heart pressures is dramatic, right ventricular failure may occur.

CLINICAL MANIFESTATIONS

Communicative patients are very likely to report symptoms of acute dyspnea, pleuritic chest pain, apprehension, or cough. The minority of patients will present with signs or symptoms of deep venous thrombosis (DVT), hemoptysis, palpitations, or syncope. On examination, 90 percent of patients are tachypneic, about one half of patents will have fever, tachycardia, or increased P_2. Only one-third of patients will have signs of a DVT and 5 percent will present with shock.

The chest x-ray usually shows nonspecific findings. Its principle use is to rule out other diagnoses such as pneumonia, pneumothorax, or aortic dissection. Twelve-lead electrocardiography may reveal signs of right heart strain, but usually shows only sinus tachycardia. More invasive monitoring may offer more specific clues for the diagnosis of PE. Unexplained increases in $\dot{V}_E$, falls in $ETCO_2$, or a widening difference between $ETCO_2$ and $PaCO_2$ should suggest the diagnosis of PE. Muscle relaxed patients with a fixed minute ventilation may demonstrate unexplained rises in $PaCO_2$. Pulmonary artery catheterization may reveal acute elevation in right atrial and ventricular pressure, fall in ($\dot{Q}_T$), widening difference between the pulmonary diastolic pressure and capillary wedge pressure, or a fall in the $S_{\bar{V}}O_2$. Unfortunately, each of these findings is nonspecific and they rarely appear all in concert.

Echocardiographic (transthoracic and transesophageal) findings suggestive of PE include a dilated, thin walled, poorly contractile right ventricle with possible bowing of the interventricular septum to the left, reducing left ventricular filling.

DIAGNOSIS

Accurate diagnosis requires weighing the risks of PE and understanding the limitations of diagnostic tests. The index of suspicion should be raised for patients who demonstrate an unusual number of risk factors (Table 24-1). Further workup should be guided by an individualized approach given the clinical setting and the likelihood of PE (Figure 24-1). Noninvasive leg studies (impedance plethysmography, venous doppler, venous ultrasound, phleborrheography) offer a safe means to diagnose DVT of the leg and thus may justify the initiation of anticoagulation. However, almost one third of patients with proven PE have negative noninvasive leg studies. An inconclusive study should not rule out the diagnosis in patients for whom clinical suspicion is high. Perfusion lung scans have a very limited role as many common disorders may render an abnormal study. On the other hand, a normal study may be useful in eliminating the diagnosis. "High probability" $\dot{V}/\dot{Q}$ scans have a specificity of 85 percent and are therefore helpful in making the diagnosis. Intermediate and low probability studies generally warrant further workup.

TABLE 24-1 Risk Factors for Pulmonary Embolism

Epidemiologic Factors: Obesity, prior thromboembolism, advanced age, malignancy (especially adenocarcinoma), estrogens.

Venous Stasis: Immobility, paralysis, leg casts, varicose veins, congestive heart failure, prolonged travel, and use of muscle relaxants

Injury: post surgical, posttrauma, postpartum

Hypercoagulable States: Proteins C and S and antithrombin-III deficiency, lupus anticoagulant, polycythemia, macroglobulinemia

Indwelling Lines: Central venous and pulmonary artery catheters

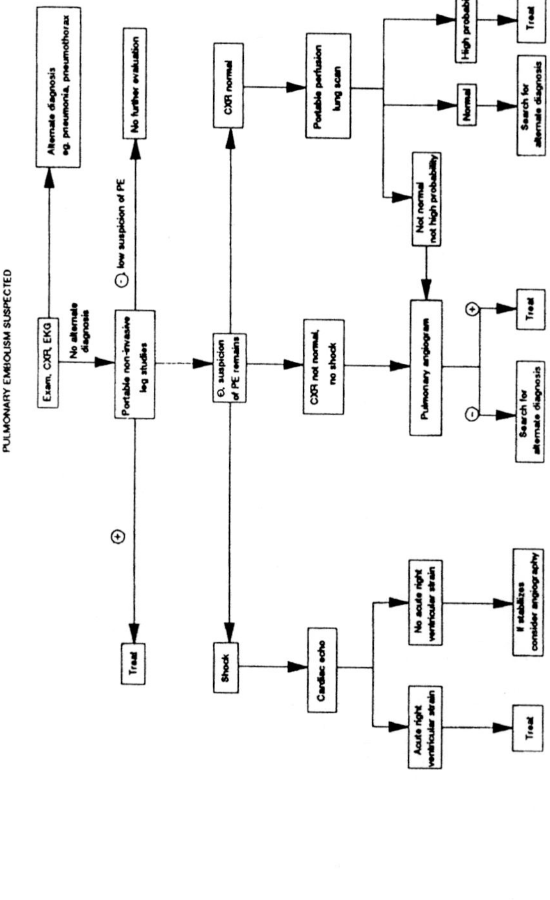
PULMONARY EMBOLISM SUSPECTED
Exam, CXR, EKG
Alternate diagnosis
eg. pneumonia, pneumothorax
No alternate diagnosis
Portable non-invasive leg studies
+
Treat
−, low suspicion of PE
No further evaluation
−, suspicion of PE remains
Shock
Cardiac echo
Acute right ventricular strain
Treat
No acute right ventricular strain
If stabilizes consider angiography
CXR not normal, no shock
Pulmonary angiogram
−
Search for alternate diagnosis
+
Treat
CXR normal
Portable perfusion lung scan
Not normal not high probability
Normal
Search for alternate diagnosis
High probability
Treat

FIG. 24-1

Pulmonary angiography remains the gold standard for the diagnosis of PE; however, it risks moving the patient to the radiology suite for an invasive test involving contrast material. Pulmonary hypertension is no longer considered to be an absolute contraindication to pulmonary angiography, and with the practice of selective angiography, mortality has been found to be approximately 2 percent in even the sickest patients.

THERAPY

Patients with suspected PE should be given supplemental oxygen and placed at bedrest to reduce oxygen consumption and decrease the possibility of dislodging an existent clot. Muscle relaxation and mechanical ventilation may be necessary to reduce O_2 consumption in patients with shock. Heparin anticoagulation is begun if not contraindicated as described below and continued for 7 to 10 days (see Figure 24-2). After two days of heparin therapy, oral warfarin is begun to allow for continued systemic anticoagulation, unless the patient is unstable. If the patient is not a candidate for prolonged systemic anticoagulation, inferior vena caval interruption is necessary. Thrombolytic agents may be useful in cases of severe PE with shock.

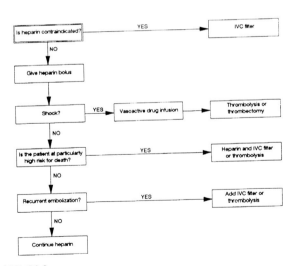

FIG. 24-2

Contraindications to Systemic Anticoagulation

Absolute contraindications include active serious bleeding, intracranial bleeding, and recent (< 2 weeks) central nervous system injury or eye surgery. Relative contraindications include recent major surgery, uncontrolled hypertension, large nonhemorrhagic stroke, bleeding diathesis, hepatic or renal failure, and heparin induced thrombocytopenia.

Anticoagulation

Heparin

Heparin is typically started with a bolus of 7,500 to 10,000 U followed by a constant infusion (e.g., 1000 U/h) to prolong the partial thromboplastin time (PTT) to 1.5 to 2.5 times its normal value. If the PTT is < 1.5 times the control value, the heparin infusion should be increased by 100 U/h and rechecked in four h. If the PTT is > 2.5 times control, the infusion should be stopped for one hour and the heparin infusion decreased 100 U/h. It should be a principle goal to have the patient therapeutically anticoagulated with heparin within several h. After thrombolytic agents heparin is begun at 1000 U/h and the PTT maintained 1.5 to 2.0 times control.

Complications of heparin use include bleeding, immune mediated thrombocytopenia, hypoaldosteronism, and rarely anaphylaxis. Heparin induced thrombocytopenia may occur three to fifteen days after the start of therapy and is not seen with highly purified low-molecular weight heparins.

Warfarin

Warfarin sodium (5 mg po qd) should be started when the patient has stabilized with the goal of elevating the prothrombin time (PT) to 1.3 to 1.5 times its normal value. It should overlap with heparin therapy for about five days. Many drugs affect the metabolism of warfarin, (e.g., antibiotics, H2 blockers, antiepileptics). Vitamin K negates the effect of warfarin and may be used to reverse anticoagulation. Complications of warfarin therapy include an increased risk of bleeding, skin necrosis, and teratogenesis during pregnancy.

Thrombolysis

Thrombolytic therapy has been shown to reduce right heart pressures due to acute PE; however, it has not been shown to improve survival. Given the risk of significant complications, thrombolytic therapy is reserved for patients with proven PE and shock. Contraindications to thrombolytic therapy are listed in Table 24-2. Protocols for the use of several thrombolytic agents are listed in Table

TABLE 24-2 Contraindications to Thrombolytic Therapy

Absolute
Trauma (including CPR) or major surgery within 10 days
Recent puncture in a noncompressible site
Active or recent internal bleeding
Hemorrhagic diathesis
Recent central nervous system surgery or active intracranial lesion
Uncontrolled hypertension (blood pressure > 180/110)
Known hypersensitivity, or for SK, use of SK within 6 months
Diabetic hemorrhagic retinopathy
Acute pericarditis
Recent obstetrical delivery
History of stroke

Relative
Pregnancy
High likelihood of left ventricular thrombus
Advanced age
Liver disease

24-3. Arterial and venous punctures should be avoided. Clinical monitoring should include serial neurologic assessments and frequent vital signs. Recent puncture sites should be frequently inspected for signs of bleeding. Pulse oximetry should be used instead of arterial blood gases to monitor oxygenation. After any of the thrombolytic agents is administered, heparin is usually started at 1000 U/h IV (no bolus) and titrated to a PTT of 1.5 to 2.0 times control.

The principle complications of thrombolytic use are bleeding and allergic reactions. There is a 20% risk of hemorrhage in patients with PE who are treated with SK or rt-PA which seems to be related to the number of vascular puncture sites, the duration of lytic therapy, and coadministration of antiplatelet agents or heparin. When serious hemorrhage occurs, the thrombolytic agent should be discontinued, multiple large bore IV catheters should be secured, and consideration given to reversing the effects of heparin with protamine. Cryoprecipitate, fresh frozen plasma, and platelets may be used to reverse the lytic state.

TABLE 24-3 Selected Thrombolytic Regimens

1. UK: 4400 U/kg bolus, followed by 4400 U/kg/h for 24 h
2. UK: 1,000,000 U bolus over 10 min., followed by 2,000,000 U over 110 min.
3. UK: 15,000 U/kg bolus over 10 min.
4. rt-PA: 0.6 mg/kg bolus over 2 min.
5. rt-PA: 100 mg over 2–3 h
6. SK: 250,000 U over 30 min., followed by 100,000 U/h for 24 h

Inferior Vena Caval Interruption

Patients who cannot tolerate anticoagulation should have a vena caval filter placed to prevent embolization of clot from leg veins to the lungs.

Fluid and Vasoactive Drug Administration

Volume administration does not usually improve hemodynamics in patients with PE and shock and may cause overfilling of the right ventricle, leading to right ventricular failure. Vasoactive drugs often improve cardiac output while lowering filling pressures. Dobutamine (5 to 10 μg/kg/min) should be tried first, as in other patients with right heart shock. Norepinephrine has been shown to be beneficial in animal models of PE and is recommended when hypoperfusion is not corrected with dobutamine. Choice of drug and infusion rate should be guided by improvement in global perfusion (cardiac output), not blood pressure.

Embolectomy

Surgical removal of the clot from the pulmonary vasculature is a potential therapy in cases of massive PE. Patients are placed on cardiopulmonary bypass while the embolus is removed. Embolectomy is indicated for cases of massive PE in patients who can not be anticoagulated. Unfortunately, most patients are moribund or stabilized on medical therapy before this complex procedure can be performed.

PROPHYLAXIS

PE is a potentially lethal disorder which is largely preventable. Subcutaneous "minidose" heparin (5000 U twice daily) has been shown to be effective in the reduction of PE in general medical, stroke, and cardiac patients. There is overwhelming evidence that routine preoperative minidose heparin saves lives without serious complications. Intermittent pneumatic compression cuffs may be employed when heparin is contraindicated. Patients with an extremely high risk of PE should be considered for elective IVC filter placement.

For further reading in *Principles of Critical Care,* see Chap 118 "Pulmonary Embolic Disorders: Thrombus, Air, and Fat" Gregory A Schmidt, Chap 119 "Anticoagulants and Thrombolytic Agents" Gregory A Schmidt

25

Rhythm Disturbances

C.A. Manthous

Successful management of rhythm disturbances in the critical care unit depends upon prompt recognition and treatment. Critically ill patients often have coexistent illnesses which predispose to arrhythmia. Furthermore, renal and hepatic dysfunction are common and impact on metabolism of drugs used to treat these disorders. Chapter 5 discusses the emergent management of arrhythmia as per ACLS (Advanced Cardiac Life Support) protocols. As a general rule arrhythmias that cause signs or symptoms require treatment. When organ hypoperfusion occurs secondary to a rhythm disturbance, electrical cardioversion, defibrillation or pacing are the treatments of choice except in a short list of rhythms described below.

BRADYCARDIA

Bradycardia may be defined as a ventricular rate less than 60 beats per min. Bradycardia, by this definition, can occur in normal healthy volunteers, but assumes more importance when it is symptomatic.

Sinus Bradycardia

Sinus bradycardia occurs when the sinus node fails to depolarize in automatic fashion or when the depolarization fails to propagate out of the sinus node. Sinus node blocks are rare and can only be diagnosed by electrophysiologic study (EPS). Failure to discharge is more common and occurs secondary to excessive vagal tone, deficient sympathetic tone, or intrinsic sinus node failure. Degenerative, ischemic, inflammatory or infiltrative processes can cause sinus node failure. In addition, common events in the ICU, including endotracheal suctioning, treatment with β or calcium channel blockers, hypothyroidism, hyperkalemia or abdominal catastrophe may cause bradycardia. When sinus bradycardia causes no symptoms it need not be treated. When hemodynamic compromise (chest pain, syncope, hypotension) occurs during sinus bradycardia, treatment should be instituted. Atropine 0.5 mg every 5 min up to 2.0 mg total is used to antagonize vagal tone that is often responsible for sinus bradycardia. When hypotension is life-threatening, epinephrine 0.5 to 1.0 mg intravenously/endotracheally, every 5 min should be used. In the rare setting of bradycardia with hypertension, isoproterenol by a constant infusion of 1 to 20 mcg/min is indicated. Cardiac pacing should be considered early when the above managements have failed to treat the bradycardia.

Atrioventricular (AV) Block

There are three main types (referred to as degrees) of AV block. First degree block is defined by a PR interval on ECG of greater than 0.2 s. This usually occurs in the AV node and is asymptomatic. Common causes include ischemic heart disease, myocarditis, beta or calcium channel blockade, and digitalis. When first degree block is associated with a widened QRS complex, about half of such patients have more serious conduction system disease warranting further evaluation.

Second degree AV block is defined as intermittent failure of supraventricular depolarizations to be propagated through the AV node. When progressive lengthening of the PR interval precedes a dropped beat the disturbance is referred to as Mobitz I or Wenckebach. Mobitz I block is usually benign but in the setting of myocardial infarction may progress to complete heart block. Mobitz II block occurs when a supraventricular depolarization fails to propagate to the ventricle without preceding PR lengthening. This is considered more severe as it connotes infranodal disease and more often goes on to complete heart block and symptoms. However, unless Mobitz II occurs in the setting of myocardial infarction, myocarditis, endocarditis or coexistent bundle-branch block, pacemaker placement is not indicated in asymptomatic patients. 2:1 AV block is a special case of Mobitz II which likewise requires treatment when symptomatic or when EPS reveals that the site of block is infranodal.

Third degree AV block, also known as complete heart block, is defined by failure of all supraventricular impulses to reach the ventricles. Tissues with automaticity below the level of block will usually depolarize the ventricles in a phenomenon termed *escape*. When the origin of escape is in the AV node the rate is 45 to 60/min, while an origin in the ventricles leads to a rate of 30 to 40/min. The most common etiologies for third degree block in the ICU are myocardial infarction, endocarditis, trauma, cardiac surgery, or drugs. Since most patients with complete heart block are symptomatic, urgent therapy is required. Atropine, epinephrine or isoproterenol may be used in the doses delineated above until external, then internal pacing is placed.

TACHYARRHYTHMIAS

Tachycardia may be generally defined as a ventricular rate exceeding 100 beats per min. Tachycardias may be divided into two main categories: wide and narrow complexes (QRS). Wide complex tachycardia (QRS>12 ms) is most often ventricular tachycardia, especially in the setting of pre-existent structural or ischemic heart disease. Narrow complex tachycardia is most often supraventricular in origin.

Supraventricular Tachycardias (SVT)

Supraventricular tachycardias are defined as arising from a focus above the ventricles. Common causes of SVT are listed in Table 25-1. We will list the more common variants and their treatments. Aside from the specific therapies listed, carotid massage should be attempted (after carotid bruits are ruled out) to aid in diagnosis and treatment of these arrhythmias. Adenosine, an ultra-short acting drug, can block AV conduction allowing proper diagnosis and in some cases, cessation of an SVT.

Sinus tachycardia is the most common rhythm abnormality in the ICU and may occur secondary to a variety of precipitants including those listed in Table 25-1. In addition, sepsis, pneumothorax, cardiac tamponade, pain, and anxiety may also cause resting tachycardia. Treatment requires investigation as to etiology and treatment of the underlying cause. In patients with thyroid storm, aortic dissection, and myocardial infarction with good ventricular function, careful treatment with β-blocking agents is indicated.

TABLE 25-1 Causes of Atrial Ectopy and Atrial Tachyarrhythmias

Hypertensive heart disease
Hyperthyroidism
Pericarditis
Congestive heart failure
Mitral valve disease (mitral stenosis, mitral regurgitation, mitral valve prolapse)
Postcardiac surgery
Sick sinus syndrome
Myocardial infarction
Pulmonary embolism
COPD
Drugs (catecholamines, theophylline, caffeine, nicotine)
Alcohol (either acute intoxication or withdrawal)
Digitalis toxicity
Cardiac contusion
Idiopathic

(Reprinted with permission from Santoro IH, Soble JS, Bump TE: Rhythm Disturbances, in Hall JB, Schmidt GA, Wood LDH: Principles of Critical Care, McGraw-Hill, New York, 1992.)

Intra-atrial reentrant tachycardia (IART) is paroxysmal, with uniform P-wave morphology, occuring secondary to a re-entrant focus in the atria related to structural heart disease and is refractory to most therapies except amiodarone, electrical cardioversion, or overdrive pacing.

Multifocal atrial tachycardia (MAT) waxes and wanes, with changing P-wave morphologies which arise from different sites as a result of atrial enlargement, hypoxia, hypercarbia, or electrolyte disturbances. Treatment of MAT rests on treatment of the underlying pulmonary, metabolic, infectious or cardiac causes. Calcium channel or β-blockers may be effective when pharmacologic therapy is indicated, while digoxin is not useful. Electrical pacing and cardioversion are not efficacious.

Automatic atrial tachycardia (AAT) results from an accelerated atrial focus (uniform P-wave morphology) which depolarizes at a rate of 120 to 200/min. It occurs during myocardial infarction, chronic obstructive pulmonary disease (COPD), alcohol ingestion or electrolyte disturbances. Treatment of the underlying disorder is the mainstay of treatment though the use of AV blocking drugs (digitalis, β-blocker, calcium blocker). Electrical therapies are generally unsuccessful.

Atrial flutter is a reentrant atrial rhythm occurring at a frequency of 250 to 350/min with variable AV conduction, though AV conduction of 150/min often occurs. Digoxin, β blockers or calcium channel blockers usually reduce AV conduction successfully in flutter, though class 1A and 1C drugs, moricizine or amiodarone (see Table 25-2) are used for pharmacologic cardioversion. In emergency situations, electrical cardioversion starting at 50 J should be attempted. Overdrive pacing, when available, may also terminate this rhythm.

Atrial fibrillation is the lack of any organized atrial electrical or mechanical activity. As with flutter, the rate of conduction to the ventricles may vary, and in the setting of a bypass tract (e.g., Wolff-Parkinson-White [WPW]), syndrome, may superconduct leading to dangerously fast tachycardias leading to ventricular fibrillation. Digoxin, β-blockers and calcium channel blockers are used to control AV conduction unless a bypass tract is detected in which case class 1A or 1 C drugs should be used. Verapamil and digoxin are contraindicated in patients with WPW and atrial fibrillation. Class 1A and 1B drugs are indicated for medical cardioversion when a patient is hemodynamically stable. Electrical cardioversion starting at 100 J is indicated for the emergent treatment of atrial fibrillation or for cases refractory to medical management.

Paroxysmal supraventricular tachycardia (PSVT) is the most common SVT other than sinus tachycardia. It results from in-

TABLE 25-2 FDA-Approved Antiarrhythmic Drugs with Their Indications

		FDA-Approved Indications
Class 1. Drugs that block the fast inward sodium channel		
Class 1A	Quinidine	Supraventricular and ventricular arrhythmias
	Procainamide	Life-threatening or symptomatic ventricular arrhythmias
	Disopyramide	Premature ventricular beats and episodes of ventricular tachycardia
Class 1B	Lidocaine	Ventricular arrhythmias
	Tocainide	Life-threatening ventricular arrhythmias
	Mexiletine	Symptomatic ventricular arrhythmias
	Moricizine	Life-threatening ventricular arrhythmias
Class 1C	Flecainide	Life-threatening ventricular arrhythmias
	Encainide	Life-threatening ventricular arrhythmias
	Propafenone	Life-threatening ventricular arrhythmias
Class 2. Drugs that block β receptors		
	Propranolol	Supraventricular and ventricular arrhythmias and inappropriate sinus tachycardia
	Acebutolol	Ventricular premature beats
	Esmolol	Control of ventricular rate in atrial flutter and fibrillation and noncompensatory sinus tachycardia
Class 3. Drugs that delay repolarization		
	Bretylium	Ventricular fibrillation and other life-threatening ventricular arrhythmias
	Amiodarone	Life-threatening recurrent ventricular arrhythmias only when other agents have failed
Class 4. Drugs that block calcium channels		
	Verapamil	Control of ventricular rate in atrial flutter and fibrillation; paroxysmal supraventricular tachycardia (SVT)
Unclassified Drugs		
	Digoxin	Control of ventricular rate in atrial flutter and fibrillation; paroxysmal SVT
	Adenosine	Paroxysmal SVT

(Reprinted with permission from Santoro IH, Soble JS, Bump TE: Rhythm Disturbances, in Hall JB, Schmidt G, Wood LDH: Principles of Critical Care, McGraw-Hill, New York, 1992.)

tranodal re-entry at a rate of 120 to 250/min and is treated with adenosine or a calcium channel blocker (most commonly vera-pamil). Electrical cardioversion can also be useful in terminating this rhythm. PSVT can then be prevented by use of β-blockers, calcium channel blockers or digoxin.

Accelerated junctional tachycardia—Increased automaticity of the AV node may lead to accelerated junctional tachycardia which occur at rates of 70 to 140/min. P waves are inverted in leads II, III, and aVF secondary to retrograde conduction of AV depolarization. This rhythm occurs secondary to a variety of illnesses, especially digitalis toxicity, theophylline toxicity or recent thoracic surgery. Therapy consists of treatment of the underlying cause, while most pharmacologic and electrical therapies are not successful.

Ventricular Arrhythmias

Premature ventricular complexes (PVC) occur commonly and, un-less hemodynamically significant or occurring in runs or salvos, need not be treated. Accelerated idioventricular rhythm is a wide-complex rhythm occurring at a rate which is greater than the normal automaticity of the ventricles occurring at 70 to 110/min, most commonly after myocardial infarction. This rhythm does not re-quire therapy.

Ventricular tachycardia (VT) is a wide complex tachycardia which always requires treatment. The precipitants of VT are listed in Table 25-3. Table 25-4 itemizes the differentiating ECG char-

TABLE 25-3 Causes of Ventricular Ectopy

Cardiac ischemia/infarction	Acid-base disorders
Cardiomyopathies	Hypoxemia
Ischemic	Drugs
Nonischemic, dilated	Digitalis
Hypertrophic	Phenothiazines
Restrictive	Antiarrhythmic agents
Arrhythmogenic right ven-	Tricyclic antidepressants
tricular dysplasia	Excess catecholamine states
Mechanical irritation	Coronary reperfusion
(catheter, pacemaker wire)	Congenital heart disease
Electrolyte disorders	Mitral valve prolapse
Hypokalemia	Idiopathic
Hypomagnesemia	
Hypocalcemia	

(Reprinted with permission from Santoro IH, Soble JS, Bump TE: Rhythm Disturbances, in Hall JB, Schmidt GA, Wood LDH: Principles of Critical Care, McGraw-Hill, New York, 1992.)

TABLE 25-4 Morphologic Criteria Favoring Ventricular Tachycardia during Wide QRS Complex Tachycardia

QRS duration >140 ms with RBBB morphology
QRS duration >160 ms with LBBB morphology
Positive QRS concordance (predominantly positive QRS in all precordial leads)
Extreme left axis deviation ($-90°$ to $\pm 180°$)
Combined LBBB with right axis deviation
Different QRS pattern during tachycardia than baseline in patients with preexisting bundle branch block

(Reprinted with permission from Santoro IH, Soble JS, Bump TE: Rhythm Disturbances, in Hall JB, Schmidt GA, Wood LDH: Principles of Critical Care, McGraw-Hill, New York, 1992.)

acteristics of VT (compared to SVT with aberrant conduction which is much less frequent). Treatment of this arrhythmia is outlined in Chapter 5. In addition, electrolyte abnormalities, hypoxia, and drug intoxications should be ruled out and treated if identified. Briefly hemodynamically stable VT is treated with lidocaine, procainamide, and synchronized cardioversion if necessary. Pulseless VT is treated with electrical defibrillation as if it were ventricular fibrillation. Torsade de pointes is a special case of wide complex tachycardia in which the QRS axis rotates around the isoelectric line. This rhythm, often associated with Class I antiarrhythmic toxicity or electrolyte disorders, is treated with withdrawal of an offending drug, correction of electrolyte disturbances, and intravenous magnesium infusion. Sustained torsades may also respond to cardioversion, overdrive ventricular pacing, or isoproterenol infusion. In some cases of neurologic catastrophe, a β-blocker may also be useful.

Ventricular fibrillation is chaotic ventricular activity leading to complete loss of cardiac output. Treatment is outlined in Chapter 5. Successful resuscitation depends upon rapid electrical defibrillation.

Antiarrhythmic Therapy

The acute management of various arrhythmias is described above. Additional agents (Table 25-2) and their common side effects (Table 25-5) and doses (Table 25-6) are provided. In general, antiarrhythmic medications possess many side effects. Effects common to most of these drugs is that they may increase the propensity to arrhythmia (proarrhythmic effect) in some patients and usually depress myocardial contractility. All of these drugs should be used with caution and only when absolutely required for the acute or chronic suppression of arrhythmia. VT or VF in the perimyocardial

TABLE 25-5 Extracardiac Side Effects of Antiarrhythmic Drugs

Class 1A		
	Quinidine	Diarrhea, hypotension, cinchonism, thrombocytopenia
	Procainamide	Lupus-like syndrome, agranulocytosis
	Disopyramide	Anticholinergic effects (dry mouth, urinary retention, exacerbation of glaucoma)
Class 1B		
	Lidocaine	Confusion, seizures, coma
	Tocainide	Confusion, seizures, coma, agranulocytosis, pulmonary fibrosis
	Mexiletine	Confusion, seizures, coma, nausea
	Moricizine	Light-headedness
Class 1C		
	Flecainide	Dizziness, headache, visual disturbance
	Encainide	Dizziness, headache, visual disturbance
	Propafenone	Dizziness, headache, visual disturbance
Class 2		
	Propranolol	Exacerbation of asthma, lethargy, exacerbation of periperal vascular disease, masking of hypoglycemia
	Acebutolol	Same as propranolol
	Esmolol	Same as propranolol
Class 3		
	Bretylium	Vasodilation and hypotension, parotid pain
	Amiodarone	Intentional tremor and ataxia, pulmonary fibrosis, dermal photosensitivity, constipation, cirrhosis, hypothyroidism or hyperthyroidism
Class 4		
	Verapamil	Constipation, vasodilation, hypotension
Unclassified		
	Digoxin	Nausea, visual disturbance, confusion
	Adenosine	Flushing

(Reprinted with permission from Santoro IH, Soble JS, Bump TE: Rhythm Disturbances, in Hall JB, Schmidt GA, Wood LDH: Principles of Critical Care, McGraw-Hill, New York, 1992.)

infarction period may not require any antiarrhythmic therapy long term.

Radiofrequency catheter ablation and surgical ventriculectomy are useful in selected cases of refractory VT when the focus has been mapped during electrophysiologic studies. Catheter ablation of the AV node has been useful in treatment of super-conducting atrial fibrillation and flutter as well as WPW syndrome. The use of implantable defibrillators for the treatment of VT that cannot be

TABLE 25-6 Doses of Antiarrhythmic Drugs

Drug	Loading Dose	Maintenance Dose	Gastrointestinal Absorption, %	Oral Bio-availability	Therapeutic Plasma Concentration
Digoxin	10–15µg/kg or 0.5–1.0 mg IV/PO then 0.25 mg prn to total 1.0–2.5 mg	0.125–0.750 mg qd IV/PO	75–90	50–80	0.5–2.0 ng/mL
Adenosine	6–12 mg IV	—	—	—	—
Verapamil	2.5–10 mg IV over 2–5 min	2.5–5.0 µg/kg/min or 120–480 mg PO qd	90	10–22	15–100 µg/L
Propranolol	0.5–1.0 mg IV q5 min to 0.1–0.2 mg/kg total dose	10–40 mg PO qid-bid to 320 mg PO total dose	95	20–50	50–100 ng/mL
Atenolol	5 mg IV over 5 min, repeat in 10 min	50 mg PO qd-bid, initiate 10 min after IV dose	50	50	0.2–0.5 µg/mL
Metoprolol	5 mg IV q 5 min to total dose 15 mg	5O mg PO bid to total dose 450 mg PO qd	95	50	50–100 ng/mL
Labetalol	0.25 mg/kg IV (or 20 mg) over 2 min, repeat 40, 80 mg IV prn	2 mg/min IV or 100–400 mg PO bid	95	25	0.7–3.0 µg/mL
Esmolol	500 µg/kg/min IV	50–300 µg/kg/min IV	—	—	—
Quinidine	5–7 mg/kg IV at 20 mg/min (gluconate) or 600–1000 mg PO (sulfate)	10–30 mg/kg total dose PO divided bid-qid depending on preparation	95	70–80	2.0–5.0 µ/mL

(continued)

TABLE 25-6 Doses of Antiarrhythmic Drugs (continued)

Drug	Loading Dose	Maintenance Dose	Gastrointestinal Absorption, %	Oral Bio-availability	Therapeutic Plasma Concentration
Procainamide	15–20 mg/kg IV at 20 mg/min to total dose 1.0 g or 1000 mg PO (standard preparation)	1–4 mg/min IV or 50–100 mg/kg total dose PO divided tid-qid depending on preparation	70–90	70–90	Procainamide 5–10 μg/mL NAPA 10–30 μg/mL
Disopyramide	300–400 mg PO (standard preparation)	Standard 100–400 mg PO qid; CR 200–300 mg PO bid	80–100	90	3–6 μg/mL
Lidocaine	1.0 mg/kg IV; 0.5 mg/kg in 10 min to total dose 3.0 mg/kg	30–50 μg/kg/min or 1–4 mg/min	—	—	1–5 μg/mL
Encainide	0.6–1.0 mg/kg IV over 15 min	25–50 mg PO tid-qid	95	7–82	1–56 ng/mL
Flecainide	1.5–2.0 mg/kg IV	100–200 mg PO bid	95	95	0.2–1.0 μg/mL
Moricizine	—	200–300 mg PO tid	—	38	0.1–0.3μg/mL
Mexiletine	0.5–1.5 mg/min IV or 400 mg PO	200–400 mg PO tid	90	88	0.5–2.0 μg/mL
Propafenone	1–2 mg/kg IV or 600–900 mg PO	150–300 mg PO tid	95	25–75	0.5–2.0 μg/mL
Bretylium	5 mg/kg IV; repeat bolus 10 mg/kg q15–30 min to total dose 30 mg/kg	0.5–2.0 mg/min IV	—	—	0.6–20.0 μg/mL
Phenytoin	1.0 g at 20 mg/min	300 mg PO qd	—	57–85	6.0–20 mg/L
Amiodarone	5–10 mg/kg IV over 5–10 min or 800–1600 mg qd PO	200–800 mg PO qd	—	22–88	1.0–2.5 μg/mL

(Reprinted with permission from Santoro IH, Soble JS, Bump TE: Rhythm Disturbances, in Hall JB, Schmidt GA, Wood LDH: Principles of Critical Care, McGraw-Hill, New York, 1992.)

pharmacologically managed prevents sudden death but is expensive and requires major surgery.

For further reading in *Principles of Critical Care*, see Chap 47 "Resuscitation and Stabilization" William F Rutherford/Edward A Panacek, Chap 120 "Rhythm Disturbances" Ian H Santoro/Jeffrey S Soble/Thomas E Bump

---

26

Pericardial Involvement in Critical Illness

Allan Garland

In any critically ill patient with an acute or subacute low cardiac output state, pericardial disease must be considered and excluded from other potential etiologies (see Chap. 22). There is a broad spectrum of pathologic conditions which affect the pericardium, and in the great majority of cases they do not cause hemodynamic embarrassment. When one of these states does result in hemodynamic compromise it does so primarily by interfering with cardiac filling, either via cardiac tamponade secondary to a hemodynamically significant pericardial effusion, constrictive pericarditis, or a combination of tamponade and constriction resulting in "effusive-constrictive" physiology.

The underlying process can develop rapidly, as effusive disease frequently does, or slowly as is most common with constrictive disease. However, even with a chronic pericardial process, a patient's clinical condition can deteriorate acutely. *Pericardial disease must be considered in all patients with low cardiac output syndromes and elevated right atrial pressures.*

NORMAL PHYSIOLOGY OF CARDIAC FILLING

Understanding the events of ventricular filling is the key to distinguishing between cardiac tamponade and constrictive pericarditis. The double layer of pericardium encloses the atria and ventricles. In principle the elastance (inverse of compliance) of the cardiac chambers is the sum of the elastances of the myocardial and pericardial elements. In health there is minimal pericardial fluid and the pericardium has relatively little effect on the pressure-volume characteristics of the cardiac chambers. Additionally, the intrapericardial pressure approximates the negative pressure that exists within the pleural space and mediastinum.

Consideration of the atrial and ventricular pressure waves, as well as of blood flow across the atrioventricular (AV) valves allows us to follow the events of cardiac filling. Early in diastole, passive flow from atrium to ventricle is especially favored by the low pressure in the relaxing ventricle; this rapid ventricular filling phase is characterized by a fall in the atrial pressure tracing, known as the *y* descent. Next, with atrial systole there is a rapid rise in atrial pressure (the *a* wave) with an increase in flow across the AV valves. With the onset of ventricular systole, the atrial pressure initially declines during the isovolumic relaxation phase of the atrium (*x* descent), and then rises as atrial filling continues while the AV valve is closed and the ventricle actively contracts (the *v* wave). Alteration in the atrial pressure waveform from the usual appearance of the sequence (*a* wave—*x* descent—*v* wave—*y* descent), is an important sign of hemodynamically significant pericardial disease.

With spontaneous inspiration, there is a fall in intrathoracic and intrapericardial (and hence extracardiac) pressures, and venous return increases. With this increased right-sided filling, and as dictated by the compliance characteristics of the right atrium and ventricle, transmural pressures increase. This is effected by a fall in intrapericardial pressure which is larger than the fall in right atrial pressure. Hence, right atrial pressure normally falls with inspiration.

PATHOPHYSIOLOGY OF ALTERED HEMODYNAMICS IN PERICARDIAL EFFUSIVE DISEASE

When intrapericardial pressures exceed 15 to 20 mmHg, cardiac tamponade is likely. In tamponade, all four cardiac chambers are enclosed within a tense bag of free flowing pericardial fluid which severely restricts cardiac filling at all chamber volumes. In this situation, the passive pressure-volume relationship (i.e., compliance) of each chamber is dominated by the mechanical properties of the pericardium and its fluid contents. Thus any attempt to increase the volume of a single chamber will be opposed by the application of increased pressure to the external surface of all chambers by the tense bag of pericardial fluid. The result is elevated diastolic pressures, equalization of simultaneously measured intrapericardial and diastolic (usually right atrial) pressures, and diastolic equalization of pressures in all chambers. As a consequence of the last of these alterations, early diastolic ventricular filling does not occur, as reflected by the absence of the *y* descent in the atrial pressure tracing (Fig. 26-1).

The increased intrapericardial pressure, along with the limited chamber filling, requires that transmyocardial diastolic pressures be reduced in tamponade. For the ventricles this means that they will be operating on the low end of their Frank-Starling function curves and ejecting small stroke volumes.

In a spontaneously breathing patient with cardiac tamponade, the fall in intrathoracic pressure with inspiration is transmitted to the pericardial surface and on through the fluid to the chambers. Consequently, the recorded right atrial diastolic pressure will decrease with inspiration, as in the normal situation. In addition, the increased venous return leads to augmented right ventricular filling with inspiration, which because of the limited intrapericardial volume, results in leftward shift of the interventricular septum, further impeding filling of the left ventricle. The Frank-Starling relation of

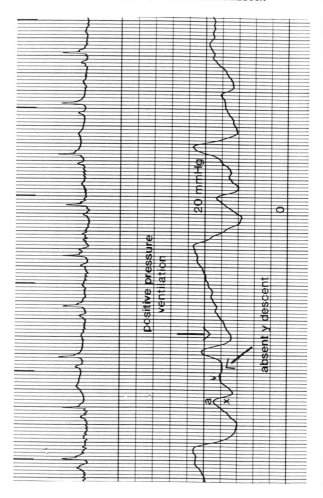

the heart then dictates that as a consequence of this, the resultant contraction generates a smaller pressure. The resultant fall in arterial blood pressure with inspiration (a fall of > 10 mmHg is considered abnormal) is the *pulsus paradoxus*.

PATHOPHYSIOLOGY OF ALTERED HEMODYNAMICS IN CONSTRICTIVE PERICARDITIS

In contrast to cardiac tamponade, in constrictive pericarditis, there is no pathologic limitation to cardiac filling at low cardiac volume. Thus the chambers fill freely in early diastole, until they suddenly come up against the limitation imposed by the thickened, rigid pericardium whose maximum volume is fixed. For the remainder of diastole the situation is essentially akin to that in tamponade, previously mentioned. These events give rise to the classic "square root" appearance of the pressure waveform of the ventricles (Fig. 26-2). The point at which there is equalization of diastolic pressures in all four chambers depends upon the intravascular volume status of the patient; there will reliably be equalization at end-diastole, with increasing intravascular volume resulting in earlier encroachment of diastolic cardiac volume upon the pericardial limitation, and thus earlier equalization.

In the atrial pressure tracing, rapid early ventricular filling (the *y* descent during passive atrial emptying) is followed by the abrupt opposition to further atrial emptying both during the balance of diastole and during atrial systole (*a* wave). Systolic emptying of the ventricles enables the subsequent release of the impediment to atrial filling causing a rapid *x* descent. The result of these events is exaggerated peaks and valleys—the classic M shape—of the right atrial tracing (Fig. 26-3).

During inspiration, diaphragmatic movement causes the intrathoracic pressure to fall and the intra-abdominal pressure to rise. This causes increased venous return which, in the face of the rigid pericardium and the inflexible limitation to diastolic atrial filling present, leads to an increase in right atrial pressure with inspiration; this is the origin of the Kussmaul sign of rising neck veins during inspiration seen in constrictive pericarditis.

PATHOPHYSIOLOGY OF ALTERED HEMODYNAMICS IN EFFUSIVE-CONSTRICTIVE DISEASE

A patient may have both a hemodynamically significant pericardial effusion, and a rigid, thickened pericardium. In these cases, most

FIG. 26-1 Right atrial pressure from a patient with cardiac tamponade during mechanical ventilation. Note the absent *y* descent and the blunting of the waveforms, especially during positive-pressure ventilation.

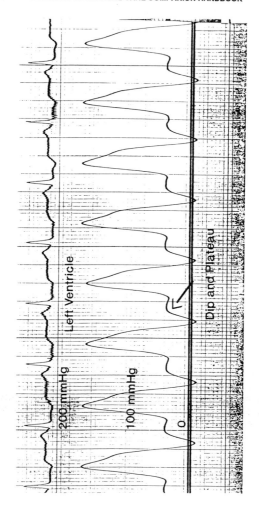

commonly seen in patients treated for malignancy, the hemodynamic presentation is of tamponade. Only after drainage of the effusion are the physiologic changes associated with constriction apparent.

ETIOLOGY

A wide variety of conditions may result in tamponade and/or constrictive pericarditis (see Table 26-1). Typically, effusions tend to be seen early in the course of these conditions, with either effusion or pericarditis seen later.

Idiopathic cases are common and are often preceeded by a viral syndrome days to weeks prior to clinical manifestations of pericardial disease.

A wide variety of infective organisms can be causative, with viruses being the most common. Amongst the viruses, Coxsackie virus Type B is the most commonly identified agent, with Coxsackie Type A, Echo Type A, influenza, mumps, Epstein-Barr, cytomegalovirus and other viruses also having been reported. Purulent pericarditis is rare, even in patients with systemic infections or with immunosuppressed states. When it does occur, it is more frequently a result of contiguous extension from an intrathoracic focus than blood borne spread from a distant site. Infection of the pericardium may occur with bacteria (a wide variety of both Gram+ and Gram− organisms), and more rarely fungi (esp. *Histoplasma*, *Coccidioides*), eubacteria (*Actinomyces*, *Nocardia*) or parasites (esp. *Entameoba*, *Echinococcus*). Tuberculous pericardial infection is usually accompanied by pulmonary tuberculosis (TB), but may occur as the sole clinical manifestation of infection; acid-fast bacteria are rarely seen in pericardial fluid and diagnosis depends upon histopathology and culture of fluid and of pericardial tissue.

Uremia may cause pericardial effusion or constriction. Intensive hemodialysis may result in resolution, but in some patients this complication of renal failure will worsen, or even first develop, while being adequately dialyzed.

Neoplastic causes are common in adults. Metastatic disease (esp. cancer of the lung and breast, lymphomas, and leukemias) is more common than primary malignant or benign tumors of the pericardium. Amongst primary neoplasms, mesothelioma is most commonly seen. It should be noted, however, that nearly half of all pericardial effusions arising in cancer patients are not malignant.

FIG. 26-2 Left ventricular pressure in a patient with constrictive pericarditis. Note the dip and plateau caused by rapid inflow of blood early in diastole, with little filling in the last two-thirds.

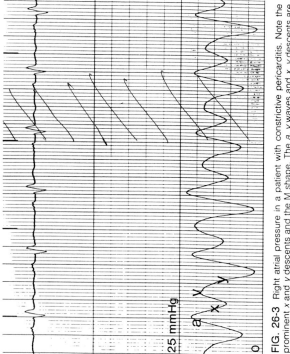

FIG. 26-3 Right atrial pressure in a patient with constrictive pericarditis. Note the prominent x and y descents and the M shape. The a, v waves and x, y descents are as described in text

25 mmHg

a v
x
y

0

TABLE 26-1 Differential Diagnosis of Hemodynamically Significant Pericardial Disease

Etiology	Effusive	Constrictive
Idiopathic	X	X
Infection[a]	X	X
early	X	
late	X	X
Renal failure	X	X
Neoplasm	X	X
Connective tissue diseases[b]	X	X
Drugs[c]	X	X
Post-irradiation		
early	X	
late	X	X
Post-myocardial infarction (Dressler's syndrome)		
early	X	
late		X
Postpericardiotomy		
early	X	
late		X
Trauma		
early	X	
late	X	X

[a]including viral, bacterial, tuberculous, fungal, parasitic
[b]including SLE, RA, MCTD, PSS, PAN, Wegener's granulomatosis, polymyositis, Reiter's syndrome, serum sickness. In children ARF.
[c]including PCN, INH, methysergide, daunorubicin, emetine, cromolyn, minoxidil, bleomycin, cyclophosphamide, and any causes of drug-induced SLE.

Most of the connective tissue diseases have been reported in association with pericardial disease. In children, acute rheumatic fever is the leading association, while in adults, systemic lupus erythematosis and rheumatoid arthritis are more common associations than are systemic sclerosis, mixed connective tissue disease, polyarteritis nodosum, and others.

Tamponade or constriction may occur after a variety of mechanical insults to the thoracic contents. Penetrating trauma to the chest may cause hemopericardium or lead to pericardial infection. In addition, when it occurs, hemodynamically significant pericardial disease typically appears weeks to months, and sometimes as much as years, after thoracic surgery (usually post-pericardiotomy but occasionally after noncardiac procedures), acute myocardial infarction (Dressler's syndrome), blunt chest trauma, or high dose radiation to the mediastinum.

Drugs can lead to pericardial disease by causing drug-induced lupus (e.g. hydralazine, procainamide), or via unknown mechanisms. In this latter category, penicillin, isoniazid, methysergide, daunorubicin, emetine, cromolyn, minoxidil, bleomycin, cyclophosphamide, and other drugs have been reported.

Among miscellaneous causes are aortic dissection, myocardial perforation, sarcoidosis, myxedema, and asbestosis.

CLINICAL AND DIAGNOSTIC ASPECTS

Signs and symptoms may be useful to suggest the presence of cardiac tamponade or pericardial constriction. However, their sensitivity is not sufficiently great and objective evaluation is always necessary. Central venous or intracardiac pressure monitoring can be useful, but echocardiography is the best noninvasive method of evaluating both the anatomic status of the pericardium and the hemodynamic significance of abnormalities.

Both effusive and constrictive disease are marked by a low cardiac output state with elevated jugular venous pulsation (usually >20 cm H_2O) and usually accompanied by systemic hypotension, a decreased pulse pressure and tachycardia. A pericardial friction rub may be present or absent in either condition.

In tamponade the heart sounds are usually muffled and palpation of the precordium demonstrates soft impulses. The jugular venous pulsations demonstrate their usual fall during inspiration but are elevated with less noticeable fluctuations than normal. A pulsus paradoxus is usually present. The chest X-ray shows the characteristic enlarged "water-bottle" heart shadow with rapid tapering toward the great vessels; this finding may be absent, however, when tamponade is due to hyperacute causes such as aortic dissection. The electrocardiogram (ECG) findings, which are relatively insensitive, include decreased QRS voltage, and a changing QRS axis from beat to beat (electrical alternans) caused by the shifting position of the heart within the pericardial fluid. Intravascular pressure and waveform monitoring demonstrates elevated diastolic pressures, equal end-diastolic pressures (i.e., the right atrial a wave, RVEDP, pulmonary wedge a wave, and LVEDP), and an absent y descent in the atrial pressure waveform (Fig. 26-1). In addition to the effusion, echocardiographic signs of tamponade include right atrial compression throughout the cardiac cycle, right ventricular compression in diastole, leftward septal shift during inspiration, and decreased transmitral and transaortic Doppler flows.

In constrictive pericarditis there may be an early diastolic knock and the precordium is often hyperdynamic on palpation. The neck veins are elevated, demonstrate a fluttering appearance, and become further elevated with inspiration (Kussmaul's sign). Rarely, a pulsus paradoxus will be present. On X-ray the cardiac silhouette can be of any size, but more than 60 percent of cases demonstrate pericardial calcification best seen on the lateral chest X-ray. Many changes may be seen on ECG in pericarditis; early in the course these include diffuse ST-segment elevations and PR-segment depressions, followed later by replacement of those abnormalities by diffuse T-wave inversions. In practice these findings are not sufficiently sensitive or specific to be of much diagnostic value in the critically ill patient. Intravascular monitoring demonstrates elevated diastolic pressures, equal end-diastolic pressure in right and left ventricles, the square root sign in the ventricular pressure waveforms (Figure 26-2), and the M-shaped appearance of the right atrial pressure tracing (Figure 26-3). In constriction the M-mode echocardiogram can be suggestive. Findings may include thickened pericardium, flattening of the left ventricular free wall during the last part of diastole, a shuttering motion of the interventricular septum as diastolic filling suddenly stops, premature opening of the pulmonic valve, and pericardial calcifications.

The newer modalities of rapid-sequence computed tomography (CT) or magnetic resonance imaging (MRI) have high sensitivity for detecting pericardial thickening or effusion, and in addition can provide data on the hemodynamic significance of the changes.

ACUTE THERAPY OF HEMODYNAMIC COMPROMISE

Tamponade

The prime consideration in acute therapy is relief of hemodynamic compromise via a drainage procedure. Immediate medical management prior to drainage consists of intravenous fluid administration, which will often improve the stroke volume of both ventricles despite accentuating pulsus paradoxus. There is no evidence that inotropic agents or vasodilators in any way alter the hemodynamics of tamponade.

There is not a consensus as to the best drainage procedure. It is believed that long-term survival depends on the underlying disease rather than the type of drainage procedure performed.

Pericardiocentesis is a lifesaving procedure which can be performed safely and quickly at the bedside; electrocardiography, fluoroscopy, or echocardiography to guide needle placement is extremely useful and increases the success and safety of the procedure. Often, removal of just a small amount of the pericardial effusion will result in rapid hemodynamic improvement. Any bloody fluid obtained should be tested for clotting; nonclotting blood confirms that aspiration from the pericardium has occurred while clotting blood signals ventricular puncture. Using the Seldinger technique, a catheter can be left in place for ongoing drainage. Complications are not uncommon, are seen more frequently with smaller effusions, and include arrhythmias, ventricular perforation, coronary artery or internal mammary artery laceration, pneumothorax, and phrenic nerve injury. The immediate success rate of this technique is high, but the recurrence rate is greater than 50% and frequently patients require subsequent, more definitive, surgical therapy. However, *in patients with clear hemodynamic compromise, needle drainage is the procedure of choice.*

Subxiphoid pericardiostomy can be performed under local or general anesthesia and has a high rate of success. The immediate success rate is nearly 100 percent, but about one-third of patients develop recurrent effusion or constriction. Contrary to common understanding, this technique does not create a permanent route for fluid drainage as all mesothelial defects heal quickly. Rather, when successful the procedure leads to obliteration of the pericardial space. This technique is usually the treatment of choice when the hemodynamic compromise is not immediately life-threatening. Formal pericardiectomy clearly increases the short term risks of therapy and is rarely necessary in treating effusive disease.

Rare episodes of pulmonary edema have been reported post-drainage and are probably related to the sudden increase in right ventricular output in patients who have already received large fluid volumes.

Constriction

Constrictive pericarditis needs to be treated with wide surgical pericardiectomy. Patients usually improve quickly, although some degree of diastolic abnormality may persist for months as the epicardium remodels.

For further reading in *Principles of Critical Care,* see Chap 121 "Pericardial Involvement in Critical Illness" Kerry Teplinsky

---

27

Valvular Heart Disease

David Olson

The clinical impact of valvular heart disease is different during critical illness than in the resting state. A valvular lesion which is insignificant at rest may become clinically important under physiologic stress. Assuming optimized hemoglobin and oxygen saturation, four major hemodyamic parameters affecting cardiac output must be addressed in proper management of critically ill patients with valvular disease.

Preload is the force that stretches the cardiac muscle to its precontraction volume and is clinically estimated as the pulmonary capillary wedge pressure (PCWP) or the left ventricular end-diastolic pressure (LVEDP). Preload is related to a patient's volume status and ventricular compliance. *Afterload* is the force opposing contraction and is estimated clinically as the mean aortic pressure. Afterload is largely a function of the systemic vascular resistance. *Contractility* refers to the intrinsic ability of the heart to generate the force and velocity necessary for contraction. *Heart rate* is the final relevant parameter and in conjunction with stroke volume, directly determines cardiac output.

Valvular lesions are clinically important because they limit cardiac output, create abnormal chamber pressures, engender rhythm disturbances, provide a nidus for infection, predispose to systemic embolism, or generate ventricular ischemia. In patients with stenotic lesions, cardiac output is dependent on heart rate, preload, and contractility, while being less dependent on afterload. Regurgitant lesions must be defined as acute or chronic. Minor regurgitation in an acute situation is often more catastrophic than major regurgitation in a chronic setting. Decreasing afterload, increasing preload, and optimizing heart rate are the mainstays of treatment for regurgitant lesions. Relative tachycardia provides too little time for forward flow, while relative bradycardia allows too much time for regurgitant flow.

Diagnosis of valvular heart disease is based on history and physical examination, electrocardiography, and invasive and noninvasive imaging modalities. The history is frequently nonspecific and typical symptoms relate to a low cardiac output state. The physical exam is directed toward cardiac auscultation and evidence of low cardiac output or congestion. The electrocardiogram (ECG) is useful in assessing the cardiac rhythm, chamber enlargement, or chamber hypertrophy. Acute valvular problems usually display nonspecific ECG findings unless ischemia is a precipitating factor. The chest radiograph is important in looking for pulmonary vascular redistribution, cardiac chamber size, and underlying pulmonary pathology. Echocardiography has revolutionized noninvasive imaging of valvular heart disease. Echocardiography can quantify regurgitant and stenotic valve lesions, assess left ventricular function, estimate pulmonary artery pressures, visualize the valves, and help direct therapy. Invasive modalities include pulmonary artery and left heart catheterization. The latter is usually indicated after all medical modalities have been exhausted and surgical intervention or valvuloplasty is planned.

General principles of management of all valvular lesions during superimposed critical illness include arterial blood pressure monitoring, pulmonary artery catheterization, and utilization of radiology and echocardiography. Underlying medical conditions must be treated aggressively. Determinants of oxygen delivery should be maximized, while oxygen consumption should be reduced (e.g., treating fever, controlling agitation, and initiating muscle relaxation and mechanical ventilation).

AORTIC STENOSIS

Aortic stenosis can involve the supravalvular, valvular or subvalvular areas. The vast majority of patients have valvular stenosis secondary to rheumatic heart disease, a bicuspid valve, or calcific valvular disease. Obstruction to flow through the aortic orifice causes stroke volume, cardiac output, and mean aortic pressure to fall, while mean left ventricular (LV) systolic pressure rises. Over time, compensatory changes produce increased preload, afterload, contractility and heart rate which combine to elevate myocardial oxygen demand. At the same time, LV coronary flow is limited by the decreased mean aortic pressure and impaired diastolic filling. In critical illness, myocardial oxygen demands outpace oxygen supply, leading to ischemia, arrhythmia, and death. Reductions in systemic vascular resistance (SVR) due to sepsis or vasodilating drugs can be potentially lethal. In chronic aortic stenosis, the reduction in ventricular compliance leads to unusual sensitivity to small changes in filling pressure. Clinically, the classic triad of aortic stenosis includes angina, dyspnea on exertion, and syncope. On physical exam, one may find pulsus parvus et tardus, a left ventricular heave, an ejection click followed by a crescendo-decrescendo murmur, a faint or absent second heart sound, and a prominent fourth heart sound. Signs of LV dysfunction (third heart sound, pulmonary edema) convey a poor prognosis.

The ECG usually reveals LV hypertrophy with a "strain" pattern, poor R wave progression and, in severe disease, left bundle branch block or anterior hemiblock. Echocardiography is the mainstay of diagnosis and should be performed immediately if the diagnosis is suspected. Right heart catheterization is useful in management but not in diagnosis.

Medical management of aortic stenosis is limited primarily to adjusting preload and contractility. The pulmonary capillary wedge pressure should be as high as clinically acceptable. Contractility may be increased with inotropes (dobutamine, dopamine), though cardiac output should be kept at the minimum necessary level so as not to further elevate myocardial oxygen consumption. Afterload reducing agents must be used with extreme caution as they are seldom helpful and can cause catastrophic hypotension. If serious arrhythmias occur, urgent mechanical intervention (surgery, valvuloplasty, or intra-aortic balloon pump [IABP] must be considered.) If angina occurs, interventions include the judicious use of intravenous nitrates, heparinization, and a reduction in the dose of inotropes. If these measures fail, IABP and mechanical intervention should be undertaken without delay.

In general, patients with aortic stenosis refractory to medical management should have valve replacement, since aortic valvuloplasty has a high short-term (< 1 year) restenosis rate. Aortic valve areas of less than 0.75 cm^2 or 0.6 cm/m^2 body surface area require replacement; a bioprosthetic valve should be used, if possible, to avoid the need for anticoagulation.

AORTIC INSUFFICIENCY

Aortic insufficiency has multiple etiologies, many of them from systemic disorders (rheumatic heart disease, connective tissue diseases). Acutely, bacterial endocarditis and aortic dissection are the most common causes of aortic insufficiency.

Clinically, even severe chronic aortic insufficiency may by asymptomatic until a critical illness occurs. Symptoms of dyspnea, angina, and fatigue are then magnified. Hypovolemia is also poorly tolerated. Acute aortic insufficiency is a medical and surgical emergency. A dramatic rise in LV end-diastolic pressure leads to pulmonary edema, hypotension, and clinical shock.

It is important to determine, as soon as possible, whether aortic insufficiency is acute or chronic. In the chronic state, left ventricular hypertrophy (LVH) and left atrial enlargement are evident on the ECG and echocardiogram, while right heart catheterization reveals normal pressures and cardiac output in asymptomatic patients. In the acute setting, the left ventricle is of normal size and the PCWP will be significantly elevated (> 20 mm Hg) with a low cardiac output.

Management of regurgitant lesions requires improving forward flow while minimizing the regurgitant fraction. Afterload reduction is the first intervention and is best accomplished acutely with nitroprusside unless refractory hypotension is present. If afterload reduction fails to improve cardiac output and reduce pulmonary edema, an inotrope (dobutamine, amrinone) should be added. Norepinephrine should be avoided unless complete cardiovascular collapse occurs. Intra-aortic balloon counterpulsation is contraindicated. Pulmonary edema may require a loop diuretic, and early intubation should be considered. Care must be taken to avoid excessive tachycardia or bradycardia. Tachycardia can be difficult to control, but increases in preload along with cautious use of digoxin may be adequate. Bradycardia is best avoided by using dobutamine or a pacemaker. Aggressive treatment of arrhythmias with lidocaine or procainamide is also necessary. In chronic lesions, all attempts at medical therapy should be tried. In acute insufficiency, the valve must be replaced at the earliest sign of hemodynamic compromise.

MITRAL STENOSIS

Mitral stenosis is resistance to diastolic flow through the mitral valve and is usually caused by rheumatic heart disease. Symptoms usually are not noticed until the valve area is reduced to approximately 1.5 cm^2, and replacement is usually not necessary until it falls further to 1 cm^2 or less. Mitral stenosis may remain subclinical until an acute illness supervenes. Dyspnea, with or without hemoptysis, secondary to pulmonary edema is a common presenting symptom. Chest pain, hoarseness or palpitations from left atrial enlargement, and evidence of clot embolization may also be present. On exam, the length of the diastolic murmur, not the loudness, determines the severity of the lesion.

The ECG may reveal left atrial enlargement or atrial fibrillation. The echocardiogram is particularly valuable in characterizing valvular mechanics, chamber size, hemodynamics, and determining the presence or absence of vegetations. The PCWP is usually in the 20 to 30 mmHg range and reflects the left atrial pressure, not the LVEDP. Cardiac output is usually normal to decreased.

Management of critically ill patients with mitral stenosis is extremely difficult. The controllable factors are preload, heart rate, and to a small extent, contractility. Patients are extremely sensitive to afterload reduction requiring extreme caution when vasodilators are used. Small changes in preload can cause pulmonary edema or hypotension. Careful diuresis or volume repletion, guided by a pulmonary artery catheter, echocardiography, and frequent exams is often necessary. Tachycardia or bradycardia can lower cardiac output. Tachycardia may be controlled with a β-blocker (esmolol), a calcium channel blocker (verapamil or diltiazem), or adenosine. Atrial fibrillation is often a catastrophic complication, thus the use of digoxin in the critically ill patient with mitral stenosis is recommended. In unstable patients, urgent electrocardioversion should be performed. If multiple premature atrial contractions occur in an unstable patient, procainamide should be considered. In addition, anticoagulation is recommended for all patients with mitral stenosis who are symptomatic, particularly in the presence of atrial fibrillation or left atrial enlargement. Inotropes are usually of little benefit. If medical measures fail, balloon valvuloplasty should be considered, as it is frequently a definitive therapy. Valve replacement should be performed if there is recurrent embolization or a contraindication to valvuloplasty.

MITRAL INSUFFICIENCY

Chronic mitral regurgitation is usually caused by rheumatic fever, mitral valve prolapse, ischemic heart disease, or LV dilation from several etiologies. Acute mitral regurgitation usually results from endocarditis or papillary muscle dysfunction due to ischemic heart disease. Decompensated chronic disease typically causes dyspnea and congestion. Phrenic nerve irritation due to the large left atrium may produce coughing or hoarseness. Neither the length or intensity of the murmur correlate with the severity of insufficiency. Patients with acute mitral regurgitation appear critically ill, with pulmonary edema, tachycardia, and hypoperfusion.

Again, echocardiography is the most important diagnostic tool. A flail mitral valve leaflet can usually be seen, as can a vegetation. Pulmonary artery catheterization is necessary in assessing the patient's volume status.

Hemodynamic management requires encouragement of forward flow and prevention of pulmonary edema. Afterload reduction should be the first intervention with the use of nitroprusside or intravenous enalaprilat. Use of these drugs in those with underlying heart disease in addition to the valve lesion may produce dramatic hypotension. Preload must also be optimized: reduction in those with adequate blood pressure and cardiac output by the use of intravenous nitroglycerin or diuretic and aggressive fluid replacement at the expense of pulmonary edema in those with poor perfusion (early ventilatory support should then be initiated).

Inotropic agents must be used with caution. Dobutamine is an ideal first choice because of its ability to reduce pulmonary venous pressures, lower systemic vascular resistance, and increase cardiac output. Intra-aortic balloon counterpulsation may also be used to lower afterload and augment coronary artery flow. Ischemic conditions should be treated with intravenous nitroglycerin and heparin. Excessive tachycardia must be avoided and atrial fibrillation prevented by the use of digoxin. Procainamide can be given in the presence of frequent premature atrial contractions. Systemic anticoagulation should be instituted during atrial fibrillation unless there is a contraindication.

HYPERTROPHIC CARDIOMYOPATHY

Hypertrophic obstructive cardiomyopathy (HOCM) is not a valvular problem, rather an inherited disorder of excess myofibrillar tissue usually located in the cardiac septum. The major hemodynamic abnormality is the inability of the ventricular muscle to relax, preventing adequate LV filling (i.e., diastolic dysfunction). In addition, the anterior leaflet of the mitral valve often does not function properly, and mitral insufficiency is common in HOCM. These problems are magnified by anything that increases contractility or reduces either preload or afterload.

Clinically, these patients often resemble those with refractory congestive heart failure (CHF). Patients tend to be young with complaints of syncope (or near syncope), chest pain, and dyspnea. A positive family history is very important. The ECG will reveal marked QRS voltage increases, marked T wave inversion, and poor R wave progression. The echocardiogram shows a large septum and mitral leaflet dysfunction. Right heart catheterization typically shows mild pulmonary hypertension and a decrement in cardiac output when afterload is reduced or contractility is augmented.

In management of patients with HOCM, first establishing the diagnosis is imperative. Once confirmed, the principles of management are to minimize contractility and maximize loading conditions. A beta-blocker (propranolol) in large doses should be the initial drug of choice. Verapamil may be used if there is a contraindication to β blockade. Paradoxically, patients with HOCM and pulmonary edema usually improve with saline administration (they can tolerate large volumes) and a calcium channel or β-blocker. Norepinephrine is the treatment of choice in refractory hypotension. Drugs which increase contractility should not be used. Nitrates may cause catastrophic hypotension. Because patients with diastolic dysfunction depend on atrial function for ventricular filling, atrial fibrillation can be a medical emergency requiring electrocardioversion (digoxin should not be used). Frequent premature atrial contractions or short runs of atrial fibrillation can be treated with a type 1A antiarrhythmic agent (disopyramide). Ventricular arrhythmias are frequent in these patients and lidocaine is the drug of choice.

PROSTHETIC VALVES

Prosthetic valves can become dysfunctional through mechanical failure, infection, thrombosis, or a sewing ring problem. Disease may present as a regurgitant lesion (valvular or paravalvular), a worsening stenotic lesion, a source of recurrent embolization, or a nidus of infection. Most paraprosthetic leaks occur within 6 months of the valvular surgery. Mechanical valves have a higher risk of thrombus occluding the valve, which is more likely to occur in valves in the mitral position than the aortic. All valves carry a high risk of endocarditis.

Clinically, presentation of prosthetic valve dysfunction is similar to any worsening valve lesion. Attention should be paid to signs of infective endocarditis and to any change in the valvular murmur. A mild hemolytic anemia is often present and the ECG may reveal a new arrhythmia. Echocardiography is technically more difficult with mechanical valves, but the transesophageal approach is especially useful in detecting thrombi or vegetations. Cardiac fluoroscopy can be used to assess proper leaflet or ball motion.

Medical management of a patient with a properly functioning prosthetic valve is similar to that of a patient with mild valvular stenosis. Management of prosthetic valve malfunction is generally surgical, especially with mechanical valves.

ANTICOAGULATION IN VALVULAR HEART DISEASE

A decision to institute anticoagulation therapy in valvular heart disease must be made on an individual case basis, with the clinician weighing the risk of bleeding against the risk of thrombus formation when critical illness supervenes. Those at high risk for thrombus are adequately anticoagulated when the partial thromboplastin time (PTT) is 1.5 to 2.0 times the control valve. If there has been a recent clot embolization, then the PTT should be raised to 2.0 to 2.5 times control.

In patients with mitral stenosis, anticoagulation is recommended in those who have symptoms of CHF, are in atrial fibrillation, or have evidence of a thrombus on echocardiography. In patients with mitral insufficiency and atrial fibrillation, anticoagulation is preferred. Patients with aortic, pulmonic, and tricuspid valvular disease do not generally require anticoagulation therapy. Abnormally functioning bioprosthetic valves should be anticoagulated like abnormally functioning native valves, especially if replacement was within the last 6 months or atrial fibrillation is present. Those with mechanical valves are at a significant risk for embolism and require anticoagulation.

ENDOCARDITIS

Critical illness can obscure many of the findings of endocarditis. The patient may present with regurgitant or stenotic lesions. Vegetations are not seen by echocardiography in 30 to 40 percent of all patients with endocarditis, and transesophageal echocardiography

TABLE 27-1 Indications for Surgery for Endocarditis
1. Intractable heart failure secondary to valve leaflet compromise.
2. Repeated embolic phenomena.
3. No response of infection despite one week of proper intensive therapy.
4. Presence of a septal abscess.
    Development of heart block.
    Aortic valve involvement.
    Persistence of block after one week of intensive medical therapy.
5. Recurrent endocarditis >6 months after a cure.
6. Relapse of infection <3 months.
7. Valvular obstruction.
8. Ruptured chordae tendonae.
9. Periprosthetic leak or unstable prosthesis.
10. Endocarditis in the sinus of valsalva.
11. Fungal endocarditis.

has proven particularly useful, especially for those patients being mechanically ventilated. In symptomatic patients, a right heart catheter should be placed to evaluate the cardiac output, loading conditions, and the presence of valvular insufficiency.

In general, the hemodynamic complications of endocarditis are those of valvular insufficiency, and the focus should be on the progression of disease. If rapid hemodynamic deterioration occurs or symptoms gradually worsen in those with mitral or aortic valvular involvement, then surgery must be performed as soon as feasible. Surgery must also be considered in those with recurrent embolization, myocardial abscess, pericarditis, or prosthetic valve endocarditis. A complete list of surgical indications for endocarditis are outlined in Table 27-1.

CATHETER BALLOON VALVULOPLASTY

Aortic Stenosis

Though surgical correction of aortic stenosis with valve replacement has an excellent record of efficacy and durability, there remain some limitations. Surgical mortality is increased for those patients over age eighty, who have severe left ventricular dysfunction, or who have other complicating illnesses such as severe lung disease or renal failure. Balloon aortic valvuloplasty has emerged as an alternative to surgical therapy. The patients are often identified in the critical care setting and are usually very old. Patients with severe left ventricular failure may be good candidates for initial valve dilation, followed by valve replacement if some recovery of left ventricular performance occurs. In addition, patients with aortic stenosis and in need of urgent noncardiac surgery are excellent candidates for valve dilation. Relative contraindications to aortic valvuloplasty include significant aortic insufficiency, a bleeding diathesis, and left main or severe three-vessel coronary artery disease. The latter group achieves no increase in prognosis with valvuloplasty but may have palliation of symptoms.

The procedure is performed after ensuring via Doppler echocardiography or aortogram that aortic insufficiency is not the predominant hemodynamic lesion. A large sheath is placed in the femoral artery and serial balloon inflations are performed. Following the procedure, valve area typically increases to 0.9 to 1.2 cm^2, cardiac output usually increases slightly, and many patients have a dramatic fall in PCWP and LVEDP. The restenosis rate at 1 year following balloon dilation is at least 50 percent. The procedure mortality is approximately one percent. Other complications include CNS embolization, femoral artery bleeding requiring transfusion, guide wire or catheter perforations of the left ventricle, and complete heart block (this usually resolves within 24 h, but occasionally a permanent pacemaker is required).

MITRAL VALVULOPLASTY

Mitral valvuloplasty has proven to be efficacious in a large segment of the population of patients with rheumatic mitral valve disease and for those who are not surgical candidates because of extremes of age or associated illnesses. Patients with symptomatic mitral stenosis and pliable mitral valve leaflets with little evidence on echocardiography for leaflet thickening, rigidity, calcification, or subvalvular thickening are ideal candidates for percutaneous mitral commisurotomy. Follow-up studies between 6 and 12 months show no significant incidence of restenosis and it is likely that they will have longterm results similar to those seen for surgical mitral valve commissurotomy. Valvuloplasty is also an excellent alternative for elderly patients with end stage mitral stenosis and severely deformed valves. Contraindications to the procedure include mitral regurgitation of more than moderate degree and those with contraindication to trans-septal puncture, including patients with severe thoracic spinal deformity which obscures essential landmarks. When possible, a patient should have warfarin anticoagulation for 4 to 6 weeks prior to the procedure (the drug is held 4 to 5 days prior to valvuloplasty).

Mitral valvuloplasty can be performed by percutaneous balloon commisurotomy via trans-septal puncture and conventionl single or double balloon commissurotomy or the newer Inoue balloon commissurotomy technique. Complications of mitral valvuloplasty are primarily represented by the transseptal puncture (into the aorta or pericardial space). In addition, a large atrial septal defect may be created, the left ventricular apex may be perforated by the guide wires or balloon tips, mitral regurgitation may be worsened, and thrombus can be dislodged creating a stroke or transient ischemic attack (one to two percent of patients).

For further reading in *Principles of Critical Care,* see Chap 26 "Cardiac Catheterization, Balloon Angioplasty, and Percutaneous Valvuloplasty" Ted Feldman/John D Carroll, Chap 122 "Valvular Heart Disease" Duane Follman/Paul Sobotka

28

Malignant Hypertension and Aortic Dissection

J. Edward Jordan

MALIGNANT HYPERTENSION

Hypertensive urgencies are defined as those disorders which require control of blood pressure within hours to days and occur in the setting of severely elevated blood pressure and have one or more of the following features:

1. Physical signs or laboratory findings suggesting subacute target organ damage
2. Recent discontinuation of antihypertensive drugs
3. Impending or recent surgical procedures
4. Occurring within the immediate postoperative period
5. Status post renal transplantation
6. Occurring after severe body burns

Hypertensive emergencies consist of those circumstances which require control of hypertension within minutes to hours to avoid end organ damage. Hypertensive encephalopathy, acute cerebrovascular accidents, acute aortic dissection, acute myocardial infarction, bleeding from vascular surgery sites, severe epistaxis, acute head injury, and states of excess catecholamines such as pheochromocytoma and monoamine oxidase crisis each constitute a hypertensive emergency.

Clinical Presentation

The diagnosis of malignant hypertension is based upon the association of extremely elevated blood pressure and signs of end organ damage by physical examination or laboratory findings. Changes in mental status indicative of hypertensive encephalopathy or an acute cerebrovascular accident require urgent control of blood pressure. Visualization of the optic fundi for papilledema or retinal hemorrhages is helpful in securing the diagnosis if either of these signs is seen. The assessment of cardiac function may suggest fluid overload, congestive heart failure secondary to excessive afterload, or myocardial ischemia. Physical examination of the abdomen may reveal abdominal bruits suggestive of renal arterial disease, palpable kidneys as seen in polycystic kidney disease, or abnormal masses raising the question of an extra-adrenal pheochromocytoma. Other clinical symptoms and signs include azotemia, headache, blurring vision, chest pain, and dyspnea.

Management

The first step in management of the hypertensive patient is to determine the urgency of blood pressure reduction. The patient with a hypertensive emergency will require significant correction of the hypertension within minutes to hours. Complete correction of blood pressure is usually not desirable since it may induce ischemia. The mean arterial pressure should be reduced by only 15 percent during the first hour (mean arterial pressure = 1/3 × systolic blood pressure + 2/3 × diastolic blood pressure) and gradually thereafter to a diastolic blood pressure between 100 and 110 mmHg (or a reduction of 25 percent compared to the initial baseline, whichever is higher). Seizures, coma, paraplegia, myocardial ischemia, renal failure, stroke, or death may ensue if blood pressure is poorly controlled.

In most situations, the drug of choice for control of blood pressure in the hypertensive emergency is sodium nitroprusside because of its short onset time, duration of action, and overall effectiveness. Nitroprusside is usually initiated at a rate of 0.5 μg/kg/min and thereafter increased by 0.5 to 1.0 μg/kg/min every 3 to 5 min until the goal of blood pressure reduction is reached. Complications of nitroprusside revolve around the toxicity associated with its metabolic byproducts of thiocyanate and cyanide. These can accumulate to toxic levels with high doses of nitroprusside (>2μ/kg/minute) or after prolonged infusion times. Symptoms of toxicity include nausea, fatigue, muscle spasms, and disorientation. A widening anion gap or rising serum lactate levels may signify toxicity. *The most common problem with nitroprusside use in patents with malignant hypertension is the failure to substitute an oral medication soon enough after the blood pressure is stabilized, leading to toxic levels of thiocyanate and cyanide.* Therefore, when an effective infusion rate is discovered, consideration of oral agents to replace the nitroprusside should begin.

Other medications which may be better suited for an individual patient include intravenous nitroglycerin which can control hypertension while simultaneously treating angina pectoris. Labetalol may be given as a constant infusion or in boluses (typically escalating in dose at 15 min intervals: e.g., 25 mg, then 50 mg, etc.) when a β-blocker is desired. Phentolamine is useful for pheochromocytoma crisis.

When patients with malignant hypertension present with an intracerebral process, blood pressure should be reduced more gradually (e.g., 10 percent reduction in mean arterial pressure) and with more careful attention to changes in neurologic status. Serial neurologic exams should be performed (including written tasks) in this setting to accurately assess for subtle changes in mental status.

Preferred oral medications will lower the blood pressure incrementally over a few hours rather than unpredictably in minutes. This will facilitate the discontinuation of nitroprusside and offer a smooth transition to oral therapy. β-blockers and calcium channel blockers have been found to be very useful in this regard.

There are several useful medications for the treatment of *hypertensive urgencies* which allow for timely control of the hypertension and yet are generally well tolerated. Nifedipine (taken sublingually or chewed and swallowed) is effective in most circumstances and allows for the administration of a second dose after 30 min if necessary. It probably should not be used in patients with congestive heart failure or volume depletion. Clonidine hydrochloride is also widely used in this setting since it is highly effective and may be given in small, repeated doses (0.1 mg PO until BP goals are reached or a total of 0.6 mg has been administered). Clonidine is associated with sedation in some patients and potentially dangerous rebound hypertension when abruptly discontinued. Captopril and enalapril are two angiotensin converting enzyme inhibitors which are effective in acutely correcting severe hypertension. These medications are not first line of therapy since they may precipitously reduce blood pressure in patients who are sensitive to afterload reduction and cause acute renal insufficiency in patients with critical renal artery stenosis.

Differential Diagnosis

Malignant hypertension may be a reflection of uncontrolled essential hypertension, or it may represent one of the secondary causes of hypertension such as renovascular hypertension, pheochromocytoma, drug ingestion (monoamine oxidase inhibitors, phenylpropanolamines, cocaine), or rebound hypertension after the discontinuation of therapy. Systemic vasculitis and renal failure are also important causes of malignant hypertension.

AORTIC DISSECTION

Dissection of the aorta represents one of the most difficult diagnoses to make clinically, and failure to recognize the signs results in formidable short term mortality. The patient's survival is dependent upon a high level of suspicion of this diagnosis and definitive therapy.

Pathogenesis

A hematoma forms as a result of an intimal tear and proceeds antero- or posterogradely along the aortic wall creating a false lumen and narrowing the true lumen. The hematoma may subsequently rupture into the pericardial space resulting in tamponade or into the pleural space with life threatening hypovolemia. Several conditions predispose to aortic dissection, including Marfan's and Ehlers-Danlos syndromes, annulo-aortic ectasia, bicuspid aortic valve, coarctation, late pregnancy, and open heart surgery. Intraluminal shear forces with a steeply rising aortic pressure may predispose to aortic aneurysms.

Classification

Aortic dissections are classified according to location and duration. Type A aneurysms are located in the ascending aorta. These are associated with the risk of sudden death due to tamponade, acute aortic insufficiency, congestive heart failure, or coronary thrombosis. Type B aneurysms are located in the descending aorta beyond the left subclavian artery, and are not associated with a high incidence of sudden death. Similarly, dissections are categorized as either being acute (<2 weeks) or chronic (>2 weeks). Acute dissections are associated with a 50 percent mortality in the first 48 h and 90 percent mortality over one month. Type A and acute dissections are handled more urgently with surgical intervention whereas Type B and chronic aneurysms may usually be handled conservatively.

Clinical Picture

Men (particularly black males) are 2 to 3 times more prone to develop a dissecting aortic aneurysm than women, and hypertension is usually a prominent part of the history. Clinical manifestations are dominated by pain, poor peripheral perfusion despite adequate (or high) blood pressure, and signs of occlusion at aortic branch sites resulting in end organ damage. The pain encountered during a dissection is usually noted for its sharp quality with sudden onset and may begin at retrosternal, interscapular, or epigastric areas. It is often very difficult to control with opiates. Patients may present with signs of shock and end organ hypoperfusion (ashen skin, poor urine output, mental status changes) yet have an elevated blood pressure. In cases of Type A aneurysm, severe aortic insufficiency, cardiac tamponade, or rupture into the pleural space may cause shock. Approximately one-third of patients will present with compromised flow to a major branch of the aorta which may occlude during aortic dissection. Vascular beds such as a lower extremity, the brain, kidney, or mesentery may become ischemic with permanent sequelae.

Investigations and Diagnosis

Standard chest radiography with antero-posterior and lateral views often reveals a widened mediastinum. Classically the aorta bulges to the right with Type A and to the left with Type B dissections. Aortography is currently believed to be the most specific and sensitive means of diagnosis and offers the best opportunity to identify the site of the intimal tear. However, aortography subjects the patient to a highly invasive procedure and exposure to intravenous contrast. CT scanning offers high specificity by a noninvasive technique and may visualize the true and false lumen of an aneurysm, as well as reveal aortic root, pericardial, and pleural involvement. Sensitivity is moderately compromised; therefore, in cases of high clinical suspicion other investigations should be performed to rule out dissection.

Echocardiography (transthoracic and transesophageal) can noninvasively, accurately, and quickly evaluate aortic dissections for extent of involvement, aortic insufficiency, and aortic arch dilation. Doppler echocardiography allows clear identification of the true and false lumens. Pericardial effusions and left ventricular wall motion abnormalities may also be evaluated.

There is limited experience with magnetic resonance imaging although it holds promise for clearly defining anatomy without the use of contrast or ionizing radiation.

The recommended workup includes transesophageal echocardiography initially (if available), proceeding to thoracic computerized tomography (CT) if necessary. If these studies are inconclusive and a strong clinical suspicion of aortic dissection remains, an arch aortogram should be obtained.

Treatment

Initial care of the patient with a dissecting aortic aneurysm should begin once the diagnosis is suspected and include extensive efforts to monitor the patient, control blood pressure, and prepare for more definitive therapy. The patient should be monitored with an electrocardiograph (ECG) monitor, arterial line, central venous pressure line, and frequent urinary output assessment. Blood samples should be sent for cross and typing should surgery become necessary.

Control of blood pressure is required to limit the extent of dissection. Both the overall elevation of blood pressure and the rate of pressure rise during systole generate excessive wall tension and shearing forces which promote extension of the ongoing dissection.

Labetalol is a nonselective β-blocker and selective α_1 blocker, reduces blood pressure and the rate of rise in aortic pressures, and thus is the drug of choice. It may be given by continuous infusion (1 to 2 mg/min) or bolus (0.25 mg/kg over 2 min; may repeat every 10 min). Its effect peaks in 5 minutes and lasts 2 to 12 hours. If Labetalol is not available, nitroprusside (continuous infusion: 0.5 to 8.0 μg/kg/min) with intravenous propranolol (bolus infusion: 1 to 3 mg over 2 to 3 min; may repeat in 2 to 3 min) may be used. Nitroprusside will reduce the overall blood pressure and propranolol will blunt the rate of rise of aortic pressure. Patients who will not tolerate β-blockers may be given trimethaphan (continuous infusion: begin with 3 to 4 mg/min); however, it is often necessary to lift the head of the patient and allow the feet to dangle over the edge of the bed to achieve proper control of the hypertension. Reserpine or guanethidine may be required with trimethaphan to control the sympathoplegic side effects which may cause precipitous drops in blood pressure.

Systolic blood pressure should be reduced to 90–100 mmHg to confine the progression of the dissection. The patient should be continually monitored for adequate organ perfusion as evidenced by a clear sensorium, good urine output, and absence of lactic acidosis.

Decisions concerning surgical intervention are often complex and must be individualized. Generally speaking, Type A aortic dissections should be offered urgent surgical correction to optimize survival. Relative contraindications to surgery include severe organ dysfunction, age greater than 80, paraplegia, and the presence of a cerebrovascular accident (controversial). Type B dissections are usually best managed conservatively with surgical therapy reserved for complications of dissection (such as occlusion of an aortic branch). Patients with Type B dissections should nevertheless be admitted to a critical care setting when the character of the aneurysm changes until the patient's blood pressure can be controlled, hemodynamics stabilized, and needed diagnostic tests completed.

For further reading in *Principles of Critical Care,* see Chap 123 "Malignant Hypertension" William J Elliott, Chap 124 "Aortic Dissection" Joseph J Austin/B William Shragge, Chap 125 "Vasoactive Drugs" William J Elliott/Daniel D Gretler

Allan Garland

The most obvious function of the lungs is to exchange oxygen and carbon dioxide between the blood and the ambient environment. Oxygen is absorbed into the blood for subsequent delivery to cells, while carbon dioxide, the gaseous byproduct of cellular metabolism, is excreted by the lungs. At its most simple functional level, *respiratory failure* may be defined as an inadequacy of one or both of these vital functions of gas exchange, leading to arterial hypoxemia and/or arterial hypercarbia. However, a completely satisfactory definition of what constitutes adequate gas exchange must be viewed in the context of the metabolism of tissues and cells; a comprehensive treatment of respiratory failure would have as its goal a review of factors which result in inadequate cellular respiration. Thus, the differential diagnosis of respiratory failure includes states in which there may be pathologic alteration in any of: the lung parenchyma, airways, abdomen or chest wall, cardiovascular system, blood, the muscles of respiration with their periperal and central nervous system control mechanisms, or cellular metabolism.

This chapter examines the causes of respiratory failure on three different levels. The first of these reviews the spectrum of fundamental physiologic mechanisms responsible for altered gas exchange at the level of the lungs. The second is a clinically relevant approach which separates causes of respiratory failure according to the mechanisms by which patients become unable to spontaneously support adequate mechanical respiratory function. The third is a practical classification based upon the way patients present clinically with respiratory failure. Seemingly separate, but in fact strongly coupled via an understanding of physiology, these different views of respiratory failure each supply a perspective on the topic which is of considerable assistance in the care of critically ill patients.

A more specific and detailed treatment of evaluation and therapy for specific types of respiratory failure may be found in Chap. 30, 31, 32 and 33. A discussion of mechanical ventilation in the patient with respiratory failure is contained in Chap. 6.

PATHOPHYSIOLOGIC CAUSES OF ALTERED GAS EXCHANGE

Causes of Arterial Hypoxemia

From the point of view of gas exchange at the alveolar-pulmonary capillary interface, the 6 basic mechanisms which can result in arterial hypoxemia are: alveolar hypoventilation, shunt, ventilation-perfusion mismatch, decreased mixed venous oxygenation, true diffusion block, and asphyxia.

In *alveolar hypoventilation*, the alveolar P_{O_2} falls because the rate of replenishment of alveolar oxygen falls below the rate of O_2 removal by the pulmonary circulation. Since alveolar ventilation equals the total minute ventilation (MV) minus the dead space ventilation, alveolar hypoventilation may occur as a result of either decreased MV, or an increase in the dead space fraction. Examples of states with decreased MV include oversedation, respiratory muscle weakness secondary to hypophosphatemia, and severe airways obstruction, while pulmonary embolism is an example of a disorder which causes increased dead-space. Hypoventilation responds promptly to measures that decrease dead-space.

In *shunt*, some alveoli are perfused but not ventilated; this occurs when alveoli are filled with fluid (e.g., pulmonary edema, pulmonary hemorrhage, pneumonia). Thus the blood effluxing from shunted alveoli has the same O_2 and CO_2 content as does mixed venous blood, and when combined with blood exiting fully arterialized from normal terminal respiratory units, this venous admixture lowers the net arterial P_{O_2}. Because increasing inspired oxygen fraction does not alter the situation in flooded alveoli, hypoxemia due to shunt is largely refractory to enriched oxygen therapy.

Ventilation-perfusion mismatch describes the situation wherein despite normal values of total alveolar ventilation and pulmonary bloodflow, an imbalance between these occurs in different lung units. Thus, some units are relatively overventilated for the amount of blood flow they receive, while others are underventilated. The result of such imbalance is both arterial hypoxemia and hypercarbia. This mechanism is the most important mechanism causing gas exchange abnormalities in many intrinsic lung diseases (e.g., chronic obstructive pulmonary disease [COPD], asthma, idiopathic pulmonary fibrosis). Unlike shunt, hypoxemia due to ventilation-perfusion mismatch responds to oxygen therapy (although the hypercarbia does not); despite the mismatch, a lung unit which is filled with 100% oxygen will fully saturate the blood with which it comes in contact.

Decreased mixed venous oxygenation normally has no influence upon arterial oxygenation; the functional reserve of normal lungs is sufficiently great that they are able to fully oxygenate the mixed venous blood that passes through them, no matter how deoxygenated it may be. However, when passed through lungs units which have shunt, or sufficiently severe ventilation-perfusion mismatching, mixed venous blood does not become fully saturated with oxygen, and thus contributes a venous admixture that results in arterial hypoxemia; the lower the mixed venous oxygen saturation, the lower the resultant arterial oxygen saturation will be. The dependence of arterial oxygenation upon mixed venous oxygenation becomes more pronounced as the amount of shunt or ventilation-perfusion mismatching increases. Any of the causes of mixed venous hypoxemia (i.e., decreased cardiac output, increased total body oxygen utilization, or any independent cause of decreased arterial oxygen content) can cause hypoxemia if the lungs are sufficiently abnormal; a typical clinical scenario is the patient with underlying COPD who was not previously hypoxemic, but becomes hypoxemic when his mixed venous oxygenation falls as a result of the onset of cor pulmonale and its attendant limitation to cardiac output.

In principle, *diffusion block*, resulting from thickening in the alveolar-capillary membrane, could appreciably alter transport of gases between blood and alveoli. In practice however, this is rarely a limiting factor; even in advanced idiopathic pulmonary fibrosis, membrane limitation to diffusion is only significant during exercise, when the time available for equilibration is reduced by the rapid passage of blood past the alveoli.

The alveolar gas equation predicts that alveolar oxygen tension depends on oxygen tension in inspired gas (P_IO_2). Even in normal lungs decreasing P_IO_2 must lead to reduced arterial P_{O_2}. *Asphyxia* describes the situation wherein inspired gas has a reduced partial pressure of oxygen. Examples include breathing within the area of a fire, which consumes the ambient oxygen, or at altitude.

Causes of Arterial Hypercarbia

In the steady state, P_{CO_2} represents the balance between the rate of CO_2 production by cellular metabolism, and the rate of pulmonary CO_2 excretion, which is proportional to the alveolar ventilation. Thus: $P_{CO_2} = \text{constant} \times \dot{V}_{CO_2}/\{MV \times [1 - (V_D/V_T)].\}$, where $\dot{V}_{CO_2}$ = metabolic CO_2 production; V_D = dead-space volume; V_T = tidal volume; and MV = minute ventilation = respiratory rate $\times$ V_T. It thus follows that hypercarbia may be caused by: **1.** increased metabolic CO_2 production in the presence of an inability to compensate by increasing alveolar ventilation, **2.** a decreased minute ventilation, or **3.** increased dead-space fraction in the presence of an inability to compensate by adequately increasing minute ventilation. Examples of states which could cause each of these abnormalities are seizures; oversedation, or respiratory muscle weakness; and severe idiopathic pulmonary fibrosis.

MECHANISMS OF RESPIRATORY FAILURE

Perhaps the most flexible and practically helpful way to view respiratory function is to separate it into the 3 basic elements of: central respiratory drive, respiratory load and respiratory strength. Even with an adequate drive to breathe, each of us must have adequate strength to bear the ongoing load of breathing. Thus respiratory failure will result from either a failure of respiratory drive, or from a relative imbalance between load vs. strength. *It is not unusual for critically ill patients to have multiple abnormalities which affect combinations of respiratory drive, load, and strength.*

Decreases in Central Respiratory Drive

Central respiratory drive, which is generated and integrated in the brainstem, is affected by numerous influences including input from: mechanoreceptors in the lungs and chest wall, central and peripheral chemoreceptors (which respond to pH, P_{CO_2}, and P_{O_2}), the cerebral cortex, and hormonal inputs. Meaningful measurement of central drive is difficult, and is rarely performed outside of the research laboratory. The parameter most often assayed is $P_{0.1}$, the (negative) pressure at the airway opening 0.1 sec after the onset of a spontaneous breath, with the airway occluded; a normal value for this parameter is 2 cm H_2O and as expected, it normally increases as P_{CO_2} rises, unless central drive is suppressed.

While most disease states which have an effect upon the neurohormonal inputs to the brainstem result in augmented respiratory drive, there are a handful of states which reduce central drive. These include drugs and toxins (e.g., narcotics, sedatives, alcohol, anesthetics), some central nervous system abnormalities (such as stupor, coma and some cerebral vascular accidents), and significant hypothyroidism. *With the exception of drugs and toxins, failure of central respiratory drive is rarely the sole cause of respiratory failure.*

Increases in Respiratory Load

The causes of increased respiratory load may be divided into those which are associated with an increased mechanical load of breathing, and those which result in an increase in ventilatory requirements (Table 29-1).

In order to move gases in and out of the alveoli, the action of the muscles of respiration must be translated into a pressure gradient. This gradient is needed to overcome both the resistance to airflow within airways, and the elastic forces of the lungs, chest wall and abdomen. Thus, an increased mechanical load of breathing will result from any state which causes airways obstruction, or decreases compliance of the lung or the chest wall. Examples of the former include bronchoconstrictive diseases, and secretions or foreign bodies impacted in the airways; of the many states included in the latter category are pulmonary edema, atelectasis, hyperinflation, pleural effusion and tense ascites (which decreases chest wall compliance by pushing up on the diaphragms from below).

Any condition which necessitates an increased minute ventilation in order to maintain normal P_{O_2}, P_{CO_2}, and pH may precipitate ventilatory failure in a patient who has an inadequate reserve of

TABLE 29-1 Causes of Imbalance between Respiratory Load and Respiratory Strength

Increased Load	Decreased Strength
Increased Mechanical Load	*Respiratory muscle fatigue*
Airways obstruction	
Bronchoconstriction	*Respiratory muscle atrophy*
Secretions	
Increased ET tube resistance	*Circulatory insufficiency*
	hypotension
Decreased resp. system	hypoperfusion
complaince	anemia
Decreased lung compliance	hypoxemia
pneumonia	
pulmonary edema	*Toxic-metabolic neuromusular*
atelectasis	*dysfunction*
hyperinflation	decreased K^+, Ca^{++} Mg^{++}, PO_4^{-3}
increased PEEP	protein-calorie malnutrition
Decreased chest wall compliance	sepsis
pleural effusion	drugs (e.g. muscle relaxants,
pneumothorax	aminoglycosides, steroids)
intraabdominal processes	fever
(e.g. tense ascites)	
abdominal/thoracic pain with	*Neuromuscular disease*
splinting	
	Miscellaneous
Increased Ventilatory Requirements	sedation
Increased V_D/V_T	paralysis
pulmonary embolus	stupor/coma
air embolus	CVA
intrinsic lung disease	subclinical status epilepticus
increased Zone 1	hyperinflation
Increased V_{CO_2}	hypothyroidism
fever	diaphragmatic dysfunction
overfeeding	phrenic nerve dysfunction
stressed states (e.g. sepsis, burns)	
Metabolic acidosis	
Hypoxemia	

respiratory muscle strength with which to respond to that increased need. As discussed above, gas exchange is proportional to alveolar ventilation, and alveolar ventilation goes down when either the minute ventilation (MV) falls or the dead-space fraction rises. Thus, respiratory load increases in states which increase CO_2 production; these states, such as fever, severe physiologic stress, and overfeeding, usually also increase O_2 consumption. Also, both hypoxemia and metabolic acidosis call forth compensatory hyperventilation which borderline patients may not be able to maintain.

Since patients with an increased dead-space fraction require an increased MV in order to maintain their alveolar ventilation, diseases associated with pathologically increased dead space (as seen in pulmonary embolus, some intrinsic lung diseases, and situations which increase the amount of lung in West's Zone 1) also increase the effective load of breathing.

Decreases in Respiratory Strength

The muscles of respiration (diaphragms, intercostals, scalenes) must be able to indefatigably generate a force sufficient to overcome the patient's respiratory load. As an approximation, the respiratory muscles are capable of exerting roughly one-third of their maximum force generation indefinitely without fatiguing. Normal individuals have abundant functional reserve since the pressure load of tidal breathing is 5 to 10 cm H_2O, while the maximum pressure generation is >100 cm H_2O. However, any factor which impinges upon that functional reserve can contribute to respiratory insufficiency. The main categories of etiologies of decreased respiratory muscle strength are: neuromuscular diseases (e.g., amyotrophic lateral sclerosis [ALS], muscular dystrophies, myasthenia gravis), toxic-metabolic neuromuscular dysfunction (e.g., electrolyte disturbances, malnutrition, sepsis, drugs), circulatory insufficiency, respiratory muscle fatigue (as may occur in a patient with COPD who develops a superimposed pneumonia), and respiratory muscle atrophy (as may occur after prolonged mechanical ventilation). In addition a number of miscellaneous conditions, such as hypothyroidism, can contribute to weakness.

CLINICAL CLASSIFICATION OF RESPIRATORY FAILURE

Many of the cases of respiratory failure seen in the ICU can be placed into one of four clinical patterns, each having a predominant mechanism. They are set apart from each other by their different presentations, as well as by the clinical settings in which they occur.

Type I, or *acute hypoxemic respiratory failure*, is a failure of oxygenation due to airspace flooding. In this type, compensatory hyperventilation typically results in a reduced P_{CO_2} until very late in its course. Whether the alveoli are filled with edema, blood, or pus, Type I failure is signalled by evidence of focal or diffuse alveolar filling, and hypoxemia which is refractory to oxygen therapy.

In Type II or *hypoventilatory respiratory failure*, primary failure of alveolar ventilation leads to CO_2 retention associated with hypoxemia which, in contrast to Type I failure, corrects easily with O_2 therapy. The cause of this may be either decreased central respiratory drive, decreased neuromuscular coupling, or an increase in dead space fraction. This common type of failure is seen in a wide variety of lung diseases, neuromuscular disorders, and also drug overdoses and some central nervous system injuries.

In Type III, or *perioperative respiratory failure,* multiple mechanical factors reduce the end-expired lung volume (i.e., functional residual capacity, FRC) below the closing volume of some lung units. The resulting atelectasis causes ventilation-perfusion mismatch and subsequent hypoxemia and CO_2 retention. Factors which promote a decreased FRC include the supine position, anesthesia, splinting after a thoracic or abdominal incision, and if present, obesity or ascites. The closing volume increases with age, fluid overload, bronchospasm, intrabronchial secretions, and a history of cigarette smoking. While this clinical picture is common in the post-operative patient, those factors which promote atelectasis are also often present in other critically ill patients; indeed, atelectasis and lobar collapse are common in the medical ICU and not infrequently contribute to respiratory insufficiency.

Type IV, or *hypoperfusion respiratory failure* represents inability of the circulation to supply needed substrates to the respiratory muscles. This is most frequently seen in shock of any cause.

GENERAL APPROACH TO THE TREATMENT OF RESPIRATORY FAILURE

The first priority in treating patients with incipient respiratory failure is evaluation and, if needed, support of vital functions. Included in consideration of the ABCs (Airway, Breathing and Circulation) is recognition of whether intubation and mechanical ventilatory support is emergently required; this topic is covered in Chap. 4, 5 and 6. Once the patient is stabilized, attention shifts to evaluation and treatment of the underlying condition(s) responsible for the ventilatory failure.

In the ICU patients frequently have multiple factors contributing to respiratory insufficiency; for example it would not be unusual to see a patient with underlying COPD admitted for pneumonia who is obtunded, wheezing, febrile, and hypomagnesemic. *Careful attention to detail in recognizing and treating all the contributing factors, even when they are not part of the primary problem (the pneumonia in this case), results in superior care of the patient with respiratory insufficiency.*

For further reading in *Principles of Critical Care,* see Chap 1 "The Respiratory System" LDH Wood, Chap 128 "Acute Hypoxemic Respiratory Failure" Jesse B Hall/Lawrence DH Wood, Chap 129 "Acute on Chronic Respiratory Failure" Gregory A Schmidt/Jesse B Hall

Edward T. Naureckas

PATHOPHYSIOLOGY

Acute hypoxemic respiratory failure (AHRF) is characterized by severe hypoxemia that is relatively refractory to oxygen therapy. It is caused by any process that results in alveolar collapse or filling (Table 30-1). Conceptually the causes of hypoxemia can be roughly divided into homogeneous lung lesions such as pulmonary edema, and focal lung lesions such as bacterial lobar pneumonia.

Cardiogenic Pulmonary Edema

Homogeneous lung lesions are most commonly due to cardiogenic pulmonary edema or low pressure pulmonary edema. Both cases are characterized by an accumulation of excess lung fluid. In the case of cardiogenic pulmonary edema the driving force for fluid accumulation is an increase in hydrostatic pressure due to any of the causes listed on Table 30-1. Fluid accumulates initially in the interstitial region where an increase in interstitial pressure and a dilution of interstitial oncotic pressures help to limit further fluid flux. If these mechanisms are overwhelmed, however, fluid accumulation continues and eventually the alveolar tight junctions are disrupted resulting in alveolar flooding.

Low Pressure Pulmonary Edema

Low pressure pulmonary edema, also termed pulmonary capillary leak or adult respiratory distress syndrome (ARDS), results from an increase in capillary permeability to fluid due to injury. This injury may be a result of direct lung injury such as aspiration of gastric acid, or indirectly from systemic processes such as sepsis. The cascade of events leading to ARDS is still not completely elucidated but may involve the complement system, neutrophils and macrophage activation, oxygen free radicals, cytokines such as tumor necrosis factor, and many other mediators.

The early phase of acute lung injury has been classified as the exudative phase. On pathology, there is flooding of the lung interstitium and alveoli with proteinaceous fluid with little evidence of cellular injury initially. As lung injury progresses over the next few days hyaline membranes, representing precipitated serum proteins, are seen along with extensive necrosis of type I alveolar epithelial

TABLE 30-1 Causes of Acute Hypoxemic Respiratory Failure

Homogenous Lung Lesions (Producing Pulmonary Edema)

Cardiogenic or hydrostatic edema
  Left ventricular failure
  Acute ischemia
  Mitral regurgitation
  Mitral stenosis
  Ball-valve thrombus
  Volume overload, particularly with coexisting renal and cardiac disease
Permeability or low pressure edema (ARDS)
  Most common
    Sepsis and sepsis syndrome
    Acid aspiration
    Multiple transfusions for hypovolemic shock
  Less common
    Near-drowning
    Pancreatitis
    Air or fat emboli
    Cardiopulmonary bypass
    Pneumonia
    Drug reaction or overdose
    Leukoagglutination
    Inhalation injury
    Infusion of biologics (e.g., interleukin-2)
Edema of unclear or "mixed" etiology
  Reexpansion
  Neurogenic
  Postictal
  Tocolysis-associated

Focal Lung Lesions

Lobar pneumonia
Lung contusion
Lobar atelectasis (acutely)

cells. Inflammatory cells also become more numerous in the interstitium.

The latter, or proliferative phase, is dominated by disordered healing which can occur as early as 7 to 10 days. In some cases this phase may be rapidly progressive resulting in massive pulmonary fibrosis with honeycombing seen on chest x-ray (CXR). The areas where type I cells have been lost are replaced with proliferating type II cells. Within the alveolar wall fibroblasts and myoblasts become more prominent.

Nonhomogeneous AHRF

A typical form of nonhomogeneous AHRF is lobar bacterial pneumonia. Although pneumonias involving a single lobe involve approximately 20 percent of alveoli, shunt fraction may reach 40 percent of total cardiac output. One hypothesis for this large shunt fraction is the paralysis of hypoxic vasoconstriction. An element of V/Q mismatch is also present in pneumonia due to hypoventilation of adjacent areas as a result of their mechanical interdependence with the consolidated regions. Consequently, about half of the hypoxemia during air breathing is due to low ventilation perfusion ratios and is very responsive to oxygen therapy.

Another focal lung lesion that can result in significant hypoxemia is lung contusion. These lesions emerge within minutes to hours of blunt chest trauma as a result of hemorrhage and mechanical injury to the pulmonary arterial circulation. The hypoxemia seen is largely due to low V/Q areas in the surrounding lung as a result of mechanical interdependence. Thus these patients respond well to oxygen and strategies such as pain control to increase ventilation, and often do not require intubation. Positive end-expiratory pressure (PEEP) and positive pressure ventilation tend to increase the degree of injury.

CLINICAL PRESENTATION

In the alert patient, the presentation of AHRF is characterized by marked dyspnea and tachypnea with a respiratory rate greater than 30. On physical exam, diffuse crackles are heard with pulmonary edema. Wheezes may sometimes be heard as well. It has been observed that the secretions of patients with noncardiogenic edema are copious, frothy and resemble plasma due to the high permeability to proteins. In fact, it has been shown that total protein content 50 percent of serum protein or greater, indicates noncardiogenic pulmonary edema. Other means for distinguishing between cardiogenic and noncardiogenic pulmonary edema include echocardiography and invasive hemodynamic monitoring to determine the pulmonary capillary wedge pressure (Ppw). One set of criteria for the diagnosis of ARDS is shown in Table 30-2.

Radiographic findings may be helpful in determining the etiology of AHRF. Lobar pneumonia will, of course, present as an area of focal consolidation with or without pleural effusion. Cardiogenic pulmonary edema may demonstrate an enlarged cardiac size, pulmonary vascular redistribution, septal (Kerley B) lines, and a perihilar or "bat's wing" distribution of infiltrates. The lack of these findings in the setting of pulmonary edema may suggest noncardiogenic pulmonary edema, but there is a considerable degree of radiologic overlap.

Failure to visualize an obvious alveolar abnormality on chest radiographic in a patient whose blood gas analysis suggests AHRF should prompt reassessment of the accuracy of the data (e.g. effec-

TABLE 30-2 Criteria for Diagnosis of ARDS

Clinical presentation
Tachypnea and dyspnea
Crackles on auscultation
Clinical setting
Direct lung insult (e.g., aspiration) or systemic process with potential for lung injury (e.g., sepsis)
Radiologic appearance
Three or four quadrant alveolar flooding
Lung mechanics
Diminished compliance (<40 mL/cmH$_2$O)
Gas exchange
Severe hypoxemia refractory to oxygen therapy (Pa$_{O_2}$/F$_{IO_2}$ < 150)
Normal pulmonary vascular pressures PW < 16 mmHg

tive fraction of inspired oxygen and true Pa$_{O_2}$) and the possibility of other types of right to left shunt such as intacardiac shunts or pulmonary venous malformations.

TREATMENT

While the majority of the therapy in AHRF is supportive, the underlying cause of the lung failure must be searched for and treated, as supportive therapy alone will ultimately result in mounting complications and irreversible organ failure.

Initial therapy for all patients includes supplemental oxygen in the highest concentration available, understanding that the maximal FIO$_2$ attainable with high flow masks and rebreathing devices is 0.6 to 0.7 under most clinical conditions. The failure to achieve full arterial saturation using this therapy confirms the presence of a large shunt fraction.

Cardiogenic Pulmonary Edema

Correction of hypoxemia should be attempted immediately with nasal cannula or mask, titrated against oximetry or arterial blood gas measurements. Thereafter the goal of therapy is to reduce the left atrial and pulmonary vascular pressures responsible for cardiogenic pulmonary edema. This can be done by reducing preload and afterload and by increasing cardiac contractility.

Preload reduction can be accomplished in many ways. Positioning of the patient in an upright position, even after intubation, is preferable if arterial blood pressure allows and is most comfortable for the patient. Morphine in doses of 2 to 4 mg IV followed by equivalent doses every 5 to 10 min, titrated to the patient's level of anxiety and conciousness, will reduce preload by decreasing tone in the venous capacitance vessels. Further preload reduction can be achieved using furosemide with an initial dose of 20 to 40mg IV (in a patient with normal renal function) which can be doubled if no response is noted within 30 to 90 min. Nitroglycerin, either topical, sublingual, or IV may also be used to reduce preload and may be especially helpful in settings where cardiac dysfunction is due to ischemia. Rotating tourniquets and phlebotomy have also been used in extreme circumstances.

Afterload reduction, especially in the setting of hypertension not responsive to the above measures, may be helpful. Calcium channel blockers, such as nifedipine, may be used but they are negatively ionotropic. Substantial elevations of blood pressure may be treated with nitroprusside. Be aware that this drug may lead to increased shunting due to decreased hypoxic vasoconstriction.

In a subset of patients, inotropic support with drugs such as dobutamine may be warranted. As the above measures are instituted any underlying cause such as ischemia or valvular disease should be found and corrected.

The vast majority of patients respond to the above measures and do not require intubation. Indications for intubation in cardiogenic pulmonary edema include hypotension precluding the use of vaso-active drugs, complex or persistent arrhythmias, and failure to respond to therapy within the first few hours.

Noncardiogenic Pulmonary Edema

Many experimental therapies have been investigated for the treatment of ARDS. These include corticosteroids, prostaglandin administration and inhibition, surfactant, and pentoxifylline (an inhibitor of neutrophil activation). While many of these agents have shown encouraging results in animal models, they have not been shown to be efficacious in the clinical setting, with the exception of surfactant in neonates. Thus, therapy for ARDS is focused on support and treatment of underlying conditions.

In contrast to patients with cardiogenic pulmonary edema, patients with ARDS typically require early, elective intubation since the duration of AHRF is usually greater. Exceptions to this generalization are postictal pulmonary edema, heroin associated pulmonary edema, transfusion related pulmonary edema, air embolism and AHRF associated with tocolysis which all tend to have a more benign course.

Ventilator management of patients in the exudative phase of ARDS should begin with an $F_{I_{O_2}}$ of 1.0, tidal volumes of 6 to 7 ml/kg and a respiratory rate of 20 to 28. During the initial phase of ventilator management, sedation, and often muscle relaxation, may be required to minimize oxygen consumption and airway pressures. Most patients will achieve adequate saturation on these settings.

Subsequent management should be directed at achieving the least possible PEEP achieving 90 percent saturation on an FI_{O_2} of less than 0.6. The use of low tidal volumes as recommended above may help reduce lung injury induced by overdistention of alveoli during positive pressure breathing. As multiple blood gas determinations are common during this phase of management, the insertion of an arterial line is advisable.

Novel forms of ventilatory management such as high frequency ventilation have failed to show an improvement in outcome in controlled trials. This does not preclude their use in individual situations when available.

Circulatory management directed at reduction of the pulmonary capillary wedge pressure to the least level consistent with adequate cardiac output and oxygen delivery may reduce edemagenesis and thus decrease the morbidity and mortality inherent in supportive care. Adequate cardiac output is best measured by observation of nailbed perfusion, urine output, mental status, and blood pressure, as well as the absence of a lactic acidosis. Tissue hypoxia and lactic acidosis can be ameliorated by increasing oxygen delivery (such as with dobutamine in selected patients with left ventricular dysfunction), maintenance of adequate hemoglobin level (14 g/dl) and saturation (90 percent). Sepsis may complicate the determination of adequate oxygen delivery due to extraction defects.

Monitoring and manipulation of the circulation in these patients must take into account the fact that altered perfusion may significantly impact on arterial saturation via the effects of shunted mixed venous blood. In addition vasoactive drugs may have varying arteriolar, venous and pulmonary arteriolar effects on preload, afterload and pulmonary shunt fraction. For these reasons right heart catheterization may be useful, but should never be performed as a matter of routine. Right heart catheterization should be used with a specific question in mind and should be discontinued when those questions have been answered.

Late or proliferative phase ARDS is characterized by a large dead space fraction, high airway pressures, pulmonary hypertension and a "honeycomb" appearance radiographically. Edema may be minimal in this phase, and since hypovolemia is poorly tolerated due to adverse effects on dead space and venous return, the continued reduction of the Ppw should no longer be pursued.

Focal Lung Lesions

In focal lung disease producing AHRF such as lobar pneumonia or contusion, PEEP therapy may increase pulmonary shunt. When a trial of PEEP is applied to these patients, frequent determinations of benefit should be made. Focal lung diseases confer increased permeability on apparently noninvolved lung vessels. So, as in noncardiogenic pulmonary edema, wedge pressure should be maintained at the lowest level consistent with adequate cardiac output and oxygen delivery. In addition other measures such as patient positioning with the unaffected lung placed in a dependent position and split lung ventilation, may be helpful in patients with AHRF due to focal lung lesions.

For further reading in *Principles of Critical Care,* see Chap 54 "Adult Respiratory Distress Syndrome" Jean E Rinaldo, Chap 128 "Acute Hypoxemic Respiratory Failure" Jesse B Hall/Lawrence DH Wood, Chap 136 "Aspiration Syndromes" Aaron R Zucker/Jacob Iasha Sznajder

31 | Acute On Chronic Respiratory Failure

Shannon Carson

Even minor insults to the respiratory system of a patient with chronic obstructive pulmonary disease (COPD) can precipitate respiratory failure. This acute deterioration superimposed on stable disease is termed *acute on chronic respiratory failure (ACRF)*.

PATHOPHYSIOLOGY

A primary determinant of ACRF is thought to be inspiratory muscle fatigue which develops when respiratory system load exceeds neuromuscular competence. (See Figure 31-1). In patients with COPD, the respiratory system load may be chronically elevated due to increased airway resistance and increased elastance associated with dynamic hyperinflation. Even minor additional increments in load or decrements in neuromuscular competence are sufficient to precipitate inspiratory muscle fatigue and respiratory failure.

Increased Load

Causes of increased respiratory system load are depicted in Fig. 31-1. The most significant contributor to the elastic load is dynamic hyperinflation. The rate of lung emptying in patients with COPD is slowed and expiration may not be completed before the ensuing inspiration. At end expiration, there remains a positive elastic recoil pressure, called intrinsic positive end-expiratory pressure (PEEPi), which opposes the inspiratory muscles on the subsequent breath (see Fig. 31-2). The phenomenon of PEEPi is easily demonstrated when a patient with COPD is mechanically ventilated, but it is present during spontaneous breathing as well.

Decreased Neuromuscular Competence

At the same time that the respiratory system load is elevated in these patients, the inspiratory muscle function is often impaired because of hyperexpansion (placing the muscles in a disadvantgeous position for force generation) and chronic protein-calorie malnutrition. Additional causes of decreased neuromuscular competence are shown in Fig. 31-1.

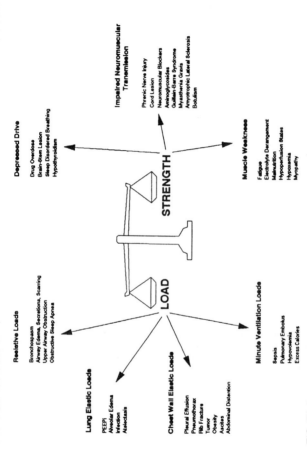

Depressed Drive

Drug Overdose
Brain-Stem Lesion
Sleep Disordered Breathing
Hypothyroidism

Impaired Neuromuscular Transmission

Phrenic Nerve Injury
Cord Lesion
Neuromuscular Blockers
Aminoglycosides
Guillain-Barre Syndrome
Myasthenia Gravis
Amyotrophic Lateral Sclerosis
Botulism

STRENGTH

LOAD

Muscle Weakness

Fatigue
Electrolyte Derangement
Malnutrition
Hypoperfusion States
Hypoxemia
Myopathy

Resistive Loads

Bronchospasm
Airway Edema, Secretions, Scarring
Upper Airway Obstruction
Obstructive Sleep Apnea

Lung Elastic Loads

PEEPi
Alveolar Edema
Infarction
Atelectasis

Chest Wall Elastic Loads

Pleural Effusion
Pneumothorax
Rib Fracture
Tumor
Obesity
Ascites
Abdominal Distention

Minute Ventilation Loads

Sepsis
Pulmonary Embolus
Hypovolemia
Excess Calories

FIG. 31-1 The balance between load upon and strength of the respiratory system determines progression to and a resolution of ACRF.

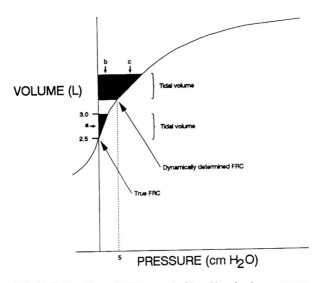

FIG. 31-2 The effects of PEEPi on work of breathing. A volume-pressure curve for the respiratory system is shown. Under normal conditions, alveolar pressure is atmospheric at end expiration (shown as True FRC). As transpulmonary pressure is generated by the respiratory muscles, there is a V_T change (here from 2.5 to 3.0L, a V_T of 0.5L). The pressure-volume product or the external work is shown by shaded area **a**. With gas trapping due to airflow obstruction, FRC can become dynamically determined. In this example the end-expiratory pressure (PEEPi) is 5 cm H_2O, which raises the end-expired lung volume. Now for the same V_T generation the respiratory muscles must overcome the positive alveolar pressure (PEEPi) before flow occurs, and the work of breathing is increased accordingly (**b** and **c**). In addition, the V_T change can occur on a flatter portion of the volume-pressure curve, resulting in yet another increment in elastic load. The addition of continuous positive airway pressure (CPAP) in an amount to counterbalance the PEEPi has the ability to reduce the work of breathing from **b** and **c** to **c** only.

APPROACH TO THE PATIENT

Phase 1: Before Intubation

The goals of management in the patient not yet intubated are to forestall mechanical ventilation when this is possible and recognize progressive respiratory failure when it is not. Avoiding mechanical ventilation nearly always depends on discerning the cause of ACRF and reversing it. Thus the first step is to review each of the potential causes discussed above in light of the clinical presentation. The treatments of many of these precipitants are discussed elsewhere in the text; here, the use of oxygen, pharmacotherapy, and continuous positive airway pressure (CPAP) will be discussed.

One of the most pervasive myths surrounding the treatment of ACRF is that these patients rely on hypoxic drive to breathe. Since these patients are typically hypoxemic on presentation, failure to supply adequate oxygen is a potentially devastating treatment error. In several studies performed over the past decade, patients with COPD have been convincingly shown to nearly maintain $\dot{V}_E$ despite treatment with 100 percent oxygen, and to augment their drive in response to hypercapnia. The goal of oxygen therapy is to maintain 90 percent saturation of an adequate circulating hemoglobin. High concentrations of inspired oxygen are not usually necessary in ACRF, unless pneumonia or pulmonary edema is present.

Bronchodilators are an essential part of early management. (Table 31-1). While much of the airflow obstruction of COPD is irreversible, most patients will have some reversible component. Inhaled β_2-selective agonists (albuterol, bitolterol, terbutaline, metaproterenol) should be given by metered dose inhaler (MDI) unless patient distress makes this impractical. A handheld nebulizer may be useful in patients who cannot use an MDI reliably, but otherwise, this route confers no additional efficacy. Parenteral agents (e.g., epinephrine 0.3 mg subcutaneously), and their concomitant toxicity, can nearly always be avoided. The anticholinergic agent, ipratroprium bromide, is as effective as metaproterenol in

TABLE 31-1 Bronchodilator Therapy in ACRF

Beta agonists	
	Albuterol or Metaproterenol by MDI (Three puffs q 30 to 60 mins) or Albuterol or Metaproterenol by nebulizer (.5 cc albuterol or .3 mL metaproterenol in 2.5 mL normal saline)
Ipratroprium	
	Three puffs q 6 h by MDI Consider high doses (100–600 μg q six h) in the intubated patient
Aminophylline	
	Loading dose is 5 mg/kg Maintenance dose is approximately .5 mg/kg/h Must be titrated against serum levels
Corticosteroids	
	Methylprednisolone, .5–2 mg/kg q 6 h Assess ongoing need after 72 h

treatment of ACRF, and may even be better in stable COPD. Until there is more solid evidence that the combination of ipratroprium and β-agonists is no better than either agent alone, we advise the use of both drugs. Aminophylline is a mildly effective bronchodilator in patients with COPD. In combination with β-agonists, a synergistic effect has been noted. It is therefore indicated in the treatment of ACRF. The toxicity of these drugs is substantial, including arrhythmogenesis and CNS effects. Daily serum levels are necessary for safe use, especially in light of the significant interactions with other drugs. Patients with ACRF given methylprednisolone in addition to standard bronchodilators show greater improvement in spirometric values than patients who are not. Therefore, any patient with ACRF should be given methylprednisolone, 0.5 to 2 mg/kg every 6 h. The benefit of corticosteroids beyond the first few days is not known. Since these drugs have important detrimental effects on metabolic and immune function, their continued use should be re-evaluated after the first 72 h. Bronchitis is a common precipitant of ACRF. Therefore, empiric therapy with an inexpensive broad spectrum antibiotic (e.g., ampicillin, doxycycline, cotrimoxazole) should be considered.

Continuous positive airway pressure by means of a tight fitting mask over the face of a nonintubated patient is an approach under investigation. This could potentially help patients with ACRF overcome the elastic forces generated by PEEPi and, therefore, decrease their work of breathing (see Fig. 31-2).

In recognizing impending respiratory failure, the decision to intubate requires clinical judgment and should be assessed by a physician present at the bedside. Assessment of respiratory failure cannot be based solely upon arterial blood gas results. Useful bedside parameters of impending respiratory arrest include respiratory rate, mentation, pattern of breathing, and the patient's own assessment. The goal at this stage of management is to intubate the patient *electively* once mechanical ventilation becomes unavoidable. Respiratory arrest may be complicated by aspiration or cardiovascular instability, compromising future efforts to return the patient to spontaneous breathing.

In a small number of patients with ACRF, face mask ventilation has been described as an alternative to endotracheal intubation. A tight-fitting mask allows substantial ventilatory assistance, yet provides for brief periods off of the ventilator. Complications of the mask have been minor and few.

Phase 2: Following Intubation

This phase consists of the immediate peri-intubation management and the first few days of mechanical ventilation. Care consists of stabilizing the patient on the ventilator, ensuring rest of the patient and respiratory muscles, improving neuromuscular competence, reducing load, and giving prophylaxis against complications.

There are two common pitfalls in the postintubation period: life threatening alkalosis and hypotension. These are both related to overzealous ventilation. Ventilator settings with $\dot{V}E$ levels > 10 L/min or excessive tidal volumes often precipitate a serious alkalemia, especially in the setting of decreased $\dot{V}CO_2$ as the work of breathing is assumed by the ventilator. This scenario can be avoided by approximating the patient's own pattern of breathing. Our own practice is to select a $\dot{V}T$ of 8 mL/kg and rate of about 20/min on an assist-control (A/C) mode of ventilation. There is no need to attempt to normalize pH, a maneuver which merely serves to waste the bicarbonate that has been conserved during evolution of respiratory fatigue. Hypotension is a consequence of escalating PEEPi following intubation. Again, the key to avoiding this pitfall is to prevent excessive ventilation. When hypotension occurs, the circulation can usually be promptly restored by simply ceasing ventilation for 30 s, then reinstituting ventilation along with measures to reduce PEEPi. Volume resuscitation is usually required to maintain venous return in the face of dynamic hyperinflation.

The respiratory muscles will require 48 to 72 h of rest before substantial recovery, so resumption of breathing efforts before that is counterproductive and likely to lead to recurrence of respiratory muscle fatigue. We continue to encourage rest by maintaining ventilation, and adding sedation when necessary. Rest can be achieved using any mode of ventilation, as long as settings are chosen which minimize patient effort. CPAP has been used to counter balance PEEPi lowering the effort required to trigger a breath (see Fig. 31-2).

Each of the factors discussed in phase 1 which contribute to depressed neuromuscular competence should be reviewed daily in the ventilated patient. The importance of nutrition must be emphasized. Excessive refeeding should be avoided, however, since unnecessarily high levels of carbon dioxide production ($\dot{V}CO_2$) may result.

Efforts to decrease resistive and elastic load should continue (e.g., reducing PEEPi, or using bronchodilators). Other contributors to increased load, such as congestive heart failure, pulmonary embolization, or respiratory infection may be easier to discern once the patient is mechanically ventilated, and should be sought during this phase.

Once the respiratory muscles are rested, a program of exercise should be initiated that will allow the patient to assume nonfatiguing breathing. This can be achieved using any ventilator mode, e.g., progressively lowering the triggered sensitivity on A/C, reducing the backup rate on intermittent mandatory ventilation (IMV), or lowering the inspiratory pressure on pressure support. After a period of work, the patient is returned to full rest to facilitate sleep at night. As strength improves, the amount of exercise can be increased in step, until full spontaneous breathing can be sustained.

The prevention of complications is an essential component of the management plan. As for most other bedridden, critically ill patients, subcutaneous heparin and antacids or sucralfate should be routine. Prophylaxis against pneumonia using nonabsorbable antibiotics is under active investigation, but cannot be considered routine.

Phase 3: Liberation From The Ventilator

A strategy for successfully discontinuing mechanical ventilation emphasizes increasing the strength and decreasing the load in ways already described. The specifics of ventilator management, such as the mode chosen or the device used, are largely irrelevant details if the compensated balance of strength and load can be restored. This issue is more fully elaborated in Chap. 6.

The progress of the patient can be easily followed by measuring respiratory parameters (negative inspiratory force [NIF], peak pressure [Ppk], static pressure [Pst], PEEPi, see Chap. 6) on a daily basis. The impact of therapeutic maneuvers can be assessed in this way as well. Finally, these parameters provide clues to the ability of the patient to sustain independent ventilation. For example, while PEEPi remains at 10 cmH$_2$O, there is little point in trying to make the patient breathe. On the other hand, when PEEPi has resolved and strength is adequate, mechanical ventilation is no longer necessary. One should choose a pattern of mechanical ventilation that approximates spontaneous respiration (e.g., A/C mode, V$_T$ 450 mL, rate 18) when discontinuation of mechanical ventilation is imminent.

Following extubation, careful serial assessments are in order. In the uncomplicated patient, the respiratory rate falls slightly through the first day, most often into the mid twenties to low thirties. Deterioration in the hours just following extubation suggests upper airway edema.

For further reading in *Principles of Critical Care*, see Chap 129 "Acute on Chronic Respiratory Failure" Gregory A Schmidt/Jesse B Hall

32

Status Asthmaticus and Bronchodilator Therapy

Ikeadi Maurice Ndukwu

Status asthmaticus is an asthmatic attack that is severe at its onset or progresses despite standard therapy and may result in respiratory failure and death. Any patient with asthma has the potential to develop status asthmaticus.

PATHOPHYSIOLOGY

Abnormalities of gas exchange result from airway obstruction caused by smooth muscle-mediated bronchoconstriction and airway inflammation. Mucus plugging of both large and small airways is found at autopsy. Dead space increases probably due to hypoperfusion of regions of hyperinflated lung.

Lung mechanical abnormalities include marked elevation of airways resistance; inspiratory transpulmonary pressure during quiet tidal breathing increases to as high as 50 cmH$_2$O and expiration becomes active. Despite increased work of breathing, FEV$_1$ is reduced (to 10 to 20 percent of normal) and peak expiratory flow rate (PEFR) is less than 100 L/min in severe asthma. Expiratory times are prolonged and alveolar emptying is not complete at the end of expiration. Intrinsic or occult positive-end expiratory pressure (PEEPi) is the consequence of alveolar pressure not reaching atmospheric pressure under the condition of prolonged expiratory time.

Abnormal circulatory effects of severe airway obstruction result mostly from pleural pressure excursions associated with breathing. During expiration, increases in intrathoracic pressure diminish blood return to the right heart. During inspiration, right ventricular volume may increase sufficiently to shift the interventricular septum toward the left ventricle compromising the volume of this chamber and resulting in incomplete filling. *Pulsus paradoxus* is the net effect of these cyclic events. During quiet breathing without airway obstruction, the pulsus, measured as the maximal drop in systolic blood pressure during inspiration, is typically less than 10 mmHg. During severe asthma the pulsus is greater than 15 mmHg, and can be used to gauge the severity of airflow obstruction, unless the patient ceases making sufficient effort to cause large intrathoracic pressure swings.

Progression to ventilatory failure in status asthmaticus may result from respiratory muscle fatigue; increased work of breathing (due to increased airways resistance), diaphragm failure as a force generator (because of dynamic hyperventilation), and PEEPi (associated with dynamic gas trapping) all may contribute to fatigue of respiratory muscles. Lactate excess in status asthmaticus is thought to be due to increased muscle production, the action of catecholamines used during treatment, or diminished clearance related to hypoperfusion. Regardless of etiology, lactic acidosis is a metabolic marker which may be used to predict an increased risk of progression to ventilatory failure.

CLINICAL PRESENTATION AND DIFFERENTIAL DIAGNOSIS

Clinical signs of severe asthma include tachypnea, tachycardia, hyperinflation, wheeze, accessory respiratory muscle use, pulsus paradoxus, and diaphoresis. The absence of wheezing does not exclude a diagnosis of asthma, and in the period immediately preceeding respiratory arrest the chest may be completely silent.

The differential diagnosis of severe dyspnea with wheezing includes status asthmaticus, upper airway obstruction, foreign body aspiration, left ventricular failure or ischemia, chronic obstructive pulmonary disease, and asthma complicated by pulmonary embolus, pneumonia, or barotrauma. History and physical findings usually help to distinguish many of these disorders. Assessment of severity of a patient's acute asthma attack is important in answering when and where to admit, and if intubation is required immediately. Asthma that worsens over days despite aggressive outpatient pharmacologic therapy is likely to respond slowly. Extreme interruption of sleep for two or more evenings is likely to lead to exhaustion. Dyspnea precluding speech or permitting only monosyllabic responses, heart rate $\geq$ 120, respiratory rate $\geq$ 35, accessory muscle use, diaphoresis, pulsus paradoxus greater than 20 mmHg, PEFR less than 120 L/min, and FEV_1 less than 50 percent of predicted all indicate severe asthma. If patients with these signs and symptoms do not respond to therapy within one hour, or if any deterioration is noted, the patient should be admitted to the intensive care unit.

THERAPY

Oxygen is used to relieve hypoxemia thus improving oxygen delivery to the respiratory muscles, reversing hypoxia-mediated pulmonary vasoconstriction, protecting against a paradoxical worsening of gas exchange with bronchodilator therapy, and may have some bronchodilator effect.

Inhalation of β-adrenergic receptor agonists is the bronchodilator therapy of choice. Table 32-1 contains suggested bronchodilator therapy for status asthmaticus. Tremors, nervousness, insomnia, palpitations, and tachycardia are the major adverse effects associated with β-adrenergic receptor agonists. Cardiac stimulation and vasodilation may increase myocardial oxygen demand or aggravate cardiac arrhythmias. Use of several β-agonists, or in combination with aminophylline, may increase the incidence of cardiac arrhythmias.

Anticholinergic agents such as atropine sulfate, glycopyrrolate, and ipratropium bromide are effective bronchodilators. Ipratropium bromide is the only anticholinergic drug available in metered-dose inhaler (see Table 32-1) and is relatively free of atropine-like adverse effects because it is charged and not systemically absorbed. The potential reduction in mucocillary clearance with these agents does not appear to be a clinical problem.

Theophylline may also be useful in these patients. To initiate and maintain theophylline follow the guidelines recommended in Table 32-2. Unwanted effects and drug interactions are major clinical problems which require close monitoring. Theophylline has a narrow therapeutic window and its clearance is variable. Theophylline is hepatically metabolized and excreted by the kidney. The half life in healthy adults ranges from 7 to 9 h. This is reduced in smokers to 4 h and increased to 12 h or more in patients with liver disease or any condition which decreases liver blood flow. In addition, a number of drugs are known to alter theophylline clearance (Table 32-3). Theophylline can produce nausea, vomiting, headaches, diarrhea, and insomnia. Hyperglycemia, seizures, and cardiac arrhythmias may occur at extreme serum levels. Theophylline-induced seizures may occur without prior symptoms, may be refractory to current antiseizure therapy, and have a mortality rate as high as 50 percent. Theophylline may produce tachycardia, exacerbate pre-existing supraventricular arrhythmias, and, with rapid infusion, may cause profound hypotension and cardiovascular collapse. Serum theophylline monitoring is the only reliable means of preventing serious theophylline toxicity. The incidence of serious theophylline side effects should be near zero below 15 μg/mL, uncommon below 20 μg/mL, and 75 percent at > 25 μg/mL. Levels up to 40 μg/mL warrant discontinuation of the drug (with administration of activated char-

---

TABLE 32-1 Bronchodilator Therapy for Status Asthmaticus

Inhaled β-agonists titrated to undesirable side effects, (e.g., albuterol 5 mg by nebulization q 20 min)

If inhaled β-agonists are not tolerated, consider parenteral epinephrine or terbutaline

High-dose corticosteroids for the first 24–48 h, (e.g., methylprednisolone 250 mg IV q 6 h)

Theophylline titrated to serum level of approximately 15 μg/ml

Ipratropium bromide may be of benefit in some patients, (e.g., 200–500 μg by inhalation alternating with β-agonist administration)

(Reproduced with permission from Hall JB, Wood LDH: Status Asthmaticus, in Hall JB, Schmidt GA, and Wood LDH, eds: Principles of Critical Care, McGraw-Hill, New York, 1992.)

TABLE 32-2 Intravenous Theophylline Guidelines

Loading Dose

No previous theophylline: 6 mg/kg of aminophylline (lean body weight) infused over 30 min. If already on theophylline, reduce theophylline dose based on serum level (Cs mg/L):

Vol. of distribution (Vd) = .5L/Kg × Wt (kg)
Loading dose = Vd × desired changed in serum level (mg/L)
= Vd (Cs desired–Cs known)
For 50 kg patient with Cs of 8 mg/L and desired Cs of 18 mg/L:
Loading dose = $.54_{Kg} \times 50_{Kg} \times (18_{mg/L} - 8_{ng/L}) = 250mg$

Initial Maintenance Dose

Group	Infusion Rate (mg/kg/h)
Adults	0.5
Smokers (60% Cl increase)	0.8
Liver disease (50% Cl decrease)	0.4
Severe COPD (cor pulmonale etc.)	0.4
Congestive Failure (60% Cl decrease)	0.2
Viral Illness (probable hepatic dysfunction)	0.4
Children	0.9–1.2
Subsequent adjustment as per Table 4.	

(Reproduced with permission from Foulke G, Albertson T: Bronchodilators, in Hall JB, Schmidt GA, and Wood LDH, eds: Principles of Critical Care, McGraw-Hill, New York, 1992.)

coal for acute ingestions) and supportive care. Charcoal hemoperfusion should be considered for levels above 40 µg/mL with severe symptoms (seizures, ventricular arrhythmia) and above 60 µg/mL even in the absence of symptoms.

Assessment of need for mechanical ventilation should be ongoing. It is important to recognize those signs that herald respiratory arrest. These include: exhaustion as suggested by easy distraction, slow response, and inappropriateness; marked diaphoresis and assumption of a recumbent position despite continued worsening of airflow obstruction; absence of breath sounds; a rising P_{CO_2}; and an increasing pulsus paradoxus (or a rapid fall in pulsus in a patient with failing respiratory muscles).

Intubation should be planned prospectively, not when respiratory arrest occurs. Pretreatment with atropine and topical anesthesia minimizes the risk of worsened airflow obstruction. A short-acting benzodiazepine, e.g., midazolam, in small doses of 1 to 2 mg intravenously should be given until the patient allows inspection of the airway. If muscle relaxation is required, an agent that does not result in histamine release, such as vecuronium at a dose of 0.1 mg/kg should be used. Opiates, especially morphine, should

TABLE 32-3 Theophylline Drug Interactions

Drug/Group	Potential interaction(s)	Alterations
Cimetidine	Theo. Cl decreased 25–40%	Monitor level, may need dose reduction
Erythromycin (and other macrolide antibiotics)	Theo. Cl decreased ~ 25%	Monitor level, may need 25% dose reduction or change in antibiotic
Ciprofloxacin (and other fluroquinolones)	Theo. Cl decreased ≤ 30%	Monitor level
Allopurinol	Theo. cl decreased ~ 25% if ≥ 600mg/day	Monitor level, may need 25% dose reduction
Oral contraceptives/ Estrogens	Theo. Cl decrease ≤ 30%	Monitor level
Propranolol	Theo. Cl decreased 20–40%	β-blocker contraindicated in bronchospactic disease
Troleandomycin	Theo. Cl decreased 40–60%	Reduce Theo. (50% minimum) monitor level, better–avoid troleandomycin
Isoproterenol (intravenous)	Theo. Cl increased ≤ 40%	Monitor level, may need increased dosage
Phenobarbitol	Theo. Cl increased 10–60% after ≥ 30 days	Monitor level, may need dose increase
Rifampin	Theo. Cl increased ≤ 25%	Monitor level
Phenytoin	Theo. Cl increased ~ 75% after ≥ days Phenytoin absorption may decrease	Monitor level, may need increased Monitor level, better– avoid Phenytoin Theo. combination
Lithium	Theo. Cl may increase	Monitor levels of both drugs

Theo. Cl, Theophylline Clearance.
(Reproduced with permission from Foulke G, Albertson T: Bronchodilators, in Hall JB, Schmidt GA, and Wood LDH, eds: Principles of Critical Care, McGraw-Hill, New York, 1992.)

be avoided because of deleterious effects on venous return, possible induction of vomiting, and the potential for histamine release, which could worsen bronchospasm.

Hypotension and hypoperfusion often follow intubation and positive pressure ventilation with either a bag or mechanical ventilator. Slowly bagging (4 to 6 breaths/min) with 100% O_2 for about 1 min will allow for prolonged expiratory time to decrease PEEPi, resulting in a rise in blood pressure. If this occurs, a fluid bolus of 0.5-1.0 L normal saline should be given every 10 to 20 min until an adequate circulation is restored.

The goals of mechanical ventilation are to achieve adequate alveolar ventilation, low levels of PEEPi, minimal circulatory compromise, and low risk of barotrauma. The patient should initially be fully sedated and muscle-relaxed to minimize airway pressures, allow determination of PEEPi, and lower CO_2 production. Dynamic hyperinflation is often seen in patients with status asthmaticus mechanically ventilated to eucapnea and can be minimized by using small tidal volumes and high inspiratory flow. Mechanical ventilation should be initiated with a tidal volume of 8 ml/kg, rate of 12 to 15, and inspiratory flow rate 60 L/min. To measure PEEPi in the sedated and muscle-relaxed patient, occlude the expiratory limb of the ventilator at end expiration while omitting the subsequent breath (Fig. 32-1). The proximal airway pressure rises to a plateau (the PEEPi). If peak airway pressures exceed 55 cmH_2O and PEEPi is greater than 15 cmH_2O despite full sedation and muscle relaxtion, tidal volume can be varied in 100-ml increments with corresponding changes in rate and flow to attempt to optimize peak airway pressure (Ppk), PEEPi, and P_{CO_2}. In some patients, accepting a high P_{CO_2} (70 to 90 mmHg) is the only way to bring Ppk below 55 cmH_2O and PEEPi below 10 to 15 cmH_2O. This controlled hypoventilation is preferable to the risk of barotrauma incurred by normalizing P_{CO_2}. If the associated acute respiratory acidosis is severe (pH < 7.2), bicarbonate can be infused to achieve a serum pH of approximately 7.25.

General anesthesia with halothane or enflurane has been used to reverse status asthmaticus. This therapeutic maneuver is rarely employed and then only when the aggressive conventional management plan outlined above fails. External PEEP should not be used during ventilation of patients with status asthmaticus since it can result in dangerous increases in lung volumes and airway pressures.

Liberation from mechanical ventilation of the patient with status asthmaticus requires thoughtful prospective planning. The paralyzing agents should be discontinued briefly every several hours (q 4 h) and readministered only if evidence of muscle activity is seen. While some patients with very labile asthma may respond to therapy within hours, more typically the patient will require 24 to 48 h of aggressive bronchodilator therapy until airway pressures and PEEPi fall. Once this begins, improvement is often rapid, with resolution of all dynamic hyperinflation usually within 12 h. As airway pressures fall, sedatives, muscle relaxants, and bicarbonate infusions can be reduced to prepare the patient for a brief period of spontaneous ventilation and then extubation. Assessment of respiratory muscle strength should be made by determination of negative

NORMAL

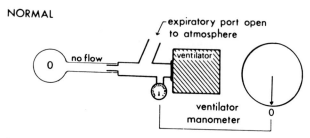

SEVERE OBSTRUCTION
expiratory port open

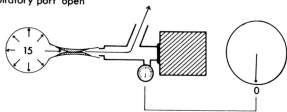

SEVERE OBSTRUCTION
expiratory port occluded

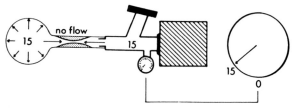

FIG. 32-1 Measurement of PEEPi in mechanically ventilated patients. (*a*) Under normal conditions alveolar pressure is atmospheric at the end of passive exhalation. (*b*) With severe airflow obstruction, alveolar pressure may not equilibrate with atmospheric pressure at end expiration (i.e., there is positive PEEPi). However, this will not be reflected by pressure measurement at the airway opening if the expiratory limb of the ventilator is open, allowing pressure downstream from the site of the obstruction to approach atmospheric. (*c*) When the expiratory limb is occluded at end expiration in the muscle-relaxed patient, alveolar emptying is complete and proximal airway pressure rises as gas is discharged to the central airways. The rise in proximal airway pressures gives PEEPi. (Reproduced with permission from Pepe PE, Marini JJ. Occult positive end-expiratory pressure in mechanically ventilated patients with airflow obstruction. Am Rev Respir Dis 126:166, 1982.

inspiratory pressure (see Chap. 29). If the patient has adequate muscle strength and no signs of ventilatory failure emerge during the brief period of spontaneous breathing, extubation should be performed since the endotracheal tube itself may perpetuate bronchospasm. Vigorous bronchodilator and chest physiotherapy should be continued in the ICU until at least the next day. During this period and following discharge from the ICU, a careful program of education should be implemented to help the patient identify signs of worsening asthma and optimize the drug regimen to obviate future episodes of life-threatening asthma.

For further reading in *Principle of Critical Care,* see Chap 130 "Status Asthmaticus" Jesse B Hall/Lawrence DH Wood, Chap 131 "Bronchodilators" Garrett Foulke/Timothy Albertson

33

Neuromuscular and Restrictive Disease

Ikeadi Maurice Ndukwu

NEUROMUSCULAR DISORDERS (See Table 33-1)

Central Nervous System Disease

Hemiplegic patients exhibit decreased chest wall motion on the side of their extremity weakness and reduced activity during voluntary inspiration in both the parasternal intercostal muscles and the hemidiaphragm on electromyography (EMG). In some cases the reduction of hemidiaphragmatic activity may be sufficient to limit regional lung ventilation and cause hypoxemia.

Quadriplegia results from acute cervical spinal cord trauma, spinal artery infarction, or cord compression by tumor. Damage at or above cord segments C3 to C5 involves the phrenic nerves. Partial or complete bilateral hemidiaphragmatic paralysis is associated with lack of lower rib cage expansion during inspiration, paralysis of intercostal muscles below the lesion, and intact accessory muscles. The contraction of the accessory muscles causes an increase in the anterior-posterior dimensions of the upper rib cage and pulls the hemidiaphragms toward the head. Abdominal paradox, in which the abdominal wall is sucked in by the negative abdominal pressure as the hemidiaphragms ascend, is a sign of diaphragmatic dysfunction in patients who inspire only with their accessory muscles. The ventilatory consequences of high-cervical quadriplegia include inability to generate an adequate tidal volume leading to hypercapnea, and a low PO_2. The hypoxemia results from both hypoventilation and from microatelectasis.

Lower cervical spinal cord lesions spare the phrenic nerves but the intercostal muscle activity necessary to stabilize the rib cage so that the hemidiaphragm can function properly is lost. Hemidiaphragmatic contraction, therefore, results in paradoxical inward motion of the upper and middle rib cage during inspiration, until the chest wall stiffens due to spasticity or fibrosis of muscles. Vital capacity (VC) and total lung capacity (TLC) are reduced and are worse in the upright position. The combination of expiratory and inspiratory weakness prevents these patients from coughing and clearing secretions, putting them at an increased risk for respiratory tract infection.

Poliomyelitis

Poliomyelitis is an acute febrile illness that may produce signs of meningeal irritation and flaccid paralysis. Paralysis may develop within hours of acute infection, or may take an indolent course.

Muscle weakness usually is asymmetric, may be widely distributed, and tends to involve the lower extremities and lower trunk. Patients with upper cord and brain stem lesions usually lose diaphragmatic function. Bulbar poliomyelitis also may cause paralysis of the muscles involved in swallowing and speech. Weakness of the laryngeal muscles may precipitate upper airway obstruction, and aspiration may occur if the gag reflex is lost. The diagnosis is based on clinical presentation, cerebrospinal fluid (CSF) findings of mild pleocytosis and minimal protein elevation, and the demonstration of denervation potentials on EMG. The therapy is supportive. Prognosis is excellent except in the elderly and those with the bulbar form of the disease. Most recover some, if not all, motor functions, except in the areas of total paralysis.

Amyotrophic Lateral Sclerosis

Amyotrophic lateral sclerosis (ALS) is the most common lower motor neuron disorder in the advanced countries. Its etiology is unknown. Patients may present with progressive muscle weakness and wasting that often involves the distal muscles initially. Although the extraocular muscles are spared in ALS, bulbar involvement may lead to impairment of the gag reflex, lingual atrophy and fasciculations, and laryngeal dysfunction. Signs of upper motor neuron disease such as spasticity and hyperreflexia may occur but after lower motor neuron damage has been present for over one year. The coexistence of upper and lower motor signs should strongly suggest the diagnosis. No specific therapy is available for ALS and more than 50 percent of patients die from complications such as aspiration and pneumonia within 3 years of diagnosis. Severe hypercapnea and hypoxemia can be corrected only by mechanical ventilatory support.

Disorders of the Peripheral Nerves

Damage to the peripheral nervous system results in a variable combination of muscle weakness, sensory changes, autonomic dysfunction, and reflex loss.

Guillain-Barré syndrome (GBS; acute postinfectious polyneuropathy) is characterized by a widespread, patchy, inflammatory demyelination of the peripheral and autonomic systems that is thought to result from a hypersensitivity reaction. Predisposing factors include antecedent upper respiratory infection or gastrointestinal illness within 1 month of onset, surgery, pregnancy, malignancy, and acute seroconversion to the human immunodeficiency virus. Characteristic features are progressive, usually symmetric, weakness that often includes facial and bulbar paresis and external ophthalmoplegia. This is accompanied by areflexia; mild sensory changes,

TABLE 33-1 Disorders of Neuromuscular Function

Level	Examples	Clinical characteristics	Cerebrospinal fluid	Nerve conduction	Electromyography
Upper motor neurons	Hemiplegia Quadriplegia	Weakness Spasticity Hyperreflexia Many have sensory and autonomic changes	Normal	Normal	Normal
Lower motor neurons	Paralytic poliomyelitis Amyotrophic lateral sclerosis	Weakness Atrophy Flaccidity Hyporeflexia Fasciculations Bulbar involvement No sensory changes	Little or no inflammation	Normal	Denervation potentials
Peripheral neurons	Guillain-Barré syndrome Diphtheria	Weakness Flaccidity Hyporeflexia Bulbar involvement Sensory and autonomic changes	Increased protein	Reduced	Denervation potentials late in course

					Changes in muscle action potential during repetitive stimulation
Myoneural junction	Myasthenia gravis Botulism Eaton Lambert Syndrome Organophosphate poisoning Tick paralysis	Fluctuating weakness Fatiguability Normal reflexes Bulbar involvement (esp. eyes) No sensory changes May have autonomic changes May respond to cholinergic agents	Normal	Normal	
Muscles	Muscular dystrophies Polymyositis Trichinosis Endocrinological disease	Weakness Normal reflexes No sensory or autonomic changes May have pain	Normal	Normal	Small motor units

(Reproduced with permission from John A Luce: Neuromuscular diseases leading to respiratory failure in Hall JB, Schmidt GA, and Wood LDH, eds: Principles of Critical Care, McGraw-Hill, New York, 1992.)

such as distal paresthesias; and autonomic abnormalities, such as tachycardia, arrhythmias, and postural hypotension. The EMG is normal early but becomes abnormal with time. The CSF protein starts normal but steadily rises within several months.

Respiratory failure does not occur in all GBS patients. Daily bedside evaluation of VC and respiratory muscle strength is necessary and patients with decreasing respiratory reserve should be transferred to the intensive care unit (ICU) before hypercapnea occurs. Elective intubation and ventilation should be performed with signs of respiratory distress and before the Pa_{CO_2} becomes elevated or the VC falls below 10 mL/kg. Plasmapheresis reduces hospital stay and the time spent on the ventilator if it is given to patients who do not improve or who worsen within 7 days. Corticosteroids are of no proven value in treating GBS. Recovery usually begins within 2 to 4 weeks after progression ceases. Although some patients recover complete motor function, about 15 percent remain handicapped by weakness.

Disorders of the Myoneural Junction

Myasthenia gravis is the prototypical myoneural junction disorder, resulting from circulating antibodies directed against acetylcholine (ACh) receptors in the myoneural junction. Cell-mediated immunity, involving sensitized lymphocytes and the thymus gland, is also involved. The result is that potential interactions between ACh and receptor molecules are reduced, leading to low-amplitude motor end-plate potentials that may fail to trigger strong muscle contractions, causing weakness and fatigability superficially resembling that seen in poisoning by botulinum toxin.

The most common presenting symptom is weakness of the eye muscles, manifested by diplopia or ptosis. Dysarthria and dysphagia also are common, as is proximal weakness of the upper and lower extremities. Myasthenia can be diagnosed on clinical grounds and by giving short-acting acetylcholinesterase-inhibiting agents that increase the interaction between ACh and its receptors. Transiently increased strength should be seen within seconds following the intravenous injection of edrophonium (Tensilon). Antibodies to the ACh receptor can also be detected in 90 percent of patients with unequivocal generalized myasthenia gravis. A rapid decline in muscle action potentials on repetitive stimulation is seen on the EMG.

Myasthenia is treated on a chronic basis with relatively long-acting anticholinesterase agents, such as pyridostigmine (Mestinon), at a dosage that improves muscle weakness with a minimum of cholinergic side effects. Plasmapheresis may improve motor function for longer periods. Thymectomy leads to complete remission or substantial improvement in about 85 percent of myasthenia patients. Corticosteroids and other immunosuppressive agents are routinely given to patients with generalized disease, and mechanical ventilation is needed in approximately 10 percent of patients, precipitated by infection, surgical stress, or the administration of aminoglycosides, neuromuscular blocking agents, or cholinergic agents.

Botulism is a disorder of the myoneural junction caused by a sporulating, gram-positive anaerobic bacterium, *Clostridium botulinum*. This organism produces potent neurotoxins, designated A through G, that bind irreversibly to the presynaptic terminal and inhibit ACh release. Neuromuscular symptoms follow exposure to *C. botulinum* neurotoxin within 2 to 24 h. The bulbar musculature is affected first, with resultant diplopia and dysphagia. Ptosis, extraocular muscle weakness, and diminution of the gag reflex are also common. Because the neurotoxin also involves the autonomic nervous system, nausea, vomiting and ileus may occur, and the pupils may be dilated. Mentation remains normal, and there is no fever. Severe respiratory muscle involvement is paralleled by decreases in VC and an increase in residual volume (RV), reflected in hyperpnea, hypoxemia, and the need for mechanical ventilation. Diagnosis is confirmed by detection of the neurotoxin in serum, stool, or contaminated food. Differential diagnosis from myasthenia gravis is made by EMG that shows small evoked muscle action potentials that increase in amplitude after repetitive stimulation. Botulism therapy involves elimination of unabsorbed neurotoxin from the gut by means of enemas and gastric lavage; administration of trivalent antitoxin to neutralize circulating neurotoxin in the serum; administration of high-dose penicillin (3 million units intravenously every 4 h) to kill *C. botulinum* organisms; and surgical debridement of offending wounds. Only about one-third of patients with botulism have respiratory failure severe enough to require mechanical ventilation, although aspiration is common.

Disorders of Muscle

Muscular dystrophies are a subgroup of myopathies with hereditary transmission, progressive weakness, and biopsy evidence of muscle degeneration without evidence of stored material or structural abnormality. The Duchenne type is associated with an X-chromosomal deficiency of the protein dystrophin that produces progressive proximal weakness starting in childhood. Expiratory muscle weakness that limits cough, and later inspiratory weakness that reduces RV and TLC are seen. Hypercapnea and hypoxemia may be due primarily to reduced innervation of the intercostal and accessory muscles during rapid eye movement (REM) sleep. There is no specific treatment beyond the possible use of corticosteroids, which increase muscle strength but do not reduce wheelchair requirements. Infections should be treated, and acute mechanical ventilation may be called for. Eventually patients become unable to walk and develop muscle contractures and kyphoscoliosis. These thoracic cage abnormalities then combine with respiratory muscle weakness to cause severe respiratory failure. Respiratory tract infections become progressively more frequent, and most patients die in the third decade.

RESTRICTIVE DISEASES OF THE CHEST WALL AND LUNGS

Kyphoscoliosis

Kyphoscoliosis, a combination of scoliosis (a lateral deformity of the spine) and kyphosis (a posterior deformity of the spine) is the prototypical restrictive disease of the chest. Most cases are idiopathic. Others result from congenital defects, poliomyelitis, thoracoplasty, syringomyelia, and tuberculosis.

Clinical symptoms and signs depend on the degree of spinal curvature. In patients with kyphoscoliosis, a scoliotic curve less than 70° rarely results in cardiopulmonary sequelae, whereas angles above 70° place the patient at risk of respiratory failure. Angles above 100° are associated with dyspnea, and angles of 120° or more may result in alveolar hypoventilation and cor pulmonale.

Kyphoscoliosis patients have abnormal gas exchange. Nocturnal hypercapnea and hypoxemia occur early, particularly during REM sleep, and may contribute to the cardiovascular deterioration in some patients. Alveolar-arterial gradients $[(A-a)Po_2]$ are usually no more than 25 mmHg. This increase in $(A-a)Po_2$ is due to ventilation-perfusion inequality caused by atelectasis or underventilation of one hemithorax. The dead space (V_D) to tidal volume (V_T) ratio is increased because small V_T (indicating inspiratory muscle dysfunction) is used to minimize the work of breathing. The increase in V_D/V_T results in alveolar hypoventilation. As inspiratory muscle strength falls, the arterial partial pressure of carbon dioxide ($Paco_2$) rises.

Pulmonary hypertension and cor pulmonale are complications of severe kyphoscoliosis that may lead to death in the untreated patient within a year. Pulmonary hypertension results from increased pulmonary vascular resistance (PVR) due to hypoxic pulmonary vasoconstriction or anatomic abnormalities and not from elevated left atrial pressure. In many kyphoscoliotic patients, progression to irreversible pulmonary hypertension occurs in association with proliferation of the media in smaller, precapillary pulmonary vessels. Potential causes of irreversible pulmonary hypertension include normal blood flow through vessels narrowed by low lung volumes, the vascular effects of chronic hypoxia and hypercapnea, failure of portions of blood vessels to grow in compressed areas during childhood, or kinking of larger vessels as they travel through deformed lung.

Acute respiratory failure (ARF) in patients with severe thoracic deformity is most often precipitated by pneumonia, upper respiratory tract infection, or congestive heart failure. The early correction of arterial hypoxemia with supplemental oxygen while seeking the diagnosis will yield the most favorable outcome. If near normal arterial oxygen saturation cannot be acheived with high fractional inspired oxygen, early intubation and mechanical ventilation are recommended. The hemodynamic status should be monitored very closely because these patients with kyphoscoliosis and pulmonary hypertension may not mount the usual hyperdynamic response to hypoxemia. Most patients survive the initial episode of ARF and may have up to 9 years median survival after the first episode of ARF.

Ventilator Management of the Patient with Restrictive Chest Wall Disease

Intubation is indicated for refractory hypoxemia, progressive ventilatory failure, shock, or a deteriorating mental status. Intubation can be difficult because of curvature of the cervical spine, distorted trachea, and higher risk of early desaturation during intubation due to smaller lungs containing less oxygen. During the peri-intubation period, a fraction of inspired oxygen (F_{IO_2}) of 1.0 is desired but should be decreased to less than 0.6 as soon as the patient is stable on the ventilator. Intubated patients with chronic hypercapnea should be ventilated to a Pa_{CO_2} similar to their baseline value to achieve a normal pH. Small V_T (6 to 7 mL/kg) and high respiratory rates (20 to 30 breaths per minute) should be used to minimize the hemodynamic effects of positive-pressure ventilation and the risk of barotrauma. The peak airway pressure should be reduced to less than 40 cmH_2O by using the least V_T needed to achieve correction of respiratory acidemia. While ventilating with small V_T, use sighs and positive end-expiratory pressure (PEEP) to decrease the risk of atelectasis. The PEEP should be started at 5 cmH_2O and increased only if atelectasis is apparent or if 90 percent saturation of the arterial blood cannot be achieved with F_{IO_2} of 0.6.

Respiratory muscle fatigue is best treated with 72 h of complete rest on the ventilator, with early nutritional supplementation and correction of metabolic irregularities. Trigger sensitivity should be low (-1 or -2 cmH_2O), and adequate sedation given. Theophylline titrated to a serum level of 10 mcg/mL can be used to increase respiratory muscle strength, help clear secretions, and treat bronchospasm. If bronchospasm is significant, then inhaled bronchodilators and systemic steroids should be added. The goals during ventilator management are to increase strength with many interventions including nutrition, rest, and theophylline while decreasing load with bronchodilators, antibiotics, or diuresis. Difficult to wean patients or those on prolonged ventilatory support may be helped with CPAP, a T-piece for several hours, and decreasing of dead space with tracheostomy.

Pulmonary Fibrosis

Pulmonary fibrosis is a condition of the lung in which normal air spaces and blood vessels are replaced predominantly by extensive fibrosis. Gas exchanging units are thickened, deformed, and dysfunctional, and the lungs are small and stiff. The etiologies of pulmonary fibrosis are numerous (see Table 33-2). Dyspnea is the

TABLE 33-2 Etiologies of Pulmonary Fibrosis

Acute (hours to days)	Chronic (weeks to years)
Oxygen toxicity	Idiopathic pulmonary fibrosis
Adult respiratory distress syndrome	Collagen vascular disease
Hypersensitivity pneumonitis	Hypersensitivity pneumonitis
Aspiration	Asbestosis
Drug-induced pneumonitis	Silicosis
Infection	Berylliosis
Inhalation injury	Coal dust disease (progressive massive fibrosis)
	Sarcoidosis
	Lymphangioleiomyomatosis
	Tuberous sclerosis
	Histiocytosis X
	Drug-induced pneumonitis
	Chronic aspiration
	Cystic fibrosis
	Talcosis
	Wegener's granulomatosis
	Bronchiolitis obliterans organizing pneumonia
	Goodpasture's syndrome
	Radiation pneumonitis
	Idiopathic pulmonary hemosiderosis
	Mitral stenosis
	Allergic bronchopulmonary aspergillosis
	Infection (Tb, fungus)

(Reproduced with permission from Thomas Corbridge, Lawrence DH Wood: *Restrictive Limitation to Breathing: Management of Patients with Thoracic Cage Deformity and Pulmonary Fibrosis,* in Hall JB, Schmidt GA, and Wood LDH, eds: *Principles of Critical Care,* McGraw-Hill, New York, 1992.)

most common symptom and may be associated with nonproductive cough. Other symptoms include fatigue, malaise, weight loss, arthralgias, and sleep-disordered breathing. Resting hypoxemia and mild respiratory alkalosis are common as patients progress to end-stage fibrosis. The chest radiographic pattern is dependent on the underlying etiology of the fibrosis. The respiratory mechanics of pulmonary fibrosis resemble those of kyphoscoliosis. Pulmonary hypertension and cor pulmonale are common in patients with end-stage fibrosis, correlating with a $D_L CO$ less than 45 percent of predicted and a VC less than 50 percent of predicted. Pulmonary hypertension occurs when blood vessels are destroyed by inflammation and progressive fibrosis, and when hypoxemia results in pulmonary vasoconstriction.

Ventilator Management of the Patient with Restrictive Lung Disease

When mechanical ventilation is needed for refractory hypoxemia or shock, a strategy that minimizes the risk of lung injury and circulatory compromise is desirable. When the usual practice of delivering tidal volumes of 10 to 12 mL/kg is followed or high levels of PEEP are used, patients with small fibrotic lungs generate high alveolar pressures. The adverse consequences of overexpansion in these patients are many. Pneumothorax and bronchopleural fistula are more likely to occur in the presence of fibrotic, honeycombed lungs. To avoid excessive tidal volume excursions and high airway pressures we use small tidal volumes (6 to 7 mL/kg) and fast respiratory rates (25 to 30 breaths per minute) when ventilating patients with pulmonary fibrosis with the goal of maintaining peak airway pressures below 40 cmH$_2$O. The approach to liberation from mechanical ventilation is similar to that used for kyphoscoliosis.

For further reading in *Principles of Critical Care,* see Chap 132 "Restrictive Limitation to Breathing: Management of Patients with Thoracic Cage Deformity and Pulmonary Fibrosis" Thomas Corbridge/Lawrence DH Wood, Chap 143 "Neuromuscular Diseases Leading to Respiratory Failure" John M Luce

---

34 | Massive Hemoptysis

Manu Jain

Massive hemoptysis is considered to be production of more than 300 to 600 mL of blood in 12 to 24 h. If the chest radiograph shows a diffuse, fine reticular pattern, patients are considered to have a pulmonary hemorrhage syndrome (Table 34-1). Blood from the lungs is generally bright red, has an alkaline pH, contains alveolar macrophages, and is frequently mixed with frothy or purulent sputum. These qualities distinguish true hemoptysis from aspirated nasal, pharyngeal or gastric blood.

STABILIZATION

As with any acutely ill patient, initial effort should be directed at assuring airway patency to prevent asphyxia. Clearance of bleeding may be facilitated by placing the patient in the Trendelenburg position or, alternatively if the site of bleeding is known, placing the bleeding lung in the dependent position. Additional maneuvers include intubation of the mainstem bronchus to the non-bleeding lung to protect the good lung and tamponade the lung that is bleeding.

After the airway has been secured volume resuscitation and transfusion should be administered as needed. One should then measure all bleeding parameters including platelet count, prothrombin time, partial thromboplastin time, thrombin time, and a bleeding time. Appropriate therapy should be initiated for any abnormality (see Chap. 51). Additionally, codeine or morphine should be used to blunt the cough reflex.

Once the patient has stabilized, underlying causes should be explored. In addition to routine lab studies, blood should be sent for antiglomerular basement antibodies, antineutrophil cytoplasmic antibodies (ANCA), antinuclear antibodies (ANA), rheumatoid factor, complement, circulating immune complexes and cryoglobulins.

SURGERY OR EMBOLIZATION

Most clinicians believe that patients with massive hemoptysis should be considered for immediate surgery. Since the definition of massive hemoptysis has varied and there are no randomized studies comparing surgical versus nonsurgical intervention the wisdom of early surgical intervention is not entirely clear. Before surgery can be considered it must be determined if the patient's pulmonary reserve is sufficient to tolerate resection and whether the underlying

TABLE 34-1 Causes of Hemoptysis and Pulmonary Hemorrhage
Hemoptysis
  Infections
    Bronchitis
    Bacterial mycobacterial pneumonia
    Mycetoma (*Aspergillus, Candida*)
    Lung abscess
    Bronchiectasis
  Tumors (suspect in patients greater than 40 years old)
    Carcinoma
    Bronchial adenoma
  Cardiovascular
    Mitral stenosis
    Pulmonary infarction
    Arteriovenous malformation
  Trauma
  Drug- and toxin-induced
    Anticoagulants
    D-penicillamine (few cases, Wilson's disease treated for 2–3 years)
    Trimellitic anhydride (exposure in the manufacture of plastics, paint,
      and epoxy resins)
  Other
    Sarcoidosis
      Endobronchial granulomas
      Mycetomatous colonization of cysts
    Blood dyscrasia
      TTP
      Hemophilia
      Leukemia
      Thrombocytopenia from other causes
    Ankylosing spondylitis
      Traction bronchiectasis
      Spontaneous pneumothorax
      Mycetoma
    Broncholithiasis
Pulmonary hemorrhage
  Pulmonary-renal syndromes
    Anti-basement membrane antibody-induced
      (Goodpasture's syndrome)
    Presumed immune complex-induced
      Associated with systemic vasculitis
        Cryoglobulinemia
        Polyarteritis
        Wegener's granulomatosis
        Lymphomatoid granulomatosis
        Churg-Strauss syndrome
        Hypersensitivity angiitis
        Behçet's syndrome
        Henoch-Schönlein purpura
        Necrotizing vasculitis
      Associated with connective tissue disease

TABLE 34-1 Causes of Hemoptysis and Pulmonary Hemorrhage *(continued)*

Systemic lupus erythematosus
Rheumatoid arthritis
Progressive systemic sclerosis
Mixed connective tissue disease
Idiopathic (alveolar hemorrhage + glomerulonephritis without immune complex deposition and without systemic vasculitis)
Hemosiderosis

(Reprinted with permission from Albert RK: Lung Hemorrhage and Hemoptysis, in Hall JB, Schmidt GA, Wood LDH, eds: Principles of Critical Care, McGraw-Hill, New York, 1992.)

cause is amenable to surgical correction. If the patient is deemed a candidate for surgery based on these criteria a "conservative" approach might be to perform surgery on most, if not all, patients producing more than 200 to 300 mL of blood in 24 h. An alternative to surgery is bronchial artery embolization which has a high success rate and low rate of recurrence. Unfortunately, in many instances the vascular anatomy precludes doing the procedure, so this cannot be considered the treatment of choice.

ROLE OF BRONCHOSCOPY AND OTHER DIAGNOSTIC TESTS

Bronchoscopy allows the site of bleeding to be determined in most patients with hemoptysis. It can also determine some specific causes of bleeding. The ability to determine the site of bleeding is markedly improved when the procedure is done early. The choice between fiberoptic bronchoscopy or rigid bronchoscopy is dependent on rate of bleeding and logistical considerations.

In many instances a specific cause for hemoptysis cannot be determined after bronchoscopy. Computerized axial tomography (CAT) scanning, pulmonary arteriography, bronchography or red blood cell scanning can be considered as alternative diagnostic tests but are rarely indicated. Patients with hemoptysis, a normal chest x-ray and a normal bronchoscopy generally have an excellent prognosis and generally do not require additional evaluation.

For further reading in *Principles of Critical Care,* see Chap 137 "Lung Hemorrhage and Hemoptysis" Richard K Albert

Manu Jain

PRESENTATION OF PLEURAL EFFUSIONS

Conscious patients in the ICU who develop a new pleural effusion may complain of dyspnea, cough and/or chest pain. In the critically ill patient the most prominent "signs" may be those of impaired gas exchange or decreased compliance of the respiratory system. Physical examination typically reveals dullness to percussion over the effusion and egophony near the upper level of the border between dull and resonant areas. The presence of a pleural effusion is confirmed radiologically, usually by a chest x-ray. At other times an ultrasound or computerized axial tomography (CAT) scan may be more useful (see Chap. 7).

The mechanical effects of pleural effusion on the respiratory system include restriction of lung volumes and outward displacement of the chest cage. By removal of pleural fluid not only are inspiratory muscles allowed to operate more effectively, but the concurrent reduction in pleural pressure may facilitate venous return and so increase cardiac output.

Pleural effusions cause an increase in the pulmonary shunt and thus may decrease the P_{O_2}. This improves after thoracentesis although sometimes removal of large effusions may worsen gas exchange secondary to re-expansion pulmonary edema.

THORACENTESIS

Thoracentesis is performed for diagnostic and therapeutic reasons. It is indicated to diagnose most newly discovered pleural effusions. It is especially important in patients with fever to rule out empyema. Only when a pleural effusion is small and the cause obvious is it permissable not to perform a thoracentesis. Alternatively a therapeutic thoracentesis is often performed when a large pleural effusion is felt to be a contributing cause of the patient's dyspnea or gas exchange abnormalities.

Important preliminary tests before performing thoracentesis include prothrombin time, PTT and platelet count or estimate. Abnormalities should be corrected by vitamin K, FFP or platelet transfusions. If the patient is uremic with a blood urea nitrogen (BUN) >60, it may be prudent to perform the thoracentesis after dialysis. In some cases it is reasonable to administer DDAVP to patients with a uremic thrombocytopathy.

If a pleural effusion is large enough, choosing a site on the chest wall for needle insertion may be made on the basis of the physical exam. For small or loculated collections, however, one should rely on ultrasonography. The decision to use ultrasonography should depend on the experience of the operator and the risks of the procedure to the patient.

Before beginning a thoracentesis the patient should be positioned next to edge of the mattress and the bed raised to a level that is comfortable. The patient's arm should be held out of the way by an assistant and the breast taped to keep it out of the midaxillary line if this is an issue. An exposure site that works well in the critically ill is the midaxillary line high enough to decrease the likelihood of inadvertent splenic or hepatic injury. When using an ultrasonographer the best site is dictated by the thickest layer of pleural fluid distant from the liver or spleen.

After selecting a puncture site, the skin should be cleaned with antiseptic solution and allowed to dry. Then the skin, periostium of nearby ribs and parietal pleura should be anesthetized using up to 20 mL of 1% lidocaine. The lower rib margin should be avoided since the neurovascular bundle is located there. After allowing 10 min for the anesthetic to work, a pleural fluid sample should be collected for pH and Pco_2 in a separate 5 mL heparinized syringe. Following collection of this sample, a larger sample is collected. All instruments and receptacles that will come into contact with the pleural fluid must be adequately heparinized. Additionally one confirms the adequacy of the length of the needle in relation to the chest wall thickness and the safety of the site chosen. Following completion of the procedure a chest x-ray (CXR) should be obtained to check for pneumothorax or hemothorax.

PLEURAL FLUID ANALYSIS

Pleural fluid from critically ill patients should be sent for analysis of pH and Pco_2, total protein, LDH, amylase, glucose, white blood cell (WBC) count and differential, red blood cell (RBC) count, cytologic studies, gram stain, aerobic cultures, anaerobic cultures, and cultures for mycobacteria and fungi. A tube should be stored for additional tests as necessary. Pleural fluid protein and lactate dehydrogenase (LDH) values are used to categorize the effusion as either a transudate or an exudate. A pleural fluid is an exudate if it satisfies at least *one* of the following criteria: **1.** Pleural fluid protein is greater than 50 percent of serum protein. **2.** Pleural LDH is greater than two-thirds of upper limit of normal serum LDH in the laboratory. **3.** Pleural fluid LDH is 60 percent (or greater) of the serum LDH. A pleural effusion which meets none of these criteria is considered a transudate.

Bloody pleural fluid should have a hematocrit determination. The closer the hematocrit of the pleural fluid to that of peripheral blood, the more likely one is dealing with hemothorax. If the fluid appears milky and chylothorax is suspected a determination of the presence of chylomicrons is diagnostic.

COMPLICATIONS

Generally less than 1.5 liters of pleural fluid should be collected to avoid the complication of re-expansion pulmonary edema. A second common complication is inadvertent puncture of the lung resulting in a pneumothorax or hemothorax. Rarely air embolism has complicated thoracentesis. Other complications include hemoptysis, laceration of liver or spleen, and an extreme vagal response resulting in bradycardia and hypotension.

TYPES OF PLEURAL EFFUSION

The differential diagnosis of a transudative pleural effusion is limited. The most common causes are congestive heart failure, nephrotic syndrome, cirrhosis of the liver, and hypoalbuminemia from other causes. Rarely does pulmonary embolus cause a transudative effusion.

There are many etiologies of an exudative pleural effusion. Some are listed in Table 35-1. The diagnosis is made based on the pleural fluid results and the clinical situation.

TABLE 35-1 Causes of Exudative Pleural Effusion in Critically Ill Patients

Venous thromboembolism
Adult Respiratory Distress Syndrome (ARDS)
Pulmonary embolus from intravascular catheter
Superior vena cava obstruction
Congestive heart failure
Empyema or complicated parapneumonic effusion
Simple parapneumonic effusion
Exudative ascites from abdominal or pelvic disease
Malignancy in the pleura or mediastinal lymph nodes
Tuberculous pleurisy
Amebiasis
Fungal disease
Acute exacerbation of systemic lupus erythematosus
Postoperative pleural effusion after thoracic surgery
Postoperative pleural effusion after abdominal or pelvic surgery
Postpartum state
Pancreatitis
Hydronephrosis
Myxedema

Recently the concept of a complicated pleural effusion has been put forward. It is defined as an effusion with a pH <7.10, a glucose of <40 mg/dL and LDH value of >1000 μ/L. Empyema can then be defined simply as the presence of frank pus in the pleural space. Both are considered emergencies and require a thoracostomy tube for drainage. For patients who are suspected of having multiple loculations of pus, multiple chest tubes or thoracotomy with surgical drainage are indicated, depending on the clinical situation.

Chylothorax is the presence of chyle in the pleural space and should be suspected when the pleural fluid appears milky. A chylous effusion contains chylomicrons, high levels of triglycerides and a predominance of lymphocytes. This differentiates it from a pseudochylous effusion which contains cholesterol crystals, smaller amounts of triglycerides but no chylomicrons. Chylothorax can result from laceration of the thoracic duct by central line placement or surgery, or by infiltrative processes such as cancer. A chylothorax can be managed conservatively initially with repeated thoracenteses or thoracostomy tube. If these measures fail operative ligation of the thoracic duct or surgical obliteration of the pleural space should be considered.

When bloody fluid is obtained from the pleural space two studies should be obtained. One is a hematocrit and the other is a clotting study. A bloody pleural effusion with a hematocrit low compared to circulating blood does not represent an emergency. It is most often caused by pleural metastases. Pulmonary embolus, pancreatitis and tuberculosis (Tb) are other causes.

A pleural effusion with a high hematocrit is a relative emergency. The rate of ongoing bleeding becomes the most important variable to assess and usually requires insertion of a thoracostomy tube. Rapid bleeding is defined as >200 ml/h or any rate that results in hypotension. Important causes of pleural hemorrhage include anticoagulation, polyarteritis nodosa, trauma, surgery, dissecting aortic aneurysm or an iatrogenic complication.

If blood drawn from the pleural space does not clot when allowed to stand, it indicates that the blood was not the result of the procedure itself but represents instead the result of pathologic bleeding of many hours to days duration. In most cases of esophageal sclerotherapy for variceal bleeding one will see a post procedure pleural effusion which is often associated with a fever. Fever 48 h post procedure with an enlarging effusion should be investigated with a thoracentesis. Patients with severe vomiting or those undergoing esophageal instrumentation may rupture their esophagus with spillage of bacteria and other contents into the mediastinum. Analysis of pleural fluid classically shows a very low pH (<6) and elevated amylase of salivary origin.

TREATMENT OF PLEURAL EFFUSIONS

Pleuritic Pain

Most forms of pleuritic chest pain can be relieved with nonsteroidal anti-inflammatory drugs. An alternative to control of severe pain is local nerve block. In addition to relieving suffering, the relief of pain plays an important role in enabling the patient to cough and take deep breaths.

High volume thoracentesis will often relieve the dyspnea of pleural effusions. The relief of dyspnea results from a decrease in the size of the thoracic cage which allows the inspiratory muscles to operate more effectively. Indications for tube thoracostomy may be classified as prophylactic or therapeutic, the latter being sub-classified into emergent or elective (Table 35-2).

All thoracostomy tubes for drainage of the entire pleural space or evacuation of a non loculated pneumothorax should be placed posteriorly and directed toward the apex. Complicated and sub-pulmonic effusions are best drained following ultrasound or computerized tomography (CT) localization. In general, no tube smaller than No. 28 French should be used and for a hemothorax; No. 32 to 40 French tubes are required. Once inserted the catheter is attached

---

TABLE 35-2 Indications for Tube Thoracostomy

A. Prophylactic
    Multiple rib fractures and large pulmonary contusion in patients
    requiring mechanical ventilation and PEEP in excess of 20 cm of water.
B. Therapeutic
    1. Emergent
        a. Traumatic
            1. Pneumothorax
                open
                closed
                    simple
                    tension
            2. Hemothorax
            3. Hemopneumothorax
            4. Crash protocols
            5. Electromechanical dissociation
        b. Nontraumatic
            1. Spontaneous pneumothorax
                a. tension
                b. simple
    2. Elective
        a. Pleural effusion
            1. Non-neoplastic
            2. Neoplastic
        b. Empyema
        c. Chylothorax

to underwater seal drainage or suction. Suction is required whenever the underwater seal system alone does not maintain evacuation of the pleural space. Failure to re-expand the lung despite an adequately functioning chest tube with suction is an indication for insertion of a second chest tube. If a second chest tube fails to re-expand the lung a major bronchial tear, a large bronchopleural fistula or a clotted hemothorax should be suspected. The definitive treatment for these complications is surgical.

When managing a thoracostomy tube an intermittent or continuous air leak mandates complete examination of the chest tube drainage circuit to ensure it is airtight. Transient clamping of the chest tube will abolish an air leak if it is intrathoracic or from the thoracostomy site, whereas a continuing leak denotes a connector system leak.

Determining the correct time to remove a chest tube is important. A general rule is that the chest tube is removed when the original indication for its use no longer exists. In a hydrothorax or hemothorax the tube may be removed if there is less than 100ml drainage in 24 h. Absence of an air leak and resolved CXR are indications for a chest-tube removal in a pneumothorax.

The incidence of complications of tube thoracostomy ranges from 5 to 25%. They may be classified as those related to therapeutic failure or an iatrogenic complication of the tube itself. Early therapeutic failure may be related to incorrect tube placement or may signal endotracheal, pneumonic or pleural pathology. This may require bronchoscopy and or thoracoscopy.

PLEURODESIS AND SHUNTS

In situations where tube thoracostomy is ineffective pleurodesis should be considered (Table 35-3). Pleurodesis, or obliteration of the pleural space can be achieved chemically or surgically. Effective drainage of the pleural space and early instillation of the sclerosant are vital for pleurodesis to be effective. Tetracycline, bleomycin and talc are the commonest sclerosants used. Pleurodesis can be repeated if an effusion recurs. Side effects of all the agents are similar and include pain, fever and morbidity of hospitalization. The indi-

---

TABLE 35-3 Indications for Chemical Pleurodesis

1. Malignant pleural effusion with good therapeutic result following thoracentesis.
2. Failure of response to standard tumor therapy and 1.
3. Metastatic pneumothorax.
4. Pulmonary blebs less than 2 cm at pleuroscopy for spontaneous pneumothorax.
5. Pneumothorax or persistent air leak in poor operative risk patients.

TABLE 35-4 Indications for Surgical Pleurodesis
1. Recurrent unilateral spontaneous pneumothorax.
2. Synchronous or metachronous bilateral pneumothorax.
3. Persistent air leak or pneumothorax.
4. Failure of chemical pleurodesis with favorable longterm prognosis.

cations for surgical pleurodesis are presented in Table 35-4. The two techniques of surgical pleurodesis are pleural abrasions and partial pleurectomy. Malignant effusions refractory to a second pleurodesis may be considered for pleuroperitoneal shunting. The shunt is also useful in nonmalignant conditions such as chylothorax.

PLEURAL BIOPSY

A closed pleural biopsy is a procedure for which there are no emergency indications. The place of closed pleural biopsy in the ICU is in the patient who is hemodynamically stable and in whom it becomes important to document the presence of Tb or coccidiomycosis of the pleura without delay.

For further reading in *Principles of Critical Care,* see Chap 15 "Thoracentesis and Pleural Biopsy" Eugene F Geppert, Chap 138 "Pleural Disease" Eugene F Geppert

36

Approach to Sepsis of Unknown Origin

Stephen R. Amesbury

Not infrequently infection is suspected in a critically ill patient on the basis of a constellation of clinical features consistent with sepsis, but without an immediately obvious focus. Two broad categories of patient presentation can be defined. Primary sepsis is acute sepsis syndrome or septic shock leading to intensive care admission in a patient without an obvious source of infection. Secondary sepsis refers to newly developing or persistent hemodynamic instability or features of the sepsis syndrome in a patient already being treated for a serious illness in the intensive care unit.

APPROACH TO PRIMARY SEPSIS

Sepsis Due to Bacterial Infections

Hypotension or frank shock with features of sepsis in the absence of localizing findings is a common problem confronting the intensivist. Once circulatory and respiratory stability are achieved and appropriate monitoring is established, the next step is to review the physical examination, history, and basic laboratory data. If this is unrevealing, one must next think about a common problem presenting in an uncommon manner. Severe intravascular volume depletion may delay the appearance of an infiltrate on chest radiograph in a patient with pneumonia. Head computerized tomography (CT) and lumbar puncture may be indicated for mild symptoms of confusion or moderate obtundation to rule out central nervous system infection in cases without the usual meningeal signs. Urinary tract infection with sepsis but no localizing signs may occur, especially in the elderly, if there is ureteral obstruction, perinephric abscess, or prostatitis. Many intra-abdominal processes, including mesenteric ischemia, may not be easily identifiable at the time of the initial evaluation. Repeated physical examination of the abdomen at frequent intervals is important. Even relatively subtle abdominal findings should prompt the intensivist to obtain abdominal radiographs and consultation with a general surgeon. Ultrasound or CT of the abdomen and angiography are further imaging studies to be considered. In the absence of one of the initially missed diagnoses noted above, sepsis in previously well individuals is most commonly due to one of the primary bacteremia syndromes or to acute bacterial endocarditis.

Staphylococcus remains the most common cause of primary sepsis in most hospitals. Diabetes mellitus, chronic renal failure, and parenteral drug abuse are associated with increased risk of this infection. Endocarditis must always be considered in staphylococcal bacteremia. Because of its frequency and poor prognosis if untreated, empiric antimicrobial therapy for life-threatening sepsis of unknown origin should always include coverage for this organism.

Meningococcemia, pneumococcal bacteremia and salmonella bacteremia are other important causes of sepsis which may not be evident from initial evaluation.

Nonbacterial Causes of Sepsis

Most of the nonbacterial pathogens causing primary sepsis occur in geographically definable areas, so travel history from the patient or family is important. Malaria, Rocky Mountain spotted fever, viral hemorrhagic fever, and viral hepatitis are examples of such pathogens.

Noninfectious Causes of Apparent Sepsis

Drug-related syndromes (acute intoxications or poisonings, drug withdrawal, neuroleptic malignant syndrome, allergic drug reactions), anaphylaxis, systemic vasculitides (hypersensitivity angiitis, systemic lupus erythematosus, polyarteritis nodosa), acute pancreatitis, extensive tissue injury (crush injury, rhabdomyolysis, vascular occlusion with tissue necrosis), and heat stroke are processes which mimic sepsis in critically ill patients.

Occult Sepsis in Patients with Underlying Medical Illness

The patient's underlying medical illness is often the single most important determinant of the clinical approach to sepsis of unknown origin. Diabetes mellitus predisposes to staphylococcal bacteremia, gram-negative sepsis, rhinocerebral mucormycosis, and candidemia. Chronic renal disease predisposes to staphylococcal bacteremia and pyogenic infections due to encapsulated organisms such as pneumococcus and *Haemophilus influenzae*. Asplenia is strongly associated with increased risk of primary bacteremia, particularly due to pneumococcus, *H. influenzae*, and to a lesser extent meningococcus and *Staph. aureus*. Functional asplenia in sickle cell anemia also increases risk of primary sepsis with these organisms and also with *Salmonella*.

EMPIRIC ANTIMICROBIAL THERAPY

Suspected infection producing life-threatening illness leading to intensive care admission should be treated early with effective antimicrobial therapy to avoid septic shock and its complications. In most cases, the basic medical evaluation outlined above will point in the direction of one or more of the categories shown in Table 36-1, and

TABLE 36-1 Antimicrobial Therapy for Sepsis of Unknown Etiology

Suspected source of sepsis	Usual pathogens	Suggested antimicrobial regimens	Alternative antimicrobial regimens
None evident Normal host	*Staph. aureus*, streptococci, Enterobacteriaceae, meningococci	Cefuroxime 1.5 g IV q8h and gentamicin 1.5 mg/kg IV q8h *or* cefotaxime 2 g IV q6h *or* ceftriaxone 2 g IV q24h	Imipenem/cilastatin 1 g IV q6h *or* chloramphenicol 750 mg IV q6h
Immuno-compromised host	Enterobacteriaceae, *Pseudomonas* spp., *Staph. aureus*, *Staph. epidermidis*, streptococci	Piperacillin 3 g IV q4h and gentamicin 1.5 mg/kg q8h	Ceftazidime 2 g IV q8h and vancomycin 500 mg IV q6h
Skin: (cellulitis, IV drug abuse)	*Staph. aureus*, streptococci, *Pseudomonas* spp.	Nafcillin 2 g IV q4h and gentamicin 1.5 mg/kg IV q8h	Clindamycin 600 mg IV q8h *or* vancomycin 500 mg IV q6h *and* gentamicin 1.5 mg/kg IV q8h *or* ceftazidime 2 g IV q8h
Lung	*Streptococcus pneumoniae*, *Staph. aureus*, Enterobacteriaceae, *Legionella pneumophila*	Cefuroxime 1.5 g IV q8h or cefotaxime 2 g IV q6h or ceftriaxone 2 g IV q24h and erythromycin 1 g IV q6h	Cotrimoxazole: 2.5 mg/kg TMP + 12.5 mg/kg SMX IV q6h and erythromycin 1 g IV q6h
Intracranial Meningitis	*Strep. pneumoniae*, meningococcus, *Listeria monocytogenes*, *Haemophilus influenzae*, Enterobacteriaceae	Ampicillin 2 g IV q4h	Ceftriaxone 2 g IV q12h *or* cefotaxime 2 g IV q6h

Abscess	Bacteroides spp. and other anaerobes, Enterobacteriaceae, Staph. aureus	Metronidazole 500 mg IV q8h and ceftriaxone 2 g IV q24h	Chloramphenicol 750 mg IV q6h
Intraabdominal and female genital tract	Enterobacteriaceae, Bacteroides fragilis and other anaerobes	Metronidazole 500 mg IV q8h and ampicillin 2 g IV q6h and gentamicin 1.5 mg/kg IV q8h or clindamycin 600 mg IV q8h and gentamicin 1.5 mg/kg IV q8h or ceftriaxone 2 g IV q24h	Imipenem/cilastatin 1 g IV q6h
Urinary tract	Enterobacteriaceae, enterococcus, coagulase negative staphylococci	Ampicillin 1 g IV q4h or cefazolin 2 g IV q8h and gentamicin 1.5 mg/kg IV q8h	Cotrimoxazole 2.5 mg/kg TMP + 12.5 mg/kg SMX IV q6h or cefotaxime 2 g IV q6h
Nonbacterial Sepsis Suspected	Rocky Mountain spotted fever	Doxycycline 100 mg IV q12h	Chloramphenicol 750 mg IV q6h
	Viral sepsis	Acyclovir or ganciclovir	
	Herpes viruses	Ribavirin	
	Hemorrhagic fever	Ribavirin	
	Influenza		
	Malaria	Quinine	

NOTE: Abbreviations: q4h, q6h, q8h, q12h, q24h, every 4, 6, 8, 12, or 24 h. (Reproduced with permission from Light, R Bruce: Approach to Sepsis of Unknown Origin, in Hall JB, Schmidt, GA and Wood LDH, eds: Principles of Critical Care, McGraw-Hill, New York, 1992.)

TABLE 36-2 Major Nosocomial Infections Complicating Intensive Care for Critical Illness

Site	Diagnosis	Usual pathogens	Predisposing factors
Head and neck	Maxillary or frontal sinusitis	*Staph. aureus*, Enterobacteriaceae, *Haemophilus influenzae*	Nasotracheal endotracheal tube, large-bore NG tube, facial trauma
	Suppurative parotitis	*Staph. aureus*, Enterobacteriaceae	Dehydration, poor oral hygiene
	Intracranial pressure monitor infection	Coagulase negative staphylococci, *Staph. aureus*	Long-duration intracranial pressure monitoring, frequent line manipulation
Chest	Pneumonia	Enterobacteriaceae, *Staph. aureus*, *Pseudomonas* spp.	Endotracheal intubation, depressed level of consciousness, use of antacids or H_2 blockers, aspiration
Skin and Vascular access sites	Vascular catheter infection and suppurative phlebitis	Coagulase negative staphylococci, *Staph. aureus*, Enterobacteriaceae	Poor aseptic technique; occlusive site dressing; frequent catheter manipulation; location: groin, axilla, antecubital fossa; skin infection/contamination: burns, impetiginized rash
	Wound infection		
	Clean surgery	*Staph. aureus*, *Strep. pyogenes*, coagulase negative staphylococci, *Candida* spp.	Protracted surgery; aseptic technique breaks; hematoma, prostheses
	Contaminated abdominal surgery	Enterobacteriaceae, *Bacteroides fragilis* and other anaerobes	Gross contamination, no antibiotic prophylaxis, inadequate drainage/debridement, malnutrition
	Infected decubiti	Enterobacteriaceae, *B. fragilis* and other anaerobes, *Staph. aureus*	Fecal soilage, poor perfusion or venous stasis, necrotic tissue not debrided

	Infection	Organisms	Predisposing factors
Abdomen	Pseudomembranous colitis	*Clostridium difficile*	Prior antimicrobial therapy
	Acalculous cholecystitis	Enterobacteriaceae, group D streptococci, *B. fragilis* and other anaerobes	Protracted critical illness
	Intraabdominal abscess	Enterobacteriaceae, *B. fragilis* and other anaerobes	Perforated viscus, contaminated abdominal surgery, pancreatitis, malnutrition
Musculoskeletal	Posttraumatic osteomyelitis	*Staph. aureus*, Enterobacteriaceae, mixed anaerobic bacteria	Compound fracture, frank wound contamination, foreign body, poor arterial perfusion, prostheses used for fixation within contaminated wound
	Septic arthritis	*Staph. aureus*, Enterobacteriaceae	Prior bacteremia, overlying cellulitis or skin breakdown, joint surgery or prosthesis in place
Urinary tract infection	Acute pyelonephritis	Enterobacteriaceae, enterococcus	Indwelling urinary catheter, diabetes mellitus, anatomic urologic abnormality or nephrolithiasis

(Reproduced with permission from Light, R Bruce: Approach to Sepsis of Unknown Origin, in Hall JB, Schmidt, GA and Wood LDH, eds: Principles of Critical Care, McGraw-Hill, New York, 1992.)

based on this, an antimicrobial regimen can be selected. When a probable source is not found, a second generation cephalosporin is generally advised. Extension of this regimen can then be considered by examining the possibility of central nervous system (CNS) infection, anaerobic infection, infection with a relatively resistant gram-negative bacillus, or infection with an organism not susceptible to conventional antimicrobials, mandating addition of erythromycin, a tetracycline or quinine.

APPROACH TO SECONDARY SEPSIS

Persistent Fever in Patients on Antimicrobial Therapy

Persistent fever despite antimicrobial and sometimes surgical therapy is a common problem which requires a systematic approach. Fever may take longer to resolve when the mass of inflamed tissue is larger. While fever due to infected intravascular catheters usually resolves within 24 h of catheter removal and institution of appropriate therapy, fever from severe systemic infections such as staphylococcal endocarditis may persist for 5 to 7 days. The clinician should reevaluate all the manifestations of sepsis present (white blood cell [WBC] count, platelet count, temperature, level of consciousness, hemodynamic stability). This evaluation should also include consideration of potential noninfectious causes of fever and the possibility of a new infection at another site.

The most important cause of antimicrobial treatment failure is lack of penetration of the antimicrobial to the site of the infection. The most important factor causing poor penetration is absence of blood supply to the site of infection as occurs with abscess, necrotic tissue, and bony sequestra. Incorrect initial choice of drugs and development of secondary antimicrobial resistance are the other causes of failure of antibiotic therapy. If there is no demonstrable resistant pathogen based on all culture results, and if the original regimen chosen was in fact appropriate to the clinical situation (see Table 36-1), it is generally not useful to simply change drugs; they are at least as likely to be the wrong ones as the initial choice. Obtaining repeat bacteriology from the site of the infection to guide antimicrobial therapy is usually a better approach.

Infectious Complications of Critical Illness

There are a number of infections which are either peculiar to the critical care unit or particularly difficult to diagnose in the critically ill. These require a systematic and directed approach which comes from specifically considering these entities and excluding them in turn. The usual pathogens and predisposing factors are listed in Table 36-2.

Noninfectious Causes of Fever or Sepsis Syndrome

The most common noninfectious cause of persistent low-grade fever, elevation of the WBC count, and mild-to-moderate "septic" hemodynamics is the host response to tissue injury. Large hematomas, traumatic injury to soft tissue, tissue ischemia, and pulmonary contusion, atelectasis, or chemical pneumonitis are examples of this. Drug fever may also be a diagnosis of exclusion which follows a careful evaluation for infection, and the diagnosis must be reconsidered at least daily.

Empiric Antimicrobial Therapy

In secondary sepsis, there are usually one or more candidate sources for the sepsis. Antimicrobial coverage should include *Staph. aureus* and enteric aerobic gram-negative bacilli regardless of the suspected source of sepsis, while coverage for other bacteria (anaerobes, *Legionella* spp., etc.) will depend on the suspected sources of sepsis. Entirely empiric therapy for fungi is generally not warranted except in neutropenic patients in whom antibacterial therapy is failing or in cases in which there is some evidence to support a diagnosis of invasive fungal infection.

For further reading in *Principles of Critical Care,* see Chap 97 "Approach to Sepsis of Unknown Origin" R Bruce Light

---

37

Sepsis, Sepsin Syndrome and Septic Shock

Constantine A. Manthous

Each year 300,000 to 400,000 patients in the United States will develop sepsis, up to half of whom will progress to shock, with a mortality of 50 percent for those in septic shock. Septic shock is the leading cause of death in many intensive care units. Accumulated data have suggested that early recognition and treatment of sepsis, before it progresses to shock, may improve this outcome. While our understanding of the pathogenesis of sepsis is still evolving, it is nevertheless essential to identify the septic patient early so that appropriate management may be promptly initiated. Early identification is in part implemented by rigorous, yet clinically applicable definitions of sepsis, sepsis syndrome and septic shock.

DEFINITIONS

Sepsis may be defined as the systemic response of a host to infectious organisms or their toxins, and is usually signalled by simple abnormalities in the vital signs—tachycardia, tachypnea, and thermodysregulation, all occurring on a background of clinically significant infection. The term *sepsis syndrome* implies progression of simple sepsis to include evidence of end organ dysfunction or injury (see Table 37-1). Note that recovery of an organism from the blood is unnecessary, and "culture negative" sepsis may be the most common form encountered in the modern hospital.

Septic shock is the extreme of sepsis syndrome, in which increasing end-organ dysfunctions (e.g., lung, kidneys, liver) are associated with a reduced blood pressure, usually defined as a systolic pressure

TABLE 37-1 Definition of the Septic Syndrome

Clinical evidence of infection
Fever or hypothermia
Tachypnea
Tachycardia
Impaired organ system function or perfusion
Altered mentation
Hypoxemia
Elevated plasma lactate
Oliguria

of < 90 mmHg or decrease of > 40 mmHg from baseline. The distinction of where shock begins in the septic syndrome is necessarily arbitrary, and end-organ failure or dysfunction is probably a more reasonable clinical delineation of hypoperfusion than any given blood pressure. Accordingly, therapy is best titrated against end-organ function rather than simply arterial blood pressure (vide infra).

ETIOLOGY

Classically, it has been taught that sepsis is caused by pyogenic bacteria, especially gram negative rods (GNR). It has become apparent that gram negative cocci, gram positive organisms, mycobacteria, rickettsia, protozoans, viruses, and fungi can all cause sepsis. So, more accurately, sepsis arises as a consequence of the host response to microbes and/or their toxins. GNRs elaborate endotoxin as part of their cell wall. Gram positive cocci elaborate a number of toxins including that responsible for toxic shock syndrome. Glutan is thought to be a toxin made by fungi which leads to activation of host responses and subsequent sepsis. Though it is controversial, processes such as pancreatitis or burns also lead to a syndrome that is indistinguishable from sepsis, likely via microbes and their toxins or through activation of host mechanisms similar to the response to infection.

PATHOPHYSIOLOGY

The Humoral Cascade

The abnormalities of sepsis are mediated by numerous host substances that normally act in wound healing and in defense against infection. A broad array of substances such as endorphins, bradykinin, kallikrein, catechols, cortisol, angiotensin, and histamine have been demonstrated to be present in the circulation in increased amounts in septic shock. Leukotrienes and cellular activating factors are also increased. Endotoxin, tumor necrosis factor, prostaglandins, and interleukins are also present in increased amounts in some patients with sepsis, and appear to be mediators which initiate and amplify the cascades underlying the pathophysiology of sepsis (see Fig. 15-1). Many of these substances appear to contribute to the capillary leak, vasodilation and intravascular thrombosis which lead to organ damage. Monoclonal antibodies to endotoxin and tumor necrosis factor and receptor antagonists for interleukin-1 have recently been or are currently being evaluated in clinical trials. Results of the antiendotoxin trials appear promising for some patients with GNR infection, while the utility of other interventions requires further definition.

Systemic and End-Organ Effects of Sepsis

Arterial and venous dilation are prominent hemodynamic responses in sepsis. The arteriolar response appears to be in excess of what is required to meet metabolic demands in many tissues and may be caused by mediators in the cascade described above, conceivably leading to the elaboration of endothelial derived relaxing factor as a common pathway to vasodilation. The arteriovenous oxygen content difference narrows in sepsis supporting the concept of supply in excess of demand. Another hypothesis is that peripheral oxygen utilization or extraction fails leading to anaerobic metabolism in some tissue beds. The lactic acidosis of sepsis has been interpreted as a marker of anaerobiosis, though clinical studies have suggested that pyruvate increases in sepsis secondary to skeletal muscle catabolism and the consequent rise in lactate may reflect this protein catabolism rather than anaerobic metabolism. This issue remains controversial.

The circulation in sepsis is typified by an increased cardiac output in response to the vasodilation and hypermetabolic state. Following volume resuscitation, cardiac output may be in excess of two to three times baseline. There is often a mild depression of myocardial contractility in sepsis, though its contribution to the end-organ failures is uncertain. Concurrent coronary artery disease may also contribute to inappropriately low cardiac output.

Adult respiratory distress syndrome (ARDS) is the most common lung abnormality that complicates sepsis. It is typified by low-pressure pulmonary edema with hyaline membrane formation and deposition of neutrophils in the early exudative phase. The lungs of early ARDS are usually stiff secondary to this edema and inflammation, and alveolar flooding causes intrapulmonary shunting with arterial hypoxemia that is relatively refractory to oxygen therapy. The administration of positive end-expiratory pressure (PEEP) reduces the shunt fraction and improves gas exchange by redistributing lung water from alveolus to interstitium, but does not affect total lung water. Therefore early use of intermittent positive pressure ventilation and PEEP may aid in improving oxygenation but does not prevent capillary leak. The use of newer ventilator modes, extracorporeal membrane oxygenation and anti-inflammatory therapies for ARDS are discussed in Chap. 30.

The hallmark of sepsis in the kidneys is prerenal azotemia leading to acute tubular necrosis (ATN). Animal studies have suggested that ATN might be attenuated or prevented by aggressive volume resuscitation. Low-dose dopamine in the range of 2 to 3 mcg/kg/min is also commonly used, though data to support this therapy are scant.

Up to 30 percent of patients with septic shock will experience encephalopathy. Alterations of the blood brain barrier or amino acid metabolism may be related to the encephalopathy which is typified by slowing on the electroencephalogram without focal lesions. Septic encephalopathy is associated with a poor prognosis.

Alterations in intestinal permeability to luminal bacterial endotoxins and liver synthetic abnormalities appear to occur commonly in sepsis. Normally, the gut serves as a barrier between luminal bacteria and the circulation. The data suggest that during sepsis the barrier function fails, possibly related to mild gut ischemia, leading to translocation of bacterial toxins. Liver cellular abnormalities including decreased production of albumin, occur related to uptake of these toxins or through ischemic damage.

SIGNS

Patients with sepsis are generally tachycardic, tachypneic, warm, well-perfused, with good capillary refill, bounding pulses and a wide pulse pressure due mainly to reduction of diastolic pressure. In untreated sepsis, the systolic pressure also drops and the clinician must utilize the above signs to differentiate between high- and low-output shock (see Chap. 22). Altered mentation and oliguria are not uncommon. In addition, signs of focal infection in lungs, urinary tract, abdomen, central nervous system, joints, and soft-tissues must be sought, so as to identify a potential source for the sepsis.

LABORATORY ABNORMALITIES

Increased blood urea nitrogen and creatinine often accompany sepsis, first with low urinary sodiums, then with inappropriately high urine sodiums after tubular ischemia has occurred. Early sepsis is accompanied by a respiratory alkalosis. Later, a concomitant anion gap metabolic acidosis develops. The anion gap is usually composed of lactate and other organic acids (e.g., pyruvate). Hypoxemia occurs when sepsis is caused by pneumonia or complicated by ARDS. Leukocytosis, leukopenia, hypoglycemia and hyperglycemia are also seen in sepsis. Disseminated intravascular coagulation and thrombocytopenia are the most common coagulation abnormalities of sepsis.

TREATMENT

One must define the source of infection and treat early with antibiotics and surgical drainage when appropriate. Antibiotics are chosen based upon gram stain (or other pathology) results of all relevant body fluids. Broad coverage of the category of organisms that is felt to be pathogenic, based upon the clinical and gram stain data, should be instituted until culture results return, usually 24 to 48 h later. Some classic clinical presentations also guide appropriate antibiosis. For example, patients presenting with meningismus, altered mental status and a petechial rash after an upper respiratory prodrome should be treated for meningococcemia. High fevers, dark urine, hemolysis, and an appropriate travel history suggest malaria. Fevers, rash, and travel to endemic areas may suggest Rocky Mountain Spotted Fever. Such classic histories can guide appropriate fluid examination and early treatment. In the cases in which history and body fluid examinations are unhelpful in the face of sepsis, broad, empiric antibiotic coverage is indicated, with all available specimens sent to the lab for culture. Table 37-2 suggests empiric coverage for sepsis from various sites of infection. An exhaustive search for an infected collection (abscess) must be part of the initial evaluation of the septic patient as antibiotics alone are very unlikely to adequately treat such infections. The abdomen, reproductive tract, bones, and soft tissues are most likely to harbor abscesses. Computed tomography (CT) or other modalities should be used to image such foci when appropriate. Prompt surgical drainage or debridement of such infections is considered part of the primary management. Gynecologic examination is especially important in patients with sepsis and a rash suggestive of toxic shock syndrome, since removal of foreign debri and retained tampons is essential to treatment of this syndrome.

When all gram stain and culture data are negative but the sepsis persists despite appropriate management, non-infectious causes of sepsis syndrome must be considered. Thermal injuries are evident, but occult liver disease, pancreatitis and ischemic bowel disease can all cause sepsis syndrome (and shock) in the absence of positive blood and body fluid cultures. Beri beri, adrenal insufficiency, thyroid storm, and severe salicylate overdosage can also mimic sepsis.

Supportive therapy includes aggressive fluid resuscitation since fluid is both sequestered in the dilated venous system and lost to the extravascular space by capillary leak. Large volumes, in excess of several liters per hour, may be required in early septic shock. The quantity and type of fluid used may vary between patients. Packed red blood cells are preferred for intravascular volume replacement (up to a hematocrit of 40) because blood provides both effective intravascular volume and oxygen carrying capacity which aides in treatment of the shock and hypoxemia when sepsis is complicated by ARDS. Albumin and hetastarch are more efficacious intravascular expanders than crystalloids, but they are expensive and have risks with no proven benefit over saline or other crytalloid. Pulmonary hydrostatic pressures should be kept at the minimal acceptable level. This means that volume should be administered to maintain the lowest possible left ventricular diastolic pressure to allow a cardiac output sufficient to meet metabolic demands as judged by total body arteriovenous oxygen content difference (less than 5 percent vol) and end-organ function. This titration is best performed using a right heart catheter, though no studies have demonstrated that use of these catheters improves morbidity or mortality.

Positive inotropes are utilized to augment oxygen delivery ($\dot{Q}_{O_2}$) after volume resuscitation. Since all patients do not respond the same to the various agents/dosages, empiric trials with hemodynamic monitoring are often required to gauge the response to these agents. Dopamine is used in renal vasodilating doses (2 to 3 mcg/kg/min) and if increased $\dot{Q}_{O_2}$ is required to meet metabolic demands, up to 25 mcg/kg/min of dobutamine is added. Dobutamine is often utilized to increase cardiac output which can allow a lower filling pressure and hence decreases hydrostatic forces contributing to pulmonary edema. Only if the patient remains hypotensive (mean arterial pressure < 50 to 55), will the addition of vasoconstrictors be considered. Norepinephrine offers both α (vasoconstricting) and β (inotropic agonist) properties. Phenylephrine or pseudoephedrine can also be used for α-agonist effect. The use of vasoconstricting agents is recommended only when all else has failed because they can cause profound vasoconstriction and end-organ ischemia. No study has shown an improvement in mortality by the use of positive inotropes or vasoconstrictors.

Reversible causes of increased oxygen demand ($\dot{V}_{O_2}$) should be treated. A substantial fraction of cardiac output and oxygen delivery can be spent by the respiratory muscles in nonventilated patients with septic shock. The early respiratory alkalosis and later metabolic acidosis lead to increased ventilatory requirements and hence work. In addition, respiratory muscles contribute significantly to the lactic acidosis which typifies septic shock. In adequately sedated (and paralyzed) patients, mechanical ventilation can effectively eliminate this respiratory work. Furthermore, volume resuscitation of the septic patient often leads to hypoxemic respiratory failure which itself requires intubation. Intermittent positive pressure ventilation with tidal volumes adjusted to the degree of alveolar flooding minimizes barotrauma of non-flooded units and can effectively reduce $\dot{V}_{O_2}$. Oxygen demand can be further reduced by controlling hyperthermia. Hyperthermia increases oxygen demand by approximately 10 percent for each degree centigrade above 37° C. Therefore antipyrexia should also be instituted to reduce $\dot{V}_{O_2}$. The use of cooling blankets in

TABLE 37-2 Empiric antimicrobial therapy for septic shock.

Suspected source of sepsis	Recommended antimicrobial regimen	Alternative agents
Primary bacteremia (no source evident)		
Normal Host	3d gen. cephalosporin: cefotaxime 2g IV q6h or ceftriaxone 2g IV q12h or ceftizoxime 2g IV q8h	nafcillin & gentamicin, chloramphenicol & gentamicin, imipenem
IV drug user	ceftazidime 2g IV q8h and nafcillin 2g IV q4h	piperacillin & gentamicin, imipenem
Immunocompromised Host	piperacillin 3g IV q4h and gentamicin 1.5 mg/kg IV q8h	ceftazidime & nafcillin, imipenem & gentamicin
Bacteremic meningitis	as for bacteremia, normal host	
Cellulitis/erysipelas	nafcillin 2g IV q4h	cefazolin, vancomycin, clindamycin
Acute bacterial pneumonia Community-acquired	3d gen. cephalosporin as above plus or minus erythromycin 1g IV q6h	clindamycin & cotrimoxazole, imipenem plus or minus erythromycin

312

Hospital acquired	3d gen. cephalosporin as above and gentamicin 1.5 mg/kg IV q8h plus or minus erythromycin 1g IV q6h	as above
Mixed aerobic/anaerobic infections Intra-abdominal infections Mediastinitis Fulminant aspiration pneumonia Necrotizing cellulitides & fasciitis Septic abortion, endometritis	3d gen. cephalosporin and clindamycin 600 mg IV q8h *or* metronidazole 500 mg IV q8h and ampicillin 2g IV q4h and gentamicin 1.5 mg/kg IV q8h	imipenem & gentamicin, piperacillin & gentamicin, cefoxitin & gentamicin, clindamycin & cotrimoxazole
Urinary tract infection	ampicillin 2g IV q4h and gentamicin 1.5 mg/kg IV q8h	3d gen. cephalosporin, plus or minus gentamicin

(Reprinted with permission from Light RB: Septic Shock, in Hall JB, Schmidt GA, Wood LDH: Principles of Critical Care. McGraw-Hill, New York, 1992.)

nonparalyzed and sedated patients can precipitate shivering with a net increase in $\dot{V}_{O_2}$.

Further supportive care should include treatment of electrolyte abnormalities and the coagulopathy of sepsis. Several studies have suggested that bicarbonate therapy for treatment of the anion-gap acidosis does not improve the morbidity and mortality in sepsis. Gastric ulcer and deep venous thrombosis prophylaxis should begin early in treatment. Early feeding so as to prevent excess catabolism is also advisable. Theoretically, enteral nutrition is preferred to hyperalimentation so as to prevent intestinal villus atrophy and the accompanying increased propensity for the translocation of bacterial toxins. Dialysis should be performed when acute tubular necrosis and renal failure complicate sepsis.

Finally, recent investigations have centered on interventions to interrupt the humoral cascade described earlier. In a large multicenter trial of over 500 patients prospectively randomized to receive a monoclonal anti-endotoxin antibody or routine care, treated patients with gram negative bacteremia experienced a 15 percent reduction in mortality. However there was no overall benefit for all patients presenting with sepsis syndrome and septic shock. Another large trial showed a reduction in mortality only in those patients with gram negative infections without shock. This therapy appears to have promise in patients with GNR sepsis, though it is impossible to predict which patients are gram negative bacteremic on presentation. Trials of anti-tumor necrosis factor antibodies and interleukin-1 receptor antagonists for sepsis are currently ongoing. Non-steroidal anti-inflammatory drugs have been shown, in small studies, to offer some benefit. Several large studies have concluded that steroids do not have a role in the treatment of septic shock. The role for mediator-blocking therapies will become more clear as further studies evaluate the efficacy of the various agents.

To summarize, sepsis is a constellation of clinical signs arising as a result of the host response to microbes. Early recognition of this syndrome is quintessential to interrupting the cascade which, if left untreated, will lead to organ failures and death. Treatment objectives can be summarized as follows:

1. Seek and eradicate foci of infection.
2. Volume resuscitation and inotropic support to provide a $\dot{Q}_{O_2}$ adequate to meet $\dot{V}_{O_2}$ at the lowest possible cardiac filling pressures.
3. Ventilatory support, sedation or paralysis (if required), and fever control, to minimize $\dot{V}_{O_2}$.
4. Routine supportive, meticulous intensive care.
5. Consider humoral therapy. Antiendotoxin antibodies may be useful in treating patients with proven GNR infections.

Prompt recognition and early, decisive treatment provide the patient with the best opportunity to avoid the morbidity and mortality of this malignant disease.

For further reading in *Principles of Critical Care,* see Chap 55 "Sepsis Syndrome" R Bruce Light, Chap 97 "Approach to Sepsis of Unknown Origin" R Bruce Light, Chap 98 "Septic Shock" R Bruce Light

---

| **The Acute Abdomen, Intraabdominal Sepsis, and Toxic Megacolon**

David Olson

THE ACUTE ABDOMEN AND INTRAABDOMINAL SEPSIS

The term "acute abdomen" refers to a patient whose chief presenting symptom is the acute onset of abdominal pain. The diagnosis is heavily dependent on a complete history and physical examination. In the ICU, however, these two sources of data may be severely limited due to patients' varying levels of consciousness, the presence of a variety of lines and tubes, and the use of masking drugs such as corticosteroids or narcotics. The physician must infer the presence of an abdominal process based on nonspecific findings such as unexplained sepsis, hypovolemia, and abdominal distention. Helpful guiding principles in approaching the acute abdomen include evaluating the patient in the context of the patient's underlying disorder, making liberal use of surgical consultants, and employing computerized tomography (CT) scan or ultrasound of the abdomen as screening tests. Patients with an acute abdomen who commonly require ICU management are those with intraabdominal sepsis (IAS). The etiologies of IAS are many, but of particular note are primary and secondary peritonitis, biliary tract sepsis, and visceral abscesses. Primary peritonitis is characterized by infection in the peritoneal cavity without an obvious source, most frequently occurring in patients with ascites secondary to an underlying disorder (cirrhosis, congestive heart failure [CHF], renal dialysis). This entity most often presents when these patients are undergoing intensive care for other reasons. Clinical presentation is usually one of fever and physical signs of peritoneal irritation, though up to one-third will have no signs or symptoms of sepsis referable to the abdomen. Diagnosis is based on clinical suspicion, patient presentation, and ascitic fluid aspiration. An ascitic fluid neutrophil count greater than $250/\mu L$ can be considered diagnostic. Gram stain and culture are confirmatory, though up to 35 percent of patients will have negative ascitic fluid cultures. In culture-negative patients, diagnosis can be confirmed by clinical improvement and decreased ascitic neutrophil count after 48 hours of appropriate antibiotic treatment. Ampicillin and an aminoglycoside or a third generation cephalosporin alone is the usual treatment of choice.

Secondary bacterial peritonitis is defined as the presence of pus or gastrointestinal contents in the peritoneal cavity. Generalized peritonitis is most commonly caused by bowel perforation; bowel infarction and perforation of an infected gall bladder or pancreatic pseudocyst are other etiologies to consider. Because of the anatomy of the peritoneal cavity, patients with generalized peritonitis may suffer massive loss of fluids into the abdomen and rapid absorption of bacterial endotoxin and inflammatory mediators into the systemic circulation. Treatment is based on rapid fluid resuscitation, initiation of antibiotic therapy, and surgical intervention. The gold standard in antibiotic therapy is the combination of an aminoglycoside and an antianaerobe agent such as metronidazole or clindamycin. In those at risk for nephrotoxicity, the use of a second generation cephalosporin (e.g., cefoxitin) as a single agent is equally efficacious. Due to the risk of drug resistance and superinfection, antibiotics should be discontinued as soon as the acute process subsides. In ICU patients, it is reasonable to stop antibiotics when the patient no longer has physical signs of peritonitis or ileus. If fever and leukocytosis persist, a CT scan should be obtained to rule out intra-abdominal abscess. If no abscess is found, antibiotics can be stopped and a search begun for an extra-peritoneal source of infection. In generalized peritonitis the mortality rate is about 30 percent, with the cause of death usually being uncontrolled sepsis.

The role of the intensivist in these patients is to guide hemodynamic, ventilatory and nutritional support, antibiotic therapy, and renal dialysis, if necessary. In addition, the critical care physician must be aware of the wide variety of possible complications (Table 38-1). In the daily patient examination, all dressings covering the abdomen should be removed and the wound inspected. Fascial dehiscence is not uncommon and most frequently occurs on postoperative days 4 to 8. It is heralded by the drainage of serosanguinous fluid through the incision. An immediate surgical consultation is required. After examining the wound, all tubes and drains should be inspected for proper position and function. The gastrointestinal tract should then be evaluated for its ability to tolerate enteral feeding. In the sedated ventilated patient, challenging with tube feedings and checking the gastric residual volume every 4 hours may be necessary. Finally, the critical care physician must determine if the patient is septic and whether the septic focus is intraabdominal. In general, if the patient is not steadily improving following surgery, or if the patient begins to deteriorate in any way, a CT scan of the abdomen should be obtained to search for a possible abscess. Such a scan may not be fruitful in the initial 5 to 7 postoperative days, as multiple, usually sterile, intraabdominal fluid collections are common. In this early period, a deteriorating patient will usually require a repeat laparotomy. Beyond this early phase, percutaneous drainage is a safe and effective method of abscess diagnosis and control.

Abnormalities of liver function tests and jaundice are quite common in the ICU patient population and may not reflect actual pathology in the biliary tree. However, when sepsis and hyperbili-

TABLE 38-1 Postoperative Complications Specifically Related to the Surgical Treatment of Peritonitis

1. Wound Complications
   wound infection
   necrotizing soft tissue infection
   fascial dehiscence/evisceration
2. GI Tract Complications
   ileus
   mechanical obstruction
   enterocutaneous fistula
   GI bleeding
   anastomotic disruption or perforation
   ischemic bowel
   antibiotic-associated colitis
3. Complications Arising in the Peritoneal Cavity
   abscess formation
   intra-abdominal bleeding
4. Miscellaneous
   post-operative pancreatitis
   septicemia
   acalculous cholecystitis

(Reprinted with permission from Mustard RA, Bohnen JMA, Schouten BD: The Acute Abdomen and Intraabdominal Sepsis, in Hall JB, Schmidt GA, and Wood LDH: Principles of Critical Care, McGraw-Hill, New York, 1992.)

rubinemia coexist, the question of biliary tract sepsis arises. Infection in the biliary tree occurs in one of three clinically distinct entities: acute calculous cholecystitis, acute cholangitis, and acute acalculous cholecystitis. Calculus cholecystitis is usually treated surgically by removal of the gall bladder and only results in ICU admission if the patient has other major medical problems. Cholangitis occurs as a bacterial infection within a partially or totally occluded bile duct system. The clinical triad is one of right upper quadrant pain, jaundice, and fever. Diagnosis may be confirmed by ultrasound, ERCP (endoscopic retrograde cholangiopancreatogram), or PTC (percutaneous transhepatic cholangiogram). Treatment consists of broad spectrum antibiotics to cover gram-negative aerobes and anaerobes, as well as adequate biliary decompression. The latter may be done surgically (placement of a T-tube), endoscopically, or percutaneously. A patient with cholangitis who does not improve clinically must be assumed to have inadequate drainage and it is essential to image the biliary tree to assess adequacy of drainage. A CT scan to look for hepatic abscesses may also be necessary.

Acute acalculous cholecystitis occurs in approximately 0.5 to 1.5 percent of longterm (> 1 week) ICU patients. The etiology is unknown, but the gall bladder wall becomes inflamed and infected with enteric organisms while the cystic duct becomes edematous and occluded. It is difficult to diagnose without resorting to laparotomy. Ultrasound and CT scan are the most valuable noninvasive tests, with findings of pericholecystic fluid, intramural gas, or sloughed mucosal membrane being virtually diagnostic. A negative biliary radionuclide scan implies cystic duct patency and effectively rules out cholecystitis. Liver function tests and percutaneous bile aspiration for culture are not helpful. Direct visualization of the gallbladder in the operating room is the only completely accurate method of diagnosis. In the rare patient who is felt to be "too sick" to undergo laparotomy significant clinical improvement may be achieved by percutaneous transhepatic drainage of the gallbladder. These patients should later undergo cholecystectomy.

Visceral abscesses of the liver and spleen are rare. Patients with hepatic abscess usually present with sepsis, right upper quadrant pain, and occasionally, peritoneal signs. Etiologies include trauma, perihepatic sepsis, systemic bacteremia, portal bacteremia, and cholangitis. Diagnosis is made by CT scan or ultrasound. The preferred treatment is percutaneous drainage of large, even multiple abscesses. Broad-spectrum antibiotics should be administered and may be the only treatment necessary for those with multiple small abscesses.

Splenic abscesses occur as a result of trauma, direct extension of a septic process (e.g., pancreatitis), infection of a splenic infarct, or secondary to bacteremia. Patients present with left upper quadrant pain, a left pleural effusion, or sepsis of unknown etiology. Again, diagnosis is established by CT scan or ultrasound. Treatment usually consists of splenectomy, though percutaneous drainage may act as a temporizing measure.

Frequently, an ICU patient will be septic or have multisystem organ failure with no obvious etiology. As other sources are ruled out, the abdomen may be considered, even if no prior gastrointestinal pathology exists. A CT scan of the abdomen is an excellent screening tool, but a negative scan (or ultrasound) does not rule out peritoneal infection. Occult causes of IAS include acute acaculous cholecystitis, interloop abscesses, a short segment of ischemic or necrotic bowel, and potentially, bacteremia from increased gut mucosal permeability as a result of critical illness. Diagnostic laparotomy is rarely helpful in preventing mortality in the absence of specific clinical or laboratory findings.

Diagnostic peritoneal lavage (DPL) is a relatively safe and useful adjunct to the physical examination and history in evaluating patients with an acute abdomen or suspected intraabdominal sepsis. Peritoneal lavage and paracentesis have been well-established in diagnosing those with intraabdominal injury following blunt trauma. More recently, these techniques have been applied to the assessment of the acute nontraumatic abdomen, especially in those patients who are unable to provide classic clinical features due to confusion, sedation, coma, mechanical ventilation, or multiple medical problems.

DPL is most often performed in an "open" manner usually through an incision in the midline below the umbilicus. Positive results include grossly bloody, cloudy, or malodorous fluid upon initial aspiration prior to instillation of lavage fluid. After instillation of one liter of lactated Ringer's solution, positive results include a WBC count >500/μL with a predominance of polymorphonuclear cells, a RBC count >100,000/μL (some studies suggest >50,000/μL), or a fluid gram stain positive for bacteria. The usefulness of bile or amylase content is questionable. Culture results of lavage fluid generally are available too late to be of use in the acute setting. DPL is not indicated in the presence of classic signs of peritoneal infection.

TOXIC MEGACOLON

Toxic megacolon, or toxic dilation of the colon, is the most dreaded and certainly most lethal complication of colitis. Toxic megacolon is most often a complication of ulcerative colitis, with 70 percent of cases occurring in patients under the age of thirty. The incidence of toxic megacolon in patients with ulcerative colitis ranges from 1.6 to 21.4 percent, with most reported frequencies in the lower range. Disease processes that can be complicated by toxic megacolon are listed in Table 38-2. Certain factors may precipitate toxic megacolon in predisposed individuals: barium enemas, opiates, anticholinergics, antidiarrheal agents, electrolyte imbalance (hypokalemia, hypocalcemia, hypomagnesemia, hypophosphatemia, and metabolic alkalosis), and possibly pregnancy.

The three features necessary to make a diagnosis of toxic megacolon are colitis, colonic dilation, and a toxic-appearing pa-

TABLE 38-2 Disease Processes That Can Be Complicated by Toxic Megacolon

Ulcerative colitis
Crohn's colitis
Amebic colitis
Salmonellosis
Cholera
Pseudomembranous colitis
Ischemic colitis
Behçet's syndrome
Methotrexate therapy

(Reprinted with permission from Reznick RK: Toxic Megacolon, in Hall JB, Schmidt GA, Wood LDH: Principles of Critical Care, McGraw-Hill, New York, 1992.)

tient. In addition, dehydration with tachycardia and hypotension, abdominal distention, and signs of peritoneal irritation are frequently present. All patients should have three views of the abdomen and an upright chest radiograph. The transverse colon is usually most prominently dilated, with 6 to 9 cm of dilation needed to label the process toxic megacolon. Workup should also include routine hematology, biochemistry, and arterial blood gas determination. A gentle and careful proctosigmoidoscopic examination using a rigid scope should be carried out. The purpose of this examination is to confirm the suspicion of active colitis, to obtain stool cultures or swabs from mucosal ulcerations, and to identify specific forms of colitis such as pseudomembranous colitis. Barium enema and total colonoscopy are contraindicated, while ultrasound and CT scan are generally not helpful.

Patients with toxic megacolon should be managed in an ICU, and often need invasive monitoring. All patients should have large bore intravenous lines, a Foley catheter, and a measure of intravascular filling pressure such as a central venous or right heart catheter. Patients should be cross-matched for at least 4 units of blood, kept n.p.o., and have nasogastric or long tube gastrointestinal decompression (with early consideration of total parenteral nutrition [TPN]).

The primary aim of therapy is urgent treatment directed at reducing dilation of the thin-walled inflamed colon, thereby reducing the chances of perforation. Aggressive medical therapy should be tried for a limited time with urgent surgical intervention for those patients who fail to show quick and dramatic improvement. Those requiring immediate surgery are patients with perforation or imminent rupture of the colon (12 cm or greater), septic shock, having at least three of the following: temperature>103°F(39.4°C), tachycardia>150, positive blood cultures, and partial loss of consciousness.

Medical management includes resuscitation, as described above, as well as directed therapy and observation. Although there is no convincing proof of efficacy, efforts at reducing the acuity of the disease process can be achieved by the administration of steroids or ACTH (100 mg hydrocortisone IV every 6 h or 40 to 180U ACTH every 24 h). The physician must be aware that high dose steroids may mask clinical signs and have been theorized to increase the risk of perforation. Intravenous steroids are essential for those patients on chronic steroid treatment for ulcerative colitis. In addition, broad spectrum antibiotics, rolling into the prone position (for 10 to 15 min every 2 to 3 h), an abdominal examination every 3 to 4 h, and a radiologic examination every 12 to 24 h are essential components of therapy.

Parameters for measurement of success of medical therapy should include: return of active bowel sounds, a decrease by at least

2 cm of colonic dilation, a measurable decrease of abdominal girth, disappearance of abdominal pain, normal temperature and pulse, and a return to normal white blood cell count. Surgical treatment is warranted in those patients who fail to manifest a majority of these parameters or are still toxic-appearing after 48 to 72 h.

Surgical intervention in toxic megacolon is challenging and demanding. Three operations currently in use are subtotal colectomy and ileostomy, total protocolectomy and ileostomy, and the Turnbull-Weakley blow hole operation.

For further reading in *Principles of Critical Care,* see Chap 85 "The Acute Abdomen and Intraabdominal Sepsis" RA Mustard/JMA Bohnen/B Schouten, Chap 166 "Toxic Megacolon" Richard K Reznick

---

| **AIDS in the Intensive Care Unit**

Phillip Cozzi

The acquired immunodeficiency syndrome (AIDS) results from the dysfunction and depletion of helper T-lymphocytes caused by chronic infection with the human immunodeficiency viruses. Because of the multiple life-threatening complications of this illness, issues of life-support should be reassessed frequently. Because of the risks of transmission of human immunodeficiency virus (HIV) through accidental needle stick or mucous membrane exposure, it is particularly important that ICU staff exercise universal precautions with all patients.

ICU admission in the AIDS population is infrequent, though rising steadily over the last decade. The causes of ICU admission in the AIDS population are limited. Acute respiratory failure due to *Pneumocystis carinii* pneumonia (PCP) is the most important due to its high frequency and mortality. Other conditions resulting in ICU admission are listed in Table 39-1.

RESPIRATORY DISEASE COMPLICATING HIV INFECTION

Although PCP is the most common respiratory disease resulting in ICU admission among HIV-infected individuals, less frequent etiologies should be considered in the diagnostic work-up of patients, including bacterial, fungal, mycobacterial, and viral infections. Kaposi's sarcoma rarely results in acute respiratory failure. Several laboratory tests are useful in the initial diagnostic evaluation. The CD4 count is particularly useful because it is unusual for patients to develop PCP with CD4 counts greater than 250 cells per μL. Lactate

TABLE 39-1 ICU Admissions in HIV-Infected Individuals* (St. Paul's Hospital 1985–1990)

Pneumocystis carinii pneumonia	92%
Cerebral Toxoplasmosis	3%
Bacterial pneumonia	2%
Gastrointestinal bleeding	2%
Kaposi's sarcoma	3%
Lymphoma	2%
Cardiomyopathy	2%

*More than one condition may be present at any given time. (Reprinted with permission from Montaner J, Phillips P, Russell JA: AIDS in the Intensive Care Unit, in Hall JB, Schmidt GA, Wood LDH: Principles of Critical Care, McGraw-Hill, New York, 1992.)

dehydrogenase is characteristically elevated in PCP, although this laboratory finding is nonspecific. The radiologic pattern is critical in formulating a differential diagnosis of lung involvement in AIDS (Table 39-2). Sputum should be screened for common bacterial pathogens as well as PCP. In the ventilated patient, bronchoscopic

TABLE 39-2 Major Radiological Differential Diagnosis of Lung Involvement in AIDS

Normal chest x-ray
PCP
CMV
MAC
Diffuse or localized interstitial pattern
PCP
CMV
MAC
M Tb
Diffuse alveolar pattern
PCP
Cardiogenic Pulmonary Edema
Miliary pattern
MTb
Consolidation
Common Bacteria
MTb
PCP
KS
Nodular Opacity
PCP
Common Bacteria
KS
Upper Lung field Involvement
PCP
MTb
Pneumothorax
PCP
Cavity
M Tb
PCP
Bacteria
Pleural Effusion
KS
Common Bacteria
Mycobacteria

PCP—Pneumocystic carinii, CMV—Cytomegalovirus, MAC—Mycobacterium avium complex, MTb—Mycobacterium tuberculosis, KS Kaposi's sarcoma *(Reprinted with permission from Montaner J, Phillips P, Russell JA: AIDS in the Intensive Care Unit, in Hall JB, Schmidt GA, Wood LDH: Principles of Critical Care, McGraw-Hill, New York, 1992.)*

bronchoalveolar lavage (BAL) may be preferred. Blood cultures should be obtained.

Pneumocystis Carinii Pneumonia

PCP is the AIDS index disease in 65 percent of cases in North America. As PCP occurs late in the evolution of HIV infection, it is recommended that all individuals with CD4 counts less than 250 cells per μL or those with a prior episode of PCP receive life-long prophylaxis. Clinical features include slow onset of dyspnea and nonproductive cough associated with fever. The onset of symptoms occurs an average of three weeks prior to diagnosis of PCP. Acute respiratory failure requiring mechanical ventilation may occur in as many of 20 percent of hospitalized patients. Chest x-ray varies from normal to a diffuse interstitial pattern to frank consolidation. Atypical radiologic presentations include pneumothorax, mass and cavity. Aerosolized pentamidine prophylaxis may be responsible for the increasingly recognized upper lung field involvement.

Diagnosis can be made through sputum analysis, bronchoalveolar lavage or lung biopsy. The utility of the induction of sputum for the diagnosis of PCP is variable from hospital to hospital, depending on the availability of trained staff and their diligence in soliciting deep sputum specimens. BAL is the usual method by which PCP is diagnosed in the ICU. Sensitivity of BAL for *P. carinii* exceeds 95 percent. The fluid should be processed to allow identification of Pneumocystis carinii, fungi, mycobacteria, and viruses. Systemic pneumocystosis involving the liver, spleen, lymph nodes, adrenals and eyes has been described.

Management of PCP in the intensive care unit includes intravenous administration of either trimethoprim-sulfamethoxasole (TMP-SMX) or pentamidine isethionate. TMP-SMX is dosed at 20 and 100 mg per kg daily, respectively, in four divided doses for not less than 14 days. Adverse drug reactions occur in 60 to 100 percent of HIV-infected patients treated with TMP-SMX, including rash, fever, liver dysfunction, renal dysfunction, leukopenia, thrombocytopenia, hyponatremia, anemia, gastrointestinal upset, and mucocutaneous reactions. Pentamidine isethionate is dosed at 4 mg/kg diluted in 250 ml of 5% dextrose and water for not less than 14 days. Common side affects include renal and liver dysfunction, neutropenia, thrombocytopenia, hyponatremia, rash, fever, gastrointestinal upset, hypertension, hyper- or hypoglycemia, ventricular arrhythmias, and pancreatitis (particularly when coadministered with ddI).

Corticosteroid use has recently been found to improve survival in acute PCP. In addition to intravenous administration of TMP-SMX or pentamidine, corticosteroids should be initiated at once in any patient whose PaO$_2$ is below 70 mmHg while breathing room air unless there is an absolute contraindication to their use. Prednisone is dosed at 40 mg by mouth twice daily for the initial 7 days followed first by 40 mg by mouth every day for 7 days then by 20 mg by mouth every other day for the final 7 days. Rapid deterioration occasionally occurs following discontinuation of corticosteroid.

With the above cited therapeutic regimen, significant improvement is anticipated within 5 to 7 days. If improvement is not seen within 7 days of therapy, a trial of an alternative agent is indicated. When properly diagnosed and treated, the first episode of PCP usually has negligible mortality. Although the mortality was initially reported as greater than 80 percent in those patients requiring mechanical ventilation, mortality has now been reduced to less than 50 percent.

Mycobacterium Tuberculosis

Tuberculosis is a common opportunistic infection in HIV-infected persons, often manifesting with unusual presentations. Pulmonary disease may be noncavitary, and extrapulmonary disease occurs with greater frequency. Critical illness associated with *M. tuberculosis* infection results from acute respiratory failure, pericarditis, meningitis or adrenocortical insufficiency.

HIV-infected persons have increased risk of developing the adult respiratory distress syndrome (ARDS) due to miliary tuberculosis or tuberculous pneumonia. Severely immunocompromised patients may develop an acute malignant form of miliary tuberculosis, known as non-reactive miliary tuberculosis, because the lesions have few typical granulomas. Respiratory failure may be complicated by non-mycobacterial sepsis, massive hemoptysis, pneumothorax, or upper airway obstruction. Acid fast bacilli are readily identifiable in the sputum of HIV-infected patients. At least three drugs are recommended for the initial treatment of tuberculosis in HIV-infected patients, and a four-drug regimen further minimizes the chances of developing drug resistance. Pharmacologic doses of corticosteroids (methylprednisolone 125 mg IV twice daily) may reduce the exudative reaction and systemic toxicity in severe tuberculosis. Corticosteroids should be used in all patients with acute respiratory failure due to tuberculosis, unless there is coincident bacterial sepsis. Blood (42 percent) and stool cultures (40 to 50 percent) have a particularly high diagnostic yield in HIV-infected patients.

Other Causes of Pulmonary Infiltrates

Streptococcus pneumoniae, Haemophilus influenzae and *Staphylococcus aureus* occur with increased frequency in HIV-infected individuals. As in other hospitalized patients, nosocomial pneumonia caused by gram-negative bacteria is associated with high mortality. Fungal pneumonias rarely cause respiratory failure among HIV-infected individuals, usually representing pulmonary epiphenomena of disseminated infection. Of patients with mucocutaneous Kaposi's sarcoma, 25 percent have pulmonary involvement. It is very rare to have pulmonary disease in the absence of mucocutaneous Kaposi's sarcoma.

NEUROLOGIC COMPLICATIONS IN HIV-INFECTED PATIENTS

Neurologic syndromes associated with HIV infection include meningitis, dementia, encephalopathy, myelopathy, peripheral neuropathy, and myopathy.

Cryptococcus neoformans is the most important cause of meningitis in the HIV-infected patient. Amphotericin B in doses of 0.4 to 0.8 mg/kg should be given intravenously daily for 2 to 10 weeks. Maintenance therapy of fluconazole 200 mg daily should be given indefinitely. Other causes of meningitis in the HIV population include *M. tuberculosis, Coccidioides immitis, Taenia pallidum, Listeria monocytogenes* and the typical bacterial agents (pneumococcus, meningococcus, and *H. influenzae*).

Although diffuse brain disease (dementia and encephalopathy), myelopathy, peripheral neuropathy and myopathy are important causes of morbidity in AIDS patients, they rarely result in ICU admission.

New or progressive focal neurologic deficits require emergent evaluation in the HIV population. CNS toxoplasmosis, lymphoma, and progressive multifocal leukoencephalopathy are the usual causative agents. Less common diagnostic considerations include neurosyphilis, cryptococcoma, tuberculoma, and herpes simplex encephalitis. If initial head CT or MRI reveals mass lesions or shift, empiric therapy for toxoplasmosis should be considered. Combination therapy should consist of pyrimethamine plus sulfadiazine or pyrimethamine plus clindamycin. A 200 mg loading dose of pyrimethamine is followed by 1.0 to 1.5 mg/kg oral daily doses for 4 to 6 weeks; sulfadiazine is given in 4 to 6 gram doses every six hours orally for the same treatment period. Smaller doses of the above cited drug should be given indefinitely. If the patient does not improve on the above cited regimen by 2 to 3 weeks, brain biopsy should be considered.

ICU ELIGIBILITY OF THE AIDS PATIENT

Since AIDS remains ultimately fatal, some physicians have wrongly restricted ICU eligibility in the HIV-infected population. ICU admission and life support are reasonable in HIV-infected patients who have a potentially reversible acute illness. These measures are inappropriate in those patients for whom there is no effective therapy. Prognostic scoring systems have been developed for AIDS patients: overall survival decreases sharply with increasing organ system involvement. Since the outlook of AIDS is changing rapidly, policies concerning ICU admission of AIDS patients should remain flexible.

For further reading in *Principles of Critical Care,* see Chap 100 "AIDS in the Intensive Care Unit" Julio SG Montaner/Peter Phillips/James A Russell

---

40

Side Effects of Chemotherapy and Immunosuppression

Shannon Carson

DEFICITS IN HOST DEFENSES RELATED TO CANCER CHEMOTHERAPY

Myelosuppression and Neutropenia

The absolute number of circulating (ANC) segmented neutrophils represents the most important single parameter predictive of the risk for life-threatening infection. As the ANC declines below 1.0 $\times$ 10^9/L the risk of infection increases, with greatest risk for bacteremic infection at neutrophil counts below 0.1×10^9/L. The duration of severe neutropenia (ANC $<0.5 \times 10^9$/L) is also related directly to infection risk.

Patients receiving pulse doses of chemotherapy for solid tissue malignancies or lymphoreticular malignancies sustain only temporary damage to the hemopoietic stem cell pool. The expected circulating neutrophil nadir occurs generally between day 10 and 14. Although the neutrophilic nadirs may be $<0.5 \times 10^9$/L, the duration of neutropenia is rarely longer than 5 to 7 days. A rise in circulating neutrophils would be expected to occur between day 15 and 21. The likelihood that this prediction is correct is increased if a relative monocytosis is observed on the differential white blood cell (WBC) count. The recovery of peripheral blood monocytes precedes that of circulating neutrophils in chemotherapy-induced aplasia and often heralds the recovery of the ANC.

In general, the more dose-intensive myelosuppressive regimens such as standard remission-induction chemotherapy for acute myloid leukemia (AML) are associated with more hemopoietic stem cell damage and longer durations of neutropenia. Circulating neutrophil counts of $<0.5 \times 10^9$/L will persist for a median of 24 days. This additional period of myelosuppression is associated with a significant increase in infectious morbidity. Periods of neutrophil recovery extending > 40 to 60 days can be encountered in heavily pretreated patients receiving high dose cytarabine for salvage therapy of relapsed or resistant leukemia.

In addition to the myelosuppressive effects of remissioninduction regimens, certain chemotherapeutic agents such as anthracyclines (e.g., doxorubicin), antimetabolites (e.g., cytarabine), and alkylating agents (e.g., cyclophosphamide) have profound suppressive effects on the numbers of circulating T and B lymphoid cells which parallel the acquired functional defects in cell-mediated and humoral immune mechanisms. The clinical consequences of T cell dysfunction vary with the underlying disease and the cytotoxic regimen. For example, *Pneumocystis carinii* infection is an intermediate risk for those undergoing bone marrow allografting or autografting. Accordingly, most centers managing these patients recommend administering primary prophylaxis for *P. carinii* in bone marrow transplantation (BMT) recipients. There does not appear to be a prognostically useful parameter of T or B cell function that predicts infection risk in neutropenic patients analogous to the predictive value of the ANC for pyogenic bacterial or fungal infection. However, presence of hypogammaglobulinemia may help identify increased risk of infection by encapsulated bacteria.

Approach to Fever Associated with Neutropenia

Febrile episodes during neutropenia are defined by an oral temperature of > 38.3°C (101°F) in the absence of other noninfectious causes of fever or pyrogenic drugs. The extent to which characteristics of the febrile episode predict a bacteremic event has been somewhat variable in different studies, however, most agree that initial oral temperatures of >39°C (102°F), shaking chills, clinical shock, initial ANC <0.1 × 10⁹/L, and initial platelet count of <10 × 10⁹/L are to some degree predictive of gram-negative bacteremia.

The incidence and magnitude of localizing findings such as exudate, fluctuance, ulceration, or fissure formation are reduced in a direct relationship to the ANC. Other localizing findings, such as erythema and focal tenderness, appear to remain as useful and reliable signs of infection regardless of the ANC. Table 40-1 lists the pertinent historical and physical clues to be sought in the clinical evaluation of a febrile neutropenic patient.

Once the relevant historical details and physical findings are established, the complete evaluation of the febrile neutropenic patient should include a series of laboratory and radiologic investigations designed to complement the clinical examination. Specimens of body fluids such as blood, urine, cerebrospinal fluid, and lower respiratory secretions should be submitted to the clinical microbiology laboratory for culture and antimicrobial susceptibility testing where appropriate. It has been recommended that for patients with multilumen indwelling central venous catheters in situ, each lumen of the catheter should be sampled in addition to blood from a peripheral venous site. Tissue obtained by biopsy of infected sites can be important in the diagnostic evaluation. It is common for pathogens to be observed histopathologically in infected tissue specimens without recovery of the organism by culture.

The empirical initial therapy for suspected infection in febrile

TABLE 40-1 Clinical Evaluation of the Febrile Neutropenic Patient

| Body System | Findings to be Sought | |
	Historical	Physical

Eye	Blurring of vision
	Double vision
	Loss of vision
	Pain
		Scleral abnormalities
		  Icterus
		  Hemorrhage
		  Local swelling
		Conjunctival abnormalities
		  Focal erythema
		  Petechiae
		Retina
		  Hemorrhage
		  "Cotton wool" exudates
		    (e.g., *candida*
		    endophthalmitis)

Skin	Skin rash
	Pruritus
	  (focal or diffuse)
	History of drug
	  reactions
	Focal pain/
	  swelling
	IV catheter site(s)
		Central venous catheters
		  Insertion site erythema/pain
		  Tunnel site erythema/pain
		  Exit site erythema/pain/exudate
		Peripheral IV catheters
		  Focal tenderness
		  Focal erythema
		  Exudate at the insertion site
		Skin rash
		  Papular/macular/vesicular
		  Ulceration
		  Focal areas of necrosis
		    (e.g., ecthyma gangrenosum)
		  Distribution

Upper respiratory	Painful ear Nasal stuffiness Sinus tenderness Epistaxis	External auditory canals Tympanic membrane erythema

Lower
respiratory
	Cough
	Increased
	  respiratory
	  secretions
	Dyspnea
	Hemoptysis
	Chest pain
		Tachypnea
		Tachycardia
		Hyperpnea
		Localized crepitations
		Consolidation

Upper
gastrointestinal
	Odynophagia
	Dysphagia
	History of
	  denture use
	History of herpes
	  stomatitis
		Gingival bleeding
		Pseudomembranous exudate
		  over buccal & gingival
		  surfaces and tongue
		Mucosal erythema
		Mucosal ulceration
		Focal pain
		Pre-existing periodontitis

TABLE 40-1 Clinical Evaluation of the Febrile Neutropenic Patient (continued)

| Body System | Findings to be Sought | |
	Historical	Physical

Lower gastrointestinal	Abdominal pain
	Constipation
	Diarrhea ±
	  Bleeding
	Perianal pain with
	  defecation
	Jaundice
		Focal abdominal pain
		  Right upper quadrant
		  (e.g., biliary tree)
		  Right lower quadrant
		  (e.g., cecum/ascending
		  colon)
		  Left lower quadrant
		  (e.g., diverticular disease)
		Perianal abnormalities
		  Focal tenderness
		  Focal/diffuse erythema
		  Fissures
		  Ulcerations
		  Hemorrhoidal tissues

(Reprinted with permission from Bow EJ: Approach to Infections In Patients Receiving Cytotoxic Chemotherapy for Malignancy, in Hall JB, Schmidt GA, Wood LDH: Principles of Critical Care, McGraw-Hill, New York, 1992.)

neutropenic patients is based on two assumptions: **1.** the majority of infections are due to bacteria, and **2.** the principal pathogens are aerobic gram-negative bacilli (*Escherichia coli, Klebsiella pneumoniae,* and *Pseudomonas aeruginosa*). Accordingly, the antibiotic regimens currently recommended for empirical therapy are designed to have excellent activity against these pathogens. With the recognition of various factors favoring infection with gram-positive organisms, the addition of agents with an improved spectrum of activity against these pathogens has also been recommended. Three classes of effective empirical regimens are available for neutropenic patients: β-lactam plus aminoglycoside combinations; double β-lactam combinations; and monotherapy (Table 40-2). The choice of the type of empirical regimen should be influenced by a number of considerations, particularly the presence of or potential for renal insufficiency, the expected pathogens, the in situ presence of indwelling central venous access devices, and the suspicion of penicillin hypersensitivity (Table 40-3).

The time until response to empirical antibacterial therapy varies with the underlying causes of neutropenia. Among patients with a short duration of neutropenia (< 7 days), the median time to defervescence is 2 days (range 1 to 7 days). Among patients with a prolonged duration of neutropenia, the median time to defervescence is 4 to 5 days. Patients with fever persisting beyond 72 h on broad-spectrum antibiotic therapy should be reevaluated carefully. Table 40-4 lists several of the possible explanations for this. When

TABLE 40-2 Antimicrobial Therapy Used for Therapy in Febrile Neutropenic Patients

β-Lactam antibiotics:	
Ticarcillin	200–300 mg/kg/day IV
Piperacillin	
Azlocillin	4–6 divided doses daily
Mezlocillin	
Cefoperazone	2 gm Q12h IV
Ceftazidime	2 gm Q8h IV
Imipenem/cilastatin	500 mg Q6h IV
Aminoglycosides:	
Gentamicin	
Netilmicin	1.6–2.0 mg/kg Q8h IV
Tobramycin	
Amikacin	7.5 mg/kg Q12h IV
Other agents	
Vancomycin	1.0 gm Q12h IV
Metronidazole	500 mg Q8h IV/PO
Erythromycin	0.5–1.0 gm Q6h IV
Trimethoprim/sulfamethoxazole	10–20 mg/50–100 mg/kg/day in 4 divided doses
Acyclovir	250–500 mg/M^2 Q8h IV
Ganciclovir	5 mg/kg Q8h–Q12h IV
Amphotericin	0.5–1.5 mg/kg/day IV
5 Flucytosine	150 mg/kg/day po in 4 divided doses

(Reprinted with permission from Bow EJ: Approach to Infections In Patients Receiving Cytotoxic Chemotherapy for Malignancy, in Hall JB, Schmidt GA, Wood LDH: Principles of Critical Care, McGraw-Hill, New York, 1992.)

TABLE 40-3 Considerations Governing the Choice of Empiric Antibacterial Regimen

β-lactam + Aminoglycoside	Risk of Pseudomonas aeruginosa infection Nosocomial infection Prolonged severe neutropenia
Double β-Lactam	Patients with renal impairment Recipients of other nephrotoxic agents Mild to moderate neutropenia
Monotherapy	Patients with renal impairment Recipients of other nephrotoxic agents Short term neutropenia
Other agents: Vancomycin	Suspect staphylococcal infection Suspect vascular catheter infection Skin or soft tissue infection
Metronidazole	Suspect intraabdominal infection Necrotising gingivitis Severe oral mucositis Suspect perianal infection

(Reprinted with permission from Bow EJ: Approach to Infections In Patients Receiving Cytotoxic Chemotherapy for Malignancy, in Hall JB, Schmidt GA, Wood LDH: Principles of Critical Care, McGraw-Hill, New York, 1992.)

TABLE 40-4 Differential Diagnosis of Fever > 72 h Despite Broad-Spectrum Antibacterial Therapy

Fever is due to a non-bacterial process
  Viral infection (*herpes simplex,* cytomegalovirus)
  Fungal infection (candidiasis, invasive aspergillosis)
  Non-infectious fever (blood products, drugs, etc.)
Bacterial infection is resistant to the antibiotic regimen
A second or subsequent infection has developed
Bacterial infection not responding because of inadequate antibiotic
  serum/tissue levels
Infection associated with an undrained focus (e.g., abscess or prosthetic
  material [eg IV catheters])

(Reprinted with permission from Bow EJ: Approach to Infections In Patients Receiving Cytotoxic Chemotherapy for Malignancy, in Hall JB, Schmidt GA, Wood LDH: Principles of Critical Care, McGraw-Hill, New York, 1992.)

reevaluation fails to identify the etiology of the persistent fever, the clinician may elect either to continue the initial empirical antibacterial regimen if the patient's condition shows no clinical change or deterioration or to modify the empirical regimen appropriate to the findings of the reevaluation (Table 40-5). If, however, defervescence has not occurred by day 7, the empirical administration of parenteral amphotericin B has been recommended.

The optimal duration of antibacterial therapy is unknown. It is generally recommended that febrile neutropenic patients receive at least 1 week of antibacterial therapy or, after fever resolves, be treated until afebrile for at least 5 days. For severely neutropenic

TABLE 40-5 Considerations for Regimen Modification: Day 5

Progressive necrotising mucositis/gingivitis	⟶ Anaerobic coverage (eg metronidazole)
Progressive ulcerating mucositis/gingivitis	⟶ Antiviral therapy (eg acyclovir)
Dysphagia	⟶ Antifungal (+/− Antiviral) therapy If pseudomembranous pharyngitis
Cellulitis or inflammatory changes at venous access sites	⟶ Anti-staphylococcal therapy (eg vancomycin)
Pulmonary infiltrates: Interstitial	⟶ Trimethoprim/sulfamethoxazole +/− erythromycin Consider bronchoalveolar lavage
Pulmonary infiltrates: Focal	⟶ Observe if ANC is recovering Consider lung biopsy Empiric amphotericin
Abdominal foci	⟶ Typhilitis Diverticular disease } Anaerobic Perirectal focus } Coverage

(Reprinted with permission from Bow EJ: Approach to Infections In Patients Receiving Cytotoxic Chemotherapy for Malignancy, in Hall JB, Schmidt GA, Wood LDH: Principles of Critical Care, McGraw-Hill, New York, 1992.)

patients, antibacterial therapy should probably be continued until marrow recovery.

Specific Infection Syndromes in Patients Undergoing Cytotoxic Chemotherapy

The natural history of oral mucositis is influenced by the cytotoxic therapy-induced neutropenia, which plays a permissive role in the clinical expression of acute or chronic periodontal infections. This process usually reaches its maximum intensity at the time of neutrophilic nadir. At this time polymicrobic infection becomes superimposed on the chemotherapy-induced mucositis. Although oropharyngeal bacterial flora probably contribute to disease in most cases of simple mucositis, fungi such as *Candida albicans* can also contribute. In addition, reactivated latent herpes simplex virus (HSV) infections of the oral cavity are common in seropositive patients undergoing remission-induction therapy or BMT with a median onset between 7 and 11 days.

Invasive enteric bacterial infections of the gut due to *Salmonella* or *Shigella* species are relatively uncommon in neutropenic patients. Two clinical entities, however must be considered in febrile neutropenic patients with abdominal pain and diarrhea, toxigenic enterocolitis due to the toxin elaborated from an overgrowth of *Clostridium difficile* and neutropenic enterocolitis (typhlitis). *C. difficile* can be cultured from stool, or the toxin can be detected in the laboratory from stool samples. In patients with a sufficiently typical clinical presentation, it is reasonable to begin therapy empirically before laboratory confirmation is available. Typhlitis is a potentially life-threatening infection of the bowel wall seen in up to 32 percent of patients undergoing remission-induction therapy for leukemia. Bacteremia with enteric microorganisms (*E. coli, Klebsiella* species) and *P. aeruginosa* is associated with typhlitis in up to 28 percent of cases.

Infections of the perirectal tissues may be life threatening in neutropenic patients. Perirectal infection must be suspected if there is focal tenderness, perirectal induration, or erythema with or without fluctuance or tissue necrosis. Current standards suggest that an appropriate antibiotic regimen should consist of a broad-spectrum antipseudomonal penicillin or a third generation antipseudomonal cephalosporin plus an aminoglycoside and an antianaerobic agent.

Invasive candidiasis encompasses deep infections of various sites with *Candida* species. When multiple organ sites are involved, the term disseminated candidiasis may be more appropriate. The most common forms of invasive candidiasis encountered in neutropenic patients are candidemia with or without associated central venous catheter infection, chronic systemic candidiasis (hepatosplenic candidiasis), endophthalmitis, hematogenously spread skin infection and renal candidiasis. Amphotericin B with or without 5-FC is the mainstay of treatment for invasive candidiasis, but fluconazole may be a useful approach for patients unable to tolerate or failing amphotericin B containing regimens.

Opportunistic filamentous fungal infections are frequently life-threatening complications among neutropenic patients undergoing remission-induction treatment for AML or BMT. These infections are most often caused by *Aspergillus* species or *Zygomycoses* (e.g., *Rhizopus, Mucor*). The definitive diagnosis of invasive aspergillosis usually requires a biopsy of involved tissue. In leukemia patients the mortality rate from invasive pulmonary aspergillosis has ranged between 13 and 100 percent whereas in BMT patients the mortality rate approaches 100 percent.

The most common microorganisms associated with intravenous site infection are gram-positive organisms such as *S. aureus*, the coagulase-negative staphylococci, *Corynebacterium* JK; gram-negative bacilli such as the Enterobacteriaceae, *P. aeruginosa* and *Acinetobacter anitratus;* and fungi such as *Candida* species. Erythema, swelling, exudate, and focal tenderness associated with a peripheral intravenous catheter site should always alert the clinician to these etiologic possibilities. Suspect catheters should be promptly and carefully removed using aseptic technique and submitted to the clinical microbiology laboratory for cultures.

Antibacterial prophylaxis with oral agents such as cotrimoxazole, norfloxacin, or ciprofloxacin can reduce the frequency of febrile episodes and bacteremic events in patients with protracted neutropenia. However, oral quinolones increase the risk of infection due to gram-positive organisms, and recipients of TMP/SMX for *Pneumocystis* prophylaxis are susceptible to coagulase-negative staphylococci, viridans streptococci, and TMP/SMX resistant *P. aeruginosa*. Patients undergoing remission-induction for AML or BMT with a history of herpetic stomatitis or who are IgG seropositive for herpes simplex virus (HSV) are at risk for severe herpetic mucositis. Such patients should be given acyclovir prophylaxis at 250 mg/m² intravenously every 12 h until marrow recovery then oral acyclovir 800 mg every 12 h for a total of 6 weeks.

TOXICITIES OF CHEMOTHERAPY

As more intensive anticancer regimens are being used to achieve cure, an increasing number of oncology patients are admitted to ICUs for complications of drug-induced toxicity that need to be distinguished from infectious complications. Drug toxicity is often a diagnosis of exclusion once infection, tumor effect, and toxicity from other drugs are eliminated from the differential diagnosis. The toxicities of a given combination of drugs with or without radiation are often more severe than the effects of the individual agents alone would suggest. Treatment is usually supportive. Specific toxicities of various agents are usually well documented except for newer agents where all toxicities are not yet known.

Gastrointestinal toxicity ranges from mild mouth sores to severe bloody diarrhea with a measurable mortality. In addition to serving as a portal of entry for infectious agents, stomatitis and diarrhea often severely compromise enteral feeding. Intravenous alimentation should be considered early.

A large number of antineoplastic drugs can cause pulmonary symptoms (Table 40-6). Syndromes reported include acute pleuritic chest pain, hypersensitivity lung disease, and noncardiogenic pulmonary edema, but the vast majority of cases fall into the pneumonitis/fibrosis category. It is classically associated with the three Bs; busulfan, bleomycin, and BCNU (carmustine) and is, for many agents, sporadic rather than dose-related. Methotrexate lung toxicity is symptomatically similar but is believed to be a form of hypersensitivity reaction. The onset may be after prolonged continuous treatment, which is typical for busulfan, after only a few cycles of therapy, as is frequently reported with the m-BACOD (methotrexate, bleomycin, doxorubicin, cyclophosphamide, vincristine, dexamethasone) regimen, or even years after therapy has ended, as can be seen with BCNU. The symptoms typically appear gradually over several weeks, but acute presentations are not unusual. The chest radiograph will generally be normal or reveal a basilar or diffuse reticulonodular pattern, but an atypical chest x-ray should not rule out a diagnosis of drug toxicity. Bleomycin is particularly notorious for occasionally producing a nodular appearance which may mimic recurrent tumor, while methotrexate may be associated with a pleural effusion or hilar adenopathy. Since the histologic findings are not specific, even a lung biopsy may not absolutely establish the diagnosis of drug-induced toxicity, although it is usually helpful.

Cardiovascular toxicity is most often associated with the anthracyclines including doxorubicin and daunorubicin and with high dose cyclophosphamide. An acute drop in ejection fraction can be seen in hours to weeks after administration of anthracyclines. This is sometimes associated with a pericardial effusion and may result in the precipitous death of the patient from severe congestive failure. It is exceedingly rare, however. A chronic cardiomyopathy, on the other hand, develops in from 1 to 10 percent of patients receiving 550 mg/m^2 of doxorubicin. Symptoms usually appear around 30 to 60 days after what appears

TABLE 40-6 Antineoplastic Drugs with Pulmonary Toxicity

Agent	Type of Toxicity	Incidence	Comments
Bleomycin	Pneumonitis/ fibrosis	2–40%	Chest x-ray may be atypical
	Hypersensitivity pneumonitis	rare	Eosinophilia may be seen on lung biopsy; steroids felt to be useful
	Acute chest pain	rare	Substernal pressure or pleuritic; self-limited over 4–72 h
Busulfan	Pneumonitis/ fibrosis	4%	Insidious onset after prolonged therapy; poor prognosis
Carmustine (BCNU)	Pneumonitis/ fibrosis	20–30%	Toxicity dose-related; common in pre-transplant regimens. May appear years after therapy has ended
Cyclophos-phamide	Pneumonitis/ fibrosis	<1%	May potentiate toxicity of bleomycin, BCNU
High-Dose Cytosine Arabinoside	Noncardiogenic pulmonary edema	4–20%	Care is supportive; prognosis variable
Methotrexate	Hypersensitivity pneumonitis	8%	Prognosis good; dramatic response to corticosteroids reported
	Acute Pleuritic pain	rare	May be associated with pleural effusion or friction rub; subsides over 3–5 days
	Noncardiogenic pulmonary edema	rare	Few reports, most with intrathecal injection
Mitomycin C	Pneumonitis/ fibrosis	3–12%	
Procarbazine	Acute hypersensitivity pneumonitis	rare	Onset within hours after drug dose; recovery rapid

(Reprinted with permission from Fleming G, Vogelzang NJ: Toxicities of Chemotherapy. In Hall JB, Schmidt GA, Wood LDH: Principles of Critical Care, McGraw-Hill, New York, 1992.)

to have been the precipitating dose of doxorubicin, but may also first be noted a year or more after the end of treatment.

The nonhematologic dose-limiting toxicity of cyclophosphamide is a severe hemorrhagic myopericarditis which is usually seen only at doses higher than 1.55 g/m². Treatment is supportive. If patients survive the acute phase, complete recovery can be expected, and there may be no residual evidence of cardiac damage even at autopsy. Pericardiocentesis often does not produce any clinical improvement.

Up to 4 percent of patients treated with 5-fluorouracil (5-FU) have been reported to suffer anginal symptoms, and a greater number have transient asymptomatic ECG changes suggestive of ischemia; prolonged infusions appear to cause more problems. Myocardial infarction may occur.

Only rarely will the neurologic toxicity (Table 40-7) of an anti-cancer drug be severe enough to be the primary reason for admission to the ICU.

Table 40-8 lists the common renal abnormalities caused by anti-neoplastic drugs. Renal injury characterized pathologically by focal necrosis of the distal tubules and collecting ducts is a dose-limiting toxicity of cisplatin. Acute renal failure can occur. Vigorous pre-treatment hydration with saline solution minimizes but does not eliminate the damage; all patients will have some decline in glomerular filtration rate with sufficient dosage. Cisplatin also causes a variety of electrolyte disorders. Renal magnesium wasting, not necessarily associated with azotemia, is seen in half the patients receiving cisplatin and may persist for years. Most patients are asymptomatic. Of particular concern in the ICU are the hypocalcemia and hypokalemia that frequently accompany the magnesium wasting, and which may be refractory to treatment if serum magnesium levels are not first corrected.

Urologic complications including bladder fibrosis, bladder cancer, and hemorrhagic cystitis are among the most troublesome side effects of cyclophosphamide and ifosfamide. Symptoms range from minimal hematuria with mild dysuria, urgency and frequency, to massive hemorrhage requiring transfusion. In serious cases vigorous hydration to promote urine flow, maintenance of adequate platelet counts (>50,000/μL), and rapid constant bladder irrigation through a large bore catheter are indicated. Intravesical instillation of certain prostaglandin analogues such as 0.2% carboprostamethamine has been reported to result in complete and lasting resolution of hemorrhage with no significant side effects. Formalin treatment produces significant pain, and must be given with the patient under anesthesia.

Venoocclusive disease of the liver (VOD) has an up to 20 percent incidence and is a common cause of death in patients given a variety of high dose chemotherapy or chemoradiotherapy combinations prior to infusion of autologous or allogeneic bone marrow. Clinically, VOD resembles Budd-Chiari syndrome. The diagnosis is based on the presence of at least two of the triad of jaundice,

TABLE 40-7 Antineoplastic Drugs With Neurologic Toxicity

Drug	Incidence	Comments
Acute Encephalopathy		
L-Asparaginase	25–50%	Ranges from drowsiness to stupor; usual onset day after start of therapy; generally resolves rapidly when therapy over
High-Dose Busulfan	15%	Acute obtundation, seizures; prophylactic anticonvulsants often used
High-Dose Carmustine (BCNU)	10%	Severe acute or chronic encephalomyelopathy; time of onset variable; not reversible; encephalopathy also seen with intracarotid therapy
Cisplatin		With intracarotid therapy only
High-Dose Cytosine Arabinoside	10–20%	Ranges from disorientation to coma; usual onset 5–7 days after start of therapy; prognosis variable
Hexamethylmelamine	variable	Investigational agent; toxicity ranges from depression to hallucinations; usually reversible when drug withdrawn
Ifosfamide	5–30%	Frequency greater with higher doses; ranges from mild somnolence to coma; onset hours after infusion, recovery usually within days
High-Dose Methotrexate	2–15%	Usual onset one week post drug; most common presentation stroke-like syndrome; usually reversible
Mitotane	40%	Lethargy, somnolence, dizziness, vertigo
Procarbazine	10%	Usually mild drowsiness or depression, rarely stupor or manic psychosis
High-Dose Thiotepa	dose-dependent	Somnolence, seizures, coma; dose-limiting extramedullary toxicity
Vincristine/Vinblastine	rare	SIADH
Acute Cerebellar Syndrome		
High-Dose Cytosine Arabinoside	10–20%	Ranges from mild dysarthria to disabling ataxia; onset 5–7 days after start of therapy; prognosis variable
5-Fluorouracil	<1%	Usually seen with large bolus doses; reversible in 1–6 weeks

TABLE 40-7 Antineoplastic Drugs With Neurologic Toxicity (continued)

Drug	Incidence	Comments
Acute Paraplegia		
Intrathecal		These are the only drugs
Cytosine Arabinoside	rare	normally given intrathecally;
Methotrexate		all cause acute reversible
Thiotepa		arachnoiditis fairly commonly,
		paralysis exceedingly rarely;
		paralysis may or may not
		be reversible
Other Neuropathies		
Cisplatin	dose-dependent	Ototoxicity; distal sensory neuropathy which may be severe enough to cause disabling ataxia
Etoposide	rare	Mild distal paresthesias; tendon reflex depression; may be synergistic with vincristine
Hexamethylmelamine	variable	Peripheral paresthesias and weakness; usually reversible when therapy discontinued
Procarbazine	10–20%	Decreased tendon reflexes, mild distal paresthesias; usually reversible when therapy discontinued
Vinca alkaloids	variable	Symmetrical areflexia and distal paresthesias; symmetrical motor weakness starting with dorsiflexors, jaw pain, cranial nerve palsies, paralytic ileus

(Adapted with permission from Fleming G, Vogelzang NJ: Toxicities of Chemotherapy. In Hall JB, Schmidt GA, Wood LDH: Principles of Critical Care, McGraw-Hill, New York, 1992.)

hepatomegaly or right upper quadrant pain, and ascites or unexplained weight gain. Hyperbilirubinemia, which generally precedes hepatomegaly and ascites by several days, is usually out of proportion to increases in transaminase concentration. Percutaneous liver biopsy to confirm the diagnosis is not advisable due to the risk of bleeding in these patients who usually have thrombocytopenia and a coagulopathy. The clinical diagnosis is 90 percent accurate. Symptoms begin at a mean of 10 days after marrow reinfusion, while graft versus host disease, one of the major differential diagnoses in patients who have had an allogeneic transplant, usually develops after day 20. The prognosis in VOD is poor, with mortality rates ranging up to 50 percent.

TABLE 40-8 Antineoplastic Drugs Producing Renal and Electrolyte Abnormalities

Agent	Toxicity	Comments
Cisplatin	Magnesium, calcium, potassium wasting; renal insufficiency	See text
Cyclophosphamide	Impaired free water excretion	Transient; seen with doses over 50 mg/kg
High-Dose Methotrexate	Acute renal failure	Usually reversible
Mithramycin	Azotemia or renal failure with tubular necrosis	Unusual at lower doses, used for hypercalcemia
Mitomycin C	Renal failure with microangiopathic hemolytic anemia	
Nitrosoureas (BCNU, CCNU, methyl-CCNU)	Progressive renal failure appearing after large cumulative doses	Decrease in renal size may be noted, effect may be years after therapy
Streptozotocin	Renal failure, proximal RTA, nephrotic syndrome	Transient proteinuria earliest manifestation

(Reprinted with permission from Fleming G, Vogelzang NJ: Toxicities of Chemotherapy. In Hall JB, Schmidt GA, Wood LDH: Principles of Critical Care, McGraw-Hill, New York, 1992.)

Biologic Agents

Most of the acute toxicity associated with IL-2 is the result of a striking capillary leak syndrome that has been compared to the early phase of septic shock. Soon after IL-2 administration the blood pressure drops; there is a decrease in systemic vascular resistance and an increase in heart rate and cardiac output. Patients develop marked prerenal azotemia. Attempts at fluid resuscitation may lead to dramatic weight gain with peripheral and pulmonary edema as a result of extravascular accumulation of the fluid.

Most of the interferon-related toxicity that would bring a patient to the ICU occurs with very high doses. In particular, doses over 100 million units produce significant acute reversible neurologic toxicity with marked lethargy, confusion, and, rarely, seizures.

IMMUNOTHERAPY IN THE TRANSPLANT PATIENT

Improvements in immunosuppression have led to dramatic expansion in organ transplantation and hence in the number of transplant recipients in the general population. These immunosuppressive drugs, however, have frequent side effects and predispose patients to infection.

The perioperative induction of immunosuppression generally involves several components (Fig. 40-1). This general strategy is altered according to changes in the clinical situation regarding infection, rejection, or toxicity. Noninfectious complications of immunosuppressive drugs are outlined in Table 40-9.

Acute rejection remains a common problem despite the best immunosuppression currently available. Most rejection episodes occur within the first year after transplantation. Rejection must be considered in any transplant patient with fever or symptoms or laboratory results suggestive of graft dysfunction or inflammation. The suspicion of rejection should initiate a thorough clinical evaluation and an immediate determination of simple parameters of graft function. These would include serum creatinine for a renal transplant, transaminases and bilirubin for a liver transplant, and so on. Liberal use should be made of relevant biopsy techniques should any suspicion of rejection remain following the initial evaluation. Because the morbidity of a single bolus dose of corticosteroids is limited, it may frequently be advisable to initiate this therapy on semiempirical grounds pending histologic confirmation of the diagnosis. OKT3 represents the current "gold standard" for highly effective reversal of acute rejection, although its use is often restricted to rejection resistant to other therapeutic modalities because of the toxicity of this agent.

Infectious Complications of Immunosuppression

Bacterial infections are most frequent in the first month after transplantation. The organisms involved reflect the flora of the transplant site. Many of these infections are more properly considered complications of surgery than of immunosuppression per se, although the adverse effects of corticosteroids on wound healing are certainly a contributing factor. Corticosteroids may also mask the symptoms of intraabdominal sepsis and contribute to dangerous delay in recognition of anastomotic leaks, abscesses, and other conditions requiring surgical intervention.

Fungal infections also usually occur within the first 1 to 2 months after transplantation. The risk of fungal infection is markedly increased by excessive corticosteroid use. Repeated courses of broad-spectrum antibiotics, multiple reoperations, and a prolonged ICU stay also predispose to fungal infections. *Candida* is the most common organism, although many other fungal pathogens are occasionally seen.

Cytomegalovirus (CMV) is the most common and important viral pathogen in transplant patients, particularly in those who have been treated extensively with OKT3 or ALG. Infections range in severity from mild to lethal. CMV infections may be caused by reactivation

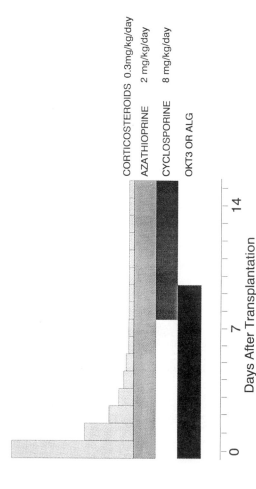

FIG. 40.1 Sample regimen for perioperative immunosuppression, illustrating the use of OKT3. *(Reprinted with permission from Bruce OS, Thistlethwaite JR: Immunotherapy in the Transplant Patient. In Hall JB, Schmidt GA, Wood LDH: Principles of Critical Care, McGraw-Hill, New York 1992.)*

CORTICOSTEROIDS 0.3mg/kg/day

AZATHIOPRINE 2 mg/kg/day

CYCLOSPORINE 8 mg/kg/day

OKT3 OR ALG

Days After Transplantation

0   7   14

TABLE 40-9 Non-infectious Complications of Immunosuppressive Drugs

Side Effects of Cyclosporine	Nephrotoxicity Hypertension Tremor Psychosis	Seizures Hypertrichosis Hyperkalemia Hepatotoxicity
Side Effects of Corticosteroids	Hyperglycemia Muscle wasting Impaired wound 　healing Gastritis Cataracts	Masking of infections Adrenal suppression Bone demineralization Cushingoid facies
Side Effects of Azathioprine	Neutropenia Hepatotoxicity	Squamous and basal cell 　skin cancer
Side Effects of ALG	Fever Chills Thrombocytopenia	Hypertension Pruritis Serum sickness
Side Effects of OKT3	Fever Bronchospasm Seizures Tachycardia Hypertension Headache	Pulmonary edema Rigors Formation of anti-OKT3 　antibodies Nausea and vomiting Diarrhea

(Reprinted with permission from Bruce OS, Thistlethwaite JR: Immunotherapy in the Transplant Patient. In Hall JB, Schmidt GA, Wood LDH: Principles of Critical Care, McGraw-Hill, New York 1992.)

of latent virus in a CMV-seropositive recipient. These reactivation infections occur 1 to 4 months after transplantation and are frequently less severe than primary infection. CMV causes several different clinical syndromes, including pneumonitis, hepatitis, nephritis, and gastrointestinal ulceration. However, the most common presentation of CMV is one of fever and leukopenia, occasionally with thrombocytopenia or atypical lymphocytes. Tissue invasion on liver or bronchoscopic biopsy serves to confirm the diagnosis. The therapy of CMV infections depends on the severity of the disease. Many minor infections resolve without specific treatment. For more severe infections, immunosuppression should be reduced and antiviral therapy begun with ganciclovir.

Other herpes viruses are commonly seen in transplant recipients including herpes simplex virus reactivation and dermatomal varicella zoster virus (shingles). These infections are troublesome to the patient but are generally not life-threatening. Low dose oral acyclovir is effective for mucocutaneous HSV lesions.

Pneumocystis carinii pneumonia is the most common parasitic infection in the transplant recipient. This typically occurs several months after transplantation and should be suspected in any transplant patient presenting with a pulmonary infiltrate. The frequency of this complication can be reduced by prophylaxis with low dose oral trimethoprim/sulfamethoxazole.

Although minor infections in transplant recipients may be managed without altering immunosuppression, severe or persistent infections often require that immunosuppression be reduced or withheld. Severe infection in the heart or liver transplant recipient presents a dilemma, as life depends on continuing function of these grafts. However, it should be noted that the discontinuation of immunosuppression does not always lead to rejection in critically ill patients, particularly those with viral infections.

PULMONARY INFILTRATES IN THE IMMUNOCOMPROMISED HOST

Immunocompromised patients with fever and new pulmonary infiltrates pose special problems for the intensive care physician. The differential diagnosis of pulmonary inflammatory processes in the immunocompromised host is wide, establishing a definitive diagnosis is often difficult, empiric antimicrobial therapy is often ineffective, and the patient's condition can deteriorate rapidly. A timely stepwise diagnostic approach at a rate determined by the rate of progression of the pneumonia should be initiated immediately.

The nature of the immunologic abnormality that is present in a given case has a major bearing on the nature of the infective processes likely to be present. The major categories of immunologic abnormality include: **1.** Deficient humoral immunity. **2.** Deficient phagocytic cell function or number. **3.** Deficient cell-mediated immune function. In Table 40-10 are listed the major pulmonary infections most strongly associated with each type of immune dysfunction. The timing of the onset of the illness, with respect to previous chemotherapy and duration of immunosuppression as discussed in the sections above, is another very helpful clue to the infectious etiology.

Approach to Diagnosis and Management

Diagnosis and management must be considered together in these patients. Initially, a presumptive diagnosis or group of potential diagnoses is formulated and empiric therapy begun while relatively noninvasive diagnostic testing is implemented. If a definitive diagnosis is necessary because of the failure of empiric therapy or the pace and severity of progression of disease, increasingly invasive diagnostic testing is performed until the diagnosis is established and definitive therapy begun.

Patients with diffuse infiltrates should receive intravenous widespectrum antimicrobials directed at hematogenous bacterial pneumonia, at least until initial culture results are available. Piperacillin

TABLE 40-10 The More Common Opportunistic Pulmonary Infections of the Immunocompromised Host

Predominant Immunodeficiency*	Most Frequent Pulmonary Infections	Clinical Setting
Humoral immunodeficiency	Pyogenic bacterial pneumonias	Hypogammaglobulinemia Chronic lymphocytic leukemia Multiple myeloma
Phagocytic cell deficiency	Bacterial pneumonia Fungal pneumonias Aspergillosis Candidemia with pulmonary involvement Cryptococcosis	Chemotherapy-induced granulocytopenia Acute myelogenous leukemia
Cell-mediated immunodeficiency	*Pneumocystis carinii* pneumonia Legionellosis Nocardiosis CMV pneumonia Cryptococcosis Mycobacteriosis	Lymphoma or acute lymphocytic leukemia undergoing chemotherapy High-dose cortico-steroid therapy Organ transplantation AIDs

*Note that these categories are not mutually exclusive. Bone marrow transplant recipients, for example, suffer mainly from bacterial and fungal infections associated with phagocytic cell deficits early after transplant; but after marrow recovery mainly develop infections related to chronic suppression of cell-mediated immunity. *(Reprinted with permission from Light BR: Pneumonia, in Hall JB, Schmidt GA, Wood LDH: Principles of Critical Care, McGraw-Hill, New York, 1992.)*

and gentamicin are usually acceptable. Erythromycin and TMP/SMX are given to cover most conventional bacteria and atypical pneumonia pathogens as well as PCP (unless the patient has been receiving TMP/SMX prophylaxis, in which case the diagnosis is essentially excluded). Investigations include blood cultures, respiratory and stool specimens for viral culture, culture of blood for CMV, respiratory secretions for Gram stain and culture, and examination for acid-fast bacilli and fungi. In patients with predominant CMI impairment (lymphoma, steroid or immunosuppressive drug therapy, or organ transplant) who have not received prophylactic TMP/SMX and have negative blood cultures, PCP is usually the leading infectious possibility, followed by CMV. Unlike what is seen in AIDS patients with PCP, the number of organisms in the lung is not large; hence sputum examination for the organism is not useful. Early bronchoscopy with BAL or a protected specimen brush is advised. For patients who are at lesser risk for PCP and CMV, for those in whom the initial investigation excludes these possibilities, and for those with rapidly progressive diffuse lung disease, open lung biopsy should be considered. In the face of progressing disease, if a biopsy is to be done it is important to make the decision to proceed before the patient has progressed to frank respiratory failure.

The diagnosis of localized pulmonary infiltrates due to conventional bacterial pneumonia can usually be established with sufficient certainty by blood cultures, respiratory secretion gram stain and culture, direct fluorescent antibody (DFA) staining and culture of respiratory secretions for *Legionella pneumophila,* and the clinical response to empiric antimicrobial therapy. *Legionellosis* should be considered in all cases where the pneumonia has atypical features, especially in hospitals where cases are being seen. If the diagnosis is not immediately forthcoming or the patient does not respond promptly to empiric therapy, bronchoscopy should be done and BAL or protected brush specimens sent for examination for bacteria, acid-fast bacilli; DFA and culture for *Legionella;* fungal elements; and cytologic examination. If there is no contraindication, transbronchial biopsy may increase the yield for invasive fungal infection and for malignancy. Culture of aspergilli from nasal scrapings or sputum can be helpful in this regard.

For further reading in *Principles of Critical Care,* see Chap 77 "Immunotherapy in the Transplant Patient" David S Bruce/J Richard Thistlethwaite, Chap 99 "Approach to Infection in Patients Receiving Cytotoxic Chemoterapy for Malignancy" Eric J Bow, Chap 102 "Pneumonia" R Bruce Light, Chap 151 "Toxicities of Chemotherapy" Gini Fleming/Nicholas J Vogelzang

---

41

Pneumonia

Manu Jain

Pneumonia remains a leading infectious cause of death in the developed world. It is also the most important nosocomial infection complicating the treatment of patients in ICUs for other problems. Pneumonias which require an ICU admission are associated with very high mortality rates, as high as 70 percent in some series.

COMMUNITY-ACQUIRED PNEUMONIAS

Pneumonia in patients presenting from outside of hospital can lead to ICU admission for respiratory failure, depressed level of consciousness or hypotension. The great majority of community-acquired pneumonias are due to *Streptococcus pneumoniae, Staphylococcus aureus,* or *Haemophilus influenza.* However, a significant minority of cases are caused by a large number of less common pathogens with widely differing anti-microbial susceptibilities (see Table 41-1).

TABLE 41-1 Infectious Etiologic Agents Implicated in Severe Community-Acquired Pneumonia Requiring Intensive Care Support

Etiologic Agent	% Of Cases Admitted*
Acute bacterial pneumonia	65
Streptococcus pneumoniae	40
Hemophilus influenzae	5
Staphylococcus aureus	10
Enterobacteriacae	10
Atypical pneumonia	20
Legionella pneumophila	10
Mycoplasma pneumoniae	5
Chlamydia psittaci	2
Coxiella burnetii	1
Viral	2
Aspiration pneumonia/lung abscess	10
Chronic pneumonia syndrome	5
Mycobacterium tuberculosis	3
Endemic dimorphic fungi	2

*The percentages shown are approximate only, based on published studies from different geographic locations and population bases. Because these percentages represent cases requiring hospital admission and ICU care, pneumonias which more commonly cause severe illness (*Staphylococcus aureus*, enteric gram-negative bacilli, *Legionella* spp. etc.) are over-represented compared to unselected community-acquired pneumonia. Also note that most published series include 20 to 50% for which no etiologic diagnosis was made and which are not included in this table. *(Reprinted with permission from Light RB: Pneumonia, in Hall JB, Schmidt GA, Wood LDH: Principles of Critical Care, McGraw-Hill, New York, 1992.)*

PATHOGENESIS

Among the different etiologic agents responsible for pneumonias there are three major routes of entry into the lung. They are aspiration of oropharyngeal or gastric contents into the lung, inhalation of aerosols or particles containing organisms and hematogenous spread of organisms into the lung from another infected site.

Aspiration accounts for the vast majority of pulmonary infections. Pneumonia due to relatively high-grade pathogens such as *S. pneumonia, Staph. aureus*, and enteric gram-negative bacilli generally occurs when patients have damaged or deficient host defense. Examples include pneumonia following a viral respiratory infection or pneumonia in a patient with chronic obstructive pulmonary disease (COPD), diabetes or renal insufficiency.

The normal flora of the upper airway have limited virulence and therefore cause pulmonary infection mainly when aspiration is massive or when there is severe local impairment of tracheobronchial clearance. Examples include epileptic seizures, abnormal motor control of the upper airway, periodontal disease, or bronchial obstruction. The infection produced by these bacteria is a subacute necrotizing pneumonia with eventual abscess formation in many cases.

The number of organisms reaching the lung is small when the route of entry is inhalation, so only organisms that are highly efficient pathogens produce infection by this mechanism. This includes most respiratory viruses, *Legionella, Mycoplasma pneumonia, Chlamydia, Coxiella burnetii, Mycobacterium tuberculosis*, and most of the endemic fungal pneumonias. They share the ability to either resist phagocytosis or to survive intracellularly within phagocytes.

For hematogenous spread of infection to the lung the organisms must gain access to the venous circulation which carries the organisms to the lung. In most cases there is an established infection elsewhere or organisms are injected directly into the blood stream. The common pathogens are *Staph. aureus* and gram-negative bacilli. Tularemia, brucellosis, and melioidosis may cause pneumonia after gaining entry directly through damaged skin.

Pathophysiology

The proliferation of microorganisms elicits the host's full acute inflammatory response. Important consequences of this include intrapulmonary shunt, impaired distribution of ventilation and decrease in lung compliance (see Chapter 30). This pathophysiology results in the constellation of clinical and radiographic signs detailed below.

Clinical and Radiographic Features

The basic features common to most forms of pneumonia include
fever, white blood cell (WBC) elevation, and pulmonary symptoms
of cough, dyspnea, and sputum production. Physical signs include
tachypnea, crackles, bronchial breath sounds, and egophony. Evidence of impaired gas exchange and an infiltrate on a chest radiograph are also typical. It has been suggested that a syndromic
approach based on the clinical, epidemiologic, and radiographic
features is useful in delineating the etiologic organism.

Acute Bacterial Pneumonia Syndrome

The typical history for community-acquired bacterial pneumonia is
acute onset of fever, with chills and rigors, associated with dyspnea
and cough productive of purulent, sometimes bloody sputum. In
severely debilitated patients or the institutionalized elderly new or
worsened confusion and tachypnea is often the only history obtain-
able. Physical examination reveals signs noted above. The chest
X-ray will usually demonstrate air space consolidation with either
a lobar or broncho-pneumonic pattern and air bronchograms. Although the WBC is usually elevated, it may be normal or even
suppressed in severely ill patients who are in shock.

All patients with pneumonia leading to an ICU admission should
have two blood cultures as well as gram stain and culture of lower
respiratory tract secretions. The utility of a gram stain can be
maximized by ensuring that there are more than 25 polymorphonuclear leucocytes per high-power field and less than 10 large
epithelial cells per high power field. A blood culture which is
positive for a recognized pathogen is usually definitive but a sputum
culture must be interpreted in light of the original gram stain. In
a patient whose condition deteriorates or the initial investigation
has been negative the next step is to repeat the sputum gram stain
and culture. If this is still negative the next step in diagnosis should
be fiberoptic bronchoscopy with protected brush specimen or
broncho-alveolar lavage with quantitative bacterial cultures. The
finding of 10^5 colony-forming units per milliliter is diagnostic of
infection.

When a specific etiologic diagnosis for bacterial pneumonia has
been established on the basis of the blood culture or sputum gram
stain and culture, antimicrobial therapy directed specifically at that
pathogen can be prescribed (see Table 41-2). However, in most
cases of pneumonia the etiologic diagnosis is not available at the
outset and empiric therapy must be directed at the most probable
bacterial etiologies in the particular patient. Some suggested empiric regimens are shown in Table 41-3.

TABLE 41-2 Antimicrobial Therapy for Acute Bacterial or Atypical Pneumonia of Known Etiology in Critically Ill Patients

Acute bacterial pneumonia	Recommended Antimicrobial Therapy*	Alternative Antimicrobial Agents
Streptococcus pneumoniae and other Streptococci	Penicillin G 1 Million units IV q4h	Cefazolin, clindamycin or vancomycin
Staphylococcus aureus		
methicillin sensitive	Nafcillin 2g IV q4h	Cefazolin, clindamycin or vancomycin
methicillin resistant	Vancomycin 500mg IV q6h	———
Hemophilus influenzae		
β-lactamase-negative	Ampicillin 2g IV q6h	Cefuroxime, co-trimoxazole
β-lactamase-positive	Cefuroxime 1.5g IV q8h	co-trimoxazole, Chloramphenicol
Branhamella catarrhalis	Cefuroxime 1.5g IV q8h	Co-trimoxazole
Enterobacteriacae (Klebsiella, E. coli Enterobacter spp. etc.)	Cefotaxime 2g IV q6h and gentamicin 1.5 mg/kg IV q8h	Imipenem, co-trimoxazole, ciprofloxacin
Pseudomonas aeruginosa	Piperacillin 3g IV q4h and tobramycin 1.5 mg/kg IV q8h	Imipenem and tobramycin, ciprofloxacin

Condition	Treatment	Alternative
Anaerobic pneumonia/ Lung abscess	Penicillin 2 MU IV q4h and metronidazole 750 mg IV q8h	Clindamycin, chloramphenicol
Legionella pneumophila	Erythromycin 1 g IV q6h and Rifampin 600 mg IV Od	—
Mycoplasma pneumoniae	Erythromycin 1 g IV q6h	Tetracycline
Chlamydia psittaci	Tetracycline 500 mg IV q6h	Erythromycin
Coxiella burnetii	Tetracycline 500 mg IV q6h ± rifampin 600 mg IV OD daily	—
Yersinia pestis	Streptomycin 30 mg/kg IM OD daily	Chloramphenicol, tetracycline
Francisella tularensis	Gentamicin 1.5 mg/kg IV q8h	Chloramphenicol, tetracycline
Influenza A or RSV (Severe with Respiratory failure)	Ribavirin aerosol 1 g/day over 12 to 18h	—
Varicella-zoster	Acyclovir 10 mg/kg IV q8h	

*Note that all drug doses cited are those for patients with normal renal function; dosage adjustment for renal insufficiency is required for a number of the agents listed. Monitoring of blood drug levels is strongly advised for the aminoglycosides, vancomycin and chloramphenicol. (Reprinted with permission from Light RB: Pneumonia, in Hall JB, Schmidt GA, Wood LDH: Principles of Critical Care, McGraw-Hill, New York, 1992.)

TABLE 41-3 Empiric Antimicrobial Therapy for Critically Ill Patients With Acute Community-Acquired Pneumonia

Clinical setting	Recommended Antimicrobial therapy*	Alternative Agents
Acute Bacterial Pneumonia Syndrome (including patients with COPD or alcohol abuse)	Cefuroxime 1.5 g IV q8h	3rd-generation cephalosporin, co-trimoxazole
Institutionalized Elderly	Cefotaxime 2g IV q6h	Imipenem, co-trimoxazole
Atypical Pneumonia Syndrome	ADD TO ABOVE Erythromycin 1g IV q6h	——
Aspiration Pneumonia/ Lung Abscess	Penicillin G 2 MU IV q4h and metronidazole 750 mg IV Q8h	Clindamycin, imipenem, chloramphenicol
Fulminant Pneumonia	Cefotaxime 2g IV q6h and Gentamicin 1.5 mg/kg IV q8h and Erythromycin 1g IV q6h	Imipenem and erythromycin

*Note that doses cited are for patients with normal renal function; dosage adjustments for renal insufficiency is required for several of these agents. Monitoring of blood levels is strongly advised for aminoglycosides and chloramphenicol. (Reprinted with permission from Light RB: Pneumonia, in Hall JB, Schmidt GA, Wood LDH: Principles of Critical Care, McGraw-Hill, New York, 1992.)

Atypical Pneumonia Syndrome

The term atypical pneumonia syndrome was coined to describe the syndrome caused by mycoplasma pneumonia. Since that description several other pulmonary infections that share atypical features have been placed in this category (see Table 41-4). Although varied in many respects, they have in common several key features: epidemiologic clues are different from usual bacterial pneumonias; extra pulmonary features are common; diagnosis is primarily by serologic methods; and treatment with conventional anti-microbials for acute bacterial pneumonia may be ineffective.

In areas with a high prevalence of legionella, many laboratories will routinely culture lower respiratory tract secretions for legionella. In low prevalence areas it should be ordered specifically for all patients in whom an etiologic diagnosis is not immediately evident from the gram stain. A direct fluorescent antibody stain is also available for legionella and can be performed on lower respiratory secretions obtained by various means. For other atypical pneumonia pathogens, acute and 14-day blood specimens for anti-

TABLE 41-4 Atypical Pneumonia Syndrome: Infectious Agents that May Produce Severe Pneumonia with an Atypical (Nonbacterial) Clinical Presentation

Mycoplasma pneumoniae
Legionella pneumophila
Chlamydia psittaci
Coxiella burnetii
Viral Pneumonia (influenza A &B, varicella-zoster, RSV, E-B virus, adenovirus)
Francisella tularensis
Pneumocystis carinii

(Reprinted with permission from Light RB: Pneumonia, in Hall JB, Schmidt GA, Wood LDH: Principles of Critical Care, McGraw-Hill, New York, 1992.)

bodies will establish the diagnosis in *M. pneumonia, Chlamydia psittaci, Coxiella burnetii* and influenza A & B infection. Serology is also valuable in diagnosing tularemia and brucellosis. Suspicion of *Pneumocystis carinii* pneumonia should prompt early consideration of fiber optic bronchoscopy with lavage although special stains of sputum is also a reasonable next step.

In a patient with suspected atypical pneumonia erythromycin has become the antimicrobial of choice. This is because it is effective against both legionella and mycoplasma. In a patient with a severe pneumonia of unknown etiology, antibiotics should include erythromycin as well as treatment for bacterial pneumonia. Tetracycline is the treatment of choice for *Coxiella* and *Chlamydia*.

ASPIRATION PNEUMONIA SYNDROMES

Large-particle aspiration causes airway obstruction with asphyxia and can lead to sub acute pneumonia with abscess formation due to impaired mucociliary clearance. Small-particle or liquid aspiration usually causes a low-grade chemical pneumonitis with a pulmonary infiltrate that resolves rapidly over a few days. When the aspirated liquid is gastric acid, a more severe chemical burn results which can lead to hypovolemic hypotension and/or hypoxemic respiratory failure. In most cases of witnessed pulmonary aspiration the number and pathogenicity of aspirated bacteria is low. A major exception to this rule is aspiration of gastric contents which have become heavily contaminated with mixed enteric organisms as can happen with bowel obstruction, following abdominal surgery, paralytic ileus, or achlorhydria.

A more common syndrome related to pulmonary aspiration is pneumonia or lung abscess due to predominantly anaerobic micro flora of the mouth. Persons who are at risk include those with depressed level of consciousness, an impaired swallowing mechanism or impaired tracheobronchial clearance mechanisms. Following aspiration a low-grade pneumonia manifests as cough, fever and malaise and begins within a few days to 1 week. The onset of production of large amounts of foul-smelling, watery sputum signals the development of a lung abscess, usually between 1 to 4 weeks. Involvement of the pleura often results in empyema.

The approach to aspiration-associated acute bacterial pneumonia due to the usual pyogenic aerobic organisms is the same as that for pneumonia due to subclinical aspiration. However, most community-acquired aspiration pneumonias are caused by normal flora of the oropharynx which are predominantly anaerobic. Culture of sputum will often show only "normal flora." In most cases it is reasonable to make a clinical diagnosis of pneumonia due to mixed oropharyngeal anaerobic bacteria and to treat accordingly. Bronchoscopy is indicated in those with no increased risk for aspiration in order to exclude an endobronchial lesion.

Most cases of recent aspiration associated with a new pulmonary infiltrate represent an acute chemical pneumonitis, which will resolve without anti-microbial therapy. Aspiration that has resulted in pneumonia, lung abscess or empyema can usually be treated with penicillin. In a critically ill patient metronidazole can be added or the patient can be treated with clindamycin alone. When both aerobic and anaerobic gram-negatives are suspected, broader spectrum anti-microbial should be used (see Table 41-3).

CHRONIC PNEUMONIA SYNDROMES

The usual definition of the chronic pneumonia syndrome is progressive pulmonary symptoms for a period of 3 weeks to several months associated with radiographic evidence of a pulmonary parenchynal process. The patient appears chronically ill and is often malnourished or cachetic.

Some of the many infectious and non infectious diseases that may present as a chronic pneumonia syndrome are listed in Table 41-5. Although there are radiographic patterns which are helpful in making a diagnosis, almost every characteristic radiologic pattern can be caused by several different disease processes. In trying to make a diagnosis several sputum samples should be obtained and sent for bacterial, mycobacterial and fungal cultures as well as cytologic studies. Testing for specific auto antibodies associated with various immunologically mediated diseases can be helpful. Examination of specimens from extra pulmonary sites of involvement can also help in making the diagnosis. If none of these procedures establishes the diagnosis open lung biopsy is usually indicated.

Empiric therapy is seldom indicated for cases of chronic pneumonia syndrome. One occasional exception is complicating infectious pneumonia in patients with extensive pneumonitis or pulmonary

TABLE 41-5 Infectious and Non-Infectious Etiologies of the Chronic Pneumonia Syndrome

Bacterial and Mycobacterial Infections
Tuberculosis
Chronic cavitary bacterial pneumonia (*Klebsiella pneumoniae, Pseudomonas aeruginosa* and others)
Actinomycosis
Nocardiosis
Melioidosis
Aspiration-induced anaerobic pneumonia & lung abscess

Fungal Infections
Blastomycosis
Coccidiodomycosis
Paracoccidioidomycosis
Histoplasmosis
Cryptococcosis
Chronic necrotizing aspergillosis

Non-Infectious Causes
Systemic vasculitides
Malignancy
Interstitial pneumonitis (fibrosing alveolitis) and other idiopathic infiltrative pulmonary diseases.
Bronchiolitis obliterans with organizing pneumonia (BOOP)
Lymphomatoid granulomatosis
Sarcoidosis
Toxic exposures and drug reactions

(Reprinted with permission from Light RB: Pneumonia, in Hall JB, Schmidt GA, Wood LDH: Principles of Critical Care, McGraw-Hill, New York, 1992.)

hemorrhage as part of a systemic inflammatory illness such as systemic lupus erythematosis (SLE), Goodpasture's syndrome, Polyarteritis Nodosa (PAN) or Wegener's granulomatosis. Treatment regimens for the most common fungal pneumonias are listed in Table 41-6.

TABLE 41-6 Treatment Regimens for Fungal Pneumonia Associated with Critical Illness in the Non-Immunocompromised Host

Etiologic Agent	Recommended Antimicrobial Therapy
Blastomyces dermatitidis	Amphotericin B 0.5–0.8 mg/kg IV OD to total dose of 2–2.5 g
Histoplasma capsulatum	as above
Coccidioides immitis (without CNS involvement)	Amphotericin B 0.5–0.8 mg/kg IV OD to total dose of 3–4 g
Cryptococcus neoformans	Amphotericin B 0.3–0.5 mg/kg IV OD and flucytosine 150 mg/kg daily in 4 divided doses, for 6 weeks

(Reprinted with permission from Light RB: Pneumonia, in Hall JB, Schmidt GA, Wood LDH: Principles of Critical Care, McGraw-Hill, New York, 1992.)

NOSOCOMIAL PNEUMONIA

The most common microbial causes of nosocomial pneumonia are listed in Table 41-7. The pathogenesis for nosocomial pneumonias is the same as that for community-acquired pneumonias, and the explanation for the distribution of the common pathogens is the pattern of colonization of the upper airway. Therefore patients who have been in the hospital for just a few days tend to get infected by organisms that affect people in the community. Patients who have chronic debilitating disease, have been hospitalized for many days or have been previously treated with antimicrobials are at increased risk of pneumonia from gram-negative bacilli. The only important nosocomial pathogen from the atypical pneumonia group is *Legionella*, which can be inhaled in aerosols from infected water supplies.

The clinical and radiographic features associated with nosocomial pneumonia are similar to those of community-acquired pneumonias. The diagnosis can be established in the same way as it is for community-acquired pneumonias.

There are several differences in antimicrobial therapy between nosocomial pneumonias and community-acquired pneumonias. Because pathogens causing nosocomial pneumonia are more likely to cause a destructive necrotizing pneumonia, the treatment should be broader spectrum, longer in duration and always parenteral, at least initially. Suggested empiric antimicrobial regimens are listed in Table 41-8.

Since nosocomial pneumonias occur by definition in the hospital, there has been interest in developing methods to prevent these

TABLE 41-7 Bacterial Causes of Nosocomial Pneumonia in Patients Requiring Intensive Care

Organism	Frequency (% Of Cases)*
Enterobacteriacae (Klebsiella, E. coli, Enterobacter, Porteus, Acinetobacter, Serratia, etc.)	30–50
Staphylococcus aureus	10–30
Pseudomonas aeruginosa	10–20
Streptococci (including *Streptococcus pneumoniae*)	10–15
Legionella spp.	5–15
Hemophilus influenzae	2–10
Branhamella catarrhalis	2–10
Anaerobes	2–5

*Ranges shown are derived from a number of studies from different geographic areas and different patient populations. Incidence of each infection varies greatly depending on local circumstances. (Reprinted with permission from Light RB: Pneumonia, in Hall JB, Schmidt GA, Wood LDH: Principles of Critical Care, McGraw-Hill, New York, 1992.)

TABLE 41-8 Empiric Antimicrobial Therapy for Nosocomial Pneumonia Associated with Critical Illness

Clinical setting	Recommended Antimicrobial Therapy*	Alternative Antimicrobial Therapy
Acute nosocomial pneumonia (Post-operative or complicating medical illness)	Cefotaxime 2g IV q6h and gentamicin 1.5 mg/kg IV q8h	Co-trimoxazole IV
Nosocomial pneumonia with increased risk of resistant aerobic gram-negatives (i.e. prior broad-spectrum antibiotics, acute leukemia, endemic resistant organisms etc.)	Piperacillin 3g IV q4h and gentamicin 1.5 mg/kg IV q8h	Imipenem, ciprofloxacin IV and ampicillin
Fulminant pneumonia following aspiration	Clindamycin 900 mg IV q8h and cefotaxime 2g IV q6h	Clindamycin and co-trimoxazole IV, and metronidazole ampicillin and gentamicin.
Suspect *Legionellosis* (endemic, organ transplant, steroid use) or undiagnosed fulminant Pneumonia	ADD Erythromycin 1g IV q6h to one of above regimens.	——

* Doses cited are for patients with normal renal function; dosage adjustments for renal insufficiency are required for a number of the listed agents. Monitoring of blood drug levels is strongly advised for aminoglycosides and choramphenicol. (Reprinted with permission from Light RB: Pneumonia, in Hall JB, Schmidt GA, Wood LDH: Principles of Critical Care, McGraw-Hill, New York, 1992.)

infections. For example, if bleeding prophylaxis is used sucralfate may be preferable to H_2-blockers since gastric acidity can be preserved with sucralfate. Another approach is administration of tube feedings only intermittently. The risk of aspiration in seriously ill patients can be decreased by nursing them on their side with the head slightly down and having them sleep in the upright position with the head of the bed up. Frequent and careful suctioning and use of small bore feeding tubes are also helpful adjunctive measures.

PULMONARY INFILTRATES IN THE IMMUNOCOMPROMISED HOST

The nature of the immunologic abnormality that is present in a given case has a major bearing on the nature of the infective processes likely to be present. The major categories of immunologic abnormality and the major pulmonary infection most strongly associated with each type are listed in Table 41-9. The timing of the illness with respect to onset of immunosuppression is often very helpful. After bone marrow transplantation or cytotoxic chemotherapy, acute bacterial infections tend to occur weeks to months later. The physical examination is only occasionally revealing in this group of patients and is usually related to extra pulmonary findings.

Chest x-ray findings in this group can be separated into two categories. Diffuse infiltrates if they are infectious, imply hematogenous spread or rapid movement along the respiratory mucosa early in the course of infection. Localized infiltrates are generally due to aspiration or inhalation.

Noninfectious causes can also cause a diffuse or focal lung lesion in the immunocompromised host (Table 41-10).

TABLE 41-9 The more common opportunistic pulmonary infections of the immunocompromised host

Predominant Immunodeficiency*	Most frequent Pulmonary Infections	Clinical Setting
Humoral immunodeficiency	Pyogenic bacterial Pneumonias	Hypogammaglobulinemia, chronic lymphocytic leukemia Multiple myeloma
Phagocytic cell deficiency	Bacterial pneumonia Fungal pneumonias Aspergillosis Candidemia with pulmonary involvement Cryptococcosis	Chemotherapy-induced granulocytopenia Acute myelogenous leukemia
Cell-mediated immunodeficiency	*Pneumocystis carinii* pneumonia *Legionellosis* CMV pneumonia *Cryptococcocis* *Mycobacteriosis* *Nocardiosis*	Lymphoma or acute lymphocytic leukemia undergoing chemotherapy, High-dose corticosteroid therapy Organ transplantation AIDS

*Note that these categories are not mutually exclusive. Bone marrow transplant recipients, for example, suffer mainly from bacterial and fungal infections associated with phagocytic cell deficits early after transplant, but after marrow recovery mainly develop infections related to chronic suppression of CMI. *(Reprinted with permission from Light RB: Pneumonia, in Hall JB, Schmidt GA, Wood LDH: Principles of Critical Care, McGraw-Hill, New York, 1992.)*

TABLE 41-10 Non-infectious Causes of Pulmonary Infiltrates in the Immunocompromised Host and the Clinical Setting in Which They Are Most Frequently Seen.

Non infectious Diagnosis	Clinical Setting
Diffuse pulmonary infiltrates	
Interstitial pneumonitis due to cytotoxic drug therapy	Bleomycin (>150mg total) or non-dose related reaction to bleomycin, cyclophosphamide, methotrexate and others.
Cardiogenic pulmonary edema	Pre-existing cardiac disease Chemotherapy with daunorubicin or adriamycin
Lymphangitic carcinomatosis	Carcinoma poorly responsive to therapy
Leukemic infiltration of lung	Uncontrolled acute leukemia
Acute low-pressure pulmonary edema (diffuse alveolar damage)	Leukemic cell lysis after chemotherapy; leukoagglutination reaction following transfusion
Focal pulmonary infiltrates	
Pulmonary metastasis	Untreated or poorly responsive primary carcinoma
Atelectasis	Endobronchial lesion Chest wall or upper abdominal pain Depressed cough or respiration (narcotics)
Pulmonary infarction (pulmonary thromboembolism)	Hypercoagulable state due to carcinoma or paraproteinemia, Immobility, venous obstruction
Radiation pneumonitis	Recent (4–12 weeks) radiotherapy with lung exposure

(Reprinted with permission from Light RB: Pneumonia, in Hall JB, Schmidt GA, Wood LDH: Principles of Critical Care, McGraw-Hill, New York, 1992.)

Diagnosis and management must be considered together, particularly for patients requiring support in an ICU. Initial investigations should include blood cultures, respiratory and stool specimens for viral culture, culture of blood for cytomegalovirus (CMV) respiratory secretions for gram stain and culture and examination for Acid-Fast Bacilli (AFB) and fungi. In patients with predominantly cell-mediated immunity impairment and who have not been on prophylaxis, *P. carinii* should be looked for aggressively with early bronchoscopy and BAL if necessary. Open lung biopsy should be considered if a diagnosis cannot be made and the patient is deteriorating.

Patients should begin empirically on broad-spectrum anti-microbials such as piperacillin and gentamicin. Erythromycin should be added in all cases where the pneumonia has atypical features or the patient is deteriorating quickly. When the diagnosis has been estab-

TABLE 41-11 Antimicrobial Therapy for Opportunistic Lung Infections in Critically Ill Immunocompromised Patients

Pulmonary Infection*	Antimicrobial Regimen
Pneumocystis carinii pneumonia	Co-trimoxazole 5 mg/kg TMP and 25 mg/kg SMX IV q6h or Pentamidine 4 mg/kg IV daily
Nocardia asteroides pneumonia or abscess	Sulfonamide 2 g Q6h (IV if available) or Cotrimoxazole (as above) ± amikacin 5 mg/kg IV q8h
Aspergillosis	Amphotericin B 0.6 to 1.0 mg/kg IV daily to total dose of 2.0 g and, if permitted by degree of myelosuppression, Flucytosine 150 mg/kg IV or PO per day initially, reducing dose to achieve 1H pre-dose blood levels of 50 to 75 ug/ml.
Candidal pneumonia due to associated Candidemia	Amphotericin B 0.3 to 0.6 mg/kg IV daily or Fluconazole 400 mg IV daily
CMV pneumonia	Ganciclovir 2.5 mg/kg IV Q8h and CMV immune globulin 400 to 500 mg/kg on alternate days (4 to 10 doses)
Varicella-zoster, disseminated, with pneumonia	Acyclovir 10 mg/kg IV q8h

*Treatment regimens for the more common acute bacterial pneumonias are shown in Tables 4 and 6, and for the dimorphic fungi in Table 6. Antituberculous drug regimens are given in Chapter 109. TMP = trimethoprim, SMX = sulfamethoxazole. (Reprinted with permission from Light RB: Pneumonia, in Hall JB, Schmidt GA, Wood LDH: Principles of Critical Care, McGraw-Hill, New York, 1992.)

lished definitive therapy can be substituted for the empiric anti-microbials. Drug regimens for the major infectious causes of opportunistic pneumonia are shown in Table 41-11.

For further reading in *Principles of Critical Care,* see Chap 102 "Pneumonia" Light RB

42

Endocarditis and Other Endovascular Infections

Ikeadi Maurice Ndukwu

The possibility of intravascular infection should be considered in all critically ill patients with bacteremia or fungemia of uncertain origin; particularly, **1.** when there are known intravascular devices, **2.** fever or hemodynamic instability of unclear origin, and **3.** signs of inflammation related to an indwelling intravascular device. Intravascular infections in the absence of any foreign device include infective endocarditis on a native valve, mycotic aneurysm, cavernous sinus thrombosis, postanginal sepsis, septic pelvic vein thrombophlebitis, and pylephlebitis. Prosthetic devices may lead to intravascular infections of the following: prosthetic valve endocarditis, cardiac pacemaker infections, peripheral and central line infections, and arterial device-induced infections.

NATIVE VALVE ENDOCARDITIS

The pathogenesis of infective endocarditis (IE) on a native valve involves transient bloodstream invasion by microorganisms followed by adherence of the organism to the endocardial surface, and multiplication of the microorganism within a layer of platelets and fibrin, which is relatively inaccessible to host phagocytic defenses. The risk of native valve infective endocarditis is related to the species, the concentration of microorganisms in the blood, the presence of antimicrobial agents at the time of bacteremia/fungemia, and characteristics of the endocardium. *Staphylococcus aureus*, enterococci, and other streptococci are very adherent to endocardium, increasing the risk of IE. *S. aureus,* commonly found on the skin, is a common cause of acute bacterial endocarditis particularly in patients without significant underlying valvular heart disease. Fever and a heart murmur are found in at least 80 percent of patients. Skin lesions include petechiae, Osler's nodes, and Janeway lesions. Roth spots in the optic fundus and splinter hemorrhages under the nails are vascular lesions of IE. Systemic consequences of IE include stroke syndrome, renosplenic infarction, and ischemic bowel disease or infarction of the small bowel. Patients with IE may also present with heart failure due to valve malfunction, embolic myocardial infarction, and myocarditis.

Diagnosis

The diagnosis of IE requires multiple blood cultures; the majority of these obtained when a patient is not receiving antimicrobial therapy will be positive. The causes of culture-negative endocarditis are prior antibiotics, and endocarditis due to fastidious organisms including anaerobes, nutritionally deficient streptococci, *Coxiella burnetti, Legionella pneumophila, Chlamydia psittaci,* members of the HACEK (*Haemophilus* species, *Actinobacillus actinomycetemcomitans, Cardiobacterium hominus, Eikenella corrodens,* and *Kingella kingae*) group, and various fungi. Echocardiography is useful in identifying vegetations or local complications of IE but cannot be used to exclude the diagnosis.

Treatment

Management of IE requires initiation of antimicrobial therapy at the earliest possible time. A patient found to have fever, murmurs, or other signs of possible IE should have multiple blood cultures obtained and antibiotic therapy initiated if the patient is critically ill, antimicrobial therapy will be necessary for some other infectious disorder, or early valve replacement is contemplated because of valve malfunction.

Critically ill patients requiring empirical therapy should be covered for the most likely organisms. Native valve endocarditis is most commonly associated with streptococci, *Staphylococcus aureus,* or enterococci. Therefore, a reasonable empiric therapy is intravenous nafcillin, 2 g every 4 h with 2 g ampicillin intravenously every 4 h and gentamicin, 1.5 mg/kg intravenously every 8 h, pending the results of blood cultures. Once the identity of the organism is established, an antibiotic regimen should be based on the minimal inhibitory concentration of that antimicrobial agent. Table 42-1 describes the recommended antimicrobial regimens for treatment of IE.

Valve replacement may be lifesaving in patients with IE. The distribution of valvular lesions are; aortic, 35 to 50 percent; mitral, 50 percent; tricuspid, 10 percent; and pulmonic, 1 percent. Indications for urgent valve replacement include severe heart failure, valvular obstruction, fungal endocarditis, ineffective antimicrobial therapy, and the presence of an unstable prosthetic device.

Prognosis

The prognosis in IE is dependent on the relative pathogenicity of the infecting organism, the location of the infected valve, and of complications of the infection. *S. aureus* typically produces a severe and destructive endocarditis that is fatal in about 50 percent of cases when the infection occurs on the aortic or mitral valve. *P. aeruginosa* carries a poor prognosis largely related to the limited activity of available antimicrobials against it. Complications associated with a worse prognosis include severe cardiac failure or shock, major

TABLE 42-1 Antimicrobial Therapy for Infective Endocarditis and Other Intravascular Infections*

Organism	Recommended Therapy	Penicillin Allergic
1. Sensitive streptococci (MIC≤ 0.1)	Penicillin G 10–20 million units IV qd for 4 weeks *plus* **Aminoglycoside for first two weeks (Streptomycin 7.5 mg/kg (≤ 500 mg) IM q12h or gentamicin 1.0 mg/kg (≤ 80 mg) IM/IV q8h)	Cephalothin 2.0 gm IV q4h for 4 weeks‡ *plus* **Aminoglycoside for 4 weeks
2. Relatively "resistant" streptococci (MIC 0.2-0.5)	Pen G 20 million units per day for 4 weeks *plus* Aminoglycoside (#) for 4 weeks	Cephalothin 2.0 gm IV q 4h for 4 weeks‡ *plus* Aminoglycoside for 4 weeks
3. Resistant streptococci (MIC >0.5) (includes enterococci)	Penicillin G 20–30 million U IV qd for 6 weeks Ampicillin 12 gm IV qd is alternative *plus* Aminoglycoside# for 6 weeks	Vancomycin 30 mg/kg (<2 gm) qd for 6 weeks *plus* Aminoglycoside# for 6 weeks
4. Staphylococci (penicillin-sensitive)	Penicillin G 20 million units IV qd for 6 weeks	Cephalothin 2.0 gm IV q4 for 6 weeks‡
5. Staphylococci (methicillin-sensitive)—in absence of prosthetic valve	Nafcillin 1.5-2.0 gm IV q4h for 4-6 weeks†	Cephalothin 2.0 gm IV q 4h for 4–6 weeks‡
6. "Methicillin-resistant" staphylococci	Vancomycin 30 mg/kg IV (<2gm) per day +/− Rifampin 300 mg po q8h for 6 weeks	Same
7. Staphylococci (methicillin-sensitive)—in presence of prosthetic valve	Nafcillin 2.0 gm IV q4h for 6–8 wks plus rifampin 300 mg*** *plus* Aminoglycoside for 2 weeks	Cephalothin 2 gm IV‡ q4h for 6–8 wks plus rifampin*** *plus* Aminoglycoside for 2 weeks

TABLE 42-1 Antimicrobial Therapy for Infective Endocarditis and Other Intravascular Infections* (continued)

Organism	Recommended Therapy	Penicillin Allergic
8. Staphylococci (methicillin-resistant)in presence of prosthetic valve	Vancomycin 30 mg/kg/24h IV (< 2 gm) for 6–8 weeks, Rifampin 300 mg for 6–8 weeks*** plus Aminoglycoside for 2 weeks	——————
9. Corynebacterium	Penicillin G 20–30 million IV qd for 6 weeks plus Aminoglycoside for 6 weeks	Vancomycin 30 mg/kg(<2 gm) qd IV for 6 weeks
10. Gram-negative bacilli		
a. Enterobacteri-aceae	Therapy should be directed by in vitro susceptibilities.	Same
b. Pseudomonas	Therapy should be directed by in vitro susceptibilities though usual regimen includes tobramycin (8 mg/kg/day) plus extended spectrum penicillin	Same though ceftazidime plus tobramycin (8 mg/kg/d) frequently used
c. HACEK group	Ampicillin 2.0 gm IV q4h is commonly used though therapy should be directed by in vitro susceptibilities. (aminoglycoside frequently used in combination)	Choice directed by in vitro suscepti-bilities.
11. Rickettsia *Coxiella burnetti*	Tetracycline 500 mg po q6h for at least one year plus Trimethoprim 480 mg plus sulfamethoxazole 2400 mg q day until there is no evidence clinically of disease or phase I antibody titer is <1:128.	Same

TABLE 42-1 Antimicrobial Therapy for Infective Endocarditis and Other Intravascular Infections* (continued)

Organism	Recommended Therapy	Penicillin Allergic
12. Fungal	Amphotericin B plus surgery	Same
13. Culture-negative endocarditis	Penicillin G 20 million U IV qd for 6 weeks *plus an* Aminoglycoside for 2 weeks	Cephalothin 2.0 gm IV‡ q4h for 6 weeks

*Duration of treatment given applies to native valve infective endocarditis only.
**Aqueous crystalline penicillin G should be used alone in patients over 65 years of age or who have renal disease or bearing impairment.
‡If patient sensitivity to penicillin is of the immediate hypersensitivity type, vancomycin is recommended.
#Choice of aminoglycoside should depend on in vitro susceptibilities.
†Addition of an aminoglycoside is optional.
***Use of rifampin in coagulase negative staphylococcal infection is recommended. The value of rifampin in coagulase positive staphylococcal infections is controversial.
(Reprinted with permission from Cobbs CG, Carr MB: Endocarditis and other Intravascular Infections in the Critically Ill, in Hall JB, Schmidt GA, and Wood LDH: Principles of Critical Care, McGraw-Hill, New York, 1992.)

arterial emboli, myocardial abscess formation, and associated major organ system failure.

Prophylaxis

Certain medical procedures and cardiac abnormalities are known to place patients at an increased risk for the development of IE. Dental extraction, periodontal surgery, lower gastrointestinal procedures, and genitourinary procedures are most frequently associated with bacteremia. Cardiac abnormalities that predispose patients to IE include aortic and mitral disease, ventricular septal defects, patent ductus arteriosis, coarctation of the aorta, prosthetic valves, and valves which previously have been infected. Mitral valve prolapse, with redundancy of the valve seen on echocardiogram or evidence of mitral regurgitation, also predisposes the patient to IE. The specific antimicrobial agents chosen for prophylaxis are dependent on the specific procedure to be performed, the cardiac abnormality present, and the presence or absence of penicillin allergy (Table 42-2).

MYCOTIC ANEURYSM

Mycotic aneurysms are aneurysmal dilations of arteries caused by infection of the vessel wall with consequent weakening of vessel

TABLE 42-2 Endocarditis Prophylaxis

Procedure	Standard Regimen	Standard Oral Regimen for PCN Allergic Patients	Alternative Parenteral Regimens
Dental or respiratory tract procedure	Amoxicillin 3.0 gm po 1 h before, then 1.5 gm 6 h later.	Erythromycin, 1.0 gm po 2 h before, then 500 mg 6 h later OR Clindamycin 300 mg po 1 h before, then 150 mg 6 h later.	Ampicillin 2.0 gm IV or IM 30 min before then 1.0 gm 6 h later OR Clindamycin 300 mg IV 30 min before, then 150 mg 6 h later OR Vancomycin 1.0 gm IV over 1 h, starting 1 h before procedure; no repeat dose necessary.
Gastrointestinal or genitourinary tract procedure	Ampicillin, 2.0 gm IV or IM, plus gentamicin 1.5 mg/kg body weight IV or IM given 30 min before, repeat 8 h later.		Vancomycin, 1.0 gm IV, slowly over 1 h, plus gentamicin, 1.5 mg/kg body weight IV or IM, given 1 h before, repeat 8 h later.

(Reprinted with permission from Cobbs CG, Carr MB: Endocarditis and other Intravascular Infections in the Critically Ill, in Hall JB, Schmidt GA, and Wood LDH: Principles of Critical Care, McGraw-Hill, New York, 1992.)

structure. This is most common in patients with IE, and usually involves vessels of smaller caliber. The proposed pathogenesis is embolic localization of a valvular vegetation with extension of suppuration from the lumen circumferentially into the vessel wall; embolization of the vasavasorum by infected material from the valve; and, in the absence of underlying IE, mycotic aneurysm following transient bacteremia with seeding of a previously damaged site in a large artery.

Clinical Features

Intracranial mycotic aneurysms most commonly are encountered in patients who already carry a diagnosis of IE. Symptoms and signs consistent with subarachnoid or intracerebral hemorrhage with sudden onset of headache, decrease in level of consciousness, and focal neurologic signs are seen with aneurysmal rupture. Mycotic aneurysms of visceral arteries have variable presentation based on the organ involved. Small bowel gives colicky abdominal pain and symptoms of small bowel obstruction. Hepatic arterial aneurysms resemble ascending cholangitis because of fever, right upper quandrant pain, and jaundice. External iliac arterial mycotic aneurysm may present with pain in the lower anterior abdomen, quadriceps wasting, diminished deep tendon reflexes, and arterial insufficiency of the ipsilateral lower extremity. Abdominal aorta mycotic aneurysms may present with chronic pain and fever. In as many as one-third of patients with abdominal aortic aneurysms there is extension into the lumbar or thoracic vertebrae with resultant osteomyelitis. Aortoenteric fistula may occur if an aneurysm erodes into the bowel lumen.

Diagnosis

In patients with IE, clinical suspicion of an intracranial mycotic aneurysm usually arises after an episode of new neurologic symptoms. Computed tomography (CT) followed by cerebral angiography is the best diagnostic strategy. The diagnosis of mycotic aneurysm of the abdominal aorta may be made with clinical suspicion, bacteremia, and radiographic examination. Abdominal CT scan, aortogram, and bone scan may be helpful.

Treatment

The management of mycotic aneurysm depends on the organ involved. For peripheral intracranial aneurysms, clipping is probably indicated. For deep lesions for which a surgical approach is felt to be hazardous, antimicrobial therapy alone is advisable because many aneurysms will resolve spontaneously with medical treatment. In the case of abdominal aortic aneurysms, surgical resection of the involved aorta is almost always necessary.

CAVERNOUS SINUS THROMBOSIS

Cavernous sinus thrombosis usually results from direct spread of bacteria from a contiguous focus of infection by several routes: septic thrombophlebitis of the angular and ophthalmic veins from facial cellulitis; along the lateral sinus and petrosal sinuses from middle ear infections via the pterygoid venous plexus; from a peritonsillar abscess following a dental infection; from osteomyelitis of the maxilla or from a cervical abscess; and along the venous plexus surrounding the internal carotid artery from the middle ear or jugular bulb.

S. aureus and streptococci represent the majority of organisms found in cavernous sinus thrombosis. Patients generally present with early onset ophthalmoplegia with decreased sensation around the eye. The physical examination reveals periorbital edema and chemosis. As the illness develops, meningismus, altered mental status, and cranial nerve palsies (especially of III, IV, and V, and VI) become evident. Examination of the fundus often reveals striking venous congestion. The differential diagnosis of cavernous sinus thrombosis includes orbital cellulitis and rhinocerebral phycomycosis (mucormycosis). Bilateral involvement, as well as fifth nerve palsy, a fixed, dilated pupil and signs of meningitis are all more likely in cavernous sinus thrombosis than orbital cellulitis.

Diagnosis may be made with ultrasound of the orbit, CT scan, carotid angiography, and orbital venography. Lumbar puncture is necessary following CT scan.

Successful management of cavernous sinus thrombosis depends on early, effective antimicrobial therapy (see Table 42-1).

PROSTHETIC VALVE ENDOCARDITIS

Prosthetic valve endocarditis (PVE) occurs in 2 percent of patients with prosthetic heart valves. One-third get infected in the first few months after valve implantation because of intraoperative inoculation or localization of microorganisms on the new device following transient bacteremia associated with indwelling lines used in the perioperative period. Increased risks for PVE include IE of the native valve prior to valve resection, use of a mechanical valve in contrast to a tissue heterograft or homograft, a history of intravenous drug abuse, male gender, and longer cardiopulmonary bypass time.

Two-thirds of cases of PVE occur sixty days or more after replacement. The pathogenesis of this late onset PVE resembles that of native valve endocarditis. *Staphylococcus epidermidis* is common in early PVE, and microorganisms found in patients with late PVE tend to be similar to those seen in native valve disease.

Cardiac complications occur readily in patients with PVE. Clinical evidence of cardiac complications include new or changing regurgitant murmur caused by paravalvular leak from dehiscence of the valve ring, intraventricular and atrioventricular conduction defects resulting from extension of a paravalvular abscess into the intraventricular septum, and muffling of prosthetic heart sounds or new stenotic murmurs related to malfunction of the valve caused by a vegetation.

Blood cultures yielding staphylococci, "diphtheroids," and yeasts are more likely to represent true prosthetic valve infection than is bacteremia with gram-negative bacilli, which is more likely due to indwelling venous catheter infection. Echocardiography and cinefluoroscopic examination may be helpful. Echocardiography may identify vegetation and local suppurative complications as well as determine ventricular function and valvular integrity. Metallic clips or devices may distort the echocardiographic image. A cinefluorogram that reveals more than a 7° rocking of the prosthesis is very suggestive of valve dehiscence.

When the infecting organism has not been identified, initial therapy should include vancomycin and gentamicin to cover the likely possibilities of *S. epidermidis, S. aureus,* and streptococci (see Table 42-1). Relative indications for valve replacement in PVE include early PVE, nonstreptococcal late PVE, and periprosthetic leak. Patients with PVE should be treated for 6 to 8 weeks regardless of valve removal. If organisms can be cultured at the time of valve replacement, an additional 6 to 8 weeks of therapy is necessary.

PACEMAKER INFECTIONS

Cardiac pacemaker infections occur at a rate of 4 percent. Generator box infections, infection of the electrode along its subcutaneous course, and bacteremic infection of the intravascular portion of the electrode, with or without associated endocarditis, each contribute approximately one-third to the overall infection problem. Predisposing factors include diabetes mellitus, cancer, corticosteroid therapy, and skin erosion adjacent to the generator pouch. Pacemaker infection may occur early (3 to 6 months) or late (more than 6 months) after implant. Early infections generally can be attributed to wound contamination by skin organisms at the time of implantation; late infection, particularly of the intravascular electrode, is often due to transient bacteremia with adherence of organisms to the surface of the device. *S. epidermidis* and *S. aureus* are the most common microorganisms isolated from the blood of patients with pacemaker infections. The usual presentation of pacemaker infection is chills, fever and other constitutional symptoms. The diagnosis of pacemaker infection is made by excluding other sources, inspecting the generator pocket and the subcutaneous electrode areas, and obtaining blood cultures. Persistent bacteremia in a patient with an intravascular pacemaker suggests intravascular electrode infection or IE. An initial trial of intravenous antimicrobial therapy (see Table 42-1) for 4 to 6 weeks is warranted if pacemaker removal is not an option. If the decision is made to remove the pacemaker, then the new transvenous generator should be located in a deeper pocket. Two weeks of antimicrobial therapy after removal of the device is probably sufficient in the case of most generator pocket infections due to pyogenic microorganisms unless there is metastatic disease or secondary native valve IE, in which case the usual duration of treatment for native valve endocarditis is given after the device is removed.

INFECTIONS OF CENTRAL VENOUS DEVICES

The incidence of bacteremia complicating central venous cannulation varies greatly depending on the type of catheter and the length of time it has been in place, but is generally about 5 percent. Local symptoms and signs are not common in central venous device infection since the vein is generally well below the skin and subcutaneous tissue layers. Fever and elevated white blood count with a left shift may be present. Blood cultures are usually positive if no antibiotics have been administered. Microorganisms responsible for central venous line infection include staphylococci, gram-negative aerobic bacilli, streptococci, enterococci, corynebacterium ("diphtheroids"), and occasionally yeasts.

The pulmonary artery catheter may be complicated by infection at a 5 percent rate. Right-sided IE risk is increased by tricuspid and pulmonic valve inflammation due to contact with the catheter. This inflammation enhances microorganism localization.

Infection of Broviac and Hickman catheters may involve the skin at the exit site only, the subcutaneous tunnel extending from the exit site to the vein entry site, or the intravascular lumen. Venography is useful in suspected infections to identify a thrombin sheath within the device, which would suggest the possibility of an infectious complication. Diagnosis is improved with local inspection, blood cultures, and semiquantitative culture of the intracutaneous portion of the suspect catheter after removal (see Fig. 42-1). Empirical therapy, based on a Gram stain if possible, is given when the infection is associated with evidence of frank systemic sepsis. When the indication for the central venous catheter is still present and additional sites for catheter placement are scarce, it is probably acceptable to change the catheter over

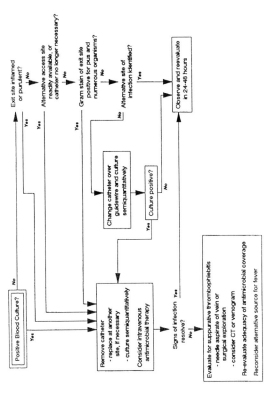

FIG. 42-1 Approach to bacteremia caused by an infected temporary intravascular device. (Reprinted with permission from Cobbs CG, Carr MB: Endocarditis and Other Intravascular Infections in the Critically Ill, in Hall JB, Schmidt GA, and Wood LDH: Principles of Critical Care, McGraw-Hill, New York, 1992.)

373

a guidewire while awaiting the result of the semiquantitative catheter culture and blood culture to determine whether the site can continue to be used. Patients with Hickman and Broviac catheters are treated for 2 weeks if the device is not removed. If relapse occurs, the device should be removed and an additional 2 weeks of therapy administered.

ARTERIAL GRAFT INFECTION

Arterial grafts have an infection rate that has varied between 2 and 6 percent with a mortality rate as high as 50 percent. The pathogenesis of graft infection resembles that of prosthetic valve disease. Graft infections present a mean of 8 months after implantation but may occur as long as 7 to 10 years after graft placement. Grafts which cross the femoral area seem to be at greatest risk for infection, possibly due to contamination by bowel flora at the time of implantation. Gram-positive microorganisms are the most common cause of graft infections particularly in the groin or popliteal area.

Intraluminal infection may present as fever and nonspecific constitutional complaints due to bacteremia. Extraluminal infection may present with evidence of local graft infection with erythema, tenderness and swelling over the graft site, with systemic inflammatory symptoms without definite localizing findings, or with graft occlusion. Rapid swelling suggests disruption of the suture line with bleeding and false aneurysm formation, and almost always implies graft infection. Graft thrombosis should be suspected when signs and symptoms of peripheral arterial insufficiency develop. Exteriorization of the graft secondary to breakdown of tissue overlying the graft is pathognomonic of infection. Abdominal aortic graft infection may lead to mass effect with evidence of ureteral obstruction of hydronephrosis, symptoms and signs of lower extremity ischemia, or development of aortoduodenal fistula. Diagnosis of graft infection can be made clinically with blood culture, scanning with indium or technetium-labelled white blood cells, or CT scanning for soft tissue edema or false aneurysm formation.

Management of an infected intravascular graft almost always requires specific antmicrobial therapy (see Table 42-1) chosen on the basis of the presumed or demonstrated infecting microorganism as well as graft removal.

AN APPROACH TO PATIENTS WITH FEVER AND SUSPECTED INTRAVASCULAR INFECTION

Patients with otherwise unexplained positive blood cultures in the presence of an intravascular device must be presumed to have an infection of the device. When the device is a temporary one, such as a peripheral intravenous line, central venous catheter, or temporary pacemaker, it should be removed. If pus can be expressed from the puncture site or there is persistent bacteremia, surgical exploration of the peripheral veins is indicated. Tunnelled central venous catheters call for a more selective approach (see Figure 42-1).

For further reading in *Principles of Critical Care,* see Chap 101 "Endocarditis and Other Intravascular Infections in the Critically Ill" C Glenn Cobbs/Mark B Carr

---

43

Central Nervous System Infections

Stephen R. Amesbury

This chapter reviews meningitis, brain abscess, subdural empyema, epidural abscess, intracranial thrombophlebitis, and encephalomyelitis.

MENINGITIS

Haemophilus influenzae accounts for only about 5 percent of total isolates after age 6 years. When isolated, other predisposing factors such as sinusitis, otitis media, epiglottitis, pneumonia, diabetes mellitus, alcoholism, asplenic states, and immune deficiency should be considered. Meningitis due to *Neisseria meningitidis* may occur in epidemics in children and young adults. Nasopharyngeal carriage accounts for initiation of infection. Pneumococcal meningitis is most common in adults over age 30 years, and is often associated with distant foci of infection such as pneumonia, otitis media, mastoiditis, sinusitis, and endocarditis. *Streptococcus pneumoniae* is the most common meningeal isolate in head trauma patients who have suffered basilar skull fracture with subsequent cerebrospinal fluid (CSF) leak.

Listeria monocytogenes accounts for only about 1.9 percent of all cases of bacterial meningitis, but carries a high mortality rate. It is more likely in neonates, the elderly, alcoholics, cancer patients, and immunosuppressed adults. Meningitis due to aerobic gram-negative bacilli occurs infrequently, but, again, the mortality rates are very high. *Staphylococcus epidermidis* is the most common cause of meningitis in persons with CSF shunts. Meningitis due to *Staph. aureus* is frequently found in the early post-neurosurgical period.

Clinical Presentation

The clinical presentation in adults with bacterial meningitis includes fever, headache, meningismus, and signs of cerebral dysfunction; these symptoms and signs are found in more than 85 percent of cases. Also common are nausea, vomiting, rigors, profuse sweating, weakness, myalgias, and photophobia. The meningismus may be accompanied by Kernig's sign and/or Brudzinski's sign. These signs are elicited in only about 50 percent of cases of bacterial meningitis in adults. Cranial nerve palsies occur in only 10 to 20 percent of cases (especially nerves III, IV, VI, and VII). Seizures occur in about 30 percent of cases. Papilledema is rare and should suggest an alternate diagnosis, such as an intracranial mass lesion.

Elderly patients, especially those with underlying conditions such as diabetes mellitus or cardiopulmonary disease, may present with insidious disease manifested only by lethargy or obtundation, variable signs of meningeal irritation, and no fever. In this subgroup, altered mental status should not be ascribed to other causes until bacterial meningitis has been excluded by CSF examination. A neurosurgical patient or a patient who has undergone head trauma also presents a unique clinical situation, since these patients already have many of the symptoms and signs of meningitis from their underlying disease processes.

Diagnosis

The diagnosis of bacterial meningitis rests on CSF examination. The opening pressure is elevated in virtually all cases; values over 600 mmH$_2$O suggest cerebral edema, presence of intracranial suppurative foci, or communicating hydrocephalus. Xanthochromia—a pale-pink to yellow-orange color of the supernatant of centrifuged CSF—is found in patients with subarachnoid hemorrhage, usually within 2 h post-hemorrhage. The CSF white cell count is usually elevated in untreated bacterial meningitis, ranging from 100 to 10,000 cells per mm^3, with a predominance of neutrophils. About 10 percent present with a lymphocytic predominance in CSF. Some patients may have a very low CSF white cell count despite high bacterial concentrations in CSF; these patients have a poor prognosis. Therefore, a gram stain and culture should be performed on all CSF specimens even with a normal cell count.

A CSF glucose concentration less than 40 mg/dl is found in about 60 percent of patients with bacterial meningitis. The CSF glucose level must always be compared to a simultaneous serum glucose concentration. The CSF protein concentration is elevated in virtually all cases of bacterial meningitis. CSF examination by gram stain permits a rapid, accurate identification in 60 to 90 percent of cases of bacterial meningitis. Cultures of CSF are positive in 70 to 80 percent of untreated cases.

Rapid diagnostic tests, such as counterimmunoelectrophoresis (CIE), detect specific antigens in CSF due to some meningococci, *H. influenzae*, pneumococci, streptococci, and *Escherichia coli*. Newer latex agglutination tests are more rapid and sensitive than CIE. One of these rapid diagnostic tests (preferably latex agglutination) should be performed on all CSF specimens from patients in whom bacterial meningitis is suspected when the gram stain is negative.

Treatment

The initial approach to the patient with suspected bacterial meningitis is to perform a lumbar puncture to determine whether the CSF findings are consistent with that diagnosis. Patients should receive empiric antimicrobial therapy based on their age and underlying disease status if no etiologic agent is identified by gram stain or rapid diagnostic tests. In patients with a focal neurologic examination, a computerized tomography (CT) scan should be performed immediately to exclude an intracranial mass lesion, since lumbar puncture is relatively contraindicated in that setting. However, since obtaining a CT scan generally entails some delay, empiric antimicrobial therapy should be started immediately and before the CT scan and lumbar puncture, because of the high mortality in patients with bacterial meningitis in whom antimicrobial therapy is delayed. Our choices for empiric antibiotic therapy in patients with presumed bacterial meningitis, based on age, are shown in Table 43-1. One situation not listed in this table deserves comment: In neurosurgical patients or patients with CSF shunts or foreign bodies, staphylococci, diptheroids, and gram-negative bacilli are likely infecting organisms. Antimicrobial therapy in these situations should consist of vancomycin plus ceftazidime pending culture results.

Once an infecting microorganism has been isolated, antimicrobial therapy can be modified for optimal treatment. Antibiotics of choice are shown in Table 43-2. Dosages for adults are listed in Table 43-3. In view of recent cases of relatively and highly resistant strains of pneumococci, susceptibility testing should be performed on all CSF isolates. For relatively resistant strains, a third-generation cephalosporin (e.g., cefotaxime or ceftriaxone) should be used; for highly resistant strains, vancomycin is the antimicrobial agent of choice.

The duration of therapy for bacterial meningitis should be 10 to

TABLE 43-1 Empiric Therapy of Purulent Meningitis

Age	Standard Therapy	Alternative Therapies
0–3 weeks	Ampicillin plus a third-generation cephalosporin*	Ampicillin plus an aminoglycoside†
4–12 weeks	Ampicillin plus a third-generation cephalosporin*	Ampicillin plus chloramphenicol
3 months–18 years	Third-generation cephalosporin*	Ampicillin plus chloramphenicol; cefuroxime
18–50 years	Penicillin G or ampicillin	Third-generation cephalosporin*
>50 years	Ampicillin plus a third-generation cephalosporin*	Ampicillin plus an aminoglycoside; † trimethoprim-sulfamethoxazole

*Cefotaxime or ceftriaxone.
†Gentamicin, tobramycin, or amikacin.
(Reproduced with permission from Tunkel AR, and Scheld MW: Bacterial Infections of the Central Nervous System, in Hall JB, Schmidt GA, and Wood LDH: Principles of Critical Care, McGraw-Hill, New York, 1992.)

TABLE 43-2 Antimicrobial Therapy of Bacterial Meningitis

Organism	Antibiotic of Choice
Neisseria meningitidis	Penicillin G or ampicillin
Streptococcus pneumoniae	Penicillin G or ampicillin
Haemophilus influenzae (β-lactamase–negative)	Ampicillin
Haemophilus influenzae (β-lactamase–positive)	Third-generation cephalosporin*
Enterobacteriaceae	Third-generation cephalosporin *
Pseudomonas aeruginosa	Ceftazidime†
Streptococcus agalactiae	Penicillin G or ampicillin†
Listeria monocytogenes	Ampicillin or penicillin G†
Staphylococcus aureus (methicillin sensitive)	Nafcillin or oxacillin
Staphylococcus aureus (methicillin-resistant)	Vancomycin
Staphylococcus epidermidis	Vancomycin‡

*Cefotaxime or ceftriaxone.
†Addition of an aminoglycoside should be considered.
‡Addition of rifampin may be indicated.
(Reproduced with permission from Tunkel AR, and Scheld MW: Bacterial Infections of the Central Nervous System, in Hall JB, Schmidt GA, and Wood LDH: Principles of Critical Care, McGraw-Hill, New York, 1992.)

TABLE 43-3 Recommended Doses of Antibiotics for Intracranial Infections in Adults with Normal Renal Function

Antibiotic	Total Daily Dose in Adults (Dosing Interval)
Penicillin G	24 million U (q 4 h)
Ampicillin	12 g (q 4 h)
Nafcillin, oxacillin	9–12 g (q 4 h)
Chloramphenicol	4–6 g* (q 6 h)
Cefotaxime	8–12 g (q 4 h)
Ceftriaxone	4–6 g† (q 12 h)
Ceftazidime	6–12 g‡ (q 8 h)
Vancomycin	2 g (q 12 h)
Gentamicin, tobramycin	3–5 mg/kg (q 8 h)
Amikacin	15 mg/kg (q 8 h)
Trimethoprim-sulfamethoxazole	10 mg/kg§ (q 12 h)
Metronidazole	30 mg/kg (q 6 h)

*Higher dose recommended for pneumococcal meningitis.
†Actual dose studied was 50 mg/kg every 12 h.
‡Not enough patients studied to make firm recommendations.
§Dosage based on trimethoprim component.
(Reproduced with permission from Tunkel AR, and Scheld MW: Bacterial Infections of the Central Nervous System, in Hall JB, Schmidt GA, and Wood LDH: Principles of Critical Care, McGraw-Hill, New York, 1992.)

14 days for most causes of nonmeningococcal meningitis, and 3 weeks for meningitis due to gram-negative enteric bacilli. Seven days of therapy appears to be adequate for meningococcal meningitis; several reports have suggested that 7 days of therapy is efficacious also for *H. influenzae* meningitis. However, therapy must be individualized, and on the basis of clinical response some patients may require longer courses of treatment.

BRAIN ABSCESS

The most common pathogenic mechanism of brain abscess formation is spread from a contiguous focus of infection, most often in the middle ear (abscess in temporal lobe or cerebellum), mastoid cells, or paranasal sinuses (infection commonly in frontal lobe). Brain abscesses due to hematogenous dissemination from a distant focus of infection are usually multiple and multiloculated, and have a higher mortality rate than abscesses that arise secondary to contiguous foci of infection. The most common source of these abscesses in adults are chronic pyogenic lung diseases—especially lung abscess, bronchiectasis, empyema, and cystic fibrosis. Trauma is a third pathogenic mechanism in the development of brain abscess, including post-neurosurgical. Finally, brain abscess is cryptogenic in about 20 percent of patients.

Overall, the most commonly isolated bacterial species in brain abscess are streptococci, present in 60 to 70 percent of cases. *Staph. aureus* accounts for 10 to 15 percent of isolates. Anaerobes are isolated in 20 to 40 percent of cases, often in mixed culture.

Clinical Presentation

Most of the clinical manifestations are due to the presence of space-occupying lesions within the brain. The most common symptom is headache, present in more than 70 percent of patients. Other findings include nausea and vomiting (about 50 percent of cases), nuchal rigidity (about 25 percent), and papilledema (about 25 percent). Mental status changes ranging from lethargy to coma occur in the majority of cases. Seizures, usually generalized, occur in 25 to 35 percent of patients. Fever appears in only 50 percent of cases; afebrile patients tend to be older, have a longer duration of illness, and have a higher mortality rate. Only about one-half of the patients present with the classic triad of fever, headache, and focal neurologic deficit.

Diagnosis

The diagnosis of brain abscess has been revolutionized by the development of CT, which not only is an excellent means to examine the brain parenchyma, but is superior to standard radiologic procedures for examination of the paranasal sinuses, mastoid cells, and middle ear. CT also yields information concerning the extent of surrounding edema, presence or absence of a midline shift, presence of hydrocephalus, and possibility of imminent ventricular rupture. After aspiration of a brain abscess, improvement in CT appearance may not be seen for up to 5 weeks or longer. Complete resolution may take 4 to 5 months. Contrast-enhanced magnetic resonance imaging (MRI) offers some benefits over CT in evaluating brain abscess, but it is not always feasible in critically ill patients. Stereotaxic CT-guided aspiration of a brain abscess can be used to facilitate bacteriologic diagnosis. At the time of aspiration, a specimen should be sent for gram stain and other special stains, routine culture, and anaerobic culture. Lumbar puncture is contraindicated in patients with suspected or proven brain abscess, because of the risk of life-threatening cerebral herniation after removal of CSF.

Treatment

When a diagnosis of brain abscess is made, either presumptively, by radiologic studies, or by aspiration of the abscess, antimicrobial therapy should be initiated. When aspiration is impractical or delayed, we recommend empiric therapy based on the likely etiologic agent, if a predisposing condition can be identified (see Table 43-4). Penicillin G should be used in high doses (20 to 24 million U/day).

TABLE 43-4 Empiric Antimicrobial Therapy for Brain Abscess

Predisposing Condition	Antimicrobial Regimen
Otitis media or mastoiditis	Metronidazole plus a third-generation cephalosporin*
Sinusitis	Nafcillin or vancomycin† plus metronidazole plus a third-generation cephalosporin*
Dental sepsis	Penicillin plus metronidazole
Cranial trauma or post-neurosurgery	Vancomycin plus a third-generation cephalosporin*
Congenital heart disease	Penicillin plus a third-generation cephalosporin*
Unknown	Nafcillin or vancomycin† plus metronidazole plus a third-generation cephalosporin*

*Cefotaxime or ceftriaxone; ceftazidime is used if *P. aeruginosa* is suspected.
†Vancomycin is used in the penicillin-allergic patient or when methicillin-resistant *Staph. aureus* is suspected.
(Reproduced with permission from Tunkel AR, and Scheld MW: Bacterial Infections of the Central Nervous System, in Hall JB, Schmidt GA, and Wood LDH: Principles of Critical Care, McGraw-Hill, New York, 1992.)

TABLE 43-5 Antimicrobial Therapy for Brain Abscess

Organism	Standard Therapy	Alternative Therapies
Streptococcus milleri and other streptococci	Penicillin G	Third-generation cephalosporin,* vancomycin
Bacteroides fragilis	Metronidazole	Chloramphenicol, clindamycin
Fusobacterium spp., *Actinomyces*	Penicillin G	Metronidazole, chloramphenicol, clindamycin
Staphylococcus aureus	Nafcillin	Vancomycin
Enterobacteriaceae	Third-generation cephalosporin*	Aztreonam†
Haemophilus sp.	Third-generation cephalosporin*	Aztreonam†
Nocardia asteroides	Trimethoprim-sulfamethoxazole	Ampicillin, erythromycin, amikacin, imipenem (all †)

*Cefotaxime or ceftriaxone.
†Limited data available for use of these agents; firm recommendations are not possible at this time.
(Reproduced with permission from Tunkel AR, and Scheld WM: Bacterial Infections of the Central Nervous System, in Hall JB, Schmidt GA, and Wood LDH: Principles of Critical Care, McGraw-Hill, New York, 1992.)

When *Bacteroides fragilis* is suspected, we recommend the addition of metronidazole (7.5 mg/kg every 6 h). In cases where ceftazidime is the third-generation cephalosporin used in empiric therapy of brain abscess, the regimen must also include penicillin G to treat a possible streptococcal infection since ceftazidime has unreliable gram-positive activity.

Once an infecting pathogen is isolated, antimicrobial therapy can be modified (see Table 43-5). Therapy with high-dose intravenous antibiotics should be continued for 4 to 6 weeks and is often followed by oral antibiotic therapy for 2 to 6 months, if an appropriate agent is available. Surgical management is required for optimal treatment of most brain abscesses. Intracranial pressure monitoring has become important in the management of brain abscess patients who have cerebral edema. The use of corticosteroids remains controversial.

SUBDURAL EMPYEMA

Subdural empyema refers to a collection of pus in the space between the dura and arachnoid. The most common predisposing conditions are otorhinologic infections and sinusitis which spread to the subdural space via valveless emissary veins or via extension of an osteomyelitis of the skull with accompanying epidural abscess. The infection is metastatic in a minority of cases.

Symptoms and signs of subdural empyema relate to the presence of increased intracranial pressure, meningeal irritation, or focal cortical inflammation. Fever above 39°C is present in most cases. Focal neurologic signs appear in 24 to 48 h and progress rapidly. Hemiparesis and hemiplegia are the most common focal signs. Seizures occur in half of patients. If the patient remains untreated, signs of increased intracranial pressure and cerebral herniation may ensue rapidly.

Subdural empyema should be suspected in any patient with meningeal signs and a focal neurologic deficit. Lumbar puncture is contraindicated in this setting, because of the risk of cerebral herniation. The diagnostic procedure of choice is either CT, with contrast enhancement, or MRI. MRI may detect empyema not clearly seen on CT. Cerebral arteriography should be utilized on an emergent basis when MRI is unavailable and subdural empyema is suspected despite a normal CT scan.

The therapy of subdural empyema optimally requires a combined medical-surgical approach. Once purulent material is aspirated, antimicrobial therapy should be initiated; it should be based on gram stain and on the site of primary infection. This consists of nafcillin or vancomycin, plus a third generation cephalosporin (cefotaxime or ceftriaxone), with or without metronidazole. The optimal surgical approach for subdural empyema is controversial, and will be determined by the neurosurgeon.

SPINAL EPIDURAL ABSCESS

Spinal epidural abscess usually follows hematogenous dissemination from foci elsewhere in the body to the epidural space, or by extension from vertebral osteomyelitis. Bacteremia is an important predisposing factor, since the incidence of spinal epidural abscess is increased in patients who use intravenous drugs or have intravenous catheters. The infecting microorganism in the vast majority of cases is *Staph. aureus.*

Spinal epidural abscess may develop within hours to days (after hematogenous seeding), or may pursue a chronic course over months (associated more often with vertebral osteomyelitis). Most abscesses pass through the following stages: focal vertebral pain; root pain; defects of motor, sensory or sphincter function; and paralysis. Fever occurs in most patients during the course of their illness. Respiratory function may be impaired if the cervical spinal cord is involved. Once there are signs of weakness, sensory deficits or disturbances of sphincter control, there may be a rapid transition to paralysis (within 24 h), indicating the need for emergent evaluation, diagnosis, and treatment.

MRI or CT should be performed in cases of suspected spinal epidural abscess, with myelography reserved for use in locations where neither MRI nor CT is available. Presumptive antimicrobial therapy for spinal epidural abscess must include a first-line antistaphylococcal agent (nafcillin or vancomycin). Coverage for gramnegative organisms is necessary in patients with a history of intravenous drug abuse or spinal procedure. Again, surgery is necessary to adequately drain the abscess.

SPINAL SUBDURAL EMPYEMA
AND CRANIAL EPIDURAL ABSCESS

Spinal subdural empyema is a rare condition occurring secondary to metastatic infection from a distant site. *Staph. aureus* is the most frequent isolate. It usually manifests itself as radicular pain and symptoms of spinal cord compression, which may occur at multiple levels. Clinically, this lesion is difficult to distinguish from a spinal epidural abscess. MRI is the diagnostic procedure of choice, because it gives more accurate information as to the extent of the lesion than does CT. Myelography may not detect the entire length of the empyema if complete blocks are present at multiple levels. Both MRI and myelography detect cord compression, block, or multiple extraaxial defects. Surgical drainage and intravenous antibiotic therapy are indicated.

Cranial epidural abscess can cross the cranial dura along emissary veins, so subdural empyema often is also present. The etiology, pathogenesis, and bacteriology of the two processes, therefore, are usually identical. The onset of symptoms in cranial epidural abscess may be insidious and overshadowed by the primary focus of infection.

Because the dura is closely apposed to the inner surface of the cranium, the abscess usually enlarges too slowly to produce sudden major neurologic deficits (in contrast to subdural empyema) unless there is deeper intracranial extension. Headache is a usual complaint. Eventually signs of increased intracranial pressure or focal neurologic signs may develop. CT and MRI are also the diagnostic procedures of choice. The therapy of cranial epidural abscess is similar to that of cranial subdural empyema.

ADJUNCTIVE THERAPY FOR EPIDURAL
AND SUBDURAL INFECTIONS

Preoperative use of mannitol, hyperventilation, and/or dexamethasone may be effective in controlling intracranial pressure prior to surgical decompression. We believe a short course of corticosteroids is appropriate in cases where surgical intervention is delayed or contraindicated. Anticonvulsants should be used in patients with seizures.

SUPPURATIVE INTRACRANIAL THROMBOPHLEBITIS

Septic intracranial thrombophlebitis may begin with veins and venous sinuses, or may follow local head and neck infections. Septic thrombophlebitis may also occur in association with epidural abscess, subdural empyema, or bacterial meningitis. The usual predisposing conditions for cavernous sinus thrombosis are paranasal sinusitis, or infection of the face or mouth. *Staph. aureus* is the most important infecting microorganism. The most common complaints in cavernous sinus thrombosis are periorbital swelling and headache, followed in frequency by drowsiness, diplopia, eye tearing, photophobia, and ptosis. Fever is present in over 90 percent of patients. Cranial nerves III, IV, and VI deficits, papilledema, meningismus, and dilated or sluggishly reactive pupils are further signs of cavernous sinus thrombosis. The diagnostic procedure of choice is MRI. Carotid arteriography with venous phase studies and orbital venography may also be useful. Empiric antimicrobial therapy should be guided by the site of the antecedent infection. Surgery may be required when antimicrobial therapy alone is ineffective. Some authors recommend operative intervention for patients who develop cavernous venous thrombosis as a complication of sinusitis. Adjunctive therapy with anticoagulants (e.g., heparin) is controversial.

ENCEPHALOMYELITIS

Most patients do not present with symptoms and signs pathognomonic of a certain cause, but rather with nonspecific problems of fever, headache, and behavioral changes or altered mental status. The approach should begin with a careful history and physical examination. The clinical features alone are not generally sufficient to establish an etiologic diagnosis but do influence the likelihood of some diagnoses. The immune status of the patient is important when considering the various etiologic possibilities. Toxoplasmosis is the most common cause of encephalitis in AIDS (acquired immunodeficiency syndrome) patients. Other causes of encephalitis in AIDS include cytomegalovirus (CMV) and other herpes viruses, fungi (especially cryptococcus), mycobacterium, and uncommon pathogens like *Nocardia* and *Listeria*.

Physical exam lends little to the diagnostic approach except in cases where a characteristic rash is present. A thorough neurologic examination is important since the presence of focal neurologic signs heightens the likelihood of treatable infectious etiologies and mandates the commencement of empirical antimicrobial therapy. The presence of focal neurologic abnormalities clearly mandates urgent diagnostic imaging with either CT scanning or MRI. A lumbar puncture is an important step in the diagnostic evaluation of encephalitis and should be performed early unless there is a specific contraindication (e.g., increased intracranial pressure). If there is concern for increased intracranial pressure (ICP), and possible herniation, a cisternal puncture should be considered. Further evaluation of all patients with encephalitis includes neurodiagnostic evaluation with an electroencephalogram (EEG), and a CT scan or MRI scan. If no specific diagnosis is established, brain biopsy should be considered.

AIDS patients are unique. The approach to management in these patients again requires a complete neurodiagnostic assessment along with toxoplasma serology. If the encephalitis is compatible with toxoplasmosis, then empirical treatment with pyrimethamine and sulfadiazine is begun.

Intensive supportive care is indicated in patients with encephalitis because these patients may make remarkable recoveries even after prolonged periods of unconsciousness.

Herpes Simplex Viral Encephalitis

Herpes simplex viral encephalitis (HSVE) is the most common fatal nonepidemic encephalitis. The patient is seldom immunocompromised. HSVE is important because untreated it has a very high mortality rate. Recent developments in antiviral therapy have significantly improved the outcome. There are no pathognomonic clinical symptoms or signs of HSVE that distinguish it from encephalitis of other etiologies. Clinical findings include fever, headache, alteration of consciousness, personality changes, dysphasia, and autonomic dysfunction. Eighty-five percent of patients have clinical findings indicative of focal neurologic disease.

The laboratory investigations are not diagnostic short of a brain biopsy. Examination of the CSF is almost always abnormal in encephalomyelitis, usually demonstrating increased leukocytes generally between 10 and 500/mm^3. The CSF glucose value is usually normal or slightly elevated. Although a completely normal CSF does not rule out encephalomyelitis, it should heighten suspicion for a toxic or metabolic encephalopathy. There are characteristic EEG findings which are more sensitive than CT scans early in the course of HSVE. The role of MRI has yet to be determined.

Definitive diagnosis of HSVE requires brain biopsy, but treatment with acyclovir should begin as soon as the diagnosis is clinically suspected. The dose of acyclovir must be adjusted according to renal function. For creatinine clearance of >50, 25 to 50, 10 to 25 or 0 to 10 mL/min/1.7m^2, the dose of acyclovir is 10 mg/kg every 8 h, 12 h, 24 h or 5 mg/kg every 24 h respectively. Patients receiving hemodialysis three times per week should receive 5 mg/kg every 24 h plus 6 mg/kg after dialysis. If a brain biopsy is not obtained, the patient must complete a full course of therapy, with ongoing investigation and surveillance to rule out other diseases mimicking HSVE.

For further reading in *Principles of Critical Care,* see Chap 103 "Bacterial Infections of the Central Nervous System" Allan R Tunkel/W Michael Scheld, Chap 104 "Encephalomyelitis" John C Galbraith/D Lorne Tyrrell

ACUTE PULMONARY TUBERCULOSIS

Mycobacterium tuberculosis causes several acute, life-threatening illnesses. Acute respiratory failure due to *M. tuberculosis* may result when a large quantity of heavily infected liquid caseum ruptures into the bronchial tree (most common) or vasculature (causing miliary tuberculosis). Massive hemoptysis from active or healed disease may similarly result in aspiration and acute hypoxemic respiratory failure.

CAVITARY PULMONARY TUBERCULOSIS

The clinical manifestations of subacute symptoms for about two weeks associated with fever (usually low grade), weight loss, and nonspecific physical findings may underestimate the extent of fibrocaseous pulmonary tuberculosis until bronchogenic spread occurs and the patient develops respiratory failure. The chest radiograph typically shows extensive chronic cavitary pneumonia with acinar shadows. A middle-aged or older person who comes from a population in which tuberculosis is endemic or one that is at increased risk of progressive disease (e.g., human immunodeficiency virus (HIV) infection) is the typical patient.

MILIARY TUBERCULOSIS

Patients who develop miliary tuberculosis are not usually critically ill. The tuberculosis organisms enter the bloodstream via the lymphatics. Adult respiratory distress syndrome (ARDS) occasionally occurs in patients with miliary tuberculosis. The quantity, dose, and type of bacillary antigen entering the bloodstream; state of host's cell-mediated immunity; and possible delayed hypersensitivity contribute to the development of ARDS. Thrombosis of small vessels in the region of the tubercles and tuberculous arteritis may lead to disseminated intravascular coagulation (DIC) in patients with miliary tuberculosis. The combination of DIC and ARDS in miliary tuberculosis signals a poor prognosis.

The complications of fibrocaseous and miliary tuberculosis include nonmycobacterial sepsis, massive hemoptysis, pneumothorax, bronchopleural fistula, endobronchial disease leading to air trapping, and upper airway obstruction.

Diagnosis

Diagnostic difficulty arises mainly because of failure to consider advanced fibrocaseous or miliary tuberculosis in someone presenting in acute respiratory failure. The differential diagnosis is extensive. Significant hypoxemia is suggestive of a nontuberculous bacterial etiology, but a relatively normal total leukocyte count should favor tuberculosis. Alternative explanations for chronic cavitary pneumonia include fungal diseases, nocardiosis, melioidosis, and *Klebsiella pneumoniae* infection. Bone marrow biopsy, lymph node biopsy, liver biopsy, lumbar puncture, or bronchoscopy with brushings and transbronchial biopsy are the definitive diagnostic procedures. The presence of caseation or acid-fast bacilli strongly suggests tuberculosis. Smear and culture of sputum or endotracheal secretions for acid-fast bacilli are negative in most cases of miliary tuberculosis but should be performed repeatedly in any case. The tuberculin skin test is not usually helpful.

Treatment

If a tuberculous etiology of respiratory failure is suspected, it is advisable to initiate therapy even before the results of diagnostic procedures are available. Three to four drugs are recommended: isoniazid (INH) with pyridoxine (50mg daily), rifampin (RIF), streptomycin (SM) or ethambutol (EMB), and pyrazinamide (PZA) (see Table 44-1). Drug resistance should be suspected in all immigrants from countries with a high prevalence of drug resistance (e.g., Southeast Asia and African countries) and in all patients thought to have acquired their infection from a known resistant case.

INH, RIF, PZA, and, rarely, EMB have all been reported to cause hepatitis. Liver disease usually occurs within the first three months of therapy and the frequency increases after age 35. Liver enzymes, specifically aspartate aminotransferase (AST), alanine aminotransferase (ALT), and alkaline phosphatase (AP) levels, and symptoms of hepatitis (nausea, vomiting, or vague abnormal discomfort), are the usual indicators of drug toxicity. INH must be stopped if enzyme elevation is progressive.

Corticosteroids (methylprednisolone, 125 mg IV twice daily) are administered to all patients with acute respiratory failure due to tuberculosis unless there is a strong suspicion of coincident bacterial sepsis. Steroid therapy is tapered over a period of 1 to 6 weeks. Reasons for steroid use are: **1.** adrenocortical insufficiency may be present and made worse by RIF induction of hepatic microsomal enzymes which leads to reduction of corticosteroid half-life and clinical efficacy; **2.** corticosteroids act to reduce the exudative reaction and systemic toxicity in severe tuberculosis; and **3.** corticosteroids may also act to hasten the resolution of tuberculosis pneumonia.

TABLE 44-1 First-Line Drugs in the Treatment of Tuberculosis

Drug	Daily dose	Route	Side effects	Monitoring
Isoniazid	5–10 mg/kg up to 300 mg	PO, IM, IV	Peripheral neuritis, hepatitis, hypersensitivity	ALT/AP/AST
Rifampin	10–20 mg/kg up to 600 mg	PO, IV	Hepatitis, febrile reaction, purpura (rare)	ALT/AP/AST
Pyrazinamide	15–30 mg/kg up to 2 g	PO	Hyperuricemia, hepatotoxicity	Uric acid, ALT/AP/AST
Streptomycin	15–30 mg/kg up to 1 g	IM	Cranial nerve VIII damage, nephrotoxicity	Vestibular function, audiograms, BUN, creatinine
Ethambutol	15 mg/kg	PO	Optic neuritis (reversible with discontinuation of drug; very rare at 15 mg/kg); skin rash	Red-green color, visual acuity

(Reprinted with permission from Long R: Critical Illness Due to Mycobacterium Tuberculosis, in Hall JB, Schmidt GA, and Wood LDH: Principles of Critical Care, McGraw-Hill, New York, 1992.)

Prevention of tuberculosis is still the most effective therapeutic measure. Heath care providers are best protected against infection when the infectious patient is kept in a maximally ventilated and ultraviolet lighted isolation room. The available face masks do not adequately prevent mycobacterium spread from the infectious patient. Whenever possible disposable circuitry should be used during mechanical ventilation, and a breathing circuit filter should be placed in the expiratory line. The circuitry and the filter should be changed every 12 h. If nondisposable equipment is used, it must be gas-sterilized before being reused.

EXTRAPULMONARY ACUTE TUBERCULOSIS

Tuberculous Pericarditis (TP) is most often due to rupture of an adjacent caseous node into the pericardial sac. Progressive hematogenous dissemination is another but less important route for TP to occur.

The clinical picture is of cardiac tamponade associated with fever or precordial pain. The diagnosis of tuberculous pericarditis is very difficult. Physical and laboratory examinations are usually nonspecific. If echocardiogram demonstrates significant pericardial effusion, then therapeutic and diagnostic pericardiocentesis or subxiphoid pericardiostomy is indicated. Fluid from pericardiocentesis is similar to the fluid of tuberculous pleurisy, but a positive acid-fast smear is very uncommon, and culture is positive in only 25 to 50 percent of the cases. Definitive diagnosis usually requires pericardial biopsy. Granulomatous pericarditis and malignant pericardial disease are part of the differential diagnosis.

Antituberculous drugs should be given to all patients, and when not contraindicated, 60 to 80 mg/day of prednisone tapered over six weeks should be administered. Serial echocardiography over a period of 6 to 8 weeks should be performed on those patients not requiring pericardiostomy initially.

Tuberculous meningitis results from the rupture of a subependymal tubercle into the subarachnoid space rather than by direct hematogenous spread. The release of a thick gelatinous inflammatory exudate may result in obliteration of the basal meningeal structures. The exudate may surround the spinal cord, spread along the pial vessels, and invade the underlying brain. Cranial nerves become involved and arteries occlude as the inflammatory exudate migrates through the subarachnoid space. Blockage of the basal cisterns frequently results in a meningeal obstructive hydrocephalus.

Examination of the cerebrospinal fluid (CSF) is the best means for diagnosis; serial lumbar puncture for CSF produces greater yield of acid-fast bacilli. Computerized tomography (CT) and magnetic resonance imaging (MRI) scanning serve to define the presence and extent of basilar arachnoid meningitis, the presence of cerebral infarction, and the presence and course of hydrocephalus. The differential diagnosis includes viral meningitis and other chronic inflammatory processes.

Management with INH, RIF, and PZA is recommended at upper mg/kg daily dose range (see Table 44.1). Corticosteroids are advised for patients with confusion or focal signs, such as cranial nerve palsies or hemiplegia, or stupor or dense paraplegia or hemiplegia.

Tuberculous adrenocortical insufficiency may result from involvement of the adrenal glands. In classic Addison's disease, tuberculosis is inactive and adrenocortical tissue is replaced with granulomas, often partially calcified. Reactivation tuberculosis may result in symptoms and signs of tuberculosis as well as chronic adrenal insufficiency. Acute or subacute adrenal failure may result from granuloma deposits during miliary tuberculosis.

Hypotension refractory to volume and vasoactive drugs, and the presence of bilateral enlarged, calcified adrenals on abdominal CT in patients with tuberculosis should suggest adrenal involvement. Adrenal insufficiency should be confirmed by an absence of response to IV corticotropin. (see Chap. 64). Note that a random cortisol level may be normal.

Treatment of adrenocortical insufficiency due to active tuberculosis is by administration of glucocorticoids (hydrocortisone 100 mg bolus, repeat every 6 to 8 h initially), maintenance doses of mineralocorticoids (Fludrocortisone acetate 0.05 to 0.1 mg PO a day), and appropriate antituberculous chemotherapy.

Tuberculosis and HIV infection are strongly associated, as HIV impairs alveolar macrophage function required for defense against tuberculosis. The hallmark of tuberculosis in the HIV-infected is the broad range of presentations. Pulmonary disease may be typical upper lobe cavitary pneumonia, but may also be noncavitary without particular distribution, and intrathoracic adenopathy may be seen. Extrapulmonary disease occurs with greater frequency in the HIV-infected population. Sputum samples for acid-fast bacilli are often positive even in the absence of cavitary disease. However, invasive procedures such as bronchoscopy or mediastinoscopy may be necessary to make the diagnosis. Tuberculosis in HIV-infected persons usually responds well to the conventional antituberculosis drugs. However, multi-drug resistant strains have recently been reported in HIV-infected patients. Therapeutic duration should be a minimum of 9 months following documented culture conversion. Tuberculosis infection in HIV-infected individuals poses significant risk of transmission to care providers. Respiratory isolation, as well as typical universal precautions, is warranted in HIV-infected patients with pulmonic processes until the diagnosis of tuberculosis is excluded.

For further reading in *Principles of Critical Care*, see Chap 109 "Critical Illness Due to *Mycobacterium Tuberculosis*" Richard Long

Shannon Carson

Tetanus is a toxin-mediated disease caused by *Clostridium tetani* and characterized by trismus, dysphagia, and localized muscle rigidity near a site of injury. It often progresses to severe generalized muscle spasms complicated by respiratory failure and cardiovascular instability. Tetanus occurs primarily in nonimmunized or inadequately immunized patients, but a history of proper immunization does not entirely exclude the diagnosis of tetanus. Tissue necrosis, foreign bodies, or concurrent anaerobic or facultative anaerobic infections allow toxin formation after inoculation of tissues. The toxin impairs inhibition of motoneurons and interneurons resulting in enhanced excitation and muscular rigidity. Paralysis is less common and usually localized to areas of high toxin concentration.

There are three clinical forms of tetanus: generalized, local, and cephalic. Generalized tetanus is the most common form and is characterized by diffuse muscle rigidity. Localized tetanus is characterized by rigidity of a group of muscles in close proximity to the site of injury. Cephalic tetanus, which is a variant of local tetanus, is defined as trismus plus paralysis of one or more cranial nerves. It is important to realize that both local and cephalic tetanus may progress to generalized tetanus, the latter occurring in approximately 65 percent of cases.

CLINICAL AND LABORATORY MANIFESTATIONS

The common means by which *C. tetani* enters the human host is through lacerations, especially if associated with tissue necrosis or foreign body. Tetanus can also follow burns or animal bites, septic abortion complicated by gangrene of the uterus, skin infections in intravenous drug users and, rarely, after otherwise uncomplicated abdominal surgery. However, in 15 to 25 percent of cases a portal of entry cannot be determined (*cryptogenic tetanus*). The interval between injury and onset of clinical symptoms is usually from 3 days to 3 weeks but occasionally is as long as several months. In general, the shorter the incubation period, the more severe the disease.

Muscle rigidity is the most prominent early symptom of tetanus. Muscular spasms are initially tonic, followed first by high frequency and then low-frequency clonic activity. In very severe tetanus, spasms may occur so frequently that status epilepticus may be suspected and may be forceful enough to cause fractures of long bones and of the spine. Spasm-induced damage to muscles can also result in rhabdomyolysis complicated by acute renal failure. Spasms may be initiated by touch, noise, lights, and swallowing, even in the sleeping patient. Spasms severe enough to require treatment may persist for up to 6 weeks. Apnea occurs when spasms involve the respiratory muscles or larynx.

Manifestations of impaired sympathetic inhibition include tachycardia, labile hypertension alternating with hypotension, peripheral vasoconstriction, fever, and profuse sweating. Overactivity of the parasympathetic nervous system causes increased bronchial and salivary gland secretions, bradycardia, and sinus arrest.

The diagnosis of tetanus is based on clinical manifestations rather than laboratory tests. The major clinical features on which the diagnosis of tetanus is based are listed in Table 45-1 along with the features of other conditions with which it can be confused.

Treatment

Patients with a presumptive diagnosis of tetanus should be admitted to an ICU. The principles of initial treatment of tetanus consist of airway management, sedation, treatment of the portal of entry, antitoxin therapy, administration of appropriate antibiotics, and general supportive measures. Drugs commonly used in the management of tetanus are listed in Table 45-2.

Appropriate management of the airway is the first priority. Patients with diffuse rigidity, especially if unresponsive to benzodiazepine therapy, should be intubated, even in the absence of respiratory compromise. All patients who have already had a generalized spasm or with evidence of respiratory compromise, including patients with severe dysphagia who are in danger of aspiration, should be intubated. An emergency cricothyroidotomy tray should be at the bedside prior to attempted intubation. If paralysis is required to facilitate intubation, a nondepolarizing agent should be used since depolarizing neuromuscular blocking agents (i.e., succinylcholine) may cause hyperkalemia and cardiac arrest in patients with tetanus.

Patients with muscular rigidity should be sedated with intravenous diazepam and morphine. Pancuronium, atracurium, and vecuronium are safe and effective in controlling tetanic spasms.

Aggressive surgical treatment of tetanus-producing wounds results in improved survival. Patients with tetanus should be treated with antitoxin as soon as possible. There is evidence that in patients who have not yet progressed to generalized rigidity and spasms, intrathecal hTIG is more effective than intramuscular hTIG in preventing generalization, and can reduce the mortality rate. They

TABLE 45-1 Differential Diagnosis of Tetanus: Clinical Features

	Tetanus	Strychnine	Neuroleptics	SMS*	Rabies	Meningitis
Trismus	+	+	+	+	–	–
Nuchal rigidity	+	+	+	+	–	+
Risus sardonicus	+	+	–	–	–	–
Opisthotonus	+	+	+	–	–	–
Muscle rigidity continuous	+	+	+	–	+	–
Muscle rigidity intermittant	–	–	–	+	+	–
Encephalopathy	–	–	–	–	+	+
Rapid course	–	+	+	–	–	–

*Stiff Man syndrome (Reprinted with permission from Gary P, Roberts D: Tetanus, in Hall JB, Schmidt GA, Wood LDH: Principles of Critical Care, McGraw-Hill, New York, 1992.)

TABLE 45-2 Drugs Used in the Medical Management of Tetanus

Medication	Indication	Dose
hTIG*	Local or cephalic tetanus	250 IU intrathecal
hTIG	Generalized tetanus	3000–6000 IU
Penicillin G	Toxin production (given in all cases)	1×10^6 units IV q6h for 10 days
Diazepam	Cardiovascular instability and sedation	2.5–20 Mg IV q2-6h
Morphine	Sedation and analgesia	2.0–10 Mg IV q1h or 1.0–2.0 Mg/Kg IV q12h.
Magnesium sulphate	Cardiovascular instability	70 Mg/Kg IV load then 1–3 Gm IV q1h.
Vecuronium	Neuromuscular Blockade for severe muscle spasms	3–4 Mg/h IV.

*Human tetanus immune globulin *(Reprinted with permission from Gray P, Roberts D: Tetanus, in Hall JB, Schmidt GA, Wood LDH: Principles of Critical Care, McGraw-Hill, New York, 1992.)*

should receive a single dose of intrathecal hTIG (250 IU) via lumbar puncture. Preparations containing no preservatives should be used for intrathecal injections to reduce the incidence of vomiting which is the most significant side effect. Intramuscular doses of hTIG ranging from 3000 to 6000 IU have been suggested for patients in whom generalization has already occurred. It is important to administer antitoxin prior to debridement because the toxin may be introduced into the blood stream during manipulation.

Antibiotics are generally given both to treat infection at the injury site and to eliminate continued toxin production. Penicillin G, 1 million units intravenously every 6 h for 10 days is the antibiotic of choice for *C. tetani*. Metronidazole, tetracycline, erythromycin, and chloramphenicol are also effective.

Treatment of cardiovascular instability consists of deep sedation, which, if not successful, is followed by morphine using doses of up to 10 mg/h. Alternately, successful control of autonomic dysfunction has been achieved using intermittent boluses of morphine, 1 to 2 mg/kg intravenously over 15 min every 12 h. If magnesium sulfate is used, it is important that diazepam and morphine be continued. A loading dose of 70 mg/kg over 5 to 20 min is followed by a continuous infusion titrated to maintain serum magnesium levels between 2.5 and 4.0 mmol/L. This usually requires infusion rates of 1 to 3 g/h. Serum calcium and magnesium levels should be measured every 4 h. Calcium supplements may be required to maintain serum calcium levels above 1.7 mmol/L. Any magnesium-induced cardiac arrhythmias should also be treated with intravenous calcium. Epidural bupivacaine has also been successfully used to control autonomic dysfunction.

Early nutrition, correction of electrolyte disturbances, subcutaneous heparin prophylaxis, and prompt treatment of nosocomial infection are crucial. Finally, it is important to remember that recovery from tetanus does not guarantee natural immunity. Patients should begin their primary immunization series prior to leaving the hospital.

For further reading in *Principles of Critical* Care, see Chap 110 "Tetanus" Perry Gray/Daniel Roberts

---

46

Miscellaneous Infections

Kevin Simpson

Infections of the gastrointestinal system, soft tissues, and urinary tract are relatively common in the ICU. Nonetheless, they are frequently overlooked and diagnosis delayed and, as such, constitute a source of significant morbidity and mortality. While the infecting organisms and clinical presentations are unique, these infections share the requirement for early diagnosis with rapid institution of antibiotics after appropriate cultures have been obtained and aggressive surgical intervention for drainage and/or debridement.

GASTROINTESTINAL INFECTIONS

Seriously ill patients with diarrhea should have an abdominal x-ray (flat and upright) to detect ileus, megacolon, peritoneal fluid, and free peritoneal air. In patients with suspected focal infections or abscess, ultrasonography and computerized tomographic examinations are useful. In some patients with inflammatory diarrhea or suspected colitis, colonoscopy and biopsy will be revealing. If intestinal ischemia is suspected, mesenteric angiography may be necessary. Finally, all patients with abdominal findings suggestive of any of these entities should be assessed by a general surgeon early in the hospital course.

In all cases of diarrhea the stool should be examined for fecal leukocytes; the presence of leukocytes denotes an inflammatory, invasive pathogenesis, while their absence denotes noninflammatory or toxigenic etiologies. Culture of stool for enteric pathogens and microscopic examination for parasites are useful diagnostic procedures for community-acquired infections but should be omitted for hospital-acquired infections. Finally, the wide use of antibiotic therapy in critically ill patients predisposes them to pseudomembranous colitis and testing the stool for toxin of *Clostridium difficile* is helpful. Therapy for intestinal infections includes rehydration with isotonic fluids and appropriate antimicrobial therapy for identified or suspected pathogens. Empiric antimicrobial therapy for diarrheal pathogens is advised only in septic patients. Noninfectious causes of diarrhea also need to be considered. In patients receiving tube feedings and elixir medications, osmotic diarrhea can be detected by measuring the stool osmotic gap. If the stool osmotic gap (stool osmolality minus twice the sum of stool sodium and potassium) is greater than 100 meq/L, the diarrhea is probably osmotic in nature. Other noninfectious factors that may cause diarrhea include partial obstruction of the intestine and hypoalbuminemia.

Noninflammatory Diarrhea

Cholera is the prototype of watery diarrheal syndromes in which intestinal fluid loss is so copious that hypovolemic shock with profound acidosis may ensue. Other, more common, noninflammatory infections include enterotoxigenic *Escherichia coli* (ETEC), *Aeromonas hydrophilia*, and the viruses rotavirus and Norwalk agent. These infections are termed "noninflammatory" because the intestinal epithelium remains structurally intact and leukocytes are absent from tissues and stool. The diarrhea is usually sudden in onset, painless, and watery. Fever is usually mild or absent although it may be prominent in viral infections. Fluid loss results in hemoconcentration and metabolic acidosis with variable electrolyte abnormalities. Bacterial cultures of stool should be performed. Management focuses on appropriate fluid resuscitation. Intravenous Ringer's lactate, or another bicarbonate containing solution, should be used, although for patients who are alert and well enough to take fluids by mouth, oral rehydration fluid may be used to quantitatively replace lost diarrhea fluid. Noninflammatory diarrheas are self-limited and do not require antibiotic treatment. Nonetheless, in the case of cholera, antibiotics should be given to shorten the course of the disease and decrease the total purging volume; tetracycline, 500 mg q 6 h by mouth or intravenously is usually adequate.

Dysentery

Acute dysentery, or inflammatory diarrhea, is a syndrome consisting of fever, abdominal pain, and frequent passage of stools containing blood and mucus. The most common causes are bacterial infections with species of *Shigella, Campylobacter, Salmonella, E. coli,* and *Yersinia* and the parasitic infection *Entamoeba histolytica* (amebiasis). Serious complications, such as sepsis, toxic megacolon, or colonic perforation, are more common than with noninflammatory diarrheas because of the invasive and inflammatory destructive character of the disease. Most patients with dysentery begin their illness with a non-specific prodrome followed by cramps, loose stools, and watery diarrhea consisting typically of small volumes of mucus and flecks of blood. Fever may be high. Examination of the stool is essential and blood and pus may be grossly apparent. Sigmoidoscopic examination reveals diffuse erythema with a mucopurulent layer and friable areas of mucosa and shallow ulceration. Definitive diagnosis depends upon isolating causative bacteria by selective media and culturing for 3 successive days is recommended. Management of inflammatory diarrhea includes appropriate fluid resuscitation and avoidance of agents that decrease intestinal motility as these agents retard intestinal clearance of the microorganisms. Trimethoprim-sulfamethoxazole, 160 and 800 mg, respectively, 2 times a day for 3 days has been shown to be effective in treating shigellosis and may decrease the duration of symptoms and duration of excretion of shigellae. In patients with dysentery due to *Campylobacter*, *Salmonella*, and *Yersinia*, antibiotics have not been shown to have any beneficial effects on the course of the intestinal disease. However, antibiotics may be advised in severe cases and in most critically ill patients because of the possibility of bacteremia and other extraintestinal manifestations.

Pseudomembranous Colitis

Virtually all antibiotics, except for vancomycin, have the potential to cause this disease, although the antibiotics most often associated with this complication are clindamycin, ampicillin, and cephalosporins. The cause of this complication is suppression of the normal colonic bacterial flora with resultant overgrowth of *C. difficile*. The organism produces toxins that damage the colonic epithelial cells and result in inflammation and impairment of normal fluid absorption by the colon. The most common presentation is watery diarrhea in a patient receiving an antibiotic. Most cases will have fever, abdominal pain, and passage of bloody stools. The worst cases of pseudomembranous colitis result in toxic megacolon, perforation, and generalized peritonitis. Stool examination often reveals leukocytes and red cells. Assay of stool for *C. difficile* toxin has become the best diagnostic test. Culture of the stool for *C. difficile* is not practical since this organism is part of the normal flora. Sigmoidoscopy should be done in suspected cases and reveals a spectrum of mucosal changes from mild erythema to a granular, friable, or hemorrhagic mucosa or the presence of a pseudomembrane. Treatment of pseudomembranous colitis includes discontinuation of the offending antibiotics, when feasible. However, in critically ill patients who require antibiotics, an alternative antibiotic regimen should be considered with the hope that other antibiotics will not allow the toxin-mediated disease to be further propagated. Specific treatment, vancomycin 125 mg orally 4 times a day or metronidazole 500 mg orally or intravenously 3 times a day, should be given to patients with moderate or severe symptoms and to patients with positive stool toxin assays whose diarrhea persists after discontinuation of the antibiotic.

SOFT TISSUE INFECTIONS

Cellulitis

Cellulitis, an acute inflammatory response of predominantly polymorphonuclear leukocytes involving to varying degrees the epidermis, dermis, adipose tissue, and superficial fascia, most often occurs in a setting of previous trauma of the skin, with local inoculation of microorganisms. The most common organisms are *Streptococcus pyogenes* and *Staphylococcus aureus*; less common organisms include *Strep. pneumoniae*, other streptococci, and gram-negative bacilli. Classic cellulitis is characterized by erythema, pain, edema, and local tenderness involving an area of the skin with ill-defined expanding borders. Occasionally there is lymphangitis and regional lymphadenopathy; systemic manifestations include fever, malaise, and rigors. Diagnosis is based primarily upon recognition of these clinical features. Needle aspiration after injection of 0.5 mL of nonbacteriostatic saline into the leading edge of the cellulitis may increase the rate of isolation of potential pathogens. However, a combination of needle aspiration, skin biopsy, and blood cultures results in isolation of pathogens in only about 25 percent of cases. For severe infections, parenteral administration of a high-dose pencillinase-resistant penicillin (i.e., nafcillin) in doses of 8 to 12 g/day, in 4 to 6 divided doses, is most appropriate. Alternate agents include a first-generation cephalosporin, vancomycin, or clindamycin. If the etiologic agent proves to be streptococcal, penicillin G (6 to 12 million U/day) should be substituted. In the immunocompromised host, or in the presence of a rapidly progressive cellulitis developing following a fresh- or salt water injury, an aminoglycoside should also be administered. Local care of cellulitis includes immobilization and elevation of the affected area with frequent inspection of the involved area to detect any area of crepitus or suppuration, which would require surgical drainage.

Anaerobic, or gangrenous, cellulitis, represents infection of already devitalized subcutaneous tissue with extensive gas formation and suppuration. Since this infection represents the local invasion of already devitalized tissue, the process does not generally have a virulent progressive course. The onset is gradual with mild-to-moderate local pain and only mild-to-moderate tissue swelling. Constitutional symptoms are not prominent. A thin, dark, malodorous discharge from the wound or inoculation site, sometimes containing fat globules, with extensive and prominent gas formation and extensive crepitus, is characteristic. Anaerobic cellulitis may be clostridial (usually *Clostridium perfringens*) or nonclostridial (most frequently *Bacteroides*, *Peptostreptococcus*, or *Peptococcus* spp). Drainage from the wound should be sent for gram stain and culture; the optimal method for obtaining anaerobic cultures is to use a needle and syringe to aseptically aspirate the crepitant area at a site removed from the wound. Radiological examination should be performed to assess the presence and extent of soft tissue gas. If gram stain reveals only large "boxcar-shaped" gram-positive bacilli, the causative microorganism is *Clostridium*, and moderate-to-high doses of parenteral penicillin G (10 to 20 million U/day in 6 to 8 divided doses) are indicated. If multiple organisms of differing morphology are present on the gram stain then one may assume that the process is polymicrobial, and an empiric broad spectrum antimicrobial regimen, such as an aminoglycoside and clindamycin, with or without penicillin G, should be instituted. The involved soft tissue must be laid open widely, devitalized tissue debrided, suppurative foci drained, and all involved fascial planes opened.

Necrotizing Fasciitis

Necrotizing fasciitis is an uncommon but severe infection involving the subcutaneous tissue and the deep fascia. It spreads rapidly in the fascial cleft, sparing the overlying skin until the later stages. The most common initiating injury leading to infection is minor trauma, followed by operative wounds and decubitis ulcers. Most patients have underlying chronic illnesses such as diabetes, cardiovascular or renal disease, or either marked obesity or marked wasting. Necrotizing fasciitis is most often a synergistic polymicrobial bacterial infection in which at least one anaerobic organism (usually a *Bacteroides*, *Peptostreptococcus*, or *Peptococcus* spp.) is isolated in combination with one or more facultative organisms (usually non-group A streptococci, *E. coli*, *Klebsiella* or *Proteus* spp., or *Staph. aureus*). The majority of cases have multiple organisms present, with an average of 3 to 4 isolates per patient. With necrotizing fasciitis, there is often a trivial injury followed by the onset of pain and swelling, after several hours or days, with chills and fever. Pain is gradually replaced by numbness or analgesia. Systemic toxicity with disorientation is often severe. In addition to gram stain and culture of fluid aspirated from the involved areas, diagnosis includes probing of the lesion through an existing drainage site or through a small incision to reveal the characteristic undermining of skin seen in necrotizing fasciitis. The principles of management include general supportive measures, antimicrobial therapy, and definitive surgery. General measures include aggressive fluid resuscitation, maintenance of adequate oxygenation, treatment of any underlying disease (e.g., correction of ketoacidosis or congestive heart failure), and attention to the patient's nutritional needs. Antibiotic coverage should be broad and include coverage for anaerobes; an aminoglyocoside plus clindamycin is adequate initial therapy. Penicillin G should be added if Gram stain suggests clostridia. The mainstay of management is surgical exploration, debridement, and drainage. Post operatively, careful and regular inspection of the wound is necessary, because initial debridement is seldom complete.

Myonecrosis

The bacterial myonecrotic syndromes all involve bacterial invasion of previously undamaged healthy muscle, resulting in its rapid destruction. The process is often referred to as gas gangrene. Clostridial myonecrosis occurs in the setting of muscle injury and concomitant soil or foreign body inoculation. Nonclostridial myonecrosis is usually polymicrobial involving a mixture of facultative and anaerobic bacteria. Intense pain, out of proportion to the extent of injury, is characteristic. The pain rapidly progresses in intensity and distribution. Although fever is not present until later in the course, severe systemic toxicity appears within hours. Early on, examination of the wound reveals tense edema and mild erythema; later, a spreading zone of woody edema appears, along with a characteristic bronzing of the skin. Although occasionally present, crepitus is not a prominent sign. Early diagnosis of myonecrosis is critical. Gram stain of the discharge or soft tissue aspirate may reveal the causative organism(s). A radiograph of the involved area may reveal gas that is not palpable and will also give an indication of the distribution of such gas. Surgical exploration is definitive and is mandated by the mere suspicion of myonecrosis. Excision of involved muscles and decompressive fasciotomies are the mainstays of surgical treatment. Antimicrobial therapy includes high dose penicillin G in the case of clostridial myonecrosis. In the presence of mixed flora on gram stain, an aminoglycoside plus clindamycin is indicated.

URINARY TRACT INFECTIONS (UTI)

The urinary tract is a frequent site of infection in critically ill patients. As with other infections in the ICU, early identification and initiation of definitive treatment, often including surgical drainage, is imperative. Significant bacteriuria implies the presence of 10^5 organisms or more per milliliter. Pyuria means the presence of five or more white blood cells per microscopic high-power field in the urine. However, the absence of such bacteriuria or pyuria does not reliably exclude UTI. For hospitalized patients, *E. coli* is a common pathogen, but *Pseudomonas* spp., *Enterococcus* spp., coagulase-negative staphylococci, and *Candida* spp. are seen with greater frequency than in the community setting.

Acute Pyelonephritis

Patients with severe urosepsis should have ultrasound examination of the kidneys, and consideration of other imaging procedures such as computed tomography (CT) to exclude obstruction and papillary necrosis and to assess for suppurative complications such as pyonephrosis or intrarenal or perinephric abscess. Ultrasound should be the initial investigation for patients with upper urinary tract infection and suspected obstruction. CT scanning more accurately defines the anatomy of the renal parenchyma than ultrasound and gives a clear cross-sectional view of the surrounding anatomy. Complications of upper urinary tract infection such as cortical abscess and perinephric abscess can be distinguished more readily by CT scan. Furthermore, accurate placement of percutaneous drains into suppurative collections may require CT scanning to delineate all structures precisely. Despite this, ultrasound is the initial investigation of choice for patients with pyelonephritis because of its lack of toxicity, ease of application, and low cost.

A number of regimens are appropriate as empiric therapy of acute pyelonephritis. These include an aminoglycoside combined with ampicillin, cefazolin, or trimethoprim-sulfamethoxazole. An aminoglycoside combined with a ureidopenicillin such as piperacillin may be preferred for hospital-acquired infection where *P. aeruginosa* and *Enterococcus faecalis* are more likely to be encountered. Initial reliance on a single agent is unwise as the patient may succumb to overwhelming septic shock during the 48 h required for antimicrobial susceptibility results to become available. The classic therapy of intrarenal abscess is incision and drainage with a nephrectomy if necessary for larger abscesses. It is now clear that a trial of intravenous antimicrobial therapy will succeed in the majority of patients once microbial etiology is established by urine, blood, or aspirate culture. Percutaneous drainage using ultrasound or CT guidance is another alternative to surgery and should be tried as initial therapy when the abscess cavity is large. Perinephric abscess generally arises from direct extension of an intrarenal abscess. Perinephric abscess is an insidious disease that has a 50 percent mortality due to delay in diagnosis. Symptoms are usually of at least 2 weeks duration and often extend for months. Most patients can be treated by a combination of intravenous antimicrobial agents and percutaneous drainage.

Urinary Tract Infection due to *Candida*

Candiduria should be assumed to reflect renal infection if the patient suffers from neutropenia, loss of mucous membrane integrity due to chemotherapy, burns, steroid use, diabetes mellitus, or is receiving total parenteral nutrition or broad-spectrum antibacterial therapy, or continues to have features of sepsis such as fever or leukocytosis. Isolation of *Candida* from other sites such as respiratory secretions, wound exudate, or throat swabs should heighten suspicion of systemic candidiasis. Renal or disseminated infection requires systemic amphotericin B therapy in a dose of 0.6 mg/kg/day to a cumulative dose of 1 gm. Fluconazole and 5-fluorocytosine are alternative, less reliable therapies. Ketoconazole is not acceptable as it is not appreciably excreted through the kidney.

A more commonly encountered situation is that of the stable ICU patient who has persistent candiduria. For such a patient amphotericin B bladder irrigation (50 mg of amphotericin B in 1000 mL of sterile water administered over 24 h by a three-way catheter) for 5 days should be considered. This will cure candiduria confined to the bladder. Daily urine cultures should be done immediately upon stopping. Immediate relapse of candiduria is indirect evidence for renal infection and should prompt initiation of systemic amphotericin B therapy.

Catheter-Associated Bacteriuria

Widespread use of urinary catheters leads to a high incidence of bacteriuria, about 5 percent per day. Fifty percent become infected by 10 days. Patients are also predisposed to candiduria. While catheterization of the bladder is unavoidable in most patients in the ICU, the necessity for the catheter should be frequently questioned and a trial of removal attempted when feasible. Once in place, there is no need for regular scheduled replacements of the catheter, which can be left indefinitely provided it is functioning well and there are no encrustations. In the ICU, where hospital-acquired bacteriuria is commonly identified early because of routine surveillance, single-dose therapy with an agent such as trimethoprim-sulfamethoxazole, an aminoglycoside, a third-generation cephalosporin, extended spectrum penicillin, or quinolone to which the organism is susceptible may be appropriate in selected patients.

For further reading in *Principles of Critical Care,* see Chap 106 "Soft Tissue Infections" John Conley, Chap 107 "Urinary Tract Infections" Gerard J Sheehan/Godfrey KM Harding, Chap 108 "Gastrointestinal Infections" Thomas Butler

47

Neuropsychiatric Disorders, Coma, and Brain Death

David Olson

In critically ill patients, mental status changes are almost always secondary to underlying physiologic problems. Those patients who develop acute agitation, confusion, or psychoses must be considered a medical emergency; without rapid diagnosis and treatment the prognosis for recovery may be poor. Importantly, the clinician should not attribute changes in mental status to an "ICU psychosis."

DELIRIUM

In the ICU, a good diagnostic rule is that any acute change in a patient's mental status is delirium until proven otherwise. Delirium can be considered as "acute brain failure" and is very common, with an incidence of up to 50 percent for medically ill patients aged 70 years or more. Of hospitalized patients who become delirious, 20 to 30 percent die during that hospitalization or soon after discharge. The morbidities associated with delirium include self-harm; harm to hospital personnel; prolonged hospitalizations; development of chronic organic brain syndromes with permanent disability; and progression to stupor, coma, seizures, or death.

Certain groups of patients are at high risk for developing delirium: children, drug-dependent patients (alcohol, barbiturates, benzodiazepines), elderly (aged 60 or older), those with HIV spectrum disorders, post-cardiotomy patients, severe burn injury patients, and those with pre-existing brain damage.

The clinical features of delirium are listed in Table 47-1. Prodromal symptoms include restlessness, irritability, anxiety, and sleep disturbance. The rapid fluctuation in mental status is an important clinical characteristic distinguishing delirium from dementia or psy-

TABLE 47-1 Clinical Features of Delirium

Prodrome	Disorganized thinking
Rapid fluctuations in mental status	and speech
Decreased attention span	Altered perceptions
Diminished memory for recent events	Neurologic abnormalities
Disorientation	Dysgraphia
Agitation or lethargy	Constructional apraxia
Emotional disturbances	Dysnomic aphasia
Sleep-wake disturbances	Motor abnormalities
	EEG slowing

(Reprinted with permission from Wise MG, Terrell CD: Delirium, Psychotic Disorders, and Anxiety, in Hall JB, Schmidt GA, Wood LDH: Principles of Critical Care, McGraw-Hill, New York, 1992.)

chotic disorders. Some patients with delirium may alternate between states of agitation and lethargy (mixed delirium). In addition, speech can become increasingly incoherent and perceptions may be altered to produce illusions or overt hallucinations; motor abnormalities such as tremor, myoclonus, or asterixis may be detected in the delirious patient as well.

If delirium is suspected, the evaluation is centered on assessment of the patient's mental and physical status and certain laboratory data (Table 47-2). The initial bedside examination of the patient's cognitive function may be accomplished by the mini-mental state examination (MMSE). Further cognitive testing includes determining the ability to perform sequential simple instructions and the presence of dysgraphia (impaired writing), dysnomia (difficulty naming objects), and constructional apraxia (difficulty drawing objects). The ability to draw a clock with the hands at a predeter-

---

TABLE 47-2 Neuropsychiatric Evaluation of the Delirious Patient

Mental status
    Interview (assess level of consciousness, psychomotor activity, appearance, affect, mood, intellect, thought processes)
    Performance tests (memory, concentration, reasoning, motor & constructional praxis)

Physical status
    Neurological exam (reflexes, limb strength, cranial nerves, gait, meningeal signs, Babinski)
    Vital signs (review past and present)
    Medical chart (review diagnoses, labs [including VDRL], behavior changes)
    Medication log (correlate abnormal behavior with medication changes)

Laboratory examination—basic
    Blood chemistries (electrolytes, glucose, calcium, albumin, ammonia, magnesium, phosphorus, liver and thyroid function tests)
    Blood count (hematocrit, MCV, WBC & differential, sedimentation rate)
    Drug levels (toxic screen, medication blood levels)
    Arterial Blood Gases
    Urinalysis
    Electrocardiogram
    Chest X-ray

Further laboratory examination—based on clinical judgment
    Electroencephalogram
    CT or MRI Scan
    Additional Blood Chemistries (heavy metals, thiamine and folate levels, LE prep, ANA, urinary porphobilinogen)
    Lumbar Puncture

Source: Reprinted from Wise, MG: Delirium, in Hales, RE and Yudofsky, SC (eds): *The American Psychiatric Press Textbook of Neuropsychiatry.* Washington, D. C., American Psychiatric Press, 1987. Copyright 1987 by The American Psychiatric Press, Inc. Reprinted by permission.

mined time is a highly sensitive test for delirium. The physical examination should include an abbreviated neurologic exam, and the basic laboratory tests listed in Table 47-2 may be supplemented by additional procedures based on clinical judgment. The electroencephalogram (EEG) demonstrates changes in virtually all cases of delirium and reflects the global cerebral dysfunction present in this disorder. Diffuse slowing of the EEG may be found in lethargic hypoactive patients while low voltage-fast activity may be seen in the hyperactive, agitated patient.

The differential diagnosis to consider when suspecting delirium includes dementia, psychosis, and depression. Dementia has a slowly progressive course, while delirium tends to present acutely, and patients are usually alert with a relatively stable clinical picture. Those with psychotic disorders, such as schizophrenia, will not have the cognitive deficits seen in delirium (normal MMSE) and are oriented. Delusions are typically well-developed and long-standing rather than the vague, rapidly changing delusions of the delirious patient. Hallucinations tend to be auditory in psychotic disorders rather than visual as in delirium. Also, new onset psychotic disorders are exceedingly rare in the elderly. Depression and mania may be differentiated from delirium by looking for the episodic waxing and waning, disorganization, disorientation, EEG slowing, or other cognitive dysfunctions characteristic of delirium yet usually absent in mania and depression.

Determining an etiology of a patient's delirium may be a difficult task, especially in the elderly who often have multi-organ system disease and are on numerous medications. The physician must first consider etiologies that can rapidly cause irreversible injury or death. These include Wernicke's encephalopathy/withdrawal, hypertensive encephalopathy, hypoglycemia, hypoperfusion of the central nervous system (CNS), hypoxemia, intracranial bleed, meningitis/encephalitis, and poisons/medications (the mnemonic WHHHHIMP is useful). After these conditions have been investigated, a more comprehensive list of etiologies may be considered, employing the mnemonic I WATCH DEATH (Table 47-3).

The primary objective in treatment of the delirious patient is to identify and treat reversible underlying causes. In addition, pharmacologic interventions are often necessary to control the agitated behavior and confusion of the delirious patient. Medications such as morphine and benzodiazepines are frequently used but carry the significant risk of sedation, decreased respiratory drive, hypotension, and worsening cognitive function. Benzodiazepines are indicated in the treatment of delirium secondary to alcohol or benzodiazepine withdrawal and, in low doses, to augment the calming effect of haloperidol in acutely agitated patients.

Haloperidol effectively reduces agitation and psychotic thought

TABLE 47-3 I Watch Death

Infections	Encephalitis, meningitis, syphilis, sepsis
Withdrawal	Alcohol, barbiturates, benzodiazepines
Acute metabolic	Acidosis, alkaloids, electrolyte disturbance, hepatic or renal failure
Trauma	Heat stroke, postoperative state, severe burns
CNS pathology	Abscesses, hemorrhage, seizures, stroke, tumor, vasculitis, normal pressure hydrocephalus
Hypoxia	Anemia, hypotension, carbon monoxide poisoning, cardiac/pulmonary failure
Deficiencies	B_{12}, niacin, thiamine
Endocrinopathies	Hyper/hypoadrenocorticalism, hyper/hypoglycemia
Acute vascular	Hypertensive encephalopathy, shock
Toxins/Drugs	Medications, pesticides, solvents
Heavy metals	Lead, manganese, mercury

Source: Reprinted from Wise MG: Delirium, in Hales, RE and Yudofsky, SC (ed): *The Amercian Psychiatric Press Textbook of Neuropsychiatry*. Washington, D. C., American Psychiatric Press, 1987. Copyright 1987 by The American Psychiatric Press, Inc. Reprinted by permission.

and sedates without further dulling awareness. It has virtually no anticholinergic or hypotensive actions. The drug may be given intravenously and in large doses without significant harmful side effects (the incidence of extra pyramidal symptoms [EPS] with IV haloperidol in the critically ill population is extremely low.) Recommended guidelines for administration of intravenous haloperidol are provided in Table 47-4. The calming action of

TABLE 47-4 Suggested Guidelines for Haloperidol Use in Acute Agitation

Level of Agitation	Starting Dose
Mild	0.5–2.0 mg
Moderate	2.0–5.0 mg
Severe	5.0–10.0 mg

1. Clear intravenous (IV) line with normal saline
2. For elderly, use starting doses in the low range
3. Allow 20 to 30 minutes between doses
4. For continued agitation, double previous dose
5. After 3 doses, give 0.5–1.0 mg of lorazepam IV concurrently, or alternate lorazepam with haloperidol every 30 minutes
6. Once patient is calm, add the total mg of haloperidol given and administer this total dose over the next 24 hours
7. Assuming the patient remains calm, reduce dose 50% every 24 hours
8. Oral dosage is twice the IV dose

Source: Reprinted from Wise MG and Rundell JR: *Concise Guide to Consultation Psychiatry*. Washington, D. C., American Psychiatric Press, 1988. Copyright 1988 by The American Psychiatric Press, Inc. Reprinted by permission.

haloperidol is not immediately seen; allow 20 to 30 min between doses. Treatment should continue for 3 to 5 days to prevent recurrence of delirium, tapering the total daily dose by no more than 50 percent every 24 h. Concurrent intravenous lorazepam (in doses from 0.5 to 2.0 mg) may be given for a synergistic calming effect.

Additional supportive measures are necessary and include monitoring of fluid balance, adequate oxygenation, and nutritional support. Attention to insomnia and reversal of the sleep-wake cycle by maintaining lighting to simulate day and night while minimizing daytime naps is also important. If haloperidol or lorazepam are used, give a large part of the dose at bedtime.

PSYCHIATRIC DISORDERS

Psychosis is characterized by impairment in the ability to interpret reality and is usually associated with dysfunctional behavior and communication, hallucinations, and delusions. Psychosis is a hallmark of certain illnesses, like schizophrenia and delusional disorders, but may also be seen in delirium, mood disorders (major depression, mania), dementia, and intoxication with certain illicit drugs (LSD, PCP). Differentiating delirium from psychotic disorder is an important part of the diagnosis. As discussed previously, delusions in chronic psychotic disorders are deeply integrated, organized, and highly resistant to change. Hallucinations tend to be auditory rather than visual. The cognitive deficits of delirium are typically not present in psychotic disorders. The past psychiatric history is also important; again schizophrenia rarely presents *de novo* in the elderly.

Treatment usually involves prescribing an antipsychotic medication to which the patient previously responded. In emergencies or when prior treatment is unknown, the guidelines for dosing haloperidol in delirium may be used (Table 47-4). Oral dosing has a higher association with EPS. These may be treated with 25 to 50 mg of diphenhydramine IM or IV.

ANXIETY

Anxiety is a physiologic and psychologic response to many conditions (illness, medication) and anxiety disorders are found in 5 to 20 percent of general medical inpatients. Anxiety can be part of a medical illness (hyperthyroidism, hypoglycemia, congestive heart failure), result from a withdrawal syndrome (alcohol, barbiturates, benzodiazepines, opiates), arise from certain medications (theophylline, thyroid supplements, epinephrine), or constitute an ongoing anxiety disorder. The physical signs and symptoms of anxiety can mimic or aggravate medical disorders, particularly those of cardiovascular origin.

Benzodiazepines are the drugs of choice for treating anxiety in critically ill patients. The choice of a particular agent is based on speed of onset, duration of action, route of administration, sedation properties, and site of metabolism. The potential for abuse of benzodiazepines in those patients with no prior history of drug abuse is very low. Initiating discussions of unknown aspects of a patient's illness and addressing their particular fears, such as those of dying, are also very useful in alleviating anxiety.

COMA

Coma is the clinical manifestation of severe, acute brain failure and can be defined as a state of "unarousable psychologic unresponsiveness." Clinically, the causes of coma can be divided into three categories based on neuroanatomy: diffuse cerebral dysfunction (usually from drug intoxication or severe metabolic derangement), primary brain stem disorders (infarction, hemorrhage, trauma, abscess, or neoplasm), and secondary brain stem compression from supratentorial mass lesions (transtentorial herniation).

Acute depression in level of consciousness is a life-threatening emergency that requires a rigorous and systematic evaluation. Most importantly, the physician must engage in an examination for systemic illness. Most cases of coma are due to metabolic derangements or drug intoxication rather than cerebral infarction or hemorrhage. Thus, physical examination and laboratory evaluation are directed toward determining the presence of sepsis, acid-base/electrolyte disturbance, or hepatic, renal, or cardiac failure. Emergency laboratory tests are listed in Table 47-5. Emergency measures aimed at stabilizing the patient, even when the diagnosis is not yet evident, are outlined in Table 47-6.

TABLE 47-5 Emergency Laboratory Tests for Metabolic Coma

1. Venous blood: hemoglobin, white blood count, platelets, glucose, electrolytes, calcium, blood urea nitrogen, creatinine, osmolality, coagulation studies, liver function tests, muscle enzymes, thyroid and adrenal functions, toxicology screen, blood cultures
2. Arterial blood: pH, P_{CO_2}, P_{O_2}, carboxyhemoglobin, ammonia
3. Urine: toxicology, microscopic examination
4. Gastric aspirate: toxicology
5. Cerebrospinal fluid: Cell count and gram stain, protein, glucose, culture, counterimmunoelectrophoresis, viral and fungal antigens and antibody titers

(Reprinted with permission from Fink ME: Coma, Persistent Vegetative State, and Brain Death, in Hall JB, Schmidt GA, Wood LDH: Principles of Critical Care, McGraw-Hill, New York, 1992.)

TABLE 47-6 Emergency Treatment for Coma

1. Protect airway and provide oxygen
2. Evaluate for trauma and stabilize spine
3. Support and maintain circulation
4. Administer glucose, thiamine, and naloxone
5. Treat intracranial hypertension
6. Stop epileptic seizures
7. Treat infections
8. Treat hyperthermia
9. Correct electrolyte and acid-base disorders
10. Give specific antidote for identified toxins

(Reprinted with permission from Fink ME: Coma, Persistent Vegetative State, and Brain Death, in Hall JB, Schmidt GA, Wood LDH: Principles of Critical Care, McGraw-Hill, New York, 1992.)

The neurologic examination in the comatose patient is limited and focuses on five physiologic variables that aid in determining the neuroanatomic correlate of coma. They are **1**. response to external stimulation, **2**. motor responses, **3**. size and reactivity of pupils, **4**. eye movements and ocular reflexes, and **5**. pattern of breathing. Details of the clinical significance of each variable may be found in the parent text.

The etiologies of coma have been mentioned previously, with toxic ingestions and metabolic causes accounting for the largest number of patients with depressed consciousness (Table 47-7). The most important sign distinguishing metabolic from structural coma is the presence of the pupillary light response. In metabolic coma, antecedent confusion and stupor as well as concurrent motor hyperactivity or seizures is common. Supratentorial mass lesions with herniation usually present with asymmetrical focal neurologic signs, usually progressing in a rostral-caudal fashion. Subtentorial lesions always have brain stem signs that precede or accompany the onset of coma. Abnormal eye movements are invariably present and cranial nerve palsies are quite common.

The sequence of diagnostic procedures in evaluating coma is guided by the differential diagnosis. Metabolic or toxic causes are identified by laboratory testing (Table 47-5). Computerized tomography (CT scanning) is the next important step, and though less sensitive than magnetic resonance imaging (MRI), is highly reliable and more easily applicable to the critically ill patient. CT scanning should precede lumbar puncture unless bacterial meningitis is strongly suspected. The EEG is helpful in the diagnosis of metabolic encephalopathies (though nonspecific) and in the rare comatose patient with nonconvulsive status epilepticus. Evoked potential studies are no more useful than clinical examination, except for the somatosensory evoked potential response, which is resistant to

TABLE 47-7 Metabolic Causes of Coma

1. Hypoxia: decreased P_{O_2}, anemia, cyanide poisoning, carbon monoxide poisoning, methemoglobinemia
2. Ischemia: Cardiac arrest, shock, blood hyperviscosity, cerebral arterial spasm after subarachnoid hemorrhage, disseminated intravascular coagulation, systemic lupus, multifocal embolism, hypertensive encephalopathy, arteritis
3. Hypoglycemia
4. Cofactor deficiency: thiamine, niacin, pyridoxine, vitamin B_{12}, folate
5. Infections: meningitis, encephalitis, postinfectious demyelinating encephalomyelitis, brain abscess
6. Hepatic or renal failure
7. Systemic diseases: septicemia, paraneoplastic syndromes, hypothyroidism, porphyria
8. Exogenous toxins and drugs: benzodiazepines, opiate analgesics, barbiturates, anticonvulsants, salicylates, ethanol, tricyclic antidepressants, anticholinergics, phenothiazines, amphetamines, cocaine, lithium, monoamine oxidase inhibitors, antihistamines, LSD, paraldehyde, methanol, ethylene glycol, cimetidine, heavy metals, organic phosphates, penicillins
9. Fluid and electrolyte disorders: hypo- and hypernatremia, hypo- and hyperosmolality, acid-base disorders, extreme values of calcium, magnesium, phosphorus
10. Hypothermia and heat stroke

(Reprinted with permission from Fink ME: Coma, Persistent Vegetative State, and Brain Death, in Hall JB, Schmidt GA, Wood LDH: Principles of Critical Care, McGraw-Hill, New York, 1992.)

sedative drug intoxication and may be present in drug overdose states that cause an "isoelectric" EEG.

Of the diverse causes of coma, hypoxic-ischemic encephalopathy, as occurs after cardiac arrest and resuscitation, is the most common and devastating in the ICU. Patients in coma less than 12 h after resuscitation usually make an excellent recovery, while those comatose longer tend to have permanent neurologic deficits. If the coma persists for 1 week, recovery is rare, and most patients remain in a persistent vegetative state. The lack of pupillary response, corneal response after one day, or purposeful motor responses after three days are all predictive of poor outcome.

The treatment of coma must be instituted immediately, even when the diagnosis is uncertain, to prevent further brain damage secondary to complications. All comatose patients should be intubated quickly to assure oxygenation and airway protection. Arterial blood pressure should be monitored closely and maintained without excessive volume replacement (thereby aggravating intracranial hypertension). Seizures, regardless of cause, must be stopped. Hypoglycemia, intracranial hypertension, systemic infections, severe acid base disorders, and hypothermia must all be addressed immediately and aggressively. Specific antidotes may be necessary in treating coma secondary to drug intoxication.

BRAIN DEATH

The Uniform Determination of Death Act states that "an individual who has sustained either irreversible cessation of circulatory and respiratory functions; or irreversible cessation of all functions of the entire brain, including the brain stem, is dead." In the diagnosis of death by neurologic criteria, a correct neurologic diagnosis is essential. This is a clinical diagnosis and requires the establishment of unresponsiveness and brain stem areflexia. The cause of coma must be known and this cause must be adequate to explain the coma.

In most states in the U.S., clinical criteria are sufficient to diagnose brain death, with confirmatory tests such as EEG and cerebral blood flow studies reserved for situations where there is uncertainty regarding cause and reversibility of coma. The patient must be in a deep coma and unresponsive to all external stimuli. Spinal reflexes and motor responses are permitted. Spontaneous movements other than of spinal origin and seizures must be absent. Decorticate and decerebrate posturing are inconsistent with the diagnosis of death as they require an intact brain stem. In certain neurologic conditions, such as "locked-in syndrome" or neuromuscular paralysis, confirmatory tests may be necessary. Pupils must be unreactive to bright light; size is unimportant. Ocular movements must be absent to passive head turning and to irrigation of patient ear canals with 30 ml of iced water with the head elevated 30°. Corneal reflexes are variable and the "gag" reflex is usually not testable due to the presence of an endotracheal tube.

Apnea testing is a critical part of brain stem assessment. The patient must have a normal blood pressure and is then ventilated with 100% oxygen for 10 min prior to testing. A maximum stimulus for breathing is attained when Pco_2 is greater than 60 torr. This level is attained during 10 to 15 min of apnea depending on the initial Pco_2. Serial arterial blood gases will confirm the appropriate level of Pco_2. The mechanical ventilator must remain connected to the patient throughout the test. Use of pulse oximetry with mechanical ventilation at low rates (2/min) with 100% oxygen will ensure hypercapnia without subjecting the patient to hypoxemia.

Irreversibility is recognized when the cause of coma is established and accounts for the loss of brain function, the possibility of recovery of brain function is excluded, and the cessation of all brain functions persists for an appropriate period of observation or trial of therapy. The combination of clinical history, neurologic examination, and cranial CT will, in most cases, identify the cause of coma. Drug screening is an essential part of every examination. The most important reversible conditions are sedative drug intoxication, hypothermia, neuromuscular paralysis (primary or drug induced), and severe hypotension. Drug-induced comas may require somatosensory evoked responses (SSER) to prove an intact brain stem. Core temperature must be above 35°C and severe hypotension must be corrected before applying the criteria for determination of death. In purely structural lesions, a 12 h period of observation is sufficient to make a diagnosis of death, while 24 h is necessary for initial treatment and observation in conditions of global brain ischemia/hypoxia.

In rare situations, the precise cause of coma cannot be immediately determined. In such cases, prolonged observation, EEG, and cerebral blood flow studies may be needed for diagnosis. EEG confirmation is not necessary when the cause of coma is clearly established from brain imaging studies and the clinical criteria are met that all brain functions are absent. Apneic coma and an isoelectric EEG in the face of normal brain imaging studies are strongly suggestive of sedative drug intoxication and appropriate toxicology studies must be performed.

Four-vessel cerebral angiography may be performed in clinically dead patients who have an uncertain diagnosis. Complete absence of cerebral circulation is an absolute confirmation of brain death. Radioisotope brain scanning, transcranial Doppler sonography, and xenon-enhanced CT are other useful modalities, but have limitations in the degree of cerebral circulation studied or availability.

For further reading in *Principles of Critical Care,* see Chap 4 "The Central Nervous System" Jesse Hall, Chap 140 "Delirium, Psychotic Disorders, and Anxiety" Michael G Wise/Clark D Terrell, Chap 144 "Coma, Persistent Vegetative State, and Brain Death" Matthew E Fink

48

Cerebrovascular Disease

Scott P. Neeley

Complications of cerebrovascular disease are common in patients admitted to intensive care units, and should be considered in any patient with new neurological findings. The suspicion of an acute cerebrovascular process should prompt rapid clinical evaluation and performance of appropriate diagnostic tests to allow formulation of an appropriate therapeutic plan. Hemodynamic monitoring is of importance in any patient with suspected acute cerebrovascular disease, since reduction of blood pressure carries a significant risk of producing further neurologic deterioration. Early neurosurgical intervention should be considered in patients with brain stem compression due to cerebellar infarction or hemorrhage and in patients with subarachnoid hemorrhage due to ruptured aneurysms.

ETIOLOGY

Cerebrovascular disease can be divided into three categories: cerebral ischemia and infarction, intracerebral hemorrhage, and subarachnoid hemorrhage.

Cerebral ischemia and infarction may occur as a result of global hypoperfusion, emboli or occlusion arising from local arterial disease such as that seen with atherosclerosis, or emboli arising from the heart. While atherosclerosis is the most common cause of cerebral ischemia and infarction in the general population, global hypoperfusion and emboli from the heart assume more importance in the critically ill patient. Global hypoperfusion may occur due to systemic hypotension or increased intracranial pressure, and may produce infarction in the distal territories of the major cerebral arteries, producing characteristic proximal arm and leg weakness, amnesia or cortical blindness. Cerebral emboli of cardiac origin occur in the settings of atrial fibrillation, rheumatic valvular heart disease, prosthetic aortic or mitral valves, infective endocarditis, nonbacterial thrombotic endocarditis, and ventricular mural thrombus secondary to acute myocardial infarction or cardiomyopathy. Rarer causes of cerebral infarction in critically ill patients include dissections of the carotid or vertebral artery after head or neck trauma, intracranial arterial or venous thrombosis secondary to meningeal or parameningeal infections, and paradoxical emboli.

Hemorrhages into the basal ganglia and cerebellum occur most commonly in middle-aged patients with long-standing hypertension, and are the most common type of intracerebral hemorrhage. Hemorrhages into the subcortical hemispheric white matter are more often due to arteriovenous malformations in younger patients, and amyloid angiopathy in the elderly. Less common causes of intracerebral hemorrhage include thrombocytopenia, hemophilia, disseminated intravascular coagulation, and rupture of intracranial aneurysms.

Spontaneous subarachnoid hemorrhage is almost always due to ruptured intracranial aneurysms, though arteriovenous malformations may rarely manifest in this manner.

CLINICAL AND LABORATORY DIAGNOSIS

The initial evaluation of the patient serves to determine whether neurologic symptoms are due to cerebrovascular disease or are caused by some other condition (infection, mass lesion, seizure disorder, hypoglycemia), and to distinguish among different types of cerebrovascular disease. Cerebrovascular disease generally produces the sudden onset of focal brain dysfunction; the exception being subarachnoid hemorrhage which may present with severe headache, with or without loss of consciousness. In addition to obvious hemiparesis, focal neurologic defects may include neglect, agnosia, aphasia, cortical blindness, and amnesia. Multiple small brain infarctions may mimic a metabolic or toxic encephalopathy with depressed consciousness and minimal focal neurologic deficits. The initial neurologic examination may provide information about the location of the lesion and provides a baseline for monitoring the subsequent course. A thorough medical evaluation is necessary to detect cardiac or systemic diseases that may be the cause of the cerebrovascular problem.

The primary role of diagnostic tests is to determine etiology; differentiation between infarction and hemorrhage is of greatest importance. Computed tomography (CT) is the diagnostic test of choice for patients with acute cerebrovascular disease. It is rapid and can be easily performed on acutely ill patients. Acute intracerebral hemorrhage is easily identified by noncontrast CT scan. Intravenous contrast administration increases sensitivity for detecting tumor, subdural hematoma, and abscess. Cerebral infarction may not be demonstrated by CT for several days, though this may not be necessary since the diagnosis can be made reliably by clinical presentation and a negative CT scan to exclude hemorrhage and other conditions. Magnetic resonance imaging (MRI) is more sensitive than CT for detection of infarction, lesions in the cerebellum and brainstem, and subacute or chronic hemorrhage. However, it is more cumbersome to perform in the acutely ill patient because of longer imaging times and requirement for non-ferromagnetic support and monitoring devices.

Lumbar puncture with cerebrospinal fluid (CSF) examination is extremely important in the diagnostic evaluation of cerebrovascular disease. It is essential to rule out meningitis with secondary stroke. CSF pleocytosis is common following septic embolism from infective endocarditis. Lumbar puncture is the most sensitive test for detection of subarachnoid hemorrhage; CT or MRI may miss this diagnosis in 10 to 20 percent of cases. In the majority of patients, cerebral edema or mass lesion can be excluded by careful history and neurologic examination. Lumbar puncture can be performed safely at the bedside without a prior brain-imaging study.

Differentiation of cerebral infarction due to atherosclerotic cerebrovascular disease from that caused by cardiac emboli may be important therapeutically. For patients over the age of 50 who present to the hospital with a cerebral infarction and who have no clinical or electrocardiographic evidence of heart disease, there is little diagnostic yield from cardiac monitoring or echocardiography. In younger patients, or those hospitalized in an ICU with underlying systemic or cardiac disease, these tests may assist in the detection of a cardiac lesion or arrhythmia that may predispose to cerebral embolism. Examination of the extracranial carotid or vertebral arteries by Doppler or ultrasound studies has little value in differentiating cardioembolic from atherosclerotic causes of brain infarction.

Cerebral arteriography may be useful in identification of nonatherosclerotic cerebrovascular diseases, such as dissection, vasculitis, and venous thrombosis. Cerebral arteriography plays an important role in the patient with subarachnoid hemorrhage by confirming the existence of an aneurysm and providing the necessary information to plan a surgical approach. In selected patients with intracerebral hemorrhage, arteriography may demonstrate vascular malformations or aneurysms.

TREATMENT

Atherothrombotic Infarction

No therapeutic intervention has been shown to be of value in reducing brain damage due to acute cerebral infarction. Trials with streptokinase and tissue plasminogen activator in acute stroke are currently under way. Cerebral edema is the major cause of early mortality following cerebral infarction, though no effective treatment is available for this complication. Mannitol and hyperventilation can temporarily reduce intracranial pressure, but have no long-term benefit. They may be of value to the patient with brain stem compression from edematous cerebellar infarction in whom craniotomy and removal of the edematous tissue is planned. This is the only situation in which surgical intervention following brain infarction is likely to provide benefit.

No benefit has been demonstrated for anticoagulation with heparin in patients with transient ischemic attack or partial stable stroke. The usefulness of heparin in acute progressing stroke has not been studied fully, and this issue is unresolved.

Therapy should, therefore, focus on prevention of complications and further neurologic damage. Patients should be mobilized as soon as possible to decrease the risk of venous thrombosis, pulmonary embolism, and pneumonia. A more gradual program of ambulation may be necessary in patients with orthostatic hypotension. In hemiplegic patients, subcutaneous heparin should be administered to prevent venous thrombosis, and vigorous pulmonary toilet should be instituted. Intermittently pumping antithrombotic stockings may provide added benefit. Some patients with stroke may have intravascular volume depletion at the time of hospitalization. Careful fluid replacement may be required, though particular care should be taken to avoid hypoosmolarity, which may exacerbate brain edema. Prior to instituting oral feeding, the patient's ability to swallow should be carefully checked in order to reduce the risk of aspiration. Incontinence also is common following acute stroke. Careful attention must be given to the prevention of decubitus ulcers in bedridden patients.

Systemic arterial hypertension is common following acute stroke. In most cases, this hypertension resolves spontaneously without treatment in a few days. There are no known hazards to the brain from this spontaneous transient elevation in systemic blood pressure. On the other hand, because of disruption of the normal mechanism of cerebral autoregulation of blood flow following stroke or intracranial hemorrhage, any reduction in systemic blood pressure is likely to cause a decrease in cerebral blood flow. This in turn may cause further damage in marginally perfused areas adjacent to the infarct. When systemic hypertension is causing organ damage elsewhere (e.g., myocardial ischemia or dissecting aortic aneurysm), careful and judicious lowering of the blood pressure, with constant monitoring of neurologic status, is indicated. It should be emphasized that *there is no level to which blood pressure can be reduced that does not carry the risk of further neurologic deterioration.*

Cardiac Emboli

The general care of the patient with cardioembolic brain infarction is the same as outlined above for atherothrombotic infarction. However, there is evidence that early anticoagulation may be of value in preventing recurrent infarction from cardiac emboli, particularly in patients with acute myocardial infarction and atrial fibrillation. Long-term anticoagulation studies in patients with cardiomyopathy, left ventricular aneurysms, and rheumatic valvular disease suggest that anticoagulation may be beneficial in these patients as well. It should be noted, however, that heparinization after cardioembolic cerebral infarction introduces a small, but real risk of producing hemorrhage into the infarction. This risk is greatest in hypertensive patients with large infarctions who are given anticoagulation within the first few days. Since recurrent stroke is rare within 2 weeks, many experts recommend postponing the institution of heparin therapy for several days in all patients, and for as much as 1 week in those at higher risk of hemorrhagic transformation.

Other Causes Of Cerebral Infarction

In general, the principles of care noted above are applicable. Specific causes may require specific definitive therapy, such as exchange transfusions for cerebral infarction due to sickle cell anemia. Anticoagulation is not indicated for patients with emboli due to nonbacterial thrombotic endocarditis. While there is evidence that anticoagulation may improve outcome in patients with cerebral venous thrombosis, patients who present with large or hemorrhagic infarctions probably should not be given anticoagulation due to the risk of brain hemorrhage.

Intracerebral Hemorrhage

The care of patients with primary intracerebral hemorrhage requires the same attention to the principles of general care, early ambulation, prophylaxis against pulmonary complications, and intravenous fluids as that of patients with cerebral infarction.

As in patients with cerebral infarction, blood pressure is often transiently elevated. Because autoregulation of blood flow is impaired, pharmacologic lowering of blood pressure may reduce blood flow to ischemic regions surrounding the hemorrhage. Increased intracranial pressure may further reduce cerebral perfusion, and vasodilation caused by systemic antihypertensive agents may cause further increases in intracranial pressure. While the dangers of reducing blood pressure are clear, benefits have not been demonstrated. Rebleeding is rare, and has not been associated with arterial hypertension.

No specific medical therapy has been shown to be of benefit in patients with acute intracerebral hemorrhage. Corticosteroids do not reduce morbidity and mortality due to edema. Mannitol and hyperventilation can be used to temporarily reduce intracranial pressure if a definitive surgical intervention is planned. The primary goal of surgery is to alleviate the effects of the hematoma acting as an intracranial mass lesion, not to reverse the effects of local tissue destruction. The value of surgery is best proven for cerebellar hemorrhages resulting in brain stem compression. Patients with large, deep hematomas arising from the basal ganglia do not benefit from surgical intervention. Those with superficial hematomas and signs of increased intracranial pressure may show improvement after surgical evacuation. In the absence of clinical signs due to mass effect, however, such operations are not indicated.

Subarachnoid Hemorrhage Due To Ruptured Intracranial Aneurysm

Following rupture of an intracranial aneurysm, three events commonly occur that can cause further brain damage: rebleeding, delayed ischemia (vasospasm), and hydrocephalus. Emergent clipping of ruptured intracranial aneurysms, acute ventricular drainage for hydrocephalus and prophylactic treatment for vasospasm by experienced neurosurgical teams is associated with improved outcome. The intensivist should recognize, however, that delayed surgery may still be appropriate for some patients when the care-providing team is not well practiced in urgent interventions for subarachnoid hemorrhage.

Preoperative Care

Cerebral angiography should be performed emergently. The Hunt-Hess clinical grade (Table 48-1), surgical accessibility of the lesion, presence of a mass effect, and presence of vasospasm should be used to determine the optimal timing of surgery. Most experienced teams operate on the majority of patients in grades I to III in the first 24 to 48 h after presentation. Preoperative prophylactic medical therapy includes anticonvulsants and calcium channel blockers. No overall benefit has been demonstrated for antifibrinolytic therapy or for medical management of blood pressure. Additional preoperative measures include bedrest, sedation, and

TABLE 48-1 Hunt-Hess Classification of Patients with Intracranial Aneurysms According to Surgical Risk

Category	Criteria
Grade I	Asymptomatic, or minimal headache and slight nuchal rigidity
Grade II	Moderate to severe headache, nuchal rigidity, no neurological deficit other than cranial nerve palsy
Grade III	Drowsiness, confusion, or mild focal deficit
Grade IV	Stupor, moderate-to-severe hemiparesis, possibly early decerebrate rigidity and vegetative disturbances
Grade V	Deep coma, decerebrate rigidity, moribund appearance

(Reprinted with permission from Powers WJ, Hanley DF: Cerebrovascular Disease, in Hall JB, Schmidt GA, Wood LDH: Principles of Critical Care, McGraw-Hill, New York 1992.)

therapy to avoid cough and Valsalva maneuvers (e.g., stool softeners).

Postoperative Care

For most ruptured aneurysms, definitive clipping can be accomplished, removing the risk of rebleeding. The focus of postoperative care then becomes prevention of vasospasm and hydrocephalus. Prophylactic use of calcium channel blockers should be continued. A second type of therapy for vasospasm is hypervolemic/hypertensive therapy. This therapy is associated with a 50 percent reduction in vasospasm-related morbidity, compared with historic controls.

Hypervolemic/hypertensive therapy is delivered by intravenous administration of saline solution and colloid to achieve pulmonary capillary wedge pressures in the range of 15 to 18 mmHg. Vasoactive and pressor agents are used; a useful combination is dopamine and phenylephrine. A practical goal is doubling of cardiac output while maintaining heart rate less than 100 beats per min. Concurrent problems that can exacerbate cerebral ischemia due to vasospasm include volume depletion secondary to diabetes insipidus or cerebral salt wasting, blood loss secondary to phlebotomy, and reduced cerebral perfusion pressure secondary to obstructive hydrocephalus. Complications of hypervolemic/hypertensive therapy include angina pectoris and congestive heart failure. The latter may occur more frequently when this therapy is administered with calcium channel blockers.

Obstructive hydrocephalus is the third process that must be prevented or managed to produce the optimal result after subarachnoid hemorrhage. Frequent use of imaging tests, such as CT or MRI, is helpful in the diagnosis of hydrocephalus. Massive intraventricular bleeding may lead to aqueductal obstruction and the acute presentation of obstructive hydrocephalus as coma. Placement of an external ventricular drain is the treatment of choice in this situation. Great care must be taken in the use of these drains to avoid complicating meningitis. In patients with unclipped aneurysms, drain placement and ventricular overdrainage may be associated with aneurysmal rupture. For patients with mildly dilated ventricles due to communicating hydrocephalus, and minimal alteration in mental state, lumbar puncture may be the best monitoring modality. For persons with surgically clipped aneurysms who have impaired mental state and clear elevation of intracranial pressure, continuous monitoring and drainage of either ventricular or lumbar cerebrospinal fluid should be performed.

Fever commonly accompanies subarachnoid hemorrhage and is usually treated symptomatically with antipyretic and anti-inflammatory drugs. The value of these drugs is ill-defined; however, since fever elevates cerebral metabolism, control of fever in patients with impaired cerebral perfusion may help to minimize ischemic damage.

For further reading in Principles of Critical Care see Chap 141, "Cerebrovascular Disease" William J Powers/Daniel F Hanley, Jr.

Edward T. Naureckas

PRESENTATION AND DIAGNOSIS

Status epilepticus (SE) is defined as a condition characterized by an epileptic seizure which is so frequently repeated or prolonged as to create a fixed and lasting condition. Untreated status epilepticus may lead to rhabdomyolysis, renal failure due to myoglobinuria, and central nervous system (CNS) damage as a direct effect of the seizure, and thus must be recognized and treated promptly. Other consequences of status epilepticus include hyperkalemia (which may lead to cardiac arrhythmias), metabolic acidosis, aspiration syndromes, hypoventilation, and in rare cases non-cardiogenic pulmonary edema.

The types of seizures which may result in status epilepticus are listed in Table 49-1. It is important to note that some types of seizures such as absence, or complex partial seizures may present as an acute confusional state and thus must always be considered in the differential diagnosis of this condition. These presentations may be subtle, but if left untreated, may have the same CNS consequences as generalized tonic-clonic status.

A large number of patients presenting to the intensive care unit (ICU) do not meet the formal definition for SE but instead present with serial seizures. The patients are subject to the same risk as patients with status epilepticus and should be treated as vigorously.

When treated properly, the mortality from status epilepticus de-

TABLE 49-1 Types of Seizures which Can Manifest as Status Epilepticus

Generalized Seizures	
Convulsive	Nonconvulsive
Tonic-clonic (grand mal)	Absence (petit mal)

Partial Seizures	
Convulsive	Nonconvulsive
Partial seizures (simple or complex) generalizing to tonic-clonic seizures	Simple partial seizures (no change in consciousness) Somatomotor (Kojevnikov's) Aphasic Complex partial seizures (altered consciousness) Confusional state

(Reproduced with permission from Leppik I: Status Epilepticus and Serial Seizures, in Hall JB, Schmidt GA, and Wood LDH: Principles of Critical Care, McGraw-Hill, New York, 1992.)

pends on the underlying etiology. Patients can be divided into two groups. Patients in group 1 have no acute CNS disorder but have epilepsy which is not under control. These patients tend to respond rapidly to a single drug and have a good prognosis rarely requiring ICU admission. Patients in group 2 have acute underlying CNS disease such as CNS hemorrhage, closed head injury, or a rapidly growing tumor. These patients may require more than one medication and have a high mortality rate due to the underlying disorder.

MANAGEMENT

The underlying principle in the treatment of SE is to rapidly end seizure activity. One protocol for treatment of SE is shown in Table 49-2. Diazepam as a single agent is no longer recommended as its redistribution into lipid stores leads to a rapid fall in serum levels resulting in recurrence of seizures. If given initially it should be followed by a loading dose of a longer acting agent such as phenytoin.

Phenytoin should be given at a loading dose of 20 mg/kg at a rate not to exceed 50 mg/min as propylene glycol in the current parenteral preparation may cause hypotension. Often it is more practical to dilute the drug to a concentration of 5 mg/ml in normal saline to allow for more uniform administration. A serum level of 25 to 30 μgm/mL should be attained.

TABLE 49-2 Treatment Protocol with Time Frame of Intervention

0–5 minutes:
  Assess cardiorespiratory function, obtain history and perform neurological and physical examination. Blood for antiepileptic drug levels, glucose, BUN, electrolytes, metabolic screen and drug screen. Insert oral airway and administer oxygen only if needed.
6–9 minutes:
  Start intravenous infusion with saline solution. Administer 25 grams of glucose and thiamine.
10–30 minutes:
  Begin infusion of phenytoin (PHT), 20 mg/kg at a rate no faster than 50 mg/minute. This may take 20–40 minutes. Monitor EKG and blood pressure. Lorazepam (4 or 8 mg) or diazepam (10 to 20 mg) may be given if convulsions occur while PHT is being infused.
31–60 minutes:
  If seizures persist, give phenobarbital, 10 mg/kg given at 100 mg/minute intravenously.
1 hour:
  If seizures persist, barbiturate coma or general anesthesia with agents with which the facility is familiar should be started.

PHT = Phenytoin
(*Reproduced with permission from Leppik I: Status Epilepticus and Serial Seizures, in Hall JB, Schmidt GA, and Wood LDH: Principles of Critical Care, McGraw-Hill, New York, 1992.*)

Phenobarbital is often used as a second line drug at a loading dose of 10 mg/kg at a rate of 100 mg/min. If seizures persist, barbiturate coma should be induced. Periodic electroencephalogram (EEG) monitoring should be used to document coma.

If seizures are persistent after institution of single drug therapy or if the patient has no previous history of seizures an EEG and a CT or MRI scan are warranted. Lumbar puncture (LP) should also be performed if the patient is febrile, keeping in mind that a mild degree of CNS pleocytosis may be seen in SE though not usually to the degree seen in meningitis. If a high degree of suspicion for meningitis exists, the patient should receive appropriate antibiotic therapy while awaiting imaging to rule out a mass lesion prior to LP.

For further reading in *Principles of Critical Care,* see Chap 142 "Status Epilepticus and Serial Seizures" Ilo E Leppik

Intracranial Hypertension

David Olson

Intracranial pressure (ICP) monitoring and control have assumed an important role in the intensive management of patients with a diversity of acute neurologic disorders. In conjunction with the mean arterial pressure (MAP), central venous pressure (CVP), and metabolic parameters such as arteriovenous oxygen content difference, monitoring of ICP can supplement the neurologic exam in determining the progression of a central nervous system (CNS) injury or the development of a new problem.

In the normal brain, cerebral blood flow (CBF) remains fairly constant, given autoregulatory control of cerebral perfusion pressure within the range of 50 to 100 mmHg (CPP=MAP-ICP). A fall in MAP may lead to cerebral ischemia, while a rise in ICP results in intracranial hypertension. Although variable among different pathologies, elevations of ICP above 20 to 25 mmHg for 10 to 15 min would generally be considered pathologic and require treatment.

INDICATIONS FOR ICP MONITORING (Table 50-1)

Severe head injuries have traditionally been the most common indication for ICP monitoring. Early detection of intracranial hypertension from a delayed expanding hematoma, increased cerebral blood volume (CBV) due to hyperemia, or massive swelling of a cerebral hemisphere after removal of an adjacent subdural or

TABLE 50-1 Conditions in Which Early Detection and Treatment of Intracranial Hypertension May Prevent Secondary Brain Ischemia

Head Injury
  Postevacuation of large subdural or epidural hematoma
  Delayed intracerebral hematoma
  Coma-producing diffuse head injury
Subarachnoid Hemorrhage (SAH)
  Pre and postoperative hydrocephalus
  Post SAH infarction
Brain Tumors
  Post-tumor removal
  Postoperative tumor-induced hydrocephalus
Fulminant Hepatic Failure
  Hepatic coma awaiting transplant
  Reye's syndrome

(Reprinted with permission from Pitts LH, Andrews BT: Intracranial Pressure Monitoring and Treatment of Intracranial Hypertension, in Hall JB, Schmidt GA, Wood LDH: Principles of Critical Care, McGraw-Hill, New York, 1992.)

epidural hematoma can be accomplished by ICP monitoring. In general, head trauma patients who are arousable can be assessed for clinical deterioration by serial neurologic examinations. However, in comatose patients (Glasgow coma scores of 8 or less) who have an abnormal computerized tomography (CT) scan or are hypotensive, older than 40 years of age, or have a Glascow motor score of less than 4, ICP monitoring should be implemented. Further CT scans should be obtained with any decrement in neurologic status, regardless of the presence of an ICP monitoring device.

In head trauma, intracranial hypertension commonly follows hyperemia and increased CBV. Vasoconstriction brought about by hyperventilation can reduce CBV in these patients. In up to a third of cases, though, elevated CBV is not present and hyperventilation may lead to cerebral ischemia. A distinction between these subsets of patients can be made by measuring the cerebral metabolic rate for oxygen or arteriovenous differences in cerebral oxygen or lactate content.

Initial surgical intervention for intracranial hematoma is a difficult clinical decision and may be based on the size of the lesion, its mass effect, or the extent of neurologic impairment. Medical management of intracranial hypertension after head injury is generally successful. Maintaining ICP< 15 to 20 mmHg seems to correlate with improved immediate outcome and less longterm neuropsychologic deficits. Pentobarbital coma and surgical subtemporal decompression can be considered in refractory cases.

Patients with subarachnoid hemorrhage typically have intracranial hypertension, and persistent elevations in ICP usually result in a poorer outcome. High pressure hydrocephalus can occur early and is related to obstruction at interventricular orifices or sites of cerebrospinal fluid (CSF) drainage at the pacchionian granulations. Diagnosis is made by measurement of rising ICP via ventriculostomy or by the discovery of progressive hydrocephalus on serial CT scans. Definitive treatment is by drainage of CSF through a ventriculostomy or by shunting if the elevated ICP persists. Shunting may also be necessary in the treatment of low pressure hydrocephalus, which typically develops weeks to months after the initial event, and is diagnosed by progressive neurologic symptoms.

Monitoring of ICP in patients with brain tumors is most useful at the time of surgical anesthesia in those patients with significant preoperative peritumor edema and in those minority of patients (13 to 18 percent) who develop increased ICP after tumor removal. In this latter group, a rise in ICP can precede a neurologic deterioration thus allowing early medical management of a postoperative complication.

Intracranial hypertension often accompanies severe liver failure, creating cerebral ischemia and subsequent neurologic dysfunction. However, hepatic encephalopathy may also produce symptoms of significant lethargy and coma, thus requiring ICP monitoring to distinguish between these two clinical states. Recognition and management of increased ICP has improved outcome in patients who might previously have suffered permanent neurologic sequelae despite recovery of native hepatic function or successful liver transplantation. Care must be given to correcting the patient's clotting components prior to placement of an ICP monitor as even mildly abnormal parameters can lead to a fatal intracranial hemorrhage.

MONITORING TECHNIQUES

Currently, the two most common ICP monitoring systems are fluid-filled catheters or rigid "bolts" attached to an electromechanical transducer or fiberoptic system. These devices can be placed in the subdural, intraventricular, or less commonly, the epidural position. The intraventricular position allows drainage of CSF when necessary to lower ICP, though a subdural catheter is required when the ventricles are compressed by brain swelling. Once placed, the ICP catheter is attached to a pressure transducer which provides continuous digital and wave form displays. A good pressure tracing will have a regular pulse pressure of 3 to 7 mmHg (greater at elevated ICP) with a baseline that varies with respiratory changes in intrathoracic pressure. A "flat" ICP tracing should not be accepted as a valid wave form and care should be given to discovering and correcting occlusion of the catheter by blood or brain tissue or a kink along the catheter's course. Relieving an occlusion can be achieved by injecting a small amount of irrigant (0.25 mL initially) and closing the system stopcock during the injection.

Two potentially devastating complications of ICP monitoring devices are intracranial infection and brain hemorrhage. The ICP catheter and transducer should be maintained as a closed system and are generally filled with an antibiotic solution containing gentamicin, 1 mg/mL. A CSF leak greatly increases the risk of infection and should be addressed immediately by resuturing the skin at the entrance site. In addition, neurosurgeons should place the ICP monitors since they are most familiar with manipulating brain tissue, thus reducing the risk of hemorrhage. Intraventricular catheters tend to be associated with a greater risk of infection or intracerebral hemorrhage than the subdural catheter, though again, the intraventricular catheters allow for withdrawal of CSF fluid and can be placed at the bedside in the ICU. Subdural catheters and bolts must be placed in the operating room, with the latter having a much higher incidence of occlusion than either catheter.

INTENSIVE CARE MANAGEMENT
OF INTRACRANIAL HYPERTENSION

Initial management of those with severe neurologic dysfunction include appropriate ventilatory and circulatory support in the acute setting, and the necessary diagnostic tests to outline further treatment strategies. If indicated (as discussed previously), an ICP monitoring device should be placed and, in conjunction with sequential neurologic assessment by physicians and nursing staff, the patient's status is followed closely, therein reflecting the efficacy of current treatment and the need for subsequent diagnostic procedures, such as cranial CT scanning.

If intracranial hypertension is present, surgical means of lowering ICP should first be evaluated. Removal of mass lesions (tumor, hematoma) or correction of hydrocephelus via ventriculostomy drainage of CSF should be attempted if appropriate. If no lesions requiring surgical intervention are present, then medical management must be undertaken, with the goal to maintain ICP less than 20 mmHg or CPP above 60 mmHg. Methods of lowering ICP are listed in Table 50-2.

Continuous arterial blood pressure monitoring and management is an extremely important adjunct to the treatment of intracranial hypertension. Systemic hypotension can lead to secondary ischemic brain injury, while unnecessary hypertension can produce a significant elevation in CPP.

Clinical manifestations of hypofusion are the most sensitive indicators of shock and thus pulse rate, skin perfusion, and urine output should be closely monitored. Volume expansion with crystalloid or colloid solutions is appropriate to maintain a MAP of 100 to 110 mmHg, while avoiding overhydration and secondary cerebral or pulmonary edema (a CVP catheter should be placed if fluid status is uncertain). Controlling blood glucose to levels of 100 to 200 mg/dl to prevent injurious effects of hypo- or hyperglycemia on damaged brain tissue, as well as optimizing oxygen carrying capacity by keeping the hematocrit at 32 to 35 percent are additional important measures.

Head injury can disrupt cerebral autoregulation and systemic hypertension can raise CBF and thus ICP. Increases in catechol levels and sympathetic activity can be managed with β-blocking agents, such as propranolol or esmolol.

A struggling patient will increase intrathoracic pressure and CVP, thereby provoking an increase in ICP. Morphine sulfate and

TABLE 50-2 Treatments for Intracranial Hypertension

Surgical removal of intracranial masses
Sedation
Paralysis
Ventricular Drainage
Controlled Hyperventilation
Hyperosmotic therapies
Diuretics
Barbiturate coma
Subtemporal decompression

(Reprinted with permission from Pitts LH, Andrews BT: Intracranial Pressure Monitoring and Treatment of Intracranial Hypertension, in Hall JB, Schmidt GA, Wood LDH: Principles of Critical Care, McGraw-Hill, New York, 1992.)

benzodiazepines are useful for sedation, though chemoparalysis may need to be employed. The benefit of these drugs must be weighed against the need for ventilatory support and the obvious effects on the neurologic exam.

Depending on the type of ICP monitor employed, drainage of CSF may provide the simplest method of lowering ICP, particularly if a relative excess is present due to obstructing tumor or hemorrhage. Even when diffuse parenchymal swelling is present, small amounts of CSF drainage in conjunction with other ICP lowering techniques can prove effective.

Controlled hyperventilation produces respiratory alkalosis and cerebral arterial vasoconstriction. The subsequent decrease in CBV and brain volume results in lowered ICP. Cerebral vasoconstriction is achieved down to a P_{CO_2} of 22 to 25 mmHg. Further reductions in P_{CO_2} can lead to cerebral ischemia. Maintaining cerebral av O_2 content difference less than 6.5 mL O_2/100 mL blood (via jugular venous bulb sampling) generally insures adequate brain tissue oxygenation while using controlled hyperventilation.

After 20 to 24 h, hyperventilation loses its effectiveness and, in fact, returning P_{CO_2} to normal levels can lead to vasodilation and increased CBV. Thus, controlled hyperventilation is most appropriately used in acute elevations of ICP, while other methods of treating intracranial hypertension are initiated. As ICP normalizes, P_{CO_2} can be returned to around 30 to 33 mmHg, thereby maintaining cerebral arteriolar responsiveness.

Osmotic therapy (mannitol, 0.25 to 0.5 g/kg body weight IV) is commonly employed in treating intracranial hypertension and has several beneficial effects. Mannitol reduces brain water, increases circulating volume and MAP, and reduces blood viscosity, both by hemodilution and increased red cell deformability. Lowered blood viscosity can induce cerebral vasoconstriction, with a concomitant reduction in ICP. The addition of furosemide may increase the effectiveness of mannitol by maintaining intravascular volume through diuresis, thus removing brain water and perhaps decreasing CSF production. Caution against dehydration must be used during hyperosmotic therapy. Mannitol should not be given when serum osmolarity exceeds 300 mM and excessive fluid losses should be replaced to maintain a CVP between 2 to 5 mmHg or a pulmonary wedge pressure of 5 to 10 mmHg.

Finally, iatrogenic barbiturate coma may be used to lower ICP when other measures have failed, though its effect on outcome is uncertain. When ICP exceeds 25 mmHg for more than 15 min, pentobarbital can be given at 10 mg/kg IV slowly, followed by 1.5 mg/kg/h to maintain serum level at about 3 mg/dL. Systemic hypotension is common with barbiturate use and hemodynamic monitoring is essential; pressor agents may be needed to support an adequate systemic blood pressure. Those patients with hypotension prior to barbiturate therapy have worse outcomes and thus its use should be avoided in this setting.

For further reading in *Principles of Critical Care,* see Chap 34 "Intracranial Pressure Monitoring and Treatment of Intracranial Hypertension" Lawrence H Pitts/Brian T Andrews

---

Scott P. Neeley

BEDSIDE AND LABORATORY DIAGNOSIS OF COAGULOPATHIES

Accurate diagnosis of the mechanism of a bleeding disorder is based on careful history and bedside evaluation along with appropriate laboratory testing. History should focus on pre-existing bleeding diathesis, medications, and organ function (e.g., hepatic or renal insufficiency). Physical examination should determine if bleeding is local or a systemic diathesis. It may be possible to distinguish a vascular or platelet disorder characterized by immediate bleeding (continued bleeding after onset and petechial/mucosal manifestations) from a fibrin generation or fibrinolysis problem typified by delayed bleeding (rebleeding after initial hemostasis and prominent ecchymoses/deep muscle and joint hemorrhage). Complex coagulopathies such as disseminated intravascular coagulation (DIC) may have features of both. The presence of splenomegaly or telangiectases may also be helpful.

Several generalizations may direct further work-up: **1.** before invoking a coagulopathy, uncomplicated vascular injury amenable to surgical hemostasis should be excluded; **2.** spontaneous hemorrhage due to a coagulopathy alone almost never causes brisk bleeding; **3.** clinically significant bleeding often is the result of the coexistence of trauma or a bleeding lesion with a coagulopathy; and **4.** laboratory screening for potential bleeding diathesis is important in predicting and preventing bleeding complications during interventions such as line placements and surgical procedures.

Appropriate laboratory evaluation for a hemostatic disorder in the critically ill patient includes a platelet count, review of peripheral smear for the presence of schistocytes and evaluation of platelet number and appearance, bleeding time (unless platelet count <50,000/μL), prothrombin time (PT), activated partial thromboplastin time (PTT), thrombin time (TT), fibrin degradation products (FDPs), and D-dimer assay. These tests should be done simultaneously.

Defects in the formation of a platelet plug in response to vessel injury cause a prolonged bleeding time. The PT and PTT are useful in detecting abnormalities in fibrin clot formation. The TT depends on the conversion of fibrinogen to fibrin and detects abnormalities in the fibrin generation cascade and inhibitors acting at this level such as heparin. Excessive fibrinolysis leading to clot instability and lysis is detected by testing for FDP and D-dimer. FDPs result from fibrinogenolysis and fibrinolysis, but D-dimer is a unique product of degradation of fibrin. Thus elevated D-dimer levels indicate that fibrin formation has taken place prior to plasmin activity.

VASCULAR DISORDERS

Patients with vasculitis may have increased risk of bleeding due to vascular fragility. The physical finding of palpable purpura suggests vasculitis in contrast to the typically flat purpura of thrombocytopenia. Cutaneous vasculitis causes a prolonged bleeding time and may increase the risk of bleeding from even small incisions. A diagnosis may be made by small punch biopsy of a purpuric lesion. Management consists of removing offending agents (e.g., drugs), treating underlying disorders, and using anti-inflammatory agents such as corticosteroids if not contraindicated.

Vascular malformations may bleed when traumatized, though there is usually no laboratory evidence of a coagulopathy. Family history and careful exam of cutaneous and mucosal sites for blanching "spiders" may be helpful.

Microcirculatory obstruction in acute nonlymphocytic leukemia due to elevated myeloblast levels may lead to microcirculatory obstruction and resulting purpura. Brain, lung, and skin are most commonly involved in this disorder which is clinically similar to the vasoocclusive bleeding seen in DIC, thrombotic thrombocytopenic purpura (TTP), and fat embolism.

THROMBOCYTOPENIAS

The platelet count is the result of the balance between production and removal of platelets from the circulation. Bone marrow normally has a six-to-eightfold reserve production capacity for platelets which can compensate for shortening of the normal platelet half-life. While not as reliable as the reticulocyte count, evaluation of Wright-stained blood smears for young (large, basophilic) platelets may aid in estimation of rate of platelet production.

Underproduction States

Hypoplastic Marrow

A variety of causes, including drugs, environmental toxins, infectious agents, immune processes, radiation injury, and idiopathic hypoplastic or aplastic marrow may result in a generalized decrease in marrow mass or a selective decrease in megakaryocyte number. This diagnosis is suggested by a finding of decreased overall marrow cellularity or selective decrease in megakaryocyte number on bone marrow examination. Care should be taken not to sample marrow in the port of prior radiation, as hypoplasia is expected and may be misleading.

Ineffective Marrow

Ineffective marrow states are characterized by normal or increased cellularity but lack of release of precursors into the blood. A common cause of ineffective marrow function is folate deficiency. The findings of hypersegmented polymorphonuclear leukocytes, ovalomacrocytes, lack of reticulocyte response and thrombocytopenia suggest this diagnosis. B_{12} deficiency may present similarly. Ineffective marrow function is also seen in myelophthisic conditions such as marrow replacement by tumor or granuloma, metabolic disturbances such as azotemia or hypothyroidism, and in primary marrow diseases such as leukemia and myeloma.

Shortened Platelet Survival

The normal half-life of platelets in the blood (5 days) is usually shortened in critically ill patients. Specific disorders causing shortened platelet survival and clinically significant thrombocytopenia are characterized by findings of purpuric or mucosal bleeding, thrombocytopenia with a peripheral blood smear showing large basophilic platelets, and normal or increased numbers of megakaryocytes on bone marrow examination.

Idiopathic Thrombocytopenic Purpura

Idiopathic (or autoimmune) thrombocytopenic purpura (ITP) is documented by finding antiplatelet antibodies in the patient's serum or on the patient's platelets. As these tests may take a number of days to perform, a decision to pursue appropriate therapy must generally be made on the basis of characteristic clinical and laboratory findings. Immune reactions to drugs are the most common etiologies of ITP. In the ICU, common offending agents include sulfonamides, furosemide, ranitidine, heparin, and rifampin, though a large number of drugs have been implicated in this disorder. Lymphoma, collagen vascular disease and viral infections (e.g., HIV) are also associated with ITP.

Therapy consists first of discontinuation of potential offending agents. Drugs which impair platelet function are also contraindicated. A response to removal of a causative drug may not be seen for several days. Administration of platelets is generally of temporary or no benefit because their survival is also shortened. If thrombocytopenia is severe (platelet count <20,000/mL) or bleeding is a problem, therapy with corticosteroids and intravenous γ-globulin, 0.4 to 1 g/kg/day for 3 to 5 days should be considered. Intravenous γ-globulin has few side effects and may result in rises in platelet counts which may be lifesaving or allow emergent surgical procedures. However, its benefit is usually temporary. Repeated doses may be effective, but cost is very high. Splenectomy may be an effective therapy for ITP but may not be possible in the critically ill patient. Other therapeutic options include splenic irradiation, danazol, colchicine and cytotoxic drugs, though these options may be more appropriate for chronic management.

Thrombotic Thrombocytopenic Purpura (TTP)

TTP is characterized by the clinical pentad of thrombocytopenia, microangiopathic hemolytic anemia (MAHA), neurologic abnormalities, fever and renal impairment. It has been suggested that the hemolytic-uremic syndromes (HUS), characterized by thrombocytopenia, MAHA, and renal failure, are part of a spectrum of thrombotic microangiopathies (TMA), including TTP with its predominant neurologic findings on one extreme, and HUS, with its predominant renal failure and lack of neurologic findings, on the other. TTP is a hematologic emergency, and patients with this disorder are at high risk for development of shock, lactic acidosis, respiratory failure and severe neurologic injury.

Neurologic symptoms and signs can be nonspecific in TTP, varying from headache and minor changes in mental status to severe focal neurologic deficits, seizures, obtundation, and coma. Fever is present in approximately two-thirds of patients. Laboratory findings in TTP include profound thrombocytopenia (counts <50,000/μL are common), MAHA with elevated total bilirubin and lactate dehydrogenase (LDH), and variable degrees of renal insufficiency. Urinalysis usually reveals proteinuria and hematuria.

It is important to differentiate TTP from other causes of MAHA such as DIC syndromes; pregnancy associated syndromes such as preeclampsia, acute fatty liver of pregnancy and HELLPS (*hy*pertension, *e*levated *l*iver enzymes, *l*ow *p*latelets *s*yndrome); and collagen vascular disease (e.g., systemic lupus erythematosus, SLE). The DIC syndromes are generally associated with a precipitating insult, such as sepsis, trauma, incompatible blood transfusion or amniotic fluid embolus. Such clinical associations are generally not seen in TTP. While DIC is also characterized by thrombocytopenia and MAHA, thrombocytopenia is less common and typically less severe. Unlike DIC, the PT, PTT, fibrinogen and FDP levels are usually normal in TTP. TTP occurs rarely in pregnancy and can appear similar to preeclampsia and HELLPS. But while these disorders can include MAHA and thrombocytopenia, fever, neurologic abnormalities and marked renal insufficiency are less commonly seen. Vasculitis associated with

SLE or other collagen vascular disease can mimic the clinical pentad of TTP. Antinuclear antibodies are positive in the majority of patients with SLE and serum complement levels are usually low. These values are typically normal in TTP, making collagen vascular disease "screening tests" useful in nearly all patients with a tentative diagnosis of TTP.

Plasma exchange is the therapy of choice for TTP, and should be instituted rapidly and performed daily until the disease is in remission. Plasma exchange can be performed either with two large bore peripheral intravenous catheters or through a double lumen dialysis catheter. Femoral vein catheter placement is preferred initially to avoid hemothorax or pneumothorax in a severely thrombocytopenic patient. Femoral vein catheters should be changed every 72 h. Complications of plasma exchange include bleeding, air embolus, hepatitis, citrate toxicity, and pulmonary edema. Aggressive supportive measures, including mechanical ventilation and hemodialysis, may be necessary to stabilize the critically ill patient with TTP, though even in these patients substantial improvement is frequently seen with plasma exchange therapy. The most sensitive indicator of response is a rising platelet count, though LDH is also a sensitive indicator of RBC turnover and can be used to monitor response to therapy. The usual course of plasma exchange is 5 to 10 days. Patients can be transferred from the ICU when mental status has normalized and hematocrit and platelet count are increasing.

Plasma infusion can be useful in patients with acute TTP, but should not delay the institution of plasma exchange nor prevent transfer to a fully equipped referral unit. High dose steroid therapy and antiplatelet agents have been advocated for therapy of TTP, but without convincing evidence of benefit. Intravenous vincristine has been reported to benefit some patients, as has splenectomy, although these should be considered second-line therapies. *Platelet transfusion is contraindicated in TTP as it may exacerbate the vasoocclusive process.*

Heparin-Induced Thrombocytopenia

While bleeding is the most common complication of heparin therapy, heparin-induced thrombocytopenia is of special interest in the ICU due to the ubiquitous exposure of patients to heparin in access and monitoring lines and 'heparin-coated' catheters. Immune-mediated heparin-induced thrombocytopenia typically occurs 5 to 7 days after first exposure, though previous sensitization may lead to earlier thrombocytopenia in some patients. Clinical findings range from no symptoms to life-threatening arterial or venous thrombotic events. Bleeding is relatively uncommon despite occasionally severe thrombocytopenia. Therapy includes immediate discontinuation of all exposure to heparin, including heparin locks, flushes of indwelling lines, and indwelling catheters that are heparin-coated. If anticoagulation is indicated for other clinical reasons, warfarin may be used, though this will necessitate a window period between discontinuation of heparin and therapeutic anticoagulation. Transfusion of platelets should be avoided unless necessitated by hemorrhage. Any history of adverse reaction to heparin should be viewed as a risk factor for serious vascular complications on reexposure to the drug.

Posttransfusion Purpura

Delayed appearance of severe thrombocytopenia may follow transfusions of blood products from P1A1-positive donors in P1A1-negative individuals. In addition to traditional therapy with whole blood or plasma exchange, recent experience suggests that infusions of intravenous γ-globulin (0.4 g/kg/day for 2 to 5 days) may be helpful in these patients (see Chap. 3).

Disseminated Intravascular Coagulation

When shortened platelet survival and thrombocytopenia are present in DIC, other manifestations, such as MAHA, hypofibrinogenemia, elevated FDPs and D-dimer levels, and prolonged clotting times are generally also present (see below).

Hypersplenism

Thrombocytopenia with or without anemia and neutropenia may be a feature of hypersplenism. Physical examination may reveal splenomegaly in this condition, though ultrasound is a noninvasive and more sensitive method for assessment of spleen size in the ICU. Conditions associated with hypersplenism include hepatic cirrhosis, splenic venous occlusion, lymphoma, leukemia, and sarcoidosis. Bone marrow evaluation generally shows increased megakaryocytes and overall hypercellularity. Splenectomy may be indicated when splenomegaly is progressive (with associated risk of rupture) or counts are particularly low. Appropriate therapy for lymphoma, leukemia or sarcoidosis can result in rapid reduction in spleen size and sequestration.

THROMBOCYTOSIS/THROMBOCYTHEMIA

Reactive thrombocytosis is commonly seen in patients with inflammatory lesions, bleeding, surgery, hemolysis, trauma or neoplasia. Platelet counts are usually $<10^6/\mu L$, and adverse effects are not seen. In contrast, patients with thrombocythemia due to myeloproliferative disorders (e.g., polycythemia vera) are at increased risk of bleeding and thrombotic sequelae, particularly when platelet counts are $>10^6/\mu L$. Efforts should be made to lower the platelet count prior to surgical or ICU procedures when possible (a platelet count of 500,000/μL is a reasonable goal). Plateletpheresis can rapidly and effectively reduce platelet counts. Chemotherapy with hydroxyurea or busulfan can be used to maintain normal platelet counts. Splenectomy should be avoided in these patients as marked platelet elevations associated with life-threatening vasoocclusive events may result.

THROMBOCYTOPATHY

Qualitative platelet abnormalities are encountered in ICU patients due to drug effects, uremia, myeloproliferative disorders, dysproteinemias (e.g., Waldenström's macroglobulinemia), effects of cardiopulmonary bypass, and DIC. Nonsteroidal anti-inflammatory drugs (NSAIDs), aspirin, alcohol and penicillins can all cause prolongations of the bleeding time. Once the offending drug is removed, the bleeding problem can be treated with administration of exogenous normal platelets, though several days may be required for the patient's own production of platelets to normalize the bleeding time. Uremic platelet dysfunction may need to be corrected prior to surgical procedures. Appropriate dialysis is of first importance; other therapies include intravenous DDAVP (0.3 mg/kg repeated at 6 to 12 h intervals in the perioperative period), infusions of cryoprecipitate, platelet transfusion and conjugated estrogens.

FIBRIN GENERATION DISORDERS

Abnormalities in fibrin generation are initially evaluated by consideration of the results of the PT and PTT in combination (Table 51-1). Prolonged clotting times should be restudied after mixing patient's plasma with an equal volume of pooled normal plasma. If the clotting time corrects with such a 1:1 mix, a deficiency is present; if the clotting time of the mix remains prolonged, an inhibitor is present.

Isolated Factor Deficiencies

Hypofibrinogenemia

Low functional fibrinogen levels usually result from either decreased hepatic synthesis or increased removal during DIC. Spontaneous hemorrhage from hypofibrinogenemia is not expected above a concentration of 100 mg/dL. Fibrinogen may be replaced with fresh frozen plasma (FFP) or, more effectively, by cryoprecipitate; 1 cryopack is expected to raise the fibrinogen level by 4 mg/dL in a 70-kg patient. In the critically ill patient, serial fibrinogen levels should be followed to determine the frequency of infusions (as often as every 6 to 12 h).

TABLE 51-1 Use of Combined PT and PTT Results to Determine Site(s) of
Fibrin Generation Cascade Defects

	PT-Normal	PT-Elevated
PTT-Normal	Result 1	Result 2
PTT-Elevated	Result 3	Result 4

Result 1: Normal screen of cascade (Factor levels at least 30–35% of
normal)
Result 2: Isolated low Factor VII level—may be due to congenital deficiency or *early* liver disease, Vitamin K deficiency or warfarin
effect.
Result 3: Intrinsic Pathway abnormality—low Factor VIII, IX, XI or XII;
typical pattern in Hemophilia A and von Willebrand's disease
Result 4: Due to common pathway abnormality (Factors I (Fibrinogen), II,
V, X) and/or combined intrinsic and extrinsic pathway defects.
Seen in *advanced* liver disease, vitamin K deficiency, full
warfarin and heparin effects, and DIC.

*(Reprinted with permission from Baron JM, Baron BW: Bleeding Disorders,
in Hall JB, Schmidt GA, Wood LDH: Principles of Critical Care, McGraw-Hill,
New York, 1992.)*

Hemophilia A and B

Critical illness in a patient with hemophilia A (factor VIII deficiency) requires careful correction of the preexisting coagulopathy,
particularly when other bleeding disorders (e.g., DIC) are present.
Treatment of bleeding or preparation of the hemophiliac for surgery or invasive procedure includes assessment for the presence of
a factor VIII inhibitor and then replacement with factor VIII concentrate to achieve the desired percent correction (100 percent
equals 1 U factor VIII/mL plasma). For major surgery or bleeding,
correction to 100 percent or higher is advisable. Further doses are
dictated by amount of bleeding and factor VIII levels. A similar
approach applies to patients with hemophilia B (factor IX deficiency, Christmas disease) except that replacement is with FFP or
factor IX concentrate in severe deficiency states.

von Willebrand's Factor

Deficiency of von Willebrand's factor (VWF) results in bleeding
similar to that seen with platelet dysfunction. Laboratory findings
include prolonged bleeding time, normal or moderately prolonged
PTT, decreased factor VIII coagulant (VIII:C) level, and decreased
ristocetin cofactor and von Willebrand's antigen levels. Patients
with type I VWF deficiency have a defect in secretion of normal
VWF from vascular endothelial cells. Less commonly, qualitative
defects in multimeric structure (type II) or severe synthetic defi-

ciency (type III) are seen. Type I patients may respond for a 2 to 3 day period to infusion of DDAVP with significant hemostatic benefit, allowing for the performance of invasive procedures. DDAVP is contraindicated in type II VWF deficiency as it may cause platelet aggregation and thrombocytopenia. Cryoprecipitate is indicated for treatment of type II and III deficiency and for prolonged therapy. In all cases, the goal of therapy is correction of the bleeding time during active bleeding and prior to surgical or invasive procedures.

Other Factor Deficiency States

Inherited deficiencies of other factors in the clotting cascade are rare, and vary in clinical significance from the trivial (factor XII) to the potentially lethal (factor XIII). In general, most of these deficiency states are treated with FFP or prothrombin complex (II, VII, X). In the ICU, acquired deficiencies of factor VII, often accompanied by deficiencies in one or more of II, V, IX and X, are the more commonly encountered abnormalities in factor levels. Acquired factor deficiency states occur most often due to vitamin K deficiency, liver disease and warfarin therapy. Risk factors for vitamin K deficiency include poor dietary intake, antibiotic therapy, and malabsorption of fat-soluble vitamins (e.g., in biliary obstruction). Vitamin K supplementation therapy may be by oral, subcutaneous, intramuscular or intravenous routes. The oral route is preferred when possible to avoid the risk of hematoma or rare anaphylaxis after intravenous dosing.

Inhibitors

Factor VIII Inhibitors

The most commonly encountered inhibitor is directed against factor VIII. It is seen most commonly in hemophiliac patients on factor replacement, but is also seen in the elderly, postpartum and in patients with autoimmune disorders or lymphoma. Factor VIII inhibitors are quantitated in Bethesda units; levels >10 U/mL signify more potent inhibitors. Patients with lower titers can be treated in the short term with infusion of factor VIII concentrate. Modes of therapy for those with high titers include prothrombin complex concentrate, porcine factor VIII concentrates, and combined immunosuppressive therapy.

Lupus Anticoagulants

The presence of a lupus anticoagulant is important to recognize, for while it is characterized by a prolonged PTT, it may be associated with a hypercoagulable state. Like other antiphospholipid antibodies (e.g., anticardiolipin), lupus anticoagulants are seen in patients with collagen vascular disease, as well as in otherwise normal individuals. Bleeding abnormalities are rare in these patients, but approximately 25 percent may demonstrate clinically important hypercoagulability.

COMPLEX COAGULOPATHIES

Disseminated Intravascular Coagulation

Disseminated intravascular coagulation (DIC) is among the most prevalent and potentially disastrous coagulopathies encountered in critical care medicine. DIC is characterized by a propensity for both fibrin deposition and increased fibrinolysis brought on by a variety of underlying disorders such as sepsis, tissue injury and neoplasm. The clinical presentation of DIC ranges from asymptomatic with laboratory abnormalities alone to a fulminant hemorrhagic diathesis accompanied by MAHA and multiple organ dysfunction due to vasoocclusion and hemorrhage.

Laboratory findings in DIC vary considerably. However, clinically evident coagulopathy is usually accompanied by increased FDP and D-dimer levels and prolonged clotting times. Other manifestations seen in severe disease include thrombocytopenia, hypofibrinogenemia, depressed circulating factor levels (particularly factor VIII), and microangiopathic changes on peripheral blood smear.

Therapy consists most importantly of treatment of the underlying condition predisposing to DIC. Judicious blood product support with RBCs, platelets, FFP and, if needed to correct hypofibrinogenemia (<100 mg/dL), cryoprecipitate, may protect the patient from hemorrhagic complications. In cases of purpura fulminans, massive thromboembolism, and acute promyelocytic leukemia, where the pace of the process is catastrophic, heparin therapy is appropriate along with blood product support. The initial dose of heparin is 5 U/kg/h by continuous infusion. If after 24 h the FDP levels have not declined, the heparin dose is increased to 10 U/kg/h. A lack of response to heparin may be due to deficiency of antithrombin III (ATIII), which can be corrected with FFP.

Massive Transfusion

Patients who have received one or more blood volumes replaced with stored RBCs may develop a complex coagulopathy due to thrombocytopenia, impaired platelet function, and decreased levels of factors VIII and V. Appropriate therapy depends on transfusion of sufficient platelets and FFP.

Liver Disease

Liver dysfunction often results in decreased synthesis of clotting factors. In addition, the presence of associated hypersplenism may result in thrombocytopenia. Finally, primary fibrinolysis secondary to liver cell injury may mimic DIC. In the differentiation of primary fibrinolysis in liver disease from DIC, the euglobulin clot lysis time and factor VIII:C level are useful. In primary fibrinolysis due to liver failure, decreased euglobulin lysis time and elevated factor VIII:C levels are seen. In DIC (secondary fibrinolysis) the euglobulin lysis time is normal, and factor VIII:C levels are low. Elevated D-dimer levels also favor DIC. Therapy consists of factor replacement and correction of vitamin K deficiency.

COAGULATION STATUS: GUIDELINES FOR INVASIVE PROCEDURES

General Considerations

Guideline 1: Perform procedures only when necessary in patients with coagulopathies.

Guideline 2: Make the intervention as limited as possible and preferably under direct vision.

Guideline 3: Define the coagulation status fully in order to anticipate potential risks and therapeutic options.

Guideline 4: If a preparatory treatment is given (e.g., infusion of FFP), check that the expected benefit has actually occurred.

Guideline 5: Coordinate the timing of procedures with suppliers of supportive products and be liberal in estimation of needs.

Guideline 6: Carefully follow the patient for both immediate and late bleeding and alert coworkers to the potential bleeding risk and appropriate therapy.

Guideline 7: Be prepared to reassess the patient's coagulation status in the face of new medications, changes in clinical status (e.g., onset of sepsis), or decreasing response to initial therapy.

Specific Coagulopathies

Thrombocytopenia

Platelet counts of 50,000 to 80,000/μL are appropriate for limited biopsies or line insertions. For major surgical procedures, or closed space needle biopsies, initial levels of 80,000 to 100,000/μL are preferred. Lumbar punctures are usually performed safely at platelet counts of 50,000/μL.

Thrombocythemia

It is advisable to lower platelet counts to ≤500,000/μL in these patients prior to invasive procedures if possible. The bleeding time may be a helpful predictor of bleeding abnormalities, though excessive bleeding can occur even with normal platelet counts and bleeding times in patients with myeloproliferative disorders. Thus, it is wise to avoid or minimize procedures in these individuals when possible.

Heparin

The heparinized patient who needs a procedure usually can be managed by discontinuation of heparin approximately 6 h beforehand. In urgent situations, neutralization with protamine can be used.

Warfarin

After discontinuation of warfarin it may take two or more days for the PT to normalize. In emergent situations the use of FFP can provide immediate correction of the coagulopathy. Oral or intravenous vitamin K has onset of its effect within 12 h. A state of warfarin resistance is likely to result from doses of vitamin K sufficient to correct the PT. During the period following the tapering of warfarin, temporary heparinization with discontinuation 6 h before the procedure will permit flexibility in planning interventions.

For further reading in *Principles of Critical Care,* see Chap 145 "Anemia, Leukopenia, and Elevated Blood Counts" R Brian Mitchell/Phillip C Hoffman, Chap 146 "Bleeding Disorders" Joseph M Baron/Beverly W Baron, Chap 147 "Thrombotic Thrombocytopenic Purpura and the Approach to Thrombotic Microangiopathies" Lawrence Tim Goodnough

---

Kevin Simpson

Acute leukemia is a malignant proliferation of bone marrow or lymphoid cells that is uniformly fatal when left untreated. However, with the use of intensive chemotherapy and skillful supportive care, many patients, particularly children and younger adults, may be cured of this devastating disease. Newly diagnosed patients deserve maximum aggressive supportive care in the medical ICU because most of the acute complications of leukemia resolve as a complete remission is achieved. The success of chemotherapy for acute leukemia depends not only on the drug susceptibility of an individual patient's particular leukemia but also on the ability of that patient to survive the rigors of treatment. This chapter focuses on the serious infectious, hematologic, infiltrative, and metabolic disorders that frequently accompany acute leukemia and its treatment.

INFECTION

Patients with leukemia are severely immunocompromised, both by their disease and by their treatment. Because chemotherapy damages mucosal barriers, these patients are prone to infection by endogenous organisms. Most common are gram-negative enteric bacteria, gram-positive cocci, and fungi such as *Candida* and *Aspergillus* species. Patients with acute lymphocytic leukemia (ALL) also are susceptible to pneumocystis, mycobacterial, and viral infections. Standard practice dictates that broad-spectrum antibiotic therapy must be initiated promptly and empirically in a granulocytopenic patient at the time of the first fever greater than 38.5°C (101.5°F). Blood, urine, and sputum cultures must be obtained, but the source of infection is rarely identified. Ceftazidime as a single agent or the combination of a semisynthetic penicillin plus an aminoglycoside is widely used, but the choice of regimen partly depends on renal function and history of allergies. Should initial cultures reveal a pathogen, antibiotic therapy should be adjusted for maximum bactericidal activity based on susceptibility testing in vitro. In general, however, broad-spectrum treatment continues until the chemotherapy is completed and the granulocyte count recovers to near normal.

Granulocyte transfusions are rarely necessary for patients receiving chemotherapy for acute leukemia. The indications for their use are generally limited to severely granulocytopenic patients who remain febrile and bacteremic despite receiving antibiotics which have bactericidal activity against the particular organism in vitro. In this situation, the phagocytic activity of exogenous granulocytes can be lifesaving. One or two leukapheresis products are transfused daily for 4 to 7 days. Complications include respiratory distress from leukoagglutination, transmission of cytomegalovirus, and rapid alloimmunization. Pulmonary infiltrates may worsen as granulocytes migrate into infected lung tissues.

Soft Silastic right atrial catheters (e.g., double-lumen Hickman or Groshong) which tunnel under the skin and enter the innominate vein can become infected. Although most gram-negative bacteremias can be treated successfully in a granulocytopenic patient by antibiotics alone without removing the catheter, gram-positive infections or candidal infections of the tunnel or vein may require catheter removal.

Typhlitis is a necrotizing enterocolitis of the terminal ileum, appendix, cecum, and right colon which occurs in granulocytopenic patients. Symptoms and signs are similar to those of inflammatory bowel disease: nausea, vomiting, abdominal pain and tenderness, profuse watery or bloody diarrhea, and fever. The intestinal mucosa is ulcerated, allowing invasion of enteric organisms into and through the bowel wall. Ileus and bowel dilation result. Plasma proteins and electrolytes are lost into the bowel lumen as occurs with toxic megacolon. Bowel perforation and peritonitis may follow. Most patients are best managed with aggressive medical treatment: broad-spectrum antibiotics, transfusion of red blood cells, platelets, and fresh frozen plasma, maintenance of normal serum electrolytes (especially potassium), and bowel rest with nasogastric suction. Narcotic analgesics and paralytic agents such as diphenoxylate should be avoided because they increase the risk of ileus. Patients with clear evidence of bowel perforation require surgery; however, a granulocytopenic patient who is otherwise doing well should not necessarily undergo laparotomy for intraperitoneal free air. Antibiotic-associated pseudomembranous colitis, radiation enteritis, and graft-versus-host-disease (GVHD) are other causes of abdominal pain and bloody diarrhea in leukemia patients.

Hyperleukocytosis

A small proportion of patients with leukemia have an extraordinary elevation of circulating leukocytes. Hyperleukocytosis ($> 100,000$ blast cells/μL) is a true medical emergency, but the risks of circulatory complications begin to rise above about $50,000/\mu$L. These patients present special problems because of the rheologic effects of blast cells in the circulation of the lung, brain, and other organs, and the metabolic consequences when massive numbers of leukemia cells are destroyed simultaneously by cytoxic drugs. Leukemic myeoloblasts are considerably larger than lymphoblasts, which are in turn larger than leukemic lymphocytes; thus, the incidence of significant leukostasis is most common in chronic myelogenous leukemia (CML) in the blast phase, followed by acute myelogenous leukemia (AML), then acute lymphoblastic leukemia (ALL). In contrast, it is rare in patients with chronic lymphocytic leukemia despite white cell counts as high as $500,000/\mu L$. The large and less deformable blast cells result in increased viscosity in the microcirculation. The high oxygen consumption and invasiveness of leukemia cells may interact with slow flow through the capillaries leading to hypoxemia and vascular damage. Leukostasis and hypoxia in the capillary beds can induce respiratory distress, cardiac arrhythmias, and central nervous system (CNS) symptoms leading to coma. Death follows rapidly unless the circulation can be restored. Emergency measures include leukapheresis to remove a large mass of tumor cells directly from the bloodstream. A single efficient leukapheresis can decrease the leukocyte count by approximately 50 percent within 2 to 3 h. Prompt use of antimetabolite drugs such as oral hydroxyurea or intravenous cytarabine can rapidly reduce cell proliferation and transiently decrease the blast count. A single dose of cranial irradiation can ameliorate CNS symptoms due to leukostasis. Pulmonary infiltrates and respiratory distress may also respond to thoracic irradiation. Prophylactic platelet transfusions must be given to prevent bleeding as the circulation is restored to hypoxic tissues. Red blood cell transfusions can precipitate a hyperviscosity syndrome in a patient with hyperleukocytosis and should be delayed if possible until the white blood cell count falls.

Care must be taken to rule out "pseudohypoxemia" which results from the in vitro consumption of oxygen within an arterial blood-gas sample by blast cells in transit to the laboratory. Such blood specimens should be rapidly transported on ice. Rarely, marked thrombocytosis can produce a similar artifact in addition to pseudohyperkalemia.

ANEMIA, THROMBOCYTOPENIA, AND DISSEMINATED INTRAVASCULAR COAGULATION (DIC)

Red blood cell transfusions are given to maintain a hematocrit of approximately 30 percent. Platelets should be transfused prophylactically to maintain a platelet count $>20,000/\mu L$ to decrease the risk of spontaneous hemorrhage such as a stroke or gastrointestinal bleeding. No salicylates or other drugs which interfere with platelet function should be given nor should intramuscular injections be given to a thrombocytopenic patient. The use of single-donor platelets collected by apheresis will decrease the rate of alloimmunization in leukemia patients. Patients who become alloimmunized may require human leukocyte antigen (HLA)-matched platelets or antibody crossmatched platelets to achieve adequate post-transfusion platelet counts.

Laboratory evidence of DIC is almost always present at diagnosis in patients with acute promyelocytic leukemia (APL), but it can accompany any leukemia or infection where there is rapid cell lysis or tissue destruction. Management of DIC is always directed at correcting the underlying tissue destruction. In the meantime, the consumption of coagulation proteins by fibrin formation and its associated secondary fibrinolysis can be rapidly brought under control using heparin. A continuous infusion of heparin at 5 U/kg/h is well tolerated even in thrombocytopenic patients and allows fresh frozen plasma or cryoprecipitate to be transfused safely without concern about adding substrate for renewed intravascular coagulation.

Cryoprecipitate infusions should be used to maintain the fibrinogen concentration at 100 mg/dL. If after 24 h of heparin therapy the fibrinogen has not stabilized and the fibrin degradation products level has not decreased, the heparin infusion may be increased to 10 U/kg/h.

TISSUE INFILTRATION

When the vascular leptomeninges surrounding the brain and spinal cord are infiltrated by malignant cells, leukemia cells can often be found in the cerebrospinal fluid by lumbar puncture. Cranial neuropathy and spinal radiculopathy result from impingement upon these nerves as they traverse narrow bony foramina by an expanding mass of leukemia cells. The most frequent symptoms in patients with overt CNS leukemia are those caused by increased intracranial pressure: vomiting, headache, papilledema, and lethargy. Mass lesions within the brain substance itself or within the spinal cord are not common, and seizures are rarely present. Meningismus is also uncommon, and its presence suggests infection or subarachnoid hemorrhage. The diagnosis is established by finding leukemia cells in the CSF. Usually, the CSF pressure is elevated in symptomatic patients, the glucose concentration is low, and the protein concentration is moderately elevated. In thrombocytopenic patients, transfusion of platelets to >20,000/μL should be administered and any coagulopathy corrected prior to LP. CNS leukemia is usually rapidly responsive to irradiation or intrathecal chemotherapy. Dexamethasone (16 mg/day) can alleviate symptoms of increased intracranial pressure. Cord involvement is best treated with intrathecal methotrexate.

Renal insufficiency is a frequent complication of acute leukemia and its treatment and may result from a variety of insults including infiltration of kidneys by leukemia cells, ureteral obstruction by enlarged retroperitoneal lymph nodes, and urate nephropathy. In leukemia patients, the production of organic acids together with decreased urine formation from dehydration due to anorexia or fever frequently leads to precipitation of urates within the renal tubules and collecting system leading to obstruction. Effective management of hyperuricemia and hyperuricosuria in leukemia patients is based on reducing the production of uric acid and at the same time promoting the solubility of uric acid in the urine. An adequate urine flow (100 mL/h) should be established by oral or intravenous hydration. The blood volume must be expanded and acidosis corrected. Acetazolamide, a carbonic anhydrase inhibitor, can be given together with sodium bicarbonate to alkalinize the urine. Allopurinol (300 mg/day) will effectively inhibit the conversion of xanthine and hypoxanthine to uric acid. Once the tumor cell mass has been reduced, these measures can be safely discontinued.

The Oncologic Emergencies

Phillip Factor

Complications of malignancies are an increasingly common problem. As therapeutic advances continue and the survival of cancer patients improves management of oncologic emergencies will become increasingly common in the critical care setting. The nature and complexity of problems that arise in cancer patients require that differential diagnosis be expanded to include etiologies not otherwise seen in patients without cancer. Table 53-1 lists abbreviated differential diagnoses of common signs and symptoms seen in cancer patients.

THORACIC SYNDROMES

Superior Vena Cava Syndrome

Superior vena cava (SVC) obstruction typically occurs due to one or more of the following mechanisms: **1.** external compression, **2.**

TABLE 53-1 Differential Diagnosis for Common Signs and Symptoms in Cancer Patients

Sign/Symptom	Differential Diagnosis
Nausea and Vomiting	Hypercalcemia
	Renal failure
	Brain metastases or herniation
	Leptomeningeal carcinomatosis
	Liver metastases
Abnormal mental status	Hypercalcemia
	Hyponatremia
	Renal Failure
	Sepsis
	Leptomeningeal carcinomatosis
	Brain metastases or herniation
Hemodynamic instability	Pulmonary embolism
	Pericardial tamponade
	Pericardial constriction
	Brain herniation
	Superior vena cava syndrome
Renal failure	Hypercalcemia
	Tumor lysis syndrome; hyperuricemia
	Obstruction
	Paraneoplastic changes
	Glomerulonephritis

(Reprinted with permission from Gradishar WJ, Hoffman PC: The Oncologic Emergencies, in Hall JB, Schmidt GA, Wood LDH: Principles of Critical Care, McGraw-Hill, New York, 1992.)

invasion of the SVC wall by tumor, or **3.** external compression with subsequent luminal thrombosis. Right sided, centrally located (perihilar) lung cancers account for the majority (52 to 81 percent) of cases of SVC obstruction (most commonly anaplastic small cell carcinoma). Non-Hodgkin's lymphoma (2 to 15 percent of cases) is also a common etiology (particularly diffuse large cell and lympho-blastic lymphomas), although Hodgkin's disease is an uncommon cause. Rare causes include tumors metastatic to the mediastinum (e.g., breast) and primary mediastinal tumors (germ-cell tumors, thymomas). SVC thrombosis also can be due to central venous catheterization in these patients.

Patients with SVC obstruction most commonly complain of dyspnea, although they may also note signs of increased central venous pressure such as headache, dizziness, blurry vision and a sensation of fullness of the head. Less commonly they may com-plain of dysphagia, dysphonia, cough and chest pain. Signs of obstruction may include venous distention in the neck and chest wall, facial swelling, upper extremity edema, cyanosis and facial plethora. Signs of subtotal obstruction may be subtle, especially early in the course. Chest x-ray may show widening of the medi-astinum, a right hilar or mediastinal mass, or pleural effusions. Computed tomography with contrast infusion can delineate the site and extent of obstruction. Contrast and radionuclide venogra-phy are also useful and may provide additional information re-garding collateralization. In clinically stable patients treatment of SVC syndrome may be delayed pending definitive diagnosis. Therapeutic measures should be directed at palliation of signs and symptoms as well as cure whenever possible. Supportive measures should include treatment of hypoxemia, elevation of the head and steroids (e.g., dexamethasone 4 mg every 6 h) when malignancy is the suspected etiology. Diuretics may be useful in selected patients.

Specific treatment of SVC syndrome will depend on etiology. Small cell carcinoma frequently responds to combined chemother-apy and radiation. Chemotherapy may produce resolution of ve-nous obstruction in patients with aggressive lymphomas. In patients who either have no histologic diagnosis or a malignancy other than small cell or lymphoma, radiation is the principal form of therapy. Administration of 4000 to 6000 Gy produces symptomatic relief in 90 percent of patients. Utilization of high initial doses (e.g., 400 Gy × 3 to 4 fractions) may produce prompter symptomatic relief, but probably does not impact on survival.

SVC obstruction due to central venous catheters can be treated with thrombolytics. The catheter should be removed after systemic heparinization to ameliorate manifestations of pulmonary emboli which can be shed from the catheter tip.

The overall prognosis of this condition depends on the underlying etiology of the SVC obstruction.

Pericardial Disease

Pericardial involvement is a common complication of malignancy and its treatment and must be considered in any cancer patient with hemodynamic instability. Symptoms of pericardial disease may mimic other conditions that occur in cancer patients.

Approximately 5 percent of patients with malignancy have pericardial seeding, although the majority have no clinical evidence of pericardial disease. Lung and breast carcinoma are the most common etiologies, although esophageal carcinoma, lymphoma, leukemia (esp. lymphocytic), and melanomas also involve the pericardium. Pericardial involvement can occur by direct extension or more commonly via lymphangitic spread and rarely by hematogenous spread.

Large pericardial effusions develop slowly, allowing for gradual stretching of the pericardium. These patients may present with signs of compression of mediastinal structures (hoarseness, cough, dysphagia) or increased central venous pressures (sensation of fullness in the head, vague abdominal complaints such as fullness, nausea, pain due to stretching of the liver capsule). Dyspnea may be present if the cardiac output is diminished. Precise delineation of the cause of a patient's symptoms is important as treatment can vary greatly.

Diagnosis requires a high index of suspicion (circulatory failure in patients with malignancy). Patients with tamponade typically present with distant heart sounds, hypotension, elevated central venous pressure (Beck's triad), tachycardia, narrow arterial pulse pressure, and a pulsus paradoxus exceeding 10 mmHg. Pulmonary congestion and ventricular gallops are distinctly uncommon. A large cardiac silhouette in the absence of pulmonary edema on chest x-ray should suggest the diagnosis. Right atrial pressure tracings may demonstrate loss of the y descent and a prominent x descent suggestive of impaired venous filling.

The electrocardiogram may show signs of pericarditis, low voltage, or electrical alternans (beat to beat variation of electrical axis). Echocardiography is the most sensitive diagnostic modality and may provide data regarding hemodynamic significance of the effusion (right atrial and ventricular diastolic collapse, loss of normal respirophasic changes or enlargement of the inferior vena cava). Pulmonary artery catheterization may show equalization (< 5 mmHg variation) of the central venous pressure (CVP), right ventricular (RV) diastolic, and pulmonary capillary wedge pressures.

Treatment of patients with tamponade hinges on reduction of pericardial pressure. Hemodynamic compromise may be temporized by administration of fluids. Pressor agents may further compromise cardiac output by increasing heart rate and further limiting diastolic filling. Rapid clinical deterioration mandates emergent pericardiocentesis. Blind subxiphoid approaches can be complicated by arrhythmias, laceration of coronary arteries and sudden death. Computerized tomography (CT) or echocardiographic guidance should be employed whenever possible. Pericardial decompression should be done slowly to prevent sudden increases in right ventricular output and acute pulmonary edema. The fluid is usually exudative; in addition to cytologic analysis, culture should be performed to rule out infectious etiologies. For patients with recurring or thick effusions tube pericardiostomy should be considered. This will also allow for obliteration of the pericardial space with sclerosing agents. Patients not responding to conservative treatment and who have a relatively long life expectancy (e.g., breast cancer) should be considered for pericardiectomy.

In constrictive pericarditis, a noncompliant thickened, pericardium limits diastolic filling and cardiac output. Patients present with the gradual development of salt and water retention (ascites, edema, dyspnea, orthopnea). Radiation therapy is the most common cause in cancer patients (typically lung and breast carcinoma, Hodgkin's disease) and may develop 6 to 30 months after initiation of radiation therapy. The central venous pressure will be elevated with a rapid y descent with rapid rebound. Central veins may not collapse with inspiration (Kussmaul's sign). A large cardiac silhouette is noted in approximately 50 percent of patients. Electrocardiogram (ECG) findings are non-specific but may include atrial fibrillation in long standing cases. Echocardiography may show pericardial thickening and doppler echocardiography may reveal altered patterns of ventricular filling (rapid deceleration of filling velocity). Cardiac catheterization will show equalization of pressures and an early dip in ventricular filling pressures (square root sign) due to rapid diastolic filling. Pericardiectomy is the treatment of choice if long term survival is anticipated.

Occasionally patients will present with radiation induced effusive-constrictive pericarditis. Signs and symptoms are those of cardiac tamponade. Treatment following stabilization should include pericardiectomy.

NEUROLOGIC SYNDROMES

Spinal Cord Compression (SCC)

Clinical evidence of this condition occurs in 5 percent of oncology patients. Vague symptoms in complex patients can present a diagnostic challenge, especially in intubated, sedated ICU patients. Prevention of permanent neurologic sequelae depends on prompt diagnosis and treatment. SCC typically occurs in patients with known widespread disease. SCC is rarely a presenting manifestation. SCC occurs most frequently in the setting of lung cancer but is also seen with multiple myeloma, prostate cancer, lymphoma, melanoma, breast and cancers of unknown primary.

Cord compression usually results from direct extension of a vertebral based mass into the epidural space. Intervertebral space invasion, compromised vascular supply and vertebral body collapse are other mechanisms responsible for spinal cord injury. Pain localized to the spine or paravertebral area is the most common symptom and may precede neurologic signs by weeks or months. Dermatomal or radicular pain, weakness of the extremities, or loss of pain and temperature sensation below the level of pain should raise the specter of SCC. As compression progresses to involve autonomic fibers altered bowel and bladder function develop. These signs can be masked in ICU patients by sedation, bladder catheterization, or other causes for diarrhea and constipation. A high level of suspicion coupled with daily neurologic evaluations must be employed in this setting.

Suspicion of SCC should prompt immediate therapy and further investigation. Dexamethasone should be promptly initiated and continued until definitive therapy is completed to reduce edema surrounding the spinal cord. Routine spinal x-rays will confirm the location of epidural metastases in most patients. Magnetic resonance imaging (MRI) or CT myelography is required to confirm the diagnosis. Surgery and radiation therapy remain the mainstay for treatment of SCC. Early therapy is essential. The likelihood of response to treatment depends on neurologic function at the time of diagnosis. Patients ambulatory at presentation have a 65 to 80 percent of remaining so. Paraplegic patients have little chance of recovering neurologic function. The morbidity associated with either radiation or surgery outweighs the likelihood of regaining lower extremity function in these patients. Decompressive laminectomy is indicated for patients without confirmed malignancy, bone impinging on the cord, tumors known to be radioresistant, and in areas of previous irradiation. Radiation therapy can be used following surgical decompression or for tumors known to be radiosensitive in the setting of a stable spinal column.

Cerebral Herniation

Herniation of cerebral contents can be brought about by primary or metastatic tumors. Cancers arising from lung, breast, kidney and skin (melanoma) account for most CNS metastases. A mass lesion and surrounding edema produce increased intracranial pressure that must be offset by redistribution of intracranial contents, i.e., herniation of the brain through the tentorium or foramen magnum. Three important herniation syndromes are temporal lobe-tentorial, transtentorial, and cerebellar-foramen magnum.

Temporal lobe mass lesions can result in herniation of the uncus through the tentorium cerebri, laterally displacing the midbrain, compressing the contralateral oculomotor nerve and pyramidal tracts. As herniation progresses symptoms will become bilateral and loss of brainstem function occurs. Loss of third nerve function will affect oculovestibular and oculocephalic reflexes in comatose patients.

Transtentorial herniation results in compression of the diencephalon and brainstem. As herniation proceeds retrocaudal progression of symptoms is seen: altered levels of consciousness with progression to coma, irregular respiratory patterns (or Cheyne-Stokes), and small reactive pupils. These signs are followed by decorticate posturing, fixed midposition pupils, and loss of oculocephalic and oculovestibular reflexes. In the final stages the patient will have flaccid paralysis, fixed pupils and shallow respirations.

Cerebellar-foramen magnum herniation typically occurs in the presence of posterior fossa masses but may also be seen with large frontal lesions. Compression of the medulla results in respiratory arrest, loss of consciousness, opisthotonos, bradycardia (or tachycardia), and loss of deep tendon reflexes.

Treatment of presumed herniation syndromes should be based on clinical suspicion and not be delayed pending confirmatory studies. Lumbar puncture must be postponed to prevent acceleration of herniation. Treatment should be directed at reduction of intracranial pressure. Cautious intubation and mechanical ventilation with intentional hyperventilation (P_{CO_2} 25 to 30 mmHg) will decrease cerebral blood flow transiently (6 to 12 h) and should be continued as long as intracranial pressure (ICP) remains elevated to prevent rebound ICP elevations. Intravascular volume depletion should be employed to diminish further edema accumulation. Mannitol (0.25 to 0.50 gm/Kg as needed) has been the traditional choice although furosemide is a reasonable alternative. Dexamethasone is indicated where vasogenic edema is suspected (e.g., mass lesions). Following stabilization, the patient should be evaluated for radiation therapy and surgical decompression.

LEPTOMENINGEAL CARCINOMATOSIS

Certain lymphomas (high grade non-Hodgkin's), leukemias (ALL, AML, CLL), and solid tumors (breast, colon, gastric, melanoma) have a propensity for spread to the meninges. Meningeal involvement typically is detected in the setting of widespread disease. Symptoms may be non-specific but commonly include headache; personality changes, altered mental status, memory loss, hallucinations, confusion and dementia may be seen. Meningeal signs are common. Radiculopathies (urinary incontinence, paresthesias, weakness) and cranial neuropathies (especially CN III and VI) also occur. Cranial nerve palsies in patients with lymphoma or leukemia in the absence of other structural causes should be assumed to indicate leptomeningeal involvement.

Diagnosis is made by cytologic examination of the cerebrospinal fluid (CSF). Multiple samples (7 to 10ml $\times$ 4) may be required for diagnosis. Cytocentrifugation and filtration may facilitate detection of tumor cells. Elevated CSF pressure and protein, low CSF glucose and a monocytic pleocytosis should suggest the diagnosis. CT and MRI may be useful in demonstrating tumor implants if the CSF is without tumor cells.

Treatment consists of intrathecal administration of appropriate chemotherapeutics via repeated lumbar punctures or an Ommaya reservoir. Radiation can be used as primary or adjunctive therapy and should be directed to locations thought to be responsible for the patient's symptoms. Treatment may provide palliation in 40 to 50 percent of patients. Overall prognosis is that expected of a patient with a widespread malignancy.

METABOLIC SYNDROMES

Hypercalcemia

Hypercalcemia in malignancy occurs via direct bone metastasis, tumor cytokine production (osteoclast activating factor), secretion of parathyroid-like hormones (PTH) and tumor induced elevations of 1,25-dihydroxycholecalciferol. Differentiation from primary hyperparathyroidism can be difficult. A low or normal immunoreactive PTH level usually excludes the diagnosis of primary hyperparathyroidism.

Symptoms of this condition are often nonspecific but may include fatigue, lethargy, polydipsia, polyuria, muscle weakness, nausea, and vomiting. The extent of clinical manifestations depends on the acuity of the hypercalcemia. Patients with chronic elevations may be completely asymptomatic. Signs of hypercalcemia include long PR and short QT intervals, renal insufficiency, obtundation/coma, seizures, hyporeflexia, adynamic ileus, bradycardia, and atrial and ventricular arrhythmias.

Treatment should be directed at restoration of intravascular volume, decreasing further bone resorption, increasing renal calcium excretion and treating the underlying malignancy. Restoration of intravascular volume using normal saline will limit further proximal tubular calcium resorption and allow enhanced excretion of calcium in the distal tubule. Loop diuretics are useful in preventing hypernatremia and pulmonary edema and to enhance calciuresis. However their use should be avoided until intravascular volume has been completely restored. Table 53-2 lists currently available therapeutic agents for the treatment of hypercalcemia. Recent studies have suggested that gallium nitrate may be the most effective agent for the treatment of hypercalcemia of malignancy.

Syndrome of Inappropriate Antidiuretic Hormone Secretion (SIADH)

Hyponatremia in oncology patients is frequently multifactorial. SIADH must be considered in the presence of a euvolemic patient with hypoosmolar hyponatremia provided that there is no clinical or laboratory evidence of adrenal insufficiency, hypothyroidism, renal insufficiency, or edema forming disorders. SIADH in these patients may be due to ectopic production of ADH (small cell carcinoma), drugs that mimic ADH activity, or conditions that stimulate its release from the posterior pituitary (e.g., cyclophos-

TABLE 53-2 Currently Available Drugs for the Treatment of Hypercalcemia

1. Normal Saline infusion	250–500mL/h	1. Replace K+, Mg+ losses 2. Observe cardio-pulmonary status 3. Consider diuretics to enhance calciuresis
2. Mithramycin	25 ug/kg (bolus infusion or IV over 2–4 h)	1. Repeat dose every 3–4 days 2. Increased toxicity with multiple doses
3. Calcitonin	8 IU/kg IM or SC every 6–12 h	
4. Diphosphonates (i.e., etidronate disodium)	7.5 mg/kg/day in 250–500 mL of normal saline infused over 2–3 h for 3 days	
5. Inorganic phosphates	Not recommended	
6. Prednisone or hydrocortisone	20–40 mg PO daily 100–150 mg IV every 12 h	
7. Gallium Nitrate	200 mg/m^2/day for 5 days, continuous infusion	

Reprinted with permission from Gradishar WJ, Hoffman PC: The Oncologic Emergencies, in Hall JB, Schmidt GA, Wood LDH: Principles of Critical Care, McGraw-Hill, New York, 1992.)

phamide, vincristine). Laboratory investigations typically reveal a urine $Na^+ > 20$ meq/L and a high urine osmolality (>500 mOsm/kg) in the face of a normal or low serum osmolality (<280 mOsm/kg). Symptoms of SIADH depend on the degree of hyponatremia and the rapidity of its development and are not different from other causes of hyponatremia.

Therapy for SIADH should focus on elimination of the tumor when possible. Patients with severe, symptomatic hyponatremia (< 120 meg/L) require prompt correction to 120 to 125 meq/L. This may best be achieved by administration of 3% NaCl and a loop diuretic. The administration of 0.9% NaCl may worsen the hyponatremia. Less severe hyponatremia can be treated with free water restriction, demeclocycline, or lithium carbonate (see Chapter 56). Oral urea (10 to 60 g/day) has also proven effective.

Lactic Acidosis

Lactic acidosis is an infrequently encountered disorder in patients with large tumor burdens. It is most frequently noted in patients with leukemias, rapidly growing lymphomas and rarely solid tumors. It tends to occur in patients with significant liver involvement.

Diagnosis hinges on the exclusion of other etiologies for lactic acidosis. Treatment is controversial as bicarbonate therapy has been shown to adversely affect patient outcome in other clinical settings. The mainstay of treatment is reduction of tumor burden (e.g., chemotherapy). Lactic acidosis may be an indication for emergent administration of chemotherapy.

TUMOR LYSIS SYNDROME

The administration of chemotherapeutic agents to patients with exquisitely chemosensitive tumors (leukemias, Burkitt's lymphoma, rarely solid tumors) can result in the sudden release of tumor cell contents into the bloodstream. This is characterized by hyperuricemia, hyperkalemia, hyperphosphatemia, and hypocalcemia. The development of cardiac arrhythmias due to electrolyte imbalance and renal failure due to hyperuricemia present the principal life-threatening complications.

Management of these patients should begin prior to initiation of chemotherapy and should include: **1.** aggressive hydration to maintain urine output of at least 100 to 200 mL/h; **2.** allopurinol, 300 to 600 mg/day; and **3.** alkalinization of the urine (pH 7 to 7.5). Alkalinization should be halted once serum uric acid normalizes to prevent further calcium phosphate salt formation and aggravation of hypocalcemia. Dialysis should be initiated early for patients with worsening renal function, congestive heart failure, hyperkalemia

(>6 meq/L), hyperphosphatemia (>10 mg/dL) or hyperuricemia (>10 mg/dL).

UROLOGIC EMERGENCIES

Hematuria in oncology patients can occur from causes that affect the general population (e.g., infection, nephrolithiasis, glomerulonephritis). The clinical manifestation, evaluation and treatment of these conditions should not differ from patients without cancer.

Hematuria due to cyclophosphamide induced hemorrhagic cystitis is a frequently encountered problem (10 to 70 percent of patients receiving high dose treatment). Bleeding, due to urothelial breakdown, typically occurs during or shortly after infusion but may occur months later. Urothelial damage can be limited by prophylactic hydration to maintain urine output and frequent voiding limits exposure of the bladder to the toxic metabolites of cyclophosphamide (acrolein). An acrolein scavenger, 2-mercaptoethane sulfonate, may also be useful. Management should include discontinuation of cyclophosphamide, volume repletion, and urologic consultation.

Urinary Tract Obstruction

Obstructive uropathy must be considered in cancer patients with acute and/or progressive azotemia. Unilateral ureteral obstruction is most often asymptomatic and may not be associated with a rise in serum creatinine. Bilateral upper urinary tract (above the level of the bladder) obstruction can occur in the presence of retroperitoneal tumors (e.g., lymphomas, sarcomas), pelvic masses, bladder tumors that affect both ureters, or retroperitoneal fibrosis due to radiation or chemotherapy.

Lower urinary tract obstruction may occur secondary to urethral compression (e.g., prostate carcinoma) or bladder outlet obstruction (intra- or extra-vesicular masses).

An empty bladder and anuria suggest an upper urinary tract etiology. CT can be used to localize the level of obstruction (upper vs. lower). Cystoscopy is useful for evaluating urethral and bladder outlet obstructions.

Treatment should be directed at preservation of renal function by prompt resolution of the obstruction, often by percutaneous placement of nephrostomy tubes. Long term treatments include placement of ureteral stents or ureteral diverting procedures. Lower tract obstruction may require suprapubic cystostomy if urethral catheterization is not feasible. Ileal conduits or surgical dilation of the bladder can also be used in appropriate settings. It should be kept in mind that the obstruction may resolve in the course of treating the underlying malignancy.

Hyperuricemic Nephropathy

Massive tumor lysis can result in serum uric acid concentrations that exceed the kidneys' ability to clear uric acid. In this setting uric acid crystals may precipitate in the renal tubules, collecting ducts, and pyramids potentially leading to acute renal failure. The risk of renal failure becomes significant at a serum level of 20 mg/dL. Anticipation and prophylaxis (hydration, alkalinization, allopurinol) are the most effective therapeutic modalities for this condition. Treatment of patients who develop acute renal failure should focus on clearing uric acid stones from the urinary tract. This may entail ureteral and medullary lavage via nephrostomy tubes or ureteral cannulation. Anuric patients require dialysis pending return of renal function.

For further reading in *Principles of Critical Care,* see Chap 149 "The Oncologic Emergencies" William W. Gradishar/Philip C Hoffman

Phillip Cozzi

Acute renal failure (ARF) is the abrupt loss of the ability to clear nitrogenous waste through the kidneys. The incidence of ARF in the ICU setting is 10 to 30 percent with mortality as high as 20 to 80 percent. The differential diagnosis includes prerenal, renal, and postrenal causes.

Prerenal azotemia is the most common cause of hospital-acquired ARF, accounting for approximately 50 percent of cases. The usual contributors include hypovolemia, hypotension, and heart failure. Postrenal causes are found in 1 to 15 percent of hospital-acquired cases of ARF. It is particularly important to identify these cases because they are often potentially reversible. Nephrolithiasis, malignancy, inflammatory processes, neurogenic bladder, ureteral dysfunction, and obstructed urinary catheter are the common contributors. Intrarenal causes of obstruction (blockage of tubules) should also be considered, including Bence-Jones protein deposition, as well as crystalline deposition of uric acid, methotrexate, and acyclovir.

The remaining cases of ARF, once pre- and postrenal causes have been excluded, are due to direct injury of the renal parenchyma. Processes involving the vasculature include the hemolytic uremic syndrome, scleroderma, malignant hypertension, vasculitis and thrombus. Interstitial injury is often drug-induced or associated with infection. Acute tubular necrosis (ATN) is the most common cause of intrinsic ARF in the ICU setting. Predisposing factors include prolonged prerenal azotemia, nephrotoxins, and pigmenturia, in the common clinical settings of major surgery, trauma, and sepsis.

APPROACH TO DIAGNOSIS

In most cases, the cause of ARF can be identified by history and physical examination alone. The history should focus on the identification of predisposing conditions, as described above. A detailed drug history is essential. If thoracic complaints accompany ARF, Goodpasture's syndrome, Wegener's granulomatosis, systemic lupus erythematosis, and Churg-Strauss syndrome should be considered. Flank pain and hematuria often accompany obstructive renal disease.

Physical examination includes a careful assessment of extracellular fluid volume status with orthostatic blood pressure measurements. Mottling of extremities, dry mucous membranes and skin tenting are also useful clues to volume status. Palpably enlarged kidneys, pelvic or abdominal mass, bladder enlargement, and prostatic hypertrophy suggest an obstructive etiology of ARF.

Diagnostic tests begin with careful measurement of urine flow. In the ICU setting, this is best accomplished with use of an indwelling bladder catheter. Bladder catherization can be both diagnostic and therapeutic in patients with urethral obstruction. Urinalysis is also essential to diagnosis of ARF. Specific gravity > 1.020 suggests prerenal failure; proteinuria suggests glomerular injury; glycosuria suggests proximal tubular injury. Hematuria is consistent with a variety of diagnoses. The presence of blood on dipstick, but not microscopically, is consistent with a pigment nephropathy (hemoglobinuria or myoglobinuria). Eosinophiluria suggests drug-induced tubulointerstitial nephritis. A urine sodium less than 10 meq/L and a fractional excretion of sodium less than 1 percent are consistent with prerenal azotemia. Several radiologic studies including plain films, ultrasound, CT, radionuclide scans, and retrograde pyelography can be useful adjuncts in the diagnosis of ARF.

CLINICAL SYNDROMES OF ARF

Prerenal Azotemia

The major signs and diagnostic tests for prerenal azotemia have been mentioned previously. It is important to recognize that prerenal azotemia can occur in the setting of total body fluid overload, as in cirrhosis and hypoalbuminemia. Approach to treatment should focus on halting ongoing fluid loss and repleting intravascular volume. A diagnostic and therapeutic fluid challenge of 1L of isotonic saline over 30 min can be helpful. The utility of concomitant albumin and furosemide is limited by the short half-life of intravenously administered albumin.

Postischemic/Septic ARF

Major surgery and massive trauma are predisposing factors to this form of ARF. Hypoperfusion, pigmenturia, antibiotic use, radiographic contrast use, and vasopressors act synergistically to injure the kidneys. The clinical features include oliguria, cellular debris on urinalysis, and fractional excretion of sodium greater than 3 percent.

Nephrotoxic ARF

Risk factors for aminoglycoside nephrotoxicity include advanced age, preexisting renal disease, volume depletion, obstructive jaundice and severe infection. Drug levels should be monitored; an increase in plasma trough drug levels on a constant dose is a sensitive marker for aminoglycoside toxicity. With the expanding armamentarium of antibiotics, aminoglycosides can often be avoided.

Risk factors for radiocontrast nephrotoxicity include preexisting renal failure, diabetes mellitus, hypovolemia, high contrast dose, congestive heart failure and advanced age. The clinical course is characterized by a rapid increase in serum creatinine concentration within 24 to 48h; the fractional excretion of sodium is usually less than 1 percent. Major therapeutic emphasis is on prevention. Volume expansion using saline or mannitol should be performed prior to contrast administration in high-risk groups.

Cancer chemotherapeutics are important causes of ARF. The most common offending agents include cisplatin, the nitrosoureas, and methotrexate. Nonsteroidal anti-inflammatory drugs can result in acute renal failure through inhibition of vasodilatory prostaglandin secretion or through allergic-type tubulointerstitial nephritis.

Thrombotic Microangiopathies

Hemolytic-uremic syndrome and thrombotic thrombocytopenic purpura are associated with ARF. Disseminated intravascular coagulation is associated with cortical necrosis. Malignant hypertension results in glomerular microthrombus formation and subsequent fibrinoid necrosis.

Tumor Lysis Syndrome

When germ cell tumors or hematologic malignancies with large tumor burdens undergo tumor lysis associated with chemotherapy administration, a nephropathy may result from the toxic effects of the intracellular contents. Acute urate nephropathy and intratubular crystallization of phosphate act synergistically with acidosis and hypovolemia to injure the kidneys. Renal function improves with hemodialysis. Allopurinol and alkalinization are effective prophylactic measures.

Hepatobiliary Disease and ARF

Liver disease may result in prerenal azotemia by ascitic redistribution of intravascular volume, emesis, and excessive diuresis. A specific glomerular lesion, called cirrotic glomerulosclerosis, has been identified. Obstructive nephropathy from blood clots in the collecting system or papillary necrosis also is associated with liver injury. Hepatorenal syndrome is the most serious coexistent hepatic and renal disease. Prerenal azotemia that does not respond to volume repletion is a good operational definition of hepatorenal syndrome. Oliguria and a low fractional excretion of sodium are typical. Therapeutics have been disappointing.

PREVENTION OF ACUTE RENAL FAILURE

Prevention of acute renal failure begins with identification of patients at risk. Risk factors for ARF include preexistant chronic renal failure, hypovolemia, diabetes mellitus, advanced age, CHF, urinary tract infection, major surgery, and prior history of ARF. Pharmacologic intervention can include diuretics and low-dose dopamine. Mannitol and loop diuretics may reduce vasospasm and protect some nephron segments. High flow rates produced by these drugs may prevent nephron obstruction. Mannitol is most useful in the setting of radiocontrast administration. Once ARF is established, these drugs are less efficacious, though modest benefits have been described.

In low doses (<5 microgram/kg/min), dopamine is used in the treatment of ARF. Some patients will convert from an oliguric to a nonoliguric state. Dopamine alone, however, has not been shown to improve mortality from ARF. Furosemide in combination with dopamine is more effective in raising urine output than either agent alone.

THERAPY OF ARF

All potentially reversible causes of ARF should be excluded or treated. In addition, the patient should be carefully monitored for detection of complications. Particular attention should be paid to blood pressure, intravascular volume, electrolytes, nutrition, and acid-base status. Fluid intake should be adjusted to replace urine and insensible losses. A small reduction in weight is expected in ARF because of severe catabolism; weight gain indicates volume expansion.

Hyponatremia is common in ARF, due to administration of excessive amounts of free water. Hyperkalemia in ARF can be life threatening. Therapy should include calcium gluconate, sodium bicarbonate, glucose with 10 units of regular insulin IV, and Kayexalate®. Hyperphosphatemia is typical of oliguric ARF. Oral administration of aluminum hydroxide gels controls hyperphosphatemia. Hypocalcemia is also common, though rarely of clinical significance. Metabolic acidosis occurs commonly in ARF. Although the additional volume may be hazardous to the patient, acidosis may be cautiously treated with sodium bicarbonate; severe acidosis may mandate dialysis.

Since infection has been the cause of death in up to 70 percent of cases of ARF, monitoring for signs of infection is essential. Intraabdominal sepsis, in particular, is an important contributor to mortality in ARF patients, and must be vigorously excluded. In prior years gastrointestinal hemorrhage was a common cause of death in ARF patients. Since the advent of stress ulcer prophylaxis with antacids and histamine receptor blockers, the incidence of this complication has markedly declined.

Indications for emergent dialysis in the ICU include volume overload, refractory hyperkalemia, profound acidosis, and complications of uremia including encephalopathy and pericarditis. In the absence of these indications, prophylactic dialysis should be initiated when the BUN value exceeds 100 mg/dL or the serum creatinine level exceeds 9 mg/dL.

For further reading in *Principles of Critical Care,* see Chap 153 "Acute Renal Failure" David M Gillum/ Stephen Brennan, Chap 154 "Rhadomyolysis and Myoglobinuria" Theodore H Lewis, Jr/Jesse B Hall

INDICATIONS FOR ULTRAFILTRATION AND DIALYSIS

Ultrafiltration is commonly used to correct volume overload, a disorder which can manifest as severe hypertension, anasarca, and pulmonary edema in patients with renal insufficiency not responsive to diuretic management. This method of intravascular fluid removal has also been used to reduce pulmonary edema due to cardiogenic and noncardiogenic causes in an effort to reduce hypoxemia when other measures fail. Ultrafiltration can also facilitate the provision of large volumes of fluid required for total parental nutrition. Dialysis is used to correct volume overload, electrolyte imbalance, symptoms of uremia, multiple metabolic derangements, or to remove toxins. Hyperkalemia represents the most common reason for acute dialysis in the intensive care unit, occurring in the setting of rhabdomyolysis, sepsis, or other types of tissue necrosis. Profound acidosis or alkalosis, hypercalcemia, hypermagnesemia, hyponatremia, and hypernatremia occasionally require hemodialysis for patients with renal impairment. Dialysis may also be used to stabilize patients with multiple metabolic derangements in preparation for general anesthesia and operative procedures in the setting of electrolyte and acid-base disorders.

Uncontrolled symptomatic uremia with anorexia, nausea, vomiting, gastrointestinal bleeding, altered mental status, seizures, stupor, or coma also requires urgent dialysis. Uremic pericarditis responds to dialysis. Abnormal platelet function, identified by an elevated bleeding time, can be treated with DDAVP, conjugated estrogens, or cryoprecipitate, but dialysis remains the first line of therapy.

Dialysis may reduce the levels of several important ingested toxins and drugs. Dialysis is effective when toxic amounts of methanol, ethylene glycol, bromide, chloral hydrate, isopropyl alcohol, or lithium are ingested. Salicylate overdose, which often causes a respiratory alkalosis, profound metabolic acidosis, tinnitus, gastrointestinal bleeding, and mental status changes is also treated with dialysis when the salicylate level is greater than 80. Generally, agents that are protein bound or have a large volume of distribution are not effectively cleared by hemodialysis.

CHOICE OF EXTRACORPOREAL THERAPY

Many alternatives for dialytic therapy are available and can be adapted to the patient's needs. The choice of therapy depends upon several factors: the specific goals of therapy for the particular patient, the clinical condition of the patient, the expertise of the physician, and the available technical support. Various options are outlined here with emphasis on the advantages and disadvantages of each.

Ultrafiltration

Intravascular volume can be reduced with one of several types of ultrafiltration. This form of therapy, however, does little to relieve the burden of toxins present in uremia and should only be performed when adequate diuresis is impossible. For the patient without hemodynamic compromise, intermittent large-volume ultrafiltration is indicated. This procedure requires all the equipment and personnel necessary for hemodialysis. In a typical ultrafiltration session, up to 6 liters of fluid may be removed over one to three h.

In the face of poor cardiac function, circulatory collapse, or sepsis, large-volume ultrafiltration may worsen hypotension and be poorly tolerated. Slow continuous ultrafiltration (SCUF) has been useful in this setting. Access to the circulation is most commonly achieved with large-bore catheters placed into the femoral artery and vein and blood is directed from the arterial limb through a high flux membrane filtration device where plasma is drawn through the filter and collected in a reservoir. (see Figure 55-1) When performed in this manner, over 15 liters can be removed from the patient in a 24 h period. Disadvantages of this technique are the requirement for systemic anticoagulation to prevent clotting of the filtration device and the risk of arterial thrombosis at the site of catheter

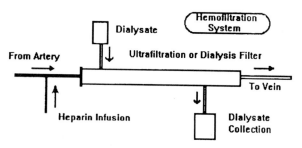

FIG. 55-1 Blood flow from the arterial limb to the venous limb is shown as it courses through the filter. Dialysate flows along the outer surface of the membrane inside the filter to create osmotic and pressure gradients to allow for the removal of intravascular volume and solutes, which are collected as demonstrated above.

placement. The filter is usually primed with 2000 IU heparin followed by a constant infusion of 10 IU/kg/h. Heparin may be omitted if there is a bleeding diathesis and good flow through the filter.

Continuous Arteriovenous Hemofiltration (CAVH)

This procedure is based upon the same principles, equipment, and personnel required for slow continuous ultrafiltration. Fluid removed during CAVH has an electrolyte composition identical to that of plasma. When euvolemia is achieved, the ultrafiltrate is replaced, on an hourly basis, with intravenous fluid. Many centers use a Ringer's solution as replacement fluid. By replacing filtered fluid, CAVH can be continued for a prolonged period in order to remove uremic toxins. Another technique, continuous arteriovenous hemofiltration dialysis (CAVHD), uses a standard artificial kidney (used for hemodialysis) instead of an ultrafiltration filter to achieve solute clearance by diffusive transport. The rate of ultrafiltration is low and not ideal for large volume removal. As each of these procedures is continued around the clock, the patient must remain in bed for long periods of time.

Hemodialysis

Hemodialysis is the most commonly used form of renal dialytic therapy in acute and chronic situations. In some clinical conditions, hemodialysis and peritoneal dialysis may be considered of equal efficacy; however, severely catabolic patients may overwhelm the clearance capabilities of peritoneal dialysis. Increased rates of urea production occur with excessive protein loads (e.g., in parenteral nutrition, gastrointestinal bleeding, or severely catabolic states, such as sepsis or multi-organ failure). In these situations, daily hemodialysis may be necessary to control azotemia, uremia, or any of the multiple electrolyte abnormalities that occur with acute renal failure. Generally, the blood urea nitrogen (BUN) concentration is reduced greater than 60 percent after a single hemodialysis session. Common complications of hemodialysis include hypotension, cardiac arrhythmias, and hypoxemia. Hypotension is thought to be secondary to volume removal, allergic reactions to the dialysis membrane, peripheral vasodilation, acute bleeding, hypocalcemia, and hypoxemia. Cardiac arrhythmias are believed to be the result of electrolyte shifts, (e.g., induced hypokalemia). Hemodialysis removes carbon dioxide thus reducing the patient's ventilatory drive. Complement is also activated as the patient's blood comes into contact with the dialysis membrane, leading to sequestration of leukocytes and release of vasoactive substances affecting ventilation/perfusion matching in the lung. Hypoventilation and $\dot{V}/\dot{Q}$

mismatch result in hypoxemia in some patients, but this is easily prevented with supplemental oxygen.

Hemodialysis requires access to the vascular space. Large-bore catheters can be placed in a femoral artery and vein for a single dialysis session and removed at the end of the procedure. Patients who require dialysis repeatedly are candidates for temporary dialysis catheters that may be inserted into the femoral, subclavian, or jugular vein at the bedside. The placement and use of these catheters is associated with a number of complications including infection, exsanguination, hemothorax, pneumothorax, and pericardial tamponade. Technical errors can also lead to potentially severe complications, such as air embolism or acute hemolysis secondary to the use of improperly prepared or contaminated dialysate. The Scribner shunt offers another form of temporary access and consists of two lengths of tubing placed within an artery and the adjacent vein and attached to dialysis apparatus. The placement of such an access requires some degree of technical expertise. These accesses function well but do have the disadvantages of destruction of the vasculature, infection, and ischemia of the distal tissue. If it is known that a patient will require hemodialysis chronically, early planning for permanent access is prudent.

Peritoneal Dialysis

Peritoneal dialysis (PD) is less efficient in the removal of small solutes and fluids than hemodialysis. It may adequately clear uremic toxins in the stable patient but the high catabolic rate of many critically ill patients as well as the formidable fluid challenges imposed upon these patients make PD less desirable. Nevertheless, in circumstances where hemodialysis cannot be safely performed, (hypotension, cardiogenic shock, acute myocardial infarction, poor vascular access), PD may be indicated. Advantages include ease of initiation and less abrupt alterations in solute concentration. Intraperitoneal catheters can be placed percutaneously by direct puncture several centimeters below the umbilicus at the midline. Chronic dialysis catheters (e.g., Tenckhoff) require placement in the operating room and are preferable to the temporary devices. The process of dialysis may be performed in one of several ways. During intermittent peritoneal dialysis, two liters of peritoneal dialysis are instilled over 10 min, permitted to dwell within the abdomen 30 min, and drained over the next 20 min. The osmolarity of the dialysate is chosen based upon the need to relieve the patient of excess intravascular volume, with a higher concentration of dextrose drawing a greater amount of intravascular volume across the peritoneum. The dwell volume may be adjusted from 1 to 3 liters as the patient tolerates. The exchanges are often performed by an automated apparatus which results in higher exchange rates than if manually performed. PD results in a urea clearance of 20 to 25 mL/min and a creatinine clearance of 12 to 20 mL/min. Once control of uremia has been obtained using this technique 24 h per day, it is sometimes possible to switch to continuous cyclic peritoneal dialysis where a cycler is used to perform exchanges over a 10 to 12 h period at night. A technique known as tidal peritoneal dialysis may improve the efficiency of intermittent peritoneal dialysis. A constant volume of dialysate remains in the peritoneal cavity and a tidal volume is circulated rapidly. Large amounts of fluid and special pumps are required which add to the expense of this modality.

Peritoneal dialysis may be made more efficient by the use of intraperitoneal or systemic vasodilators. For instance, intraperitoneal nitroprusside may double the solute clearance of larger molecules. The effect on solutes of lower molecular weight is less dramatic, and nitroprusside is rarely helpful in this application.

Complications of peritoneal dialysis include infection, (local wound and intraperitoneal), fluid leakage at the site of the catheter, metabolic derangements, and pleural effusions. Peritonitis is diagnosed by a peritoneal fluid WBC count greater than 100 per µL. Intravenous or intraperitoneal antibiotics are employed, and if there is unsatisfactory resolution over 24 to 36 h, the catheter should be removed. Hyperglycemia, postdialysis hypoglycemia, hypernatremia, and protein loss are common and should be anticipated when patients are introduced to peritoneal dialysis. Careful electrolyte and glucose monitoring is recommended for the first 4 h of dialysis and at least daily thereafter.

For further reading in *Principles of Critical Care,* see Chap 155 "Dialysis in the Critical Care Patient" Eleanor D Lederer/David M Gillum

Severe Electrolyte Disturbances

Kevin Simpson

Severe electrolyte disturbances are common in the intensive care unit and require treatment that is individualized and based upon an understanding of their pathogenesis and significance. While the various electrolyte disturbances are unique, the treatment approach to each of these disorders begins with determining if the patient is symptomatic and whether the disorder is acute or chronic.

HYPONATREMIA

Hyponatremia is of clinical importance only if it is associated with hypotonicity. Hence, serum osmolality must be directly measured and causes of pseudohyponatremia (e.g, hyperlipidemia, hyperproteinemia, and hyperglycemia) ruled out before treatment of hyponatremia is begun. Furthermore, the symptoms of hyponatremia depend on its duration and the rapidity with which it develops. Acute hyponatremia is defined as a hypotonic state that develops within 24 h, before regulation of cell volume has occurred, and is most commonly encountered in postoperative or psychiatric patients or patients receiving oxytocin or thiazide diuretics. Chronic hyponatremia is most commonly associated with diuretic use, edema-forming states, and the syndrome of inappropriate ADH secretion (SIADH). SIADH is defined as hyponatremia that occurs in the absence of any known physiologic stimulus for ADH release (especially volume depletion), and excretion of urine that is not maximally dilute (normal subjects given a water load can achieve a urinary osmolality of < 100 mOsm/l). SIADH is usually a complication of pulmonary or central nervous system diseases, or is a paraneoplastic syndrome.

The diagnostic evaluation in cases of suspected acute hyponatremia is relatively straightforward (Fig. 56-1). The most important

FIG. 56-1 Evaluation of patients with hyponatremia. Hypoosmolality must be verified by the presence of a low serum osmolality. Once true hyponatremia has been confirmed, treatment with 3% saline solution should be started in symptomatic cases. The first step in evaluation is demonstration of the presence or absence of ADH activity (i.e., high or low urinary osmolality). Once water intoxication has been excluded, appropriate causes of high ADH activity are sought. In their absence—and if thyroid, adrenal, and renal function are normal—a diagnosis of SIADH is made. *(Reprinted with permission from Brennan S, Lederer ED: Severe Electrolyte Disturbances, in Hall JB, Schmidt GA, Wood LDH: Principles of Critical Care, McGraw-Hill, New York, 1992.)*

Evaluation of Hyponatremia

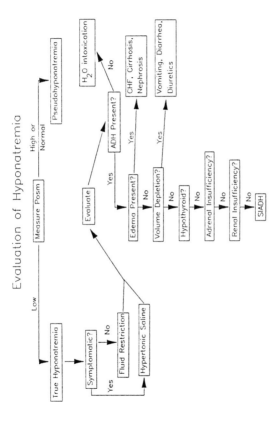

tests are the osmolality and electrolyte composition of urine and plasma. The normal range of serum osmolality is 285 to 295 mOsm/l. The documentation of a low uOsm in the face of serum hypoosmolality is virtually diagnostic of "pure" water intoxication. In SIADH, the uOsm should be less than maximally dilute (in fact, it is usually more concentrated than plasma).

Appropriate treatment of hyponatremia depends upon whether the patient is symptomatic and how quickly the hyponatremia developed. If hyponatremia is asymptomatic, appropriate treatment consists of fluid restriction and withdrawal of any offending medications. If it is symptomatic, acute hyponatremia represents a medical emergency demanding prompt therapy, even before its cause has been determined. Normal saline should be administered to correct any volume depletion, followed by hypertonic saline. Furosemide should be employed if volume overload is present. When correcting hyponatremia, the serum Na level must not be allowed to increase by more than 20 to 25 meq/L during the first 48 h of therapy under any circumstances, regardless of its initial value. A reasonable goal is to attempt to raise the serum Na concentration at the rate of 1.5 meq/L per hour. Complete correction to normal is not desirable, and hypernatremia occurring during the course of therapy is to be absolutely avoided.

HYPERNATREMIA

Acute hypernatremia is uncommon and has relatively few causes; these include water deprivation, administration of a large solute load (such as with $NaHCO_3$ administered during cardiac resuscitations), and osmotic diuretics. Chronic hypernatremia is much more common and, in addition to the causes of acute hypernatremia, includes diabetes insipidus and states of excess cortisol production. Diabetes insipidus usually presents as polyuria with plasma osmolality and sodium levels that are within, or near, the normal ranges. However, dehydration may be significant and hypernatremia extreme. Once polyuria is observed, the first task is to exclude solute diuresis. If water diuresis is identified (hypotonic polyuria), a distinction must be made between excessive water administration and a disorder of vasopressin secretion or action (primary diabetes insipidus). If the plasma sodium level is high (above 145 meq/L), primary diabetes insipidus is strongly suggested, and DDAVP should be given to distinguish neurogenic from nephrogenic forms. If DDAVP is to be administered, frequent determinations of plasma sodium and osmolality should be made to avoid water intoxication.

The diagnostic evaluation of all patients with suspected hypertonicity includes measurement of urine and plasma electrolyte levels and osmolality. Most other diagnostic testing, including water deprivation tests and hormonal determinations, can be deferred until the patient's clinical condition has stabilized.

The treatment of hypernatremia is two-pronged. The first step is to halt ongoing water losses and correct volume depletion with normal saline or blood products if indicated. This is combined with replacement of the established water deficit. The first choice of fluid should be tap water given orally or via nasogastric tube. Alternatively, 0.45% NaCl can be infused. If adequate correction does not occur with this fluid, dextrose-containing solutions may be employed. Dialysis is occasionally indicated for rapid removal of salt in patients with coexistent pulmonary edema. The desired final Na concentration (Na_f) is either 148 meq/L or a decrease from the initial sodium concentration (Na_i) of 20 to 25 meq/L, whichever is higher. The amount of water needed to induce this change is calculated as

$$\text{water (L)} = (0.6) \times (\text{weight in kg}) \times [(Na_i)/(Na_f)-1] \quad (56\text{-}1)$$

This volume can be administered at a rate predicted to decrease the plasma sodium by 1 to 1.5 meq/L per h.

HYPOKALEMIA

Hypokalemia results from either decreased intake, increased output, or shifts from the extracellular to the intracellular space. If poor intake is suspected, 24-h urinary K losses of less than 20 meq/day would be confirmatory. A random urine sample that contains less than 20 meq/L of K suggests dietary K deficiency or extrarenal K losses. Hypokalemia based on increased output, through either the urinary or the gastrointestinal tract, is more common. Gastrointestinal losses may be direct (through diarrhea), in which case the urine K excretion should be very low. The metabolic alkalosis and volume depletion accompanying vomiting will cause renal K wasting leading to urine K concentrations in excess of 20 meq/L. Other causes of renal K wasting include excess mineralocorticoid activity, diuretic use, osmotic diuresis, high urine flow rate, and alkalosis; in all these clinical settings, the spot urinary K concentration exceeds 20 meq/L and the daily K secretion exceeds 40 meq/day. In somewhat less common conditions, such as glucose and insulin infusion, β-adrenergic agonists, and bicarbonate infusion, hypokalemia results from the sudden shift of K from the extracellular to the intracellular space. In these situations the spot urine K concentration is low, indicating no evidence of renal potassium wasting. The most life-threatening potential complications of hypokalemia involve the cardiac conduction system and the neuromuscular system.

Hypokalemia characteristically produces flattening of the T wave, with the appearance of U waves on electrocardiogram (ECG), potentiates digitalis toxicity, and provokes arrhythmias. Neuromuscular complications include profound muscle weakness, occasionally resulting in respiratory failure, and rhabdomyolysis.

Treatment of hypokalemia includes K supplementation and correction of any identified underlying cause. For mild hypokalemia, oral K supplementation is generally satisfactory. For severe hypokalemia (K below 2.0 or life-threatening symptoms) intravenous K should be administered at an initial rate of 10 meq per h with frequent measurement of K levels. For life-threatening hypokalemia, intravenous K may be given at a rate of 40 meq per h, but only with continuous monitoring.

HYPERKALEMIA

An isolated elevated K value, particularly in the absence of any risk factors or clinical manifestations, should prompt a repeat K level as well as exclusion of spurious hyperkalemia secondary to in vitro hemolysis of red cells or thrombocytosis. True hyperkalemia may result from excessive intake, decreased output, and shift of K from the intracellular to the extracellular space. Excessive intake alone as a cause of hyperkalemia is extraordinarily unusual. More commonly, excessive K intake occurs in the setting of a limited capacity to excrete a K load. In these patients with decreased renal K clearance, lethal hyperkalemia may occur quickly once mechanisms of extrarenal K disposal are saturated.

The suspicion of renal excretory impairment can be confirmed by measurement of a spot urine K concentration of less than 20 meq/L in the face of hyperkalemia. Less commonly, hyperkalemia is a result of a massive shift of K from the intracellular to the extracellular space which may occur with massive cell lysis, acidosis, and severe digitalis intoxication. In these clinical conditions, the spot urine K concentration will be clearly in excess of 40 meq/L, suggesting no abnormalities in the renal excretory process.

Every clinician should recognize the ECG manifestations of hyperkalemia, as this complication is swiftly fatal. Mild degrees of hyperkalemia (5.5 to 6.0 meq/L) produce peaking of the T waves. As the degree of hyperkalemia worsens, the PR interval lengthens, the P waves disappear, and the QRS interval widens. The final event is cardiac standstill. Neuromuscular manifestations of hyperkalemia include flaccid paralysis.

Treatment of hyperkalemia depends on both the severity and the cause. For mild hyperkalemia, a thorough search for the cause of hyperkalemia, with close observation, is appropriate. Renal excretion of K can be maximized by the administration of furosemide or another loop-acting diuretic. An exchange resin such as sodium polystyrene sulfonate (Kayexalate) can be administered orally or rectally. On the other hand, severe hyperkalemia is a true medical emergency. Therapy should be directed at minimizing cardiac toxicity, enhancing K movement into the cells, and removing K from the body. Hence, treatment includes calcium (10 mL of 10% calcium gluconate), glucose and insulin (10% dextrose with 10 U/L regular insulin infused at a rate of 250 to 500 mL/h), furosemide, and Kayexalate. The practice of sodium bicarbonate administration has recently been questioned, since there is some evidence that the associated hypertoxicity may mitigate its hypokalemic effects. β-agonists have recently been shown to lower serum potassium levels but their use is still somewhat experimental. Finally, dialysis may be initiated in patients with life-threatening levels of hyperkalemia and the inability to quickly stimulate K excretion by any route.

HYPOCALCEMIA

Hypocalcemia, while commonly encountered in the ICU, is of no clinical significance unless associated with decreased ionized calcium. While calcium is frequently administered in response to either asymptomatic hypocalcemia or hypotension, there is some experimental evidence that calcium may worsen outcome. Given the present state of confusion in the literature, routine administration of calcium, in the absence of ionized hypocalcemia, appears controversial. Conditions associated with low ionized Ca concentrations include pancreatitis, rhabdomyolysis, renal failure, and administration of blood, bicarbonate, phosphate, or citrate. Tetany is the major clinical sign and may cause depression of myocardial contractility. Hypocalcemia is associated with prolongation of the QT interval on ECG and can result in ventricular arrhythmias.

Treatment of hypocalcemia depends on its severity. In addition to confirming true ionized hypocalcemia, the serum magnesium level should be checked and corrected. In mild cases, simple oral Ca supplementation is sufficient. In symptomatic cases, parenteral Ca should be administered. Generally, 100 to 200 mg of elemental Ca given intravenously, followed by a slow infusion of 0.5 to 2.0 mg/kg per h with frequent determinations of total and ionized Ca is desirable.

HYPERCALCEMIA

Hypercalcemia is common in hospitalized patients in whom it is most commonly associated with malignancy and hyperparathyroidism. Hypercalcemia may be associated with profound mental status changes, dehydration, and nephrolithiasis. Initial laboratory evaluation should include confirmation of increased ionized Ca concentration as well as serum phosphate and PTH levels.

The treatment of hypercalcemia depends on the severity of the symptoms. Mild hypercalcemia (< 12 mg/dL) can be managed by restriction of Ca intake, observation, and treatment of the underlying disorder. Severe hypercalcemia demands more aggressive treatment including prompt correction of volume depletion. Saline should continue to be infused with the goal of maintaining a urine output of at least 200 mL/h. Large doses of furosemide may be required but should not be administered until any initial volume depletion has been corrected. Frequent monitoring of electrolytes is mandatory and early consideration of placement of a central venous pressure monitoring device is prudent.

HYPOMAGNESEMIA

The consequences of hypomagnesemia are primarily related to the nervous and neuromuscular systems and include altered mental status, hyperreflexia, tetany, hypotension, respiratory failure and arrhythmias. Mild hypomagnesemia can be managed with oral Mg salts. For severe hypomagnesemia (<1.0 mg/dL or associated with severe symptoms) parenteral administration is warranted in doses of 50 meq over 4 to 6 h. Serum levels must be followed closely. Hypomagnesemia frequently accompanies hypokalemia and hypocalcemia; it may be necessary to correct the Mg deficit before the potassium and calcium levels will return to normal.

HYPERMAGNESEMIA

Hypermagnesemia is virtually unknown except in persons with renal failure. Mild degrees of hypermagnesemia, up to 5 or 6 mg/dL, are generally well tolerated. However, Mg concentrations greater than 6 mg/dL may be associated with altered mental status, hyporeflexia, weakness, and respiratory depression. Treatment includes withdrawal of Mg-containing substances and administration of calcium, 10 to 20 meq to reverse the clinical signs, and furosemide, to hasten excretion. Patients with renal failure may require dialysis.

HYPOPHOSPHATEMIA

The acute manifestations of hypophosphatemia include altered mental status, muscular weakness, rhabdomyolysis, decreased myocardial contractility, hemolysis, and respiratory depression. Mild asymptomatic cases (serum PO_4 of 1.5 to 2.5 mg/dL) can usually be managed with oral balanced sodium and potassium salts of PO_4 (Neutra-Phos-K) in a dose of 250 mg every 8 h. Patients with severe hypophosphatemia require intravenous sodium phosphate or potassium phosphate at a rate of 2 mg phosphorus per kg body weight every 6 h, until the serum PO_4 level exceeds 2.0 mg/dL, followed by continued oral repletion.

HYPERPHOSPHATEMIA

Severe hyperphosphatemia occurs almost exclusively in the setting of significant renal failure or severe cell lysis. The major clinical presentations of hyperphosphatemia are hypocalcemia due to the formation of biologically inactive calcium-phosphate complexes, acute renal failure, and ectopic deposition of calcium-phosphate crystals in the soft tissues. The first line of therapy in hyperphosphatemia is the use of enteric PO_4 binders such as calcium, magnesium, or aluminum salts, in doses of 30 mL or more every 6 h. Alkaline diuresis may be useful and, in patients with decreased renal function, dialysis may be necessary.

For further reading in *Principles of Critical Care*, see Chap 3 "Acid-Base and Electrolyte Homeostasis" Gregory A. Schmidt, Chap 156 "Severe Electrolyte Disturbances" Stephen Brennan/Eleanor D Lederer

Allan Garland

INTRODUCTION

Acid-base disorders are extremely common in the ICU. Their evaluation often seems to be an intimidating task; the chief reasons for this are lengthy differential diagnoses, and confusion engendered by mixed acid-base disorders. In fact, in critically ill patients, a relatively small subset of these lists accounts for the great majority of acid-base disturbances. In addition, straightforward regression equations exist describing the expected magnitude of renal and respiratory compensations, and using these a systematic approach will be presented at the end of this chapter which permits a thorough analysis of most acid-base disturbances.

As a general rule, the best approach to these disorders emphasizes a vigorous search for causes, rather than an immediate attempt to achieve a normal serum pH.

Two useful parameters, the anion gap and osmolal gap, will be defined in the appropriate sections below. Another parameter that is often quoted is the "base excess." This is defined as the difference between the actual level, and the normal value (i.e., 24 mEq/L) of serum bicarbonate, that would exist if the patient's blood were brought to $PCO_2 = 40$. It is often utilized as a measure of the purely metabolic portion of an acid-base disturbance. However, it embodies no additional information not contained by the combination of serum pH, serum bicarbonate, and arterial PCO_2 and is often misinterpreted in patients who have either chronic, or mixed, acid-base derangements. For this reason its use is discouraged.

PHYSIOLOGIC EFFECTS

Maintenance of normal pH is important to a wide range of biochemical and cellular functions. Powerful homeostatic mechanisms attempt to maintain extracellular pH within the normal range (i.e., 7.35 to 7.45); outside of these limits physiologic processes become deranged. Although reliable data from humans is limited, it is clear that either acidemia and alkalemia, especially when severe, may have adverse physiologic consequences. The clinical effects of these abnormalities are often most evident in the central nervous system (CNS) and cardiovascular system.

According to various investigations in human beings and in animals, acidemia may cause decreased myocardial and diaphragmatic contractility, a reduced threshold for ventricular fibrillation, complex and variable derangements in vascular smooth muscle tone, increased cerebral blood flow, and variable effects upon serum electrolyte levels (e.g., the association of hyperphosphatemia with lactic acidosis). Abrupt changes in intracellular pH, as occurs with acute respiratory acidosis, can cause headache and progressive confusion when $P_{CO_2} > 60$ mmHg; when $P_{CO_2} > 70$ mmHg seizures may occur.

Alkalemia lowers the seizure threshold and promotes coronary artery spasm, and has variable effects upon myocardial contractility and vascular tone. It produces a transient reduction in cerebral blood flow (lasting only 6 h) which is often utilized clinically to treat states of increased intracranial pressure. The maximum effect that can be realized is a 50 percent decrease in cerebral blood flow at a P_{CO_2} of approximately 20 mmHg. In addition, alkalemia lowers ionized calcium (0.03 to 0.09 mmol/L for every rise in pH of 0.1 unit), and in some clinical situation causes a small (1 to 2 mmol/L) rise in serum lactate.

METABOLIC ACIDOSIS

Metabolic acidosis is characterized by a primary decrease in serum bicarbonate concentration. The homeostatic response is compensatory hyperventilation with decreased P_{CO_2}. The expected level of respiratory compensation typically produces a $P_{CO_2} = (1.5 \times [HCO_3^-]) + 8 \pm 2$.

In the ICU, the most important causes of metabolic acidosis are diarrhea and renal tubular acidoses (normal anion gap), and lactic acidosis (elevated anion gap). Lactic acidosis is covered in Chapter 58.

Etiologies

These disorders can be divided into two groups according to whether or not the anion gap is elevated. (See Table 57-1) The anion gap is the difference between measured cations and measured anions, and since electrical neutrality must always be maintained, it also equals the difference between the "unmeasured anions" and "unmeasured cations." In the ICU this is often elevated because of the presence of excess unmeasured anions (e.g., lactate, ketone bodies). The anion gap is defined as $[Na^+] - [Cl^-] - [HCO_3^-]$, and its normal value is 8 to 14 mEq/L.

When an anion gap metabolic acidosis is discovered, a thorough search for the source of the excess unmeasured anions should be made, as this points to the specific etiology and dictates further diagnostic and therapeutic interventions. However, not infrequently, even when this is done a portion (often about one-half) of the unmeasured anions cannot be identified. On rare occasion, despite a substantially elevated anion gap and a concerted search, no uncounted anions are indentified.

TABLE 57-1 Etiologies of Metabolic Acidosis

With Increased Anion Gap	With Normal Anion Gap
renal failure	GI loss of bicarbonate
ketoacidosis	diarrhea
diabetic	urinary diversion
alcoholic	small bowel, pancreatic or biliary
starvation	fistulas, or surgical drainage
lactic acidosis (see Table 58-1)	anion-exchange resins (e.g.,
toxins	cholestyramine)
salicylates	renal loss of bicarbonate
methanol	renal tubular acidosis
ethylene glycol	(see Table 57-2)
paraldehyde	hypoaldosteronism
nonketotic hyperosmolar coma	hyperparathyroidism
inborn errors of metabolism	renal insufficiency
	acidifying substances
	HCl, NH_4 Cl, $CaCl_2$, $MgCl_2$
	Arginine HCl, Lysine HCl, TPN with
	excess cationic amino acids, sulfur
	miscellaneous
	recovery from diabetic ketoacidosis
	dilutional acidosis

The *renal tubular acidoses* (RTA) are a diverse set of disorders in which renal handling of bicarbonate is abnormal. In both Type 1 (classic distal) and Type 2 (proximal) RTA, acidosis is often accompanied by hypokalemia; while hyperkalemia is usually seen with Type 4 (hyporeninemic-hypoaldosteronemic) RTA (Table 57-2).

Alcoholic ketoacidosis is a state often accompanied by other acid-base disorders (e.g., contraction alkalosis, respiratory alkalosis or acidosis). There is a large anion gap, and ketonuria. However, because the ratio of ketone bodies greatly favors β-hydroxybutyrate over acetoacetate in this disorder, and because the usual assays (e.g., Acetest, Ketostix) measure only acetoacetate, measured ketone levels in blood and urine are falsely low. The elevated anion gap is predominantly attributable to ketones, but there is usually a contribution from the mildly elevated serum lactate present as a direct effect of ethanol. *Starvation ketoacidosis* is usually mild and self-limited.

Toxins must be suspected in any patient with an anion gap acidosis not predominantly explained by elevated lactate or ketones. Confirmation is obtained by laboratory testing for specific toxin levels, but the delay in obtaining results often necessitates beginning presumptive therapy without a definitive diagnosis. Salicylates, methanol and ethylene glycol are all common toxic ingestions, and for all three a portion of the elevated anion gap is usually due to increased serum lactate.

For *salicylates*, a serum level of 100 mg/dL results in a 7.3 mEq/L

TABLE 57-2 Etiologies of Renal Tubular Acidosis

Type 1 (Distal)	Type 4 (Distal)
primary renal disease	primary renal disease
obstructive	obstruction
nephrocalcinosis	hyporeninemia
pyelonephritis	systemic diseases
renal transplant rejection	Diabetes mellitus
systemic diseases	sickle cell disease
sickle cell disease	Addison's disease, primary
cirrhosis	hypoaldosteronism
SLE	drugs and toxins
multiple myeloma	spironolactone, triamterene,
amyloidosis	amiloride
drugs and toxins	
Amphotericin B	
lithium	
analgesic abuse	
Type 2 (Proximal)	
primary renal disease	
systemic diseases	
multiple myeloma	
amyloidosis	
SLE	
cystinosis	
Wilson's disease	
drugs and toxins	
lead, cadmium, mercury	
carbonic anhydrase inhibitors	
outdated tetracycline	

elevation in anion gap. In salicylate overdose, there is often a primary respiratory alkalosis in addition to the metabolic acidosis.

Renal failure does not result in impairment of acid-base balance until glomerular filtration rate falls below 20 mL/min. There are multiple organic and inorganic anions whose clearance is impaired in advanced renal insufficiency, leading to an increased anion gap; however these are not easily or routinely assayed, and the conclusion that renal failure is the cause of an anion gap acidosis is made in the correct clinical setting and in the absence of other identified etiologies.

Therapy

Treatment of the underlying cause should be the immediate goal of therapy for any metabolic acidosis. Many of the disorders listed in Table 57-1 have specific therapies discussed elsewhere in this volume. The special problem of metabolic acidosis caused by toxins causing an elevated osmolal gap (i.e., methanol and ethylene glycol) is discussed later in this chapter.

The anion gap acidosis caused by *salicylate* overdose is treated with aggressive alkaline diuresis; hemodialysis is instituted if acidosis, the elevation in serum salicylate levels, or symptoms of salicylate poisoning are severe.

Alcoholic ketoacidosis is treated with intravenous volume replacement, administration of glucose, and electrolyte repletion.

The administration of *sodium bicarbonate* for metabolic acidosis is one of the most controversial topics in critical care medicine today. Theoretically, by increasing CO_2 production in the extracellular space it can lead to a further decrease in intracellular pH and thus exacerbate, rather than improve, the resultant derangements in cellular metabolism; such phenomena have been shown *in vitro*. This increased CO_2 production also necessitates increased alveolar ventilation if hypercarbia is to be avoided. Studies of bicarbonate administration in human diabetic ketoacidosis have failed to show a benefit, even with arterial pH < 7.2. A variety of animal models of lactic acidosis have shown that when compared to saline infusion, bicarbonate does not improve mortality and may have adverse hemodynamic effects. A recent study in septic humans found sodium bicarbonate to result in the same, or possibly even less, improvement in patients' hemodynamic profiles, as compared to equimolar amounts of hypertonic saline. When bicarbonate infusion seems to produce salutory effects it is probably attributable to its volume expanding effect; a standard ampule containing 88 mmoles of sodium bicarbonate is the salt equivalent, and thus volume equivalent of 560 ml of normal saline. The one situation in which bicarbonate administration is clearly beneficial is in a nongap metabolic acidosis caused by ongoing bicarbonate losses which cannot readily be halted; the classic example is chronic therapy of proximal renal tubular acidosis. With this one class of exceptions, the use of bicarbonate, regardless of arterial pH is discouraged.

Carbicarb is a combination of sodium carbonate and sodium bicarbonate designed to cause a smaller increase in P_{CO_2} than does bicarbonate alone. Dichloroacetate is a promoter of substrate entry into the tricarboxylic acid cycle. Both are investigational therapies for metabolic acidosis which have shown promising results in animal models of lactic acidosis. Both are now undergoing human trials.

Severe Metabolic Acidosis with Osmolal Gap—Methanol and Ethylene Glycol Poisoning

Poisonings with methanol and ethylene glycol are common and share many similarities. Patients present as apparently drunk without an ethanol odor or ethanol in their blood, but as with ethanol intoxication CNS depression may cause a respiratory acidosis. A high anion gap metabolic acidosis is present, and in addition the "osmolal gap" = {measured plasma osmolality − calculated osmolality}, is elevated above its normal limit of < 10 mosm/L. The calculated osmolality = {2 × [Na+] + BUN(mg/dL)/2.8 + glucose(mg/dL)/18}; additional contributions to plasma osmolality by alcohols (with levels in mg/dL) are ethanol/4.6, methanol/2.9, ethylene glycol/5, and isopropanol/5.9.

The metabolic pathways of methanol and ethylene glycol begin with the action of alcohol dehydrogenase, and eventually produce toxic metabolites. Methanol ingestion results in the formation of formaldehyde and formic acid which cause retinal, gastrointestinal (GI) and CNS toxicities; ethylene glycol leads to oxalic acid and glyoxylate with subsequent renal, GI and CNS toxicities, along with hypocalcemia. The anion gap acidoses are largely a result of the production of these organic acid metabolites, however usually there is a contribution of lactic acidosis as well.

The diagnosis of methanol or ethylene glycol poisoning is sometimes obvious from a history of ingestion, but commonly an obtunded patient with a high anion gap metabolic acidosis is all that is available. A mandatory part of the laboratory evaluation is the osmolal gap; a significant elevation, with or without modest elevation in lactate, strongly suggests either methanol or ethylene glycol poisoning. As they are not included in the routine toxicology screen, specific methanol and ethylene glycol levels should be requested, but these will take many hours to be assayed and the presence of the osmolal gap dictates the need for initiation of therapy prior to this confirmation. Suggestive physical findings include a loss of the normal retinal sheen which sometimes occurs in methanol poisoning, and oxylate crystalluria often present in ethylene glycol toxicity.

Treatment should include syrup of ipecac or upper GI lavage if the patient presents within 2 to 4 h of ingestion. Definitive therapy should be initiated promptly with an intravenous infusion of ethanol with a goal of achieving a serum level of greater than 100 mg/dl. The mechanism of action is competitive inhibition of toxin generation by alcohol dehydrogenase. The usual indications for this therapy are serum methanol or ethylene glycol levels of > 20 mg/dL, significant metabolic acidemia, or any clinically significant toxicity.

With toxin levels > 50 mg/dL, serum formate (from methanol) > 20 mg/dL, severe metabolic acidemia, or visual or renal toxicity, hemodialysis should be instituted in addition to the ethanol infusion. With dialysis, the rate of ethanol infusion will need to be increased to maintain the desired serum concentration. Dialysis may be discontinued when toxicities are resolved and toxin levels decline (i.e., methanol < 25 mg/dL; ethylene glycol < 10 mg/dL).

Adjuncts to augment clearance of toxic metabolites may be

administered. For methanol poisoning, folate is given as 50 mg IV q 4 h × 4 days. For ethylene glycol, thiamine and pyridoxine are administered each as 100 mg IV q 6 h × 2 days.

An investigational inhibitor of alcohol dehydrogenase, 4-methylpyrazole, has shown promise in both methanol and ethylene glycol poisonings. There is no utility of oral charcoal, cathartics, forced diuresis or charcoal hemoperfusion.

METABOLIC ALKALOSIS

The homeostatic response to the primary increase in serum bicarbonate concentration which characterizes metabolic alkalosis is compensatory hypoventilation with increased P_{CO_2}. The expected level of respiratory compensation results in a $P_{CO_2} = (0.7 \times [HCO_3^-]) + 21 \pm 1.5$.

Since normal renal homeostatic mechanisms strongly oppose an increased serum bicarbonate, persistent metabolic alkalosis requires both an initial elevation of bicarbonate (which is usually a result of acid loss from the stomach or kidney, and may be transient and resolved by the time of evaluation), and a potent stimulus for continued renal bicarbonate reabsorption in the face of the elevated bicarbonate.

Etiologies

These disorders are usually separated into three categories (Table 57-3). "Chloride-responsive" causes have in common extracellular volume and salt (including chloride) depletion; this hypochloremic hypovolemia is the stimulus for continued renal bicarbonate reabsorbtion. In such a "contraction alkalosis," the urinary chloride concentration is usually < 10 mEq/L. In "chloride-resistant" etiologies the extracellular volume is not reduced, the alkalosis is maintained by other known mechanisms (e.g., hypokalemia or elevated mineralocorticoid activity), and urinary chloride is usually > 20 mEq/L. The third category contains a variety of miscellaneous causes in which urinary chloride is variable.

In the ICU the most important causes are vomiting, nasogastric suction, diuretics, corticosteroids, massive plasma infusion or exchange, and prolonged overventilation of patients with chronic hypercapnia. Multifactorial etiologies are common. Most patients in whom a careful search for causes is unrevealing are hypovolemic, or have multiple factors contributing to the metabolic alkalosis.

Prevention

Many cases of metabolic alkalosis occur as an adverse result of other therapies used in the ICU. Attention to detail will prevent the

TABLE 57-3 Etiologies of Metabolic Alkalosis

Chloride responsive	*Chloride resistant*
Almost any hypovolemic state, especially:	increased mineralocorticoid activity
GI disorders	primary hyperaldosteronism
vomiting, NG suction or gastric	Cushing's syndrome
drainage, villous adenoma	drugs with mineralocorticoid activity
of colon congenital	Bartter's syndrome
chloride diarrhea	licorice poisoning
diuretic therapy	renin-secreting tumor
posthypercapnia with volume	severe hypokalemia
depletion	
cystic fibrosis	

Miscellaneous
alkali administration
  acetate (e.g., TPN), citrate (e.g.,
   transfusions), bicarbonate, lactate
  nonreabsorbable alkali (e.g.,
   antacids, Milk-alkali syndrome),
   exchange resins
acute post-chronic hypercapnia
nonparathyroid hypercalcemia
refeeding after starvation
nonreabsorbable anionic antibiotics (e.g., penicillins)

advent of many cases of metabolic alkalosis. Therefore, replacement of diuretic-induced potassium losses, minimization of NG suction, use of H_2-blockers if prolonged NG suction is necessary, and resisting the temptation to "normalize" P_{CO_2} in chronically hypercarbic patients on mechanical ventilation will all contribute to improved acid-base homeostasis.

Treatment

Correction of metabolic alkalosis can almost always be accomplished safely and slowly. As always, the basic goal of therapy is correction of underlying causes.

For chloride-responsive causes, correction of hypovolemia with normal saline usually leads to resolution of the alkalosis. For patients in whom there is a worsening contraction alkalosis along with a continued need for diuresis, acetazolamide (given with KCl) may be administered.

With metabolic alkalosis in the presence of volume overload, hemodialysis coupled with replacement with a smaller volume of normal saline can be a useful strategy.

In cases of mineralocorticoid excess where the source cannot be removed, salt restriction along with potassium supplementation and administration of spironolactone or amiloride is often useful.

Rarely, rapid correction with intravenous acid infusion is warranted. The usual indication is severe alkalemia (i.e., pH > 7.6) in the presence of adverse effects of alkalemia, such as arrhythmias or CNS depression. Acid, as 0.1 to 0.2 N HCl is administered at 20 to 50 mEq/h either via a central vein, or peripherally mixed with amino acid solution and infused along with a lipid emulsion. With this therapy, arterial pH must be monitored hourly. Acid therapy should be discontinued when the indications for its institution have resolved; this does not require complete normalization of arterial pH.

RESPIRATORY ACIDOSIS

Respiratory acidosis is marked by hypercarbia which is a result of an inadequate level of alveolar ventilation for the level of tissue CO_2 production—this is respiratory failure.

In acute respiratory acidosis tissue buffers are inadequate to compensate; serum bicarbonate may rise by as much as 4 to 5 mEq/L and arterial pH falls according to the equation Δ pH $= -0.08 \times \Delta$ $Pco_2/10$). With time, the kidney retains bicarbonate. Early renal compensation occurs within 6 to 24 h and results in a rise in serum bicarbonate given by $\Delta [HCO_3^-] = (1/10) \times \Delta Pco_2$ Complete renal compensation takes 1 to 4 days with a resultant $\Delta[HCO_3^-] = (4/10) \times \Delta Pco_2$.

Etiologies

Hypercarbia will result from either decreased minute ventilation, increased carbon dioxide production with a deficient ability to compensate by hyperventilating, or an increased dead space fraction with deficient ability to compensate by hyperventilating (Table 57-4). Clinically, the states that lead to these abnormalities involve disorders of the lungs, airways, chest wall, respiratory neuromuscular system, or CNS control of respiration.

In the ICU the most important categories of causes are lung diseases, and drugs that depress respiratory drive.

Treatment

The treatment of respiratory failure is addressed in detail elsewhere in this volume. In addition to treatment of the underlying cause, prompt consideration must be given to whether these patients with respiratory failure require intubation and mechanical ventilation. In addition, therapy involves improvement of all factors that will facilitate removal of carbon dioxide by the lungs. In addition to the obvious strategy of increased alveolar ventilation, CO_2 production is lowered by treating fever and avoiding overfeeding. Dead space fraction may be lowered in some patients, especially those on

TABLE 57-4 Etiologies of Respiratory Acidosis

Reduced respiratory drive	*Neuromuscular diseases*
drugs and toxins (narcotics, sedatives, alcohols, anesthetics)	myasthenia gravis
	ALS
CNS lesions	Guillain-Barre syndrome
sleep apnea	poliomyelitis
myxedema	botulism
	multiple sclerosis
Disorders of the lung	high spinal cord injury
COPD	myopathy
asthma	brainstem injury
severe pneumonia	severe hypokalemia
severe pulmonary edema	severe hypophosphatemia
pneumothorax	periodic paralysis
ARDS	diaphragmatic paralysis
Upper airway obstruction	*Disorders of the chest wall*
foreign body	severe kyphoscoliosis
laryngospasm or laryngeal edema	morbid obesity
obstructive sleep apnea	burns with circumferential eschar
tracheal stenosis	flail chest

mechanical ventilation, by correcting hypovolemia and decreasing the level of PEEP.

RESPIRATORY ALKALOSIS

Respiratory alkalosis, marked by primary hypocarbia, is quite common in the ICU. In acute respiratory alkalosis serum bicarbonate may fall by a small amount and arterial pH rises according to the equation Δ pH $= -0.08 \times (\Delta$ $PCO_2/10)$. Within hours the kidney begins to excrete bicarbonate. Early renal compensation occurs within 1 to 2 h and reduces serum bicarbonate by Δ $[HCO_3^-] = (2/10) \times \Delta$ PCO_2 Complete renal compensation takes 2 days with a resultant Δ $[HCO_3^-] = (5/10) \times \Delta$ PCO_2.

Etiologies

Table 57-5 shows the differential diagnosis of respiratory alkalosis. In the ICU, the most important causes are pain and anxiety, fever, lung disease, excessive levels of mechanical ventilation and sepsis.

Treatment

In addition to treatment of the cause of the respiratory alkalosis, if the alkalosis is severe or intractable, use of sedation, with or without muscle relaxation, can be considered.

TABLE 57-5 Etiologies of Respiratory Alkalosis

Central stimulation of respiration	Peripheral stimulation of respiration
anxiety, pain	pneumonia
fever	pulmonary edema
sepsis	pulmonary embolus
liver disease	restrictive lung disease
hyperthyroidism	pleural effusion
CNS disease (CVA, tumor, infection, trauma)	pneumothorax
	bronchospasm
drugs (salicylates, catecholamines, progesterone)	
	Miscellaneous
	mechanical overventilation
Hypoxemia	voluntary hyperventilation
high altitude	
pulmonary disease	
severe anemia	
asphyxia (i.e., decreased P_{IO_2})	

APPROACH TO ANALYSIS OF ACID-BASE DISTURBANCES

The following stepwise approach enables one to analyze most situations, even triple disturbances:

1. Look at serum pH—is the patient acidemic (pH < 7.35) or alkalemic (pH > 7.45)?
2. Look at P_{CO_2} and $[HCO_3^-]$—is the main disturbance metabolic or respiratory?

   acidemia: P_{CO_2} > 45 mmHg identifies a respiratory acidosis
   $[HCO_3^-]$ < 20 mmol/L identifies a metabolic acidosis

   alkalemia: P_{CO_2} < 35 mmHg identifies a respiratory alkalosis
   $[HCO_3^-]$ > 28 mmol/L identifies a metabolic alkalosis

3. If there is a primary respiratory disturbance, is it acute?

   expect Δ pH = $-0.08 \times (\Delta P_{CO_2}/10)$

4. If there is a nonacute primary respiratory disturbance, is there an appropriate renal compensation?

   for acidosis expect: early (6 to 24 h) $\Delta[HCO_3^-] = (1/10) \times \Delta P_{CO_2}$
   late (1 to 4 days) $\Delta[HCO_3^-] = (4/10) \times \Delta P_{CO_2}$

   for alkalosis expect: early (1 to 2 h) $\Delta [HCO_3^-] = (2/10) \times \Delta P_{CO_2}$
   late (2 days) $\Delta[HCO_3^-] = (5/10) \times \Delta P_{CO_2}$

If not, then there is a superimposed primary metabolic disturbance, or compensation is not yet complete.

5. If there is a metabolic acidosis, is the anion gap increased?
6. If there is a metabolic disturbance, is there an appropriate respiratory compensation?

for acidosis expect: $P_{CO_2} = (1.5 \times [HCO_3^-] + 8 \pm 2$
for alkalosis expect: $P_{CO_2} = (0.7 \times [HCO_3^-] + 21 \pm 1.5$

If not, then there is a superimposed primary respiratory disturbance hidden in the numbers.

if actual P_{CO_2} > expected P_{CO_2} → then there is a hidden primary respiratory acidosis
if actual P_{CO_2} < expected P_{CO_2} → then there is a hidden primary respiratory alkalosis

7. If there is an increased anion gap acidosis, look for other metabolic disturbances by examining whether the parameter $\{[HCO_3^-] + (gap - 12)\}$ is nearly normal (i.e., 24 mEq/L in a patient who does not have a chronic respiratory acid-base disorder).

If this parameter is not nearly 24, then there is a second superimposed metabolic abnormality hidden in the data:

if the parameter < 24 → then there is another, hidden, non-gap acidosis

if the parameter > 24 → then there is another, hidden metabolic alkalosis

Step 7 is based upon the idea that since an elevated anion gap acidosis is created by the presence of a given number of milliequivalents per liter of extra hydrogen ion, and necessarily, the same concentration of uncounted anion, the resultant fall in serum bicarbonate below its usual value (caused by that extra hydrogen ion), should equal the rise in anion gap over its usual value of approximately 12 (caused by the uncounted anion).

For further reading in Principles of Critical Care, see Chap 158 "Acid-Base Disorders" V Theodore Barnett/Gregory A Schmidt

GENERAL CONSIDERATIONS

Lactic acidosis is the most important acid-base disorder encountered in critically ill patients. The acidemia has physiologic significance and, perhaps more importantly, serves as a marker for a diverse group of serious underlying conditions.

The presence, magnitude, and course of the acidosis have significant prognostic implications. Increased lactate levels correlate well with increased mortality in patients with cardiogenic shock. In other types of shock the correlation is less impressive, however the trend in lactate levels in a given patient can be helpful in gauging the effect of therapy, and assessing prognosis.

Many patients in the ICU have small elevations in serum lactate level, usually in the range of 2 to 5 mmol/L (normal 0.3 to 1.3 mmol/L), that are due to a variety of stimuli, including sympathetic activation. Mild increases in the serum lactate level may indicate early tissue hypoxia, but also may reflect the hypermetabolic state accompanying many critical illnesses. The definition of lactic acidosis is arbitrary; it is commonly defined as a lactate level greater than 5 mmol/L with an arterial pH less than 7.35.

Increased lactate levels may cause adverse physiologic effects independent of effects upon pH. Various in vitro and animal investigations have shown deleterious effects upon myocardial cell function and inotropic state, as well as upon the β-adrenergic responsiveness of various cell types. In addition, for reasons that are obscure, lactic acidosis is often accompanied by hyperphosphatemia.

ETIOLOGIES (Table 58-1)

Lactate is a dead end in human metabolism. It is interconverted to and from pyruvate by the action of lactate dehydrogenase; the normal lactate: pyruvate ratio of 1:10 being increased by inadequate tissue oxygen supply or utilization. Under aerobic conditions, some tissues (e.g., the myocardium) consume circulating lactate as an energy substrate; however, the major route of clearance of serum lactate is via hepatic uptake and subsequent entry into several metabolic pathways. Even under fully aerobic conditions when the lactate: pyruvate ratio is normal, situations which cause an increased concentration of pyruvate will necessarily produce an increased concentration of lactate. Thus lactic acidosis may result

TABLE 58-1 Etiologies of Lactic Acidosis

Increased oxygen consumption	*Toxins and Drugs*
grand mal seizure	carbon monoxide
severe asthma	ethanol, methanol, ethylene
neuroleptic malignant syndrome	glycol, propylene glycol
pheochromocytoma	salicylates
strenuous exercise	cyanide, nitroprusside
	isoniazid
	strychnine
Decreased oxygen delivery	others including: streptozocin,
decreased cardiac output	papaverine, acetaminophen,
decreased arterial oxygen content:	biguanides, nalidixic acid,
severe anemia	ritodrine, terbutaline, fructose,
severe hypoxemia	sorbitol, xylitol, epinephrine,
regional ischemia (e.g., mesenteric)	norepinephrine
microcirculatory disturbances:	
sepsis	*Congenital Enzyme Deficiencies*
	glucose-6-phosphatase, others
Decreased lactate clearance	
fulminant hepatic failure	*Miscellaneous*
	D-lactate (e.g., bacterial
Alterations in Cellular Metabolism	overgrowth)
uncontrolled Diabetes mellitus	
malignancy (esp. leukemias,	
lymphomas)	
severe alkalemia	
thiamine deficiency	
hypoglycemia	

from any cause of local or global anaerobic metabolism resulting in increased lactic acid generation; decreased lactate clearance occurring secondary to derangements in organ system (esp. hepatic), or cellular metabolic function; or diversion of alanine to gluconeogenesis leading to increased concentrations of both pyruvate and lactate.

Many conditions can cause lactic acidosis. Many drugs and toxins which cause metabolic acidosis do so, in whole or in part, by causing a lactic acidosis. However, in the ICU most cases of lactic acidosis occur secondarily to a handful of processes. Shock (cardiogenic, septic, or hypovolemic) is the predominant etiology, followed by hypoxemia, seizures, regional ischemia and toxins.

Sepsis is a common cause of lactic acidosis in the ICU. Several mechanisms may act to produce the increased lactate. Inadequate tissue oxygenation may occur, either with an obviously diminished oxygen delivery, or in the presence of a hyperdynamic circulation. In the latter situation tissue hypoxia may be related to *pathological supply dependency of oxygen utilization* (see Chap. 14), wherein alterations in cellular metabolism and/or microvascular regulation result in inadequate supply of oxygen to tissues despite a delivery of oxygen which seems to far exceed usual requirements. In addition, sepsis is a condition in which globally augmented tissue catabolism, and possibly also decreased cellular uptake and utilization of lactate, cause an increased circulating lactate level in some patients, even in the presence of aerobic conditions.

Generalized motor seizures cause tremendous muscle energy usage and glycogen breakdown, with much of the glucose converted to lactate. Normally however, within 1 h of cessation of convusions, serum lactate falls considerably and pH normalizes.

Most lactic acidoses in cancer patients are due to shock and sepsis. In patients with extensive liver involvement by their tumors, diminished hepatic lactate extraction contributes as well. However, in a variety of malignancies, most commonly leukemia and lymphoma, the malignant cells themselves produce excess lactate, apparently due to a loss of metabolic regulatory controls upon glycolytic pathways.

TREATMENT

As for all metabolic acidoses, the cornerstone of management of lactic acidosis is discovery and correction of underlying causes. When the acidemia is severe (variously defined as pH < 7.10 to 7.20), or when this approach is unsuccessful, as happens commonly in septic shock, consideration of treatment with alkalinizing agents is usually entertained. Indeed, it is in sepsis that many of the human and animal studies of such therapies of metabolic acidosis have been carried out. A more detailed discussion of this issue can be found in the discussion of therapy for metabolic acidosis in Chap. 57.

For further reading in *Principles of Critical Care,* see Chap 158
 "Acid-Base Disorders" V Theodore Barnett/Gregory A Schmidt

Diabetic Ketoacidosis, Hypergycemic Hyperosmolar Nonketotic Coma, and Hypogycemia

Manu Jain

Hypoglycemia and diabetes mellitus, with its major life-threatening complications, diabetic ketoacidosis (DKA) and hyperglycemic hyperosmolar nonketotic coma (HHNC), may precipitate or complicate critical illness. DKA is the life-threatening metabolic consequence of insulin deficiency. HHNC is the most severe presentation of a syndrome in which insulin resistance and relative insulin deficiency produce hyperglycemia. There is considerable overlap, however, between patients in DKA and HHNC when one takes into account insulin levels, secretory dynamics and tissue sensitivity.

DIFFERENTIAL DIAGNOSIS

DKA and HHNC are easily recognized when considered (Table 59-1). Metabolic decompensation develops over hours to days in DKA in which patients usually present with lethargy, Kussmaul respirations and a fruity odor. They may complain of nausea, vomiting and abdominal pain which is often quite severe. Many patients are hypotensive, tachycardiac and tachypneic with signs of mild to moderate volume depletion. Patients with HHNC have more profound dehydration and are usually stuporous. They may also manifest focal neurologic deficits such as cranial nerve abnormalities and asymmetric reflexes. These patients are also usually hypotensive and exhibit normal to diminished respirations. As in DKA hypothermia is common, but unlike in DKA cereberal edema is rare.

The sine qua non of DKA is ketoacidosis. There are two ketoacids produced in DKA; β-hydroxybutyrate and acetoacetate as well as the neutral ketone acetone. In severe DKA β-hydroxybutyrate is the predominant ketone and since the nitroprusside reaction used commonly to detect ketones does not react with β-hydroxybutyrate, it is possible to have a negative serum nitroprusside reaction in the face of severe ketosis. The arterial pH is commonly less than 7.3 and can be as low as 6.5. The serum glucose level in DKA is usually about 500 mg/dL although cases have been described where the glucose was in the normal range or only slightly elevated. One useful index to use when managing a patient is the anion-gap, which is related to the amount of unmeasured anions (here, ketoacids, and sometimes

TABLE 59-1 Signs and Symptoms of Glucose Metabolism Disorders

	Uncontrolled Diabetes		
Polyuria	Nocturia	Thirst	Polydipsia
Polyphagia	Weight loss	Blurred Vision	Dizziness
Vaginitis	Skin infection	Fatigue	Malaise
Diabetic Ketoacidosis			
Dyspnea	Nausea	Vomiting	Abdominal pain
Normotension	Tachycardia	Tachypnea	Abdominal tenderness
Hypo/hyperthermia	Lethargy to coma	Fruity breath	Orthostasis
Cerebral edema			
Hyperglycemic Hyperosmolar Nonketotic Coma			
Dehydration	Stupor to coma	Shallow respiration	Hypotension to shock
Hypo/hyperthermia	Focal neurologic signs or seizures		

(Reprinted with permission from Buse JB, Polonsky KS: Diabetic Ketoacidosis, Hyperglycemic Hyperosmolar Nonketotic Coma, and Hypoglycemia, in Hall JB, Schmidt GA, Wood LDH: Principles of Critical Care, McGraw-Hill, New York, 1992.)

lactate) in the blood. Most persons in DKA present with an anion-gap between 20 and 40.

The sine qua non of HHNC is hyperosmolality. In HHNC, the osmolality is generally greater than 350 mOsm/L and can exceed 400 mOsm/L. The glucose concentration will usually be greater than 600 mg/dL with levels over 1,000 mg/dL quite common. In pure HHNC there is usually no significant metabolic acidosis or anion gap.

Not all patients with hyperglycemia and an anion gap metabolic acidosis will have DKA. Lactic acidosis, starvation ketosis, alcoholic ketoacidosis and uremic acidosis can all increase the anion gap. The pH will be variably affected. Additional causes of anion-gap metabolic acidosis include toxic ingestions, such as salicylates and methanol. It should be noted that patients often present with combinations of these conditions which may require minor alterations in the therapy to be outlined below.

All but the mildest cases of DKA should be managed in the ICU. Initial laboratory assessment should include serum glucose, electrolytes, BUN, creatinine, calcium, magnesium, phosphate, ketones, lactate, creatinine phosphokinase and liver function tests. Additionally a urinalysis, electrocardiogram, chest X-ray, complete blood count, and an arterial blood gas should also be obtained. Subsequently, glucose and electrolyte levels should be measured hourly.

THERAPY

The optimum management of DKA and HHNC has been the object of considerable controversy over the past half century. The general approach is outlined in Table 59-2.

Volume contraction is one of the hallmarks of DKA and HHNC, where fluid deficits on the order of 5 to 10L are common. When there are physical signs of dehydration (e.g., hypotension, decreased skin turgor or dry mucous membranes) 1 liter of normal saline should be administered over the first hour and 200 to 500 mL/h in subsequent hours, until hypotension resolves and an adequate circulation is maintained. When this occurs fluid administration should be altered to replace urinary losses with one-half normal saline. In DKA and HHNC water deficits are in excess of sodium deficits. An estimated water deficit can be calculated using the corrected sodium and this water deficit should be replaced over a period of 24 to 48 h. One should give free water as necessary to correct the hypernatremia. Once the serum glucose level reaches 250 to 300 mg/dL fluids should contain 5 percent dextrose and therapy should be aimed at maintaining the serum glucose in that range for 24 h to allow slow equilibration of osmotically active substances across all membranes.

TABLE 59-2 Treatment of Severe Disorders of Glucose Metabolism

Diabetic ketoacidosis
  Fluids (usual deficit 5–10 L)
    If hypotensive: 1 L 0.90% NaCl in first hour
    If normotensive: 1 L 0.45% NaCl in first hour
    In subsequent hours:
      match urine output with 0.45% NaCl
      if hypotensive, 200–1000 mL/h 0.9% NaCl (consider pulmonary artery
        catheter and colloid solutions)
      otherwise calculate free water deficit and replace 50% over 12 h with
        5% dextrose in water
      after glucose reaches 250–300 mg/dL, add dextrose to IV fluids
        (~100 g per 24 h)
  Insulin
    10-U IV bolus
    0.1 U/kg/h IV or IM
    Check glucose hourly and adjust drip to decrease glucose 10% per h
      to a level of 250 mg/dL
  Potassium (usual deficit 200–1000 meq)
    Establish that the patient is not oliguric
    ECG monitoring for hyperkalemia and hypokalemia
    If hyperkalemic, follow hourly
    If normokalemic, 10–20 meq/h
    If hypokalemic, 20–40 meq/h
    Half as chloride and half as phosphate salts
  Bicarbonate
    None if pH >7.1
    Consider $NaHCO_3$ 1 meq/kg IV for pH <6.9
    For pH 6.9-7.1, consider for hyperkalemia or shock
    In general avoid >50 meq/h
  Search for underlying cause
  Monitor
    ECG
    Vital signs
    Hourly glucose and electrolytes
    Every 2–4 h: Calcium, magnesium, phosphate
    Every 6–24 h: BUN, creatinine, ketones
Hyperglycemic hyperosmolar nonketotic coma (HHNC)
  HHNC should be treated like DKA, though patients will generally require
    more fluids and less insulin.

(Reprinted with permission from Buse JB, Polonsky KS: Diabetic Ketoacidosis, Hyperglycemic Hyperosmolar Nonketotic Coma, and Hypoglycemia, in Hall JB, Schmidt GA, Wood LDH: Principles of Critical Care, McGraw-Hill, New York, 1992.)

Insulin is the mainstay of therapy of DKA. Studies have shown that IV insulin is as or more effective than IM or SC insulin over the first 24 h of therapy. The SC route is inappropriate in critically ill patients because of the possibility of impaired absorption. In cases where there is insufficient nursing monitoring or IV access, IM therapy is acceptable. Usually a 10 u IV priming dose of regular insulin is given to fully saturate insulin receptors. This is followed by a continuous infusion at .1u/kg/h. In those instances where the glucose level does not decrease at least 10 percent in 1 h, a second bolus of IV insulin should be administered and the infusion rate increased. After the glucose level reaches 250 mg/dL it is prudent to decrease the insulin infusion rate. It is a mistake, however, to discontinue IV insulin at this time. IV insulin must be continued until ketones are cleared from the circulation which usually takes 12 to 24 h following control of the hyperglycemia, then the patient can be switched to SC insulin.

Potassium losses during the development of DKA and HHNC are usually quite high. Initially serum levels may be normal or elevated but total body levels of potassium are always decreased. If the serum level is less than 5.5 meq/L. There are no signs of hyperkalemia on the EKG, and urine output is adequate, it is advisable to administer potassium. Since phosphate is also depleted in patients with DKA and HHNC, one should replace the potassium deficit one-half as potassium chloride and one-half as potassium phosphate.

The use of bicarbonate in the therapy of DKA is highly controversial as no benefit has ever been shown in clinical trials.

After stabilizing the patient a diagnostic strategy should be aimed at determining the precipitating event. Non-compliance with insulin and infection are the most common precipitants. Other causes which should be looked for include an acute myocardial infarction, cerebrovascular accident, pancreatitis, pregnancy or thromoembolic phenomena. Burns, hyperalimentation, dialysis, heatstroke, thyrotoxicosis and drugs have also been associated with DKA and HHNC.

The most troublesome complication of DKA and HHNC is cerebral edema. It is more common in children and can be fatal. Other complications include ARDS, bronchial mucous plugging, thromboembolic events and death.

HYPOGLYCEMIA

Hypoglycemia can be a major complication of critical illness particularly hepatic failure, drug overdose, and sepsis. The symptoms of hypoglycemia initially result from sympathoadrenal responses and consist of palpitations, anxiety, tremulousness, sweating and hunger. If hypoglycemia progresses patients may develop headaches, nightmares, confusion, hallucinations, bizarre behavior, seizures, focal neurologic deficits, coma or death.

Initial treatment should be with an IV solution of 50 percent dextrose. Then a continuous infusion of 10 percent glucose at a rate sufficient to keep the blood glucose level above 100 mg/dL should be started. If more than 200 mL/h is necessary to maintain normoglycemia, 100 mg of hydrocortisone and 1 mg of glucagon should be added to each liter of 10 percent dextrose as long as necessary.

For further reading in *Principles of Critical Care,* see Chap 159 "Diabetic Ketoacidosis, Hyperglycemic Hyperosmolar Nonketotic Coma, and Hypoglycemia" John B Buse/Kenneth S Polonsky

Manu Jain

Gastrointestinal (GI) bleeding accounts for 2 percent of all medical and surgical hospital admissions in the United States. Mortality from GI bleeding remains approximately 10 percent although this may reflect a changing population.

CLINICAL CHARACTERISTICS

The manner in which a patient bleeds may reflect the rate of bleeding and thus the outcome. Patients passing red stool with an upper GI bleed have a poorer outcome. Likewise, a nasogastric aspirate that is red predicts a higher morbidity, mortality and need for surgery than coffee-ground color or clear aspirate. The underlying pathology accounting for bleeding, although not initially evident in most cases, can be predictive of eventual outcome. Various concomitant diseases add further risk to the bleeding patient. These include congestive heart failure (CHF), arrhythmia, central nervous system (CNS) disease, and liver disease.

Regardless of the etiology and site of gastrointestinal bleeding, the initial management is similar. Adequate intravenous (IV) access, volume resuscitation with crystalloid and blood products, correction of bleeding diatheses, and nasogastric (NG) suction if the patient is vomiting are the hallmarks of initial management of GI bleeding. Once a patient is stabilized the etiology should be searched for.

UPPER GI BLEEDING

Diagnosis

Esophagogastroduodenoscopy (EGD) is the most common procedure in diagnosing upper gastrointestinal (UGI) bleeding. Although melena or hematemesis are the usual indications for EGD, hematochezia with signs of hemodynamic instability should also be initially evaluated with EGD (see Table 60-1).

Early endoscopy does not affect mortality or prevent the need for surgical intervention in patients with UGI bleeding. In certain high risk patients, however, it is possible that early endoscopy may affect management to limit mortality.

Contraindications to EGD include hemodynamic instability, GI obstruction, suspected perforation, and a combative patient. Complications of EGD are relatively rare but include respiratory depres-

TABLE 60-1 Indications for Early Esophagogastroduodenostomy

Patients over the age of 60 years

Patients with a history of chronic liver disease

Patients presenting with bright red blood or maroon stool per rectum in association with hypotension or orthostasis

Patients requiring more than 4 units of blood in 6 h

(Reprinted with permission from Hanan IM: Gastrointestinal Hemorrhage, in Hall JB, Schmidt GA, Wood LDH: Principles of Critical Care, McGraw-Hill, New York, 1992.)

sion, hypotension, aspiration of gastric contents, and perforation of the esophagus.

When EGD fails to identify the site of bleeding, several options exist. One is to repeat the endoscopy 6 to 12 h later. Alternatively, angiography or technetium labeled scanning with either colloid or red blood cells can be performed. Angiography and nuclear scanning require active bleeding at the time of the procedure (.5 mL to 1 mL/min).

Therapy

In acute variceal hemorrhage, there are several therapeutic options available although none have been shown to decrease mortality. Endoscopic variceal sclerotherapy (EVS) has become first line therapy to control acute variceal hemorrhage. EVS is indicated at the time of diagnostic endoscopy when active bleeding is seen from a varix or when large non bleeding esophageal varices are present without other obvious etiologies for bleeding. EVS should be attempted before tamponade tubes or surgical procedures. Complications from EVS include pneumonia, pleural effusions, pericarditis, esophageal rupture, and respiratory failure.

Intravenous vasopressin has long been used in variceal hemorrhage even though its efficacy has never been proven and complications are frequent. Other drug therapy includes somatostatin which produces splanchnic vasoconstriction. β-blocker therapy is never indicated in the acute management of variceal bleeding but is appropriate for chronic prophylactic use.

Balloon tamponade of esophageal varices is generally reserved for hemorrhage which is not controlled with sclerotherapy and should be viewed as a temporizing procedure until definitive therapy can be performed. The Sengstaken-Blakemore (S-B) tube with its double balloon system is most frequently used. When inserting a S-B tube one should always confirm the position of the balloon in the stomach before fully inflating it. In most patients, variceal bleeding stops after inflation of the gastric balloon. Subsequently, the esophageal balloon may be insufflated if hemorrhage is ongoing. Compression of varices for 48 h is recommended. Aspiration and esophageal perforation comprise the major complications of tamponade tube use.

Unremitting or recurrent variceal hemorrhage may require surgical intervention to relieve portal hypertension or to resect varices. The most commonly used surgical therapy for bleeding varices is the portosystemic shunt with the mesocaval shunt the preferred procedure in acute variceal hemorrhage.

When large gastric varices are present with small or absent esophageal varices splenic or portal vein thrombosis should be suspected. This is important since splenectomy is definitive therapy for recurrent bleeding rather than a porto systemic shunt.

The prognosis for nonvariceal hemorrhage is better than for variceal hemorrhage in part because of the self-limited nature of most UGI bleeding.

Mallory-Weiss tears are usually self-limited. Electrocoagulation or injection therapy can be attempted for continued bleeding but surgical intervention should only be considered if more than 10u packed cells is required to maintain the hematocrit.

Although H_2-receptor antagonists, antacids, and sucralfate are effective in healing peptic ulcers, no trial has shown benefit of these therapies in the management of acute bleeding from ulcers. If active bleeding is seen at the time of endoscopy however, both electrocoagulation and injection therapy have been shown to be effective. Angiographic therapy with intraarterial vasopressin or gel foam embolization should be reserved for high risk patients awaiting surgery. Surgical intervention should be considered when medical and endoscopic means have failed to stop life-threatening bleeding or when medical therapy has failed to heal or prevent recurrence of peptic ulceration.

Acute hemorrhagic gastritis should be treated with acid suppression or angiographic therapy. Surgery should be avoided since it carries such a high risk.

LOWER GI BLEEDING

Acute lower GI bleeding is defined as bleeding below the ligament of Treitz. As a rule the color of blood should not be used to predict the site of bleeding since the pace of bleeding will affect the color as well. Bleeding significant enough to produce orthostasis or tachycardia is generally from a vascular source rather than a polyp or carcinoma.

Diagnosis

Controversies exist regarding the diagnostic evaluation of the patient with lower GI bleeding. The three modalities most commonly

used are angiography, colonoscopy and radionuclide scanning and
have been discussed elsewhere (see Chap 7). The use of emergency
colonoscopy during severe bleeding has been largely avoided because it generally is nondiagnostic and impractical. Most en-
doscopists urge conservative support until bleeding has subsided
before proceeding with colonoscopy.

Therapy

Supportive therapy remains the mainstay for patients with lower GI
bleeding since most episodes stop spontaneously. Other options
include angiographically-guided intra-arterial vasopressin and occasionally endoscopic coagulation. Lastly, the bleeding segment can
be surgically resected if bleeding cannot be controlled or recurs.
Many consider surgery necessary if more than 6 to 8 units packed
cells are transfused over a 24 h period.

BLEEDING OF UNKNOWN ORIGIN

Occasionally a patient with significant acute GI bleeding will
undergo extensive evaluation without a source of bleeding identified. One etiology to consider in this situation is angiodysplasia
in various areas of the GI tract. A second, less common, etiology
is hemobilia from the liver, bile ducts or pancreas. Lastly, an
aortoenteric fistula can develop following abdominal vascular
surgery.

STRESS-RELATED MUCOSAL DAMAGE (SRMD)

SRMD, commonly referred to as stress ulcers, is the result of
multiple major system failure in the critically ill patient. Endoscopically, SRMD appears as multiple erosions or submucosal
hemorrhages. Therapy is supportive while attempts are made to
reverse underlying stress factors. Benefit from H_2-blockers or
antacids is unproven. Surgery should only be considered as a last
resort.

As bleeding for SRMD is difficult to treat, much attention has
been given to prophylactic therapy. Antacids, continuous H_2-
blocker infusions, and sucralfate have been tried. Sucralfate does
not raise the gastric pH, thereby lessening the degree of gram-negative colonization of the stomach. Therefore it may be the preferred
agent. In some patients combination therapy may be warranted.
Omeprazole, which achieves complete achlorhydria, is being studied as a prophylactic agent.

For further reading in *Principles of Critical Care,* see Chap 33 "Endoscopy" Ira M Hanan, Chap 163 "Gastrointestinal Hemorrhage" Ira M Hanan

Stephen R. Amesbury

Patients admitted to the ICU with severe liver disease comprise two main groups: those with fulminant hepatic failure (FHF) and those having cirrhosis. Each of these will be discussed, followed by a discussion of general supportive measures for all liver disease patients.

FULMINANT HEPATIC FAILURE

Fulminant hepatic failure is defined as the development of hepatic encephalopathy (HE) within 8 weeks of the initial presentation of liver-related symptoms. Viral hepatitis is the most common cause of FHF worldwide. Other causes include toxic ingestions (acetaminophen, tetracycline, halothane, ethanol, isoniazid), ischemia (vascular occlusion, gram-negative bacteremia and shock, low cardiac output states), and metabolic abnormalities (Wilson's disease, acute fatty liver of pregnancy).

Typical physical findings include asterixis, confusion, jaundice, and occasionally fever. Tachycardia and hypotension may be due to FHF alone or to superimposed gastrointestinal hemorrhage or sepsis. Laboratory abnormalities vary with the etiology of the hepatic injury, but it is the presence of HE which distinguishes FHF from severe hepatitis.

Complications

Complications of FHF include cerebral edema, circulatory impairment, and metabolic, renal, and pulmonary derangements. Cerebral edema complicates 50 to 80 percent of cases of FHF, may precipitate uncal or cerebellar herniation, and in some series is the leading cause of death in patients with FHF. Cerebral edema ultimately causes morbidity and mortality by increasing intracranial pressure (ICP). Volume overload or a hypooncotic state may worsen cerebral edema. Hypotension due to FHF, gastrointestinal hemorrhage, or sepsis, may reduce the cerebral perfusion pressure and further compromise brain blood flow. Cerebral edema is usually present only in those patients with significant HE (stage III or IV). Increased ICP may be evident on physical exam or may only be demonstrated by computed tomography (CT). Invasive ICP monitoring may be used to better monitor patients at high risk for increased ICP.

Two forms of therapy are effective in reducing ICP: hyperventilation and osmotic diuretics. Hyperventilation to a P_{CO_2} of 25 mmHg is only transiently useful because of renal compensation for acute hypocapnia. Mannitol (1 g/kg) may be given as often as necessary (while monitoring the ICP and serum electrolytes) as long as the serum osmolality does not exceed 320 mOsm. These therapies should be titrated to an ICP <30 mmHg or a cerebral perfusion pressure >40 mmHg.

Circulatory impairment manifested as hypotension may be due to hemorrhage or infection, but in 60 percent of instances, no explanation is found. Patients with FHF have a baseline increased cardiac output and reduced peripheral resistance.

Hypoglycemia is common and dextrose requirements may be unusually high. Commonly, 10% dextrose solutions are needed. Impaired hepatic metabolism of lactate may result in severe lactic acidosis. Sodium bicarbonate is probably not indicated in this instance. Renal failure may be due to acute tubular necrosis or may be functional in nature. Arterial hypoxemia may be due to pulmonary vascular abnormalities or pulmonary edema.

Prognosis

Survival is more likely with acetaminophen overdose (53 percent) and hepatitis A (67 percent). Survival also correlates with the severity of liver injury, as measured by prothrombin time, metabolic acidosis, ability to correct coagulopathy, and degree of HE. Orthotopic liver transplantation has improved survival of FHF patients.

CHRONIC LIVER DISEASE

Although HE is common, it is usually not the overriding complication as in FHF, since the HE of cirrhosis is more amenable to treatment and is not complicated by cerebral edema. Rather, the ICU course is dominated by variceal hemorrhage, spontaneous bacterial peritonitis (SBP), and hepatorenal syndrome (HRS).

Variceal Hemorrhage

Patients suspected of variceal hemorrhage are bleeding from other sites in about 30 percent of cases, making early definitive diagnosis with esophagogastroduodenoscopy essential. It is common for bleeding to cease spontaneously, making assessment of therapeutic interventions difficult. Despite this, rebleeding is the rule if definitive therapy is not undertaken.

Supportive management includes at least two large bore peripheral intravenous catheters and intravascular volume resuscitation, using crystalloid and adding packed red blood cells and fresh frozen plasma as needed. A central venous pressure of 10 cmH$_2$O and a pulmonary capillary wedge pressure of 12 to 16 cmH$_2$O are reasonable targets. Several units of blood should be available in the blood bank at all times. In the first few minutes of ICU stabilization, it is important to assess the need for endotracheal intubation. Airway assessment must be repeated throughout the ICU course to avoid belated, emergent intubation. Nearly all patients in whom esophageal tamponade tubes are placed should first be intubated.

Once acute resuscitation and airway control are established, attention can turn to control of bleeding. Urgent therapeutic endoscopy and sclerotherapy deserve the highest priority. Acute control of bleeding is achieved in 90 percent of patients. Balloon tamponade of varices controls bleeding in 85 percent of patients. Begin by inflating only the gastric balloon (Table 61-1) since this controls

TABLE 61-1 Use of the Sengstaken-Blakemore Tube

1. Assess the need for airway intubation. With rare exceptions (e.g., alert, cooperative, hemodynamically stable patient), an endotracheal tube (ETT) should be placed first. The sedation typically mandated by the tube itself is often an indication for airway protection in itself.

2. This three-lumen tube consists of a distal (gastric) balloon, an esophageal balloon, and a distal suction/lavage port. Before placement, the integrity of both balloons must be ensured. The gastric (distal) balloon is a "volume" balloon which is filled with 250 mL air. The esophageal balloon is a "pressure" balloon and should be tested at 40 mmHg using a mercury manometer and a three-way stopcock.

3. Deflate the balloons, lubricate the device, and insert it through the mouth and into the stomach. A cooperative patient may be able to assist passage by swallowing. Placement in the stomach should be confirmed by injecting air through the distal lumen while listening for a rush of air over the stomach.

4. The gastric balloon should be partially inflated (100 mL) and a chest radiograph obtained to confirm adequate placement in the stomach. Then the balloon is fully inflated (total volume 250 mL). The tube is gently snugged against the gastroesophageal junction and affixed to an external device to maintain traction, a maneuver which will usually stop bleeding. A conventional suction tube should be placed through the mouth, into the esophagus, to remove pooled secretions which will collect above the balloon.

5. A repeat chest radiograph should be obtained to confirm proper placement of the gastric balloon against the gastroesophageal junction.

6. If bleeding continues, the esophageal balloon should be inflated to 25 to 40 mmHg, using the least pressure which maintains hemostasis. Some advocate deflating the esophageal balloon for 30 min each 12 h to reduce the likelihood of esophageal mucosal necrosis. The gastric balloon should never be deflated while the tube is in place.

7. Plans should be made for more definitive therapy to control bleeding.

8. In an emergency, the tube can be removed after cutting across all three lumens.

bleeding in two-thirds of patients. Acute rebleeding occurs when the balloon is deflated in about half the patients so that this approach should be considered only as a bridge to one of the more definitive therapies.

Intravenous vasopressin has long been used in variceal hemorrhage, however, its efficacy has never been shown, and complications are frequent. Vasopressin is given at 40 U/h until bleeding stops, following which it is reduced to 20 U/h, then continued for 24 h or longer. Pharmacotherapy is of little efficacy and can cause serious complications so it should be used only when sclerotherapy is unavailable or has failed. Pharmacotherapy should not be used at all in patients with coronary artery disease.

Definitive therapy once acute bleeding is controlled includes liver transplantation, continued sclerotherapy, esophageal transection, and portosystemic shunting (PSS). PSS operations should be avoided in patients who are considered transplant candidates, unless transjugular intrahepatic portosystemic shunting (TIPS) is available. For patients with gastric fundal varices, PSS is the treatment of choice.

Spontaneous Bacterial Peritonitis

Clinical manifestations vary from patients who are asymptomatic to others having fulminant sepsis. Since SBP is often very subtle, paracentesis should be performed in cirrhotics with deteriorating renal function, hypothermia, new-onset diarrhea, or unexplained encephalopathy. The most sensitive indicator is a fluid PMN leukocyte count >250/mm^3. Positive ascitic fluid cultures confirm the diagnosis, but these are negative in some patients. Other causes of peritonitis, such as appendicitis and cholecystitis must be kept in mind. Empiric treatment with cefotaxime, 2 g intravenously every 6 h is preferred. Subsequent therapy should be guided by culture results. If clinical suspicion is high, continue treatment for 10 to 14 days even if cultures are negative. If the patient is unimproved in 48 h, paracentesis should be repeated to assess the effectiveness of therapy.

Hepatorenal Syndrome

Hepatorenal syndrome (HRS) is functional renal failure complicating severe hepatic disease, usually in patients with tense ascities, and may be precipitated by critical illness (hypotension, sepsis, variceal hemorrhage) or medical interventions (paracentesis, diuresis, prostaglandin inhibitors), prompting admission to the ICU. It is crucial to exclude hypovolemia, because this can mimic HRS in all respects. If hypovolemia cannot be confidently ruled out on clinical grounds, it may be necessary to place a pulmonary artery catheter or give a rapid fluid challenge (500 to 1000 mL). In HRS and prerenal azotemia, the urinary sodium concentration is low and the urine: plasma creatinine ratio is elevated. In ATN, the urine sodium content is usually higher than 20 meq/L, while the urine: plasma creatinine ratio is <20. Prostaglandin inhibitors must be avoided.

This syndrome is largely refractory to therapy short of liver transplantation, and the prognosis is poor. When the diagnosis of HRS is certain, dialysis should only be instituted as a bridge to transplantation. Vasoactive drugs and diuretics are generally ineffective.

GENERAL SUPPORTIVE MEASURES FOR HEPATIC DISEASE

Infection is common in both acute and chronic liver failure. Pneumonia and urinary tract infection are the most common. Infection is the proximate cause of death in up to one-fourth of cirrhotics. Because clinical indicators of infection may be absent (increase in temperature or white blood cell count), empirical broad-spectrum antimicrobial therapy is appropriate in any hemodynamically unstable patient.

Airway protection is important since the risk of aspiration is very high. Gastrointestinal hemorrhage, infection, drug effect, worsening of HE, endoscopy, and placement of an esophageal tamponade balloon all increase the risk of aspiration. Endotracheal intubation should be performed early, with measures taken to prevent increases in intracranial pressure related to airway manipulation.

Coagulopathy is nearly universal in patients with severe liver disease. In FHF, replacement of clotting factors has not been shown to prevent clinically significant bleeding. However, fresh frozen plasma and platelets should be transfused prior to any surgical or invasive procedure. Vitamin K (10 mg subcutaneously for 3 days) should be given to all patients with chronic liver disease. Efforts to reduce bleeding risks, such as H_2 antagonists or antacids to keep the gastric pH above 5, cannot be overemphasized. Endotracheal and nasogastric tubes should be placed through the mouth because of the risk of life-threatening epistaxis following nasotracheal intubation.

Malnutrition characterizes the patient with severe liver disease. Institution of full nutritional support should be an early priority. High concentration glucose infusion is sometimes necessary to maintain blood glucose levels. These patients must receive thiamine and folic acid because preexisting dietary inadequacy is the rule.

Drug administration may be complicated by reduced protein binding, impaired hepatic degradation or renal failure. Regular assays of drug levels and attention to adverse drug effects are important.

TABLE 61-2 Precipitants of Hepatic Encephalopathy

Gastrointestinal hemorrhage
Spontaneous bacterial peritonitis
Systemic infection
Drugs (especially benzodiazepines and barbiturates)
Acute deterioration in liver function (e.g., hepatitis, hepatotoxin)
Dietary protein load
Alkalosis
Diuretic therapy, especially with hypokalemia
Diarrhea or dehydration
Constipation
Azotemia

Hepatic encephalopathy is usually reversible in patients with cirrhosis, whereas the HE in FHF patients responds poorly, if at all, to standard treatment.

Neuropsychiatric abnormalities range from subtle findings to deep coma. The severity of HE has been stratified. Early, or stage I, encephalopathy is characterized by subtle personality changes, fine tremor, slurred speech, and disordered sleep rhythm. Stage II is easily detected when the patient is drowsy, has inappropriate behavior and is not able to maintain sphincter control. In stage III, patients sleep most of the time, speech is incoherent, and confusion is marked. Stage IV refers to coma, where the patient has minimal or no response to painful stimuli. Decerebrate posturing may be seen. In FHF, rapid progression from stage I to stage IV is common.

Other causes of impaired mentation related to underlying liver disease include hypoglycemia, subdural hematoma, meningitis, subclinical status epilepticus, hypoxemia, and Wernicke's encephalopathy. Arterial ammonia level does not correlate well with the presence or degree of encephalopathy. EEG findings may be characteristic. Precipitants of HE are listed in Table 61-2.

Treatment of HE with lactulose (30 to 45 mL/h) given by nasogastric tube to induce three loose stools per day or rectally (300 mL in saline solution as retention enema for 30 to 60 min every 6 h) is effective. Neomycin is an alternative, given as 2 g every 8 h via a nasogastric tube. Despite aggressive treatment of HE the potential for deterioration must be appreciated. Serial examinations are essential, with attention to the patient's ability to guard the airway.

For further reading in *Principles of Critical Care,* see Chap 164 "Acute and Chronic Hepatic Disease" Theodore H Lewis, Jr/Gregory A Schmidt

Acute pancreatitis in the intensive care unit is difficult to diagnose and treat. Although pancreatitis is usually self-limited, it is potentially lethal when complicated by multi-system failure and sepsis, often with complications which can make surgical intervention necessary but also increase the risks of morbidity and mortality. Accordingly, it is important to identify this lesion early, and remove precipitating factors, if possible. Acute pancreatitis present on hospitalization differs from that which develops in association with critical illness during hospitalization; the following discussion will focus on the latter.

Although alcohol and gallstones are the most common precipitants, many etiologies for acute pancreatitis are recognized (Table 62-1). An intensive inflammatory response caused by the release of activated pancreatic enzymes is the common underlying pathogenetic mechanism. A variety of illnesses precede the development of pancreatitis in the intensive care unit. After cardiopulmonary bypass, predisposing factors may include microembolism, venous

TABLE 62-1 Acute Pancreatitis—Etiologic Factors

Metabolic	Obstructive/ Mechanical	Infections	Idiopathic	Hypoperfusion
Alcohol	Gallstones	Mumps	Familial	Vascular
Hyper-calcemia	Afferent loop obstruction	Coxsackie		PAN and other collagen disorders
Drugs	Duodenal obstruction	*Mycoplasma*		embolic
Hyper-lipidemia	Periampullary tumors	Ascariasis*		†Low Flow States
	Duodenal ulcer	Clonorchiasis*		
	Pancreas divisum			
	Trauma blunt penetrating †postoperative post ERCP			

*May cause pancreatitis by an obstructive mechanism
†Aetiologic factors important in the critically ill patient who develops acute pancreatitis (*Reproduced with permission from Taylor BR: Acute Pancreatitis in the Critically Ill, in Hall JB, Schmidt GA, Wood LDH: Principles of Critical Care, McGraw-Hill, New York, 1992.*)

thrombosis, low flow states, prolonged bypass, hypothermia, and the use of narcotics. After cardiac transplantation, predisposing factors also include the use of heparin, cyclosporin A, and prednisone. Hypocalcemia, intraoperative injury, and immunosuppressive regimens may predispose to acute pancreatitis after renal and hepatic transplantation. Whether due to cardiogenic, septic, or hypovolemic mechanisms, hypoperfusion appears to be a common injury predisposing to pancreatitis. Direct injury to the organ also is common in upper abdominal surgery.

DIAGNOSIS

Early diagnosis is important because of the need for timely intervention with aggressive supportive care and consideration of surgery. Clinical symptoms and signs are variable and difficult to evaluate in the critically ill. Classically, symptoms include abdominal pain, nausea and vomiting; signs include hyperpyrexia, unexplained hemodynamic instability and abdominal tenderness. Laboratory findings include leukocytosis, elevated serum amylase, elevated random urine amylase, elevated amylase: creatinine clearance ratio, and elevated serum lipase. The serum lipase level may be the most reliable and specific indicator of acute pancreatitis.

RADIOLOGY

Abdominal x-rays may show localized jejunal or colonic ileus, widened duodenal C loop, pancreatic calcifications, radiopaque gallstones, obliteration of the psoas shadow and pleural effusions. These findings, however, are nonspecific and other radiologic techniques are needed. Ultrasound is the methodology of choice in patients with pancreatitis who respond to conservative therapy, in suspected obstructive pancreatitis, and in followup of retroperitoneal phlegmon for resolution or development of pseudocyst. Ultrasonic imaging may be limited in the presence of paralytic ileus and obesity. An advantage of this technique is that bedside evaluation can be performed. The most useful modality for assessing the retroperitoneum in complicated cases is computerized tomography. A limitation of this technique is its inconvenience to perform in critical illness, when the mechanically ventilated patient must be transported. The greatest value of computerized tomography (CT) is the recognition and follow-up of significant complications such as pancreatic abscess.

SEVERITY OF DISEASE

Ransom's criteria (Table 62-2) are useful in assessing severity and prognosis in patients presenting with pancreatitis. The utility of these criteria, however, is limited in critically ill patients who de-

TABLE 62-2 Early Objective Prognostic Signs Used to Estimate the Risk of Death or Major Complications From Acute Pancreatitis

At Admission or Diagnosis	During Initial 48 H
Age > 55	Hematocrit fall > 10
WBC > 16,000/mm^3	percentage points
Blood Glucose > 200 mg/100mL	BUN rise > 5 mg/100 mL
Serum LDH > 350 I U/L	Serum calcium level <
SGOT > 250 U/dL	8 mg/100 mL
	Arterial O_2 < 60 mmHg
	Base deficit > 4meq/L
	Estimated fluid sequestration > 6L.

From Ranson JHC et al. Surgery Gynecology Obstetrics 1976:143:209-219.

velop pancreatitis as secondary disease: They already have many of the criteria before onset of pancreatitis. In the ICU, the best indices of severity of disease include the development of abdominal tenderness, circulatory instability, or complications such as pancreatic necrosis as seen on CT.

THERAPY

If intervention to correct a precipitating factor, such as gallstone disease, is indicated, surgery may be performed forthwith. More commonly in the ICU patient, however, no immediate corrective intervention is appropriate. The principles of therapy for acute pancreatitis include careful monitoring of symptoms and physical examination, correction of metabolic and hemodynamic effects, provision of respiratory and renal support, nutrition, control of pancreatic enzyme secretion, and prevention and therapy of local complications of necrosing pancreatitis.

Patients with severe pancreatitis require close monitoring of their hemodynamic, metabolic, pulmonary and renal status. Volume replacement is necessary because of vomiting and massive peritoneal fluid loss. Requirements vary from 2 to 10 or more liters of isotonic fluid in the first 24 h. Retroperitoneal hemorrhage may necessitate transfusion. Since pancreatic hypoperfusion is postulated to worsen pancreatitis, attention to volume replacement may limit progression of injury. Metabolic abnormalities in pancreatitis include acidosis, hypoglycemia, hypocalcemia, and hypomagnesemia. Hypoalbuminemia due to a significant protein loss may confound the interpretation of serum calcium levels. Serum ionized calcium can be helpful in identifying those patients with hypocalcemia.

Aggressive ventilatory support is often needed in the setting of severe pancreatitis. Many mechanisms have been suggested for the development of adult respiratory distress syndrome (ARDS) associated with pancreatitis including breakdown of surfactant by pancreas-derived phospholipase A, increased vascular permeability due to serotonin release, or complement activation. Pancreatitis is frequently associated with acute tubular necrosis, because each may result from hypoperfusion. Fluid administration, judicious use of diuretics and hemodialysis are all used to support renal function.

Nutritional support for the critically ill patient is important because their course is often prolonged. Although the benefit of total parenteral nutrition remains unproven in pancreatitis, early institution of therapy can blunt catabolic effects. Many modalities have been tried to limit the course of acute pancreatitis by inhibiting pancreatic enzyme secretion. The efficacy of H_2 blockers, nasal gastric suctioning, somatostatin, calcitonin and glucagon remains unproven.

LOCAL COMPLICATIONS

Complications of necrosing pancreatitis include abscess and pseudocyst formation. Patients with retroperitoneal fat or pancreatic necrosis are at high risk for death; those without these complications usually survive with supportive measures only. Pancreatic and peripancreatic necrosis predispose to both local infection and sepsis. CT may identify necrosis, but it is not helpful in differentiating infected from sterile necrosis. Because debridement of the pancreas often results in the need for further surgical procedures to drain fluid sequestrations, major surgical debridement is usually avoided until sepsis is confirmed or the course is prolonged without improvement.

Although the role of antibiotics is controversial, a reasonable approach includes their use in patients with pancreatic necrosis, because they are at risk for sepsis. Antibiotic use alone, however, will not improve necrosis with infection without debridement or percutaneous drainage.

The principles of surgical treatment include wide debridement of devitalized fat and pancreatic tissue followed by generous drainage to allow passage of purulent particulate matter. Fluid collections adjoining the pancreas by the lesser sac of the stomach are extremely common. When these collections develop fibrous walls resulting from inflammatory exudate, they are referred to as pseudocysts. These lesions may be managed conservatively; however, they can grow quickly, bleed, rupture, or become infected. Enlarging or infected pseudocysts should be percutaneously decompressed; hemorrhage or free rupture require immediate surgery.

For further reading in *Principles of Critical Care,* see Chap 165 "Acute Pancreatitis in the Critically Ill" Bryce R Taylor

Edward T. Naureckas

PATHOPHYSIOLOGY

The three most common causes of mesenteric ischemia are acute arterial emboli, thrombotic events, and primary vasoconstriction.

Embolism accounts for approximately a third of cases of mesenteric ischemia and occurs most commonly in association with cardiac arrhythmias or myocardial infarction. The superior mesenteric artery (SMA) is the site of most embolic occlusions due to its oblique origin from the abdominal aorta.

Acute thrombosis at a site of atherosclerotic narrowing occurs in another one-third of cases. These pre-existing atherosclerotic lesions are often associated with prodromal symptoms. Over half of patients who die due to SMA thrombosis have had a history of postprandial abdominal pain.

Nonocclusive mesenteric ischemia involves the SMA distribution almost exclusively. The pathophysiology of this entity is multifactorial, usually involving moderate to severe mesenteric atherosclerosis, marginal cardiac reserve and the administration of vasoactive drugs. The onset usually follows an abrupt fall in cardiac output with a decreased mesenteric perfusion pressure. Catecholamines released in response to hypotension and the preceding use of drugs such as digitalis may further the vasoconstrictive process.

Venous thrombosis, a final and relatively uncommon cause of mesenteric ischemia may begin peripherally in the small veins of the mesenteric arcade or centrally in the major trunks of the portal system.

CLINICAL PRESENTATION

A high index of suspicion is required to make the diagnosis of mesenteric ischemia. If the diagnosis is made in less than 24 h, 60 percent of patients survive. If the diagnosis is delayed greater than 24 h, less than 30 percent of patients will survive. Risk factors for mesenteric ischemia include age over fifty years, severe valvular atherosclerotic disease, cardiac arrhythmias, and recent myocardial infarction.

Acute mesenteric emboli and thrombosis both classically present with severe abdominal pain localized to the mid abdomen, out of proportion to the findings on physical examination. If peritoneal signs are elicited, it is likely that intestinal infarction has already occurred. Arterial thrombosis may also mimic small bowel obstruction with a more gradual onset of symptoms including abdominal distention and vomiting.

Embolism should be suspected with an acute onset of symptoms in the setting of cardiac arrhythmias.

Nonocclusive mesenteric ischemia is also usually accompanied by periumbilical pain but may also occur with the absence of such symptoms. Clinical signs may be limited to shock, acidosis, hemoconcentration and sepsis of unknown etiology.

Mesenteric venous thrombosis generally presents with constant, diffuse abdominal pain, although symptoms may be intermittent at first. Roughly half of the patients complain of nausea with fever. Serosanguinous ascites may also be present.

Laboratory studies are nonspecific but include hemoconcentration, leukocytosis, acidosis, hyperamylasemia and hyperphosphatemia. Abdominal x-rays may be used to exclude other causes of abdominal pain such as small bowel obstruction. Other signs such as ileus, ascites, small bowel dilation and thickening of the valvulae conniventes may be positive in mesenteric ischemia, but are nonspecific. Intramural or portal air may be seen in the presence of infarction and colonization with gas forming organisms. Colonoscopy is useful mainly in detecting sigmoidal ischemia.

Barium studies are contraindicated as they interfere with the definitive diagnostic procedure which is mesenteric arteriography.

As splanchnic constriction can interfere with an adequate study, the patient must be stabilized hemodynamically, and vasoconstrictor drugs should be discontinued if possible.

THERAPY

When the diagnosis of mesenteric ischemia is considered, every effort should be made to discontinue or reduce the administration of drugs with α-adrenergic effects. In the case of nonocclusive ischemia, intraarterial administration of papaverine into the SMA at a rate of 30 to 60 mg/h for 24 to 48 h may be considered to be the primary mode of therapy, and may avert surgery if symptoms completely resolve.

In contrast all patients with suspected emboli or thrombotic occlusions should undergo urgent laparotomy. Once flow is restored via extraction of the emboli or a bypass procedure, viability of the reperfused bowel may be judged intraoperatively by a return of normal bowel color, mesenteric arterial pulsations and visible peristalsis. More objective measures of determining viability are the detection of mural blood flow by Doppler ultrasound or fluorescein injection followed by detection with a Wood's lamp.

Once resection of nonviable bowel is completed, exteriorization with cutaneous enterostomies or a "second look" procedure should be performed if there is any question of viability at the resected margins.

Careful attention to fluid management in the perioperative period is essential. Coverage with broad-spectrum antibiotics should be continued for at least five days. Unless contraindicated, heparin anticoagulation followed by 3 months of warfarin therapy is appropriate. If vascular reconstruction has been performed, postoperative angiography is prudent prior to discharge.

For further reading in *Principles of Critical Care,* see Chap 167 "Mesenteric Ischemia" Elizabeth T Clark/Bruce L Gewertz

Adrenocortical Insufficiency in the Intensive Care Unit

Stephen R. Amesbury

Adrenocortical insufficiency is classified as primary (Addison's disease) when it results from direct involvement of the adrenal gland and as secondary when it results from deficient adrenocorticotropic hormone (ACTH) production by the pituicytes or from corticotropin releasing factor (CRF) deficiency. The most common cause of adrenocortical hypofunction—that arising from glucocorticoid therapy (Table 64-1)—is an example of secondary adrenocortical insufficiency.

Autoimmune adrenalitis is the most common cause of primary adrenocortical insufficiency (Table 64-2), and is responsible for approximately 80 percent of cases. It often occurs in young white females and is often associated with other autoimmune disorders. Mycobacterium tuberculosis is the second most common cause of primary adrenocortical insufficiency, accounting for fewer than 20 percent of cases. The four most common tumors to involve the adrenals are lung cancer, breast cancer, melanoma, and lymphoma. Although adrenal metastases are common, adrenocortical insufficiency rarely results because 90 percent of the adrenal cortex must be destroyed before hypofunction occurs. Adrenal hemorrhage associated with fulminant sepsis, especially meningococcal sepsis, is an important cause of adrenocortical insufficiency in the ICU. Patients with acquired immunodeficiency syndrome (AIDS) are at risk of developing adrenocortical insufficiency from opportunistic infection, Kaposi's sarcoma, and drugs.

TABLE 64-1 Glucocorticoid and Mineralocorticoid Preparations

	Relative Glucocorticoid Potency	Relative Mineralocorticoid Potency	Equivalent Glucocorticoid Dose
Hydrocortisone (Cortef, Solu-Cortef)	1.0	1.0	100mg po, iv
Prednisone (Deltasone, Meticorten)	4.0	0.7	25mg po
Methylprednisolone (Medrol, Solu-Medrol)	5.0	0.5	20mg po, iv
Dexamethasone (Decadron, Hexadrol)	25.0	2.0	4mg po, iv
Fludrocortisone (Florinef)	10.0	400	*

*The usual mineralocorticoid replacement dose has no significant glucocorticoid activity.

TABLE 64-2 Etiology of Primary Adrenocortical Insufficiency

Autoimmune (idiopathic) (80%)
Mycobacterium tuberculosis (<20%)
Miscellaneous (<1%)
  Hemorrhage (sepsis, anticoagulants, coagulopathy, history of
    thromboembolic disease, post-surgery, trauma, "difficult" pregnancy,
    burns, leukemia, metastatic carcinoma, pancreatitis, vasculitis,
    postadrenal venography)
  AIDS (fungi, mycobacteria, CMV, Kaposi's sarcoma)
  Fungal infection (histoplasmosis, coccidioidomycosis, paracoccidioido-
    mycosis, cryptococcus, blastomycosis, candidiasis, torulopsis)
  Metastatic carcinoma
  Lymphoma
  Drugs (rifampin, ketoconazole, aminoglutethimide, metyrapone,
    trilostane, etomidate, cyproterone acetate, o p′ DDD)
  Bilateral adrenalectomy
  Irradiation
  Sarcoidosis
  Amyloidosis
  Hemochromatosis
  Congenital

TABLE 64-3 Etiology of Secondary Adrenocortical Insufficiency

Glucocorticoid therapy
Tumors (pituitary adenoma, craniopharyngioma, meningioma, glioma,
  hamartoma, pinealoma, metastatic carcinoma [breast, lung, GI],
  lymphoma, leukemia)
Vascular
  Pituitary apoplexy (almost always related to primary pituitary tumor)
  Sheehan's syndrome (postpartum)
  Intracranial aneurysm
  Cavernous sinus thrombosis
  Diabetes mellitus
  Vasculitis
  Sickle-cell disease and trait
  Arteriosclerosis
  Eclampsia
Pituitary surgery
Irradiation (to nasopharynx, sella turcica)
Head trauma
Infection (tuberculosis, fungal disease, syphilis, malaria, brucellosis,
  nocardiosis, actinomycosis, abscess, viruses)
Autoimmune
Sarcoidosis
Histiocytosis X
Hemochromatosis
Lipid storage diseases
Isolated ACTH deficiency
Congenital

The causes of secondary adrenocortical insufficiency (Table 64-3) are many, but with the exception of chronic glucocorticoid therapy, secondary is much less common than primary adrenocortical insufficiency. Most patients entering an ICU with secondary adrenocortical insufficiency are receiving glucocorticoids or have been on them in the prior year. A reasonable guideline is to consider all patients who have been on 40 mg/day of prednisone, or its equivalent, for a period longer than 2 to 3 weeks as adrenally compromised, especially if they have become cushingoid. In this setting, adrenocortical insufficiency can occur in response to stress as long as one year after steroids have been discontinued, and such patients should be considered for interim coverage with "stress doses" of steroids.

CLINICAL FEATURES OF ADRENOCORTICAL INSUFFICIENCY

The signs and symptoms of adrenocortical insufficiency are of much greater severity in the acute case. Weakness, fatigue, anorexia, hyperpigmentation, and hypotension are usually present in chronic primary adrenocortical insufficiency. Except for adrenal hemorrhage, localizing signs are usually absent. Fever is common, even without underlying infection. The classic laboratory findings of adrenocortical insufficiency (hyponatremia, hyperkalemia, hypotension) are helpful when present, but cannot be used to exclude the diagnosis when they are absent. This is because mineralocorticoid production remains unaffected in cases of secondary adrenocortical insufficiency. The presence of hypoglycemia in a hypotensive patient should immediately raise the possibility of this diagnosis.

This uncommon diagnosis demands a high index of suspicion, since its manifestations are frequently nonspecific. Because the side effects of a short course of "stress" steroids are minimal, it is better to "oversuspect" and overtreat, than to miss the diagnosis which can have grave results (Table 64-4).

DIAGNOSIS

Serum Cortisol

A random cortisol level greater than 20 μg/dL makes the diagnosis of adrenocortical insufficiency very unlikely. On the other hand, in the setting of shock, a cortisol level less than 20 μg/dL is highly suggestive of hypoadrenalism and should prompt a rapid ACTH stimulation test.

Rapid ACTH Stimulation Test

This test measures the response of the adrenal gland to stimulation by exogenous ACTH. After the drawing of samples for basal levels

TABLE 64-4 When to Consider the Diagnosis of Adrenocortical Insufficiency

History of treatment with glucocorticoids (within the past year)
Hypotension (systolic BP <110 mmHg) with a chronic history of weight loss and weakness
Hypotension with a history or evidence of tuberculosis, malignancy, AIDS, polyendocrine deficiency, vitiligo, or coagulopathy
Hyperkalemia and hyponatremia, especially in the absence of chronic renal failure
Hypotension with hypoglycemia or eosinophilia
Hypotension with hyperpigmentation
Hypotension with the absence of axillary or pubic hair in a female
Unexplained hypotension unresponsive to aggressive fluids and vasoactive drugs

of cortisol, aldosterone, and ACTH, 250 μg of synthetic ACTH (cosyntropin) is administered intravenously. Repeat samples for cortisol and aldosterone are then drawn 30 and 60 min later. A peak cortisol level greater than 20 μg/dL is a sufficient single criterion for normal adrenal function. A clearly normal response eliminates the possibility of primary adrenocortical insufficiency and makes the diagnosis of secondary hypoadrenalism unlikely. However, because patients with secondary adrenocortical insufficiency rarely show a normal response, and because there are occasional false-positives, the test results should be verified when the patient's condition stabilizes. The "gold standard" is the standard ACTH stimulation test. Other investigations to test the integrity of the hypothalamic-pituitary-adrenal axis include the metyrapone test, CRF stimulation test, and insulin-hypoglycemia test.

MANAGEMENT

Preexisting or Presumed Adrenocortical Insufficiency

Patients who are known to have adrenocortical insufficiency or who have a history of glucocorticoid treatment in the past year should be given "stress doses" of corticosteroids during severe intercurrent illness and during surgical procedures. The use of hydrocortisone sodium succinate, 100 mg intravenously every 6 to 8 h, effectively eliminates the possibility of adrenocortical insufficiency. Hydrocortisone should be promptly tapered to maintenance levels once the acute illness has resolved.

The Hemodynamically Stable Patient

Measurement of plasma cortisol and a rapid ACTH stimulation test should precede initiation of "stress doses" of steroids. Hypovolemia should be treated with glucose-containing saline solution using the usual clinical guidelines. If the diagnosis is confirmed, hydrocorti-sone sodium succinate, 100 mg intravenously every 6 to 8 h, should be instituted.

The Hemodynamically Unstable Patient

Acute adrenal insufficiency is life-threatening and requires prompt and aggressive therapy to effect an optimal outcome. Dexametha-sone sodium phosphate, 4 mg, should be given intravenously im-mediately. Dexamethasone is preferred as the initial glucocorticoid replacement because, unlike hydrocortisone, it does not interfere with the assay for cortisol, and thus will not preclude performance of the rapid ACTH stimulation test. Although dexamethasone possesses no mineralocorticoid activity, vigorous hydration with saline solution will allow the patient to tolerate this lack easily for the 1 h required to perform the rapid ACTH stimulation test. Once the diagnostic tests are concluded, hydrocortisone should be substi-tuted promptly for dexamethasone, since it has sufficient mineralocorticoid activity so as not to require concomitant mineralocorticoid replacement. The intramuscular route of admin-istration is to be avoided in hypoperfused states due to the uncer-tainty of adequate absorption. In general, persons with acute adrenocortical insufficiency have a deficit of approximately 20 per-cent of their extra cellular fluid volume and should receive at least 3 L of glucose-containing saline solution. The patient's fluid, elec-trolyte, and glucose status should be carefully monitored during resuscitation. The precipitating cause of the adrenal decompensa-tion, especially infection, should be sought.

In patients with coexistent hypothyroidism, either from hypopi-tuitarism or from autoimmune thyroiditis, glucocorticoid replace-ment should begin prior to thyroid hormone replacement. Administration of thyroid hormone increases the metabolism of glucocorticoids. Thus, treatment with thyroid hormone before glucocorticoids might worsen the hypoadrenal state, perhaps pre-cipitating a crisis.

For further reading in *Principles of Critical Care*, see Chap 160 "Adrenocortical Insufficiency in the Intensive Care Unit" Steven Koenig/Gregory A Schmidt

EUTHYROID SICK SYNDROME

The euthyroid sick syndrome, also known as nonthyroidal illness, refers to the reduction in serum T_3, T_4, and thyroid stimulating hormone (TSH) values associated with profound illness or malnutrition. Virtually all critically ill patients have reduced serum levels of T_3 and 30 to 50% also have low T_4 concentrations in association with normal or low TSH values. In the ICU population, T_4 values less than 3.0 μg/dL despite normal T_4 binding proteins are associated with a 68 to 84% mortality rate. Severe illness and malnutrition are associated with reduction in 5′-deiodinase activity, which results in low T_4 and high reverse T_3 (rT_3) levels. The nature of the perturbations resulting in low T_4 and TSH levels is less clearly understood. Several drugs, including dopamine, inhibit TSH secretion.

Because of the euthyroid sick syndrome, interpretation of thyroid function studies and the recognition of hypothyroidism in the ICU setting is particularly challenging (Table 65-1). In the absence of critical illness, low T_4 and TSH levels suggest secondary or tertiary hypothyroidism. In the ICU setting, however, primary hypothyroidism remains a consideration because of inadequate pituitary response. The strongest evidence for a primary hypothyroidism in the ICU population is elevation of TSH associated with a normal to low rT_3 value. Except in renal failure, a low T_3 value suggests hypothyroidism.

Treatment of nonthyroid illness with T_4 has not proven helpful and may lead to earlier mortality. No treatment for nonthyroidal illness is indicated unless signs of hypothyroidism, such as hyporeflexia, hypothermia, macroglossia or goiter, coexist. If the decision is made to treat, the drug of choice is T_3, which is only available in oral form.

TABLE 65-1 Interpretation of Thyroid Function Tests

Diagnosis	T_4	T_3	TSH	rT_3
1^0 hypothyroidism	dec	dec/N	inc	dec/N
Central hypothyroidism	dec	dec	N	??
Nonthyroidal illness	dec/N	dec	N/dec	N/inc

(Reproduced with permission from Weiss RE, Refetoff S: Hypothyroidism, Nonthyroidal Illness, and Myxedema Coma, in Hall JB, Schmidt GA, Wood LDH: Principles of Critical Care, McGraw-Hill, New York, 1992.)

Myxedema Coma

Myxedema coma is the profound depletion of thyroid hormones associated with defective thermoregulation, abnormal mental status and an identifiable precipitating event.

The usual precipitating factors include noncompliance with thyroid medication and intercurrent illness in patients with less severe hypothyroidism. Exacerbants include infection, surgery, stroke, occult GI bleeding, trauma, drug overdose, CHF, and exposure to cold. The common signs of myxedema are coarse skin and hair, jaundice, macroglossia, hoarseness, obtundation, delayed deep tendon reflexes, and hypothermia. The common laboratory findings include low T_4, high TSH, hypoglycemia, hyponatremia, hypokalemia, hypocortisolemia, anemia, leukocytosis, and elevated creatinine. Depressed hypoxic and hypercapnic ventilatory drives can result in alveolar hypoventilation and sleep apnea with cardiopulmonary failure may be precipitated. The cardiovascular complications of hypothyroidism include accelerated atherosclerosis, cardiomyopathy, and pericardial effusion, which can result in tamponade.

The principle of treatment is to rapidly replete the circulating pool of thyroid hormone. This is best achieved by IV administration of T_4. The active form of the hormone, T_3, is readily available to tissues and can be initiated orally, simultaneously. If only T_4 is used, a reasonable regimen is 500 μg levothyroxine initially, then 50 to 100 μg daily. If T_4 and T_3 are used, the initial bolus of levothyroxine should be followed by 25 μg T_3 per nasal gastric tube every 6 h until the intercurrent illness resolves, at which time daily T_4 is initiated. Concomitant primary hypoadrenalism is present in 5 to 10% of all patients with myxedema coma. An admission cortisol level should be obtained and glucocorticoids should be administered, 50 mg hydrocortisone every 6 h, until hypoadrenalism is ruled out. Alternatively, 2 mg dexamethasone can be given and a 1 h ACTH (Cosyntropin) stimulation test performed on admission.

Supportive care includes early intubation and mechanical ventilation. Passive warming is the best method for treating hypothermia in this setting, because external warming can to lead to peripheral vasodilation and shock. Hypothyroidism reduces the metabolism of all drugs and special attention to drug dosing is needed to avoid toxicity.

Myxedema coma is potentially fatal in approximately 50 % of patients although complete recovery can occur. Clinical indices recover over days and reduction of the TSH level is often the earliest evidence of response to therapy.

THYROTOXICOSIS

Careful history-taking and physical examination are the keys to early diagnosis of thyrotoxicosis in the ICU. Useful findings include:

1. previous diagnosis of thyrotoxicosis, 2. history of thyroid hormonal ingestion, 3. recent use of iodine containing radiologic contrast agent, and 4. presence of exophthalmos, goiter, or evidence of previous thyroid surgery.

Almost every organ system is adversely affected by thyrotoxicosis. Cardiopulmonary complications include hyperdynamic circulation, high output heart failure, myocardial ischemia, arrhythmia, respiratory muscle weakness, increased metabolic demand with increased O_2 consumption and CO_2 production. Neuromuscular complications include myopathy, ophthalmoplegia, thyrotoxic periodic paralysis, tremulousness, seizure, stupor and coma. Hypermotility with malabsorption occurs commonly and traumatic injury occurs rarely. Laboratory findings include elevated T_4, FTI, T_3, leukocytosis, anemia, hyperglycemia, hypokalemia, and hypercalcemia; hypercalcemia is the most common life-threatening electrolyte abnormality seen in thyrotoxicosis.

Autonomous hypersecretion and exogenous overdose are the most common causes of severe thyrotoxicosis. Thyroid storm, or thyrotoxic crisis, is a life-threatening complication of severe thyrotoxicosis. The hallmarks of this clinical diagnosis include tachycardia, hypertension, increased pulse pressure, hyperpyrexia, and altered mental status. Occasionally, cardiovascular collapse can result. Factors known to precipitate thyroid storm include surgery, trauma, infection, acute psychiatric illness, congestive heart failure, diabetic ketoacidosis, pulmonary embolism, bowel infarction, parturition, and use of iodide containing drugs or contrast agents.

Treatment

Therapy for severe thyrotoxicosis includes reduction of serum thyroid hormone level, reduction of action of thyroid hormone on peripheral tissues, prevention of cardiovascular collapse, and elimination of precipating factors.

To reduce circulating thyroid hormone levels, a combination of drugs to inhibit thyroid hormone synthesis and secretion is recommended. To inhibit hormone synthesis, the oral antithyroid drugs, propylthiouracil (PTU) or methimazole (MMI), are available. In addition to its inhibitory effect on hormone synthesis, PTU offers an advantage over MMI of inhibiting synthesis of T_3 in peripheral tissues. PTU is administered in 200 to 250 mg doses every 6 h; MMI is administered in 25 mg doses every 6 h. Each has the side effects of rash, agranulocytosis, and hepatic toxicity. The addition of stable iodine, as Lugol's solution or a saturated solution of potassium iodide (ssKI) 2 drops every 12 h, provides blockade of hormone secretion. Antithyroid drugs should be administered at least 1 h before iodine to avoid worsening thyrotoxicosis. The combination of an antithyroid drug and ssKI normalizes hormone levels in 1 to 5 days. In the setting of known hypersensitivity or prior adverse reaction to antithyroid drugs, iopanoate or lithium carbonate have been used.

Reduction of thyroid hormone action on body tissues is effected by inhibition of synthesis of the active thyroid hormone, T_3, or by counteracting its sympathomimetic effects. PTU, glucocorticoids, propranolol, and iopanoate have been used to inhibit T_3 synthesis; β-blockers reduce the sympathomimetic effects of T_3. Through slow IV push, 1 mg of propranolol can be administered every 5 min until the pulse rate slows. A total daily dose of 300 mg propranolol is often required. Younger patients develop a hyperadrenergic state associated with thyrotoxicosis more commonly than older patients who can present with so-called "apathetic" thyrotoxicosis, without hyperpyrexia and tachycardia. Because of cardiotoxic and bronchoconstrictive side effects, β-blockers should not be used in the elderly, asthmatic or heart failure patient.

Cardiovascular collapse can be prevented by the use of antipyretics, volume repletion with crystalloid and use of propranolol as discussed. Treatment of congestive heart failure is supportive, with judicious use of inotropic agents and diuretics. Because of accelerated metabolism of glucocorticoids in hypothyroidism, administration of 100 mg hydrocortisone every 8 h may be useful in preventing relative hypoadrenalism. Also, accelerated metabolism and clearance of many drugs, including digitalis, insulin, and antibiotics, occurs in thyrotoxicosis and dosing should be adjusted accordingly.

Finally, a scrupulous search should be performed and therapy initiated for the common precipating factors of thyrotoxicosis. Since the clinical setting often resembles sepsis, some authors recommend initiation of antibiotics pending blood and urine culture results.

Anesthesia and Surgery

The stress of surgery can precipitate thyroid storm in any thyrotoxic patient. The preoperative therapeutic goal of normalizing thyroid function using antithyroid drugs often takes 3 to 7 days. If this wait is unacceptable, an alternative approach is to block the sympathomimetic effects of thyroid hormone. Propranolol is the most commonly used drug in doses of 40 mg every 6 h.

Levothyroxine Overdose

In the United States, two to five thousand episodes of levothyroxine (L-T_4) overdose occur annually. Despite the high frequency of occurrence, there have been no deaths reported. No immediate toxic effects result; onset of symptoms begins approximately 24 h after ingestion, as the L-T_4 is converted to T_3. Treatment includes gastrointestinal decontamination using serum of ipecac and gastrointestinal lavage using charcoal. Cholestyramine will increase fecal elimination of the drug. Also recommended is the use of the prednisone, propylthiouracil, and propranolol, as needed.

For further reading in *Principles of Critical Care,* see Chap 161 "Hypothyroidism, Nonthyroidal Illness, and Myxedema Coma" Roy E Weiss/Samuel Refetoff, Chap 162 "Thyrotoxicosis" Roy E Weiss/Samuel Refetoff

GENERAL MANAGEMENT

Poisoning may be immediately apparent from history or may not be suspected until suggested by routine laboratory results or an evolving clinical course. In either case, initial management focuses on a rapid assessment of respiratory, circulatory, and central nervous system function and only then should the issue of poisoning be dealt with. All comatose patients should receive dextrose (50 mL of 50% dextrose), thiamine (100 mg), and naloxone (2 mg). Flumazenil (2.5 mg by slow IV infusion, then 0.1 mg/min up to 5 mg) may be of both diagnostic and therapeutic value in benzodiazepine overdose. Arterial blood gases, serum glucose, electrolytes, blood urea nitrogen, osmolality, and hematocrit should be included in the initial assessment of suspected poisoning. Poisons associated with hyperosmolality and an osmolar gap include ethanol, methanol, ethylene glycol, and isopropanol. Examples of poisoning causing a metabolic acidosis include cyanide, carbon monoxide, methanol, ethylene glycol, paraldehyde, and salicylates. If initial assessment suggests the presence of a poison, most laboratories can perform a toxin screen analysis on urine and blood. The clinician should be aware of the substances searched for in any given lab and should never assume that all poisons have been excluded by any given screen. It is important to remember that for intentional poisoning, history is often unreliable, and polypharmaceutical ingestion is common. Early consultation with a regional poison information center should be the rule.

After initial stabilization and while waiting confirmation of the specific diagnosis, prevention of further absorption through gastric emptying and administration of activated charcoal should be attempted. Contraindications to stomach emptying include ingestion of corrosive agents, ingestion of small amounts (less than 1 mL/kg) of petroleum distillates, ingestion of sharp objects, or history of hemorrhagic diathesis. Emptying of the stomach can be achieved by emesis or lavage. Emesis should be induced only in a fully conscious patient with normal gag reflexes. Syrup of ipecac has been used for induction of emesis at a dose of 30 to 50 mL; if vomiting has not occurred after 30 min the initial dose may be repeated. If the patient is unconscious, an endotracheal tube should be placed for airway protection and gastric aspiration and lavage via a large-bore orogastric tube should be used to empty the stomach. Emptying of the stomach should be followed by administration of activated charcoal (1 g/kg). Repeated activated charcoal administration (0.5 to 1 g/kg q 4 h) is indicated in cases of massive ingestion and in cases where significant enterohepatic recirculation of the ingested compound or of its metabolites may be present. Since charcoal may delay bowel transit and even cause impaction, sorbitol (1 g/kg) may be added to the initial dose of charcoal. Many overdoses can result in ileus, however, thereby limiting the use of the gut for detoxification.

Solute diuresis is recommended to increase elimination of substances usually excreted by the kidney with partial reabsorption by renal tubules such as lithium carbonate. Alkaline diuresis, obtained by infusing sodium bicarbonate to keep urine pH greater than 7.5, enhances the elimination of long-acting barbiturates and salicylates. Hemodialysis is the method of choice for severe methanol and ethylene glycol poisoning and should be instituted even before blood levels are known. In addition, hemodialysis should be considered when the poison is known to be removed effectively by this route and the patient exhibits acute renal failure, severe intoxication with hypotension, apnea, hypothermia unresponsive to supportive care, prolonged coma, or lethal drug levels. Charcoal/resin hemoperfusion may be considered in cases of barbiturate, phenytoin, and theophylline overdose.

The emergency treatment of corrosive ingestion is dilution and washout with fluids. Fluid washout is effective if delivered immediately after ingestion (less than 2 min) and of questionable value after 30 min. Emesis, gastric lavage, and activated charcoal administration are contraindicated after corrosive ingestion as is neutralization of the corrosives because of the generation of an exothermic reaction. Once a patient is stabilized, a chest x-ray including the upper abdomen should be performed for detection of pneumomediastinum, pneumothorax or pleural effusion due to esophageal perforation and pneumoperitoneum due to gastric or small bowel perforation. Severe hematemesis and radiographic signs of visceral perforation or signs of an acute abdomen are considered indications for immediate surgery. In all other cases, the need for surgical intervention is guided by early endoscopy.

Prolonged coma is a frequent sequela of poisoning and prevention and early treatment of complications such as hypoglycemia, aspiration pneumonia, pulmonary edema, gastrointestinal hemorrhage, rhabdomyolysis, renal failure, sepsis, hypothermia, and venous thrombosis is critical.

Poisoning due to methanol, ethylene glycol, and isopropanol and overdoses related to barbiturates, benzodiazepines, and narcotics are discussed in the following sections.

ALCOHOL POISONING

The manifestations of both acute and chronic ethanol ingestion are protean and well-known to most physicians. Acute intoxication with ethanol, even when severe enough to cause coma, usually responds to careful supportive care. Gastric emptying, cathartics and charcoal are probably not useful. Hemodialysis can increase ethanol clearance, but is rarely necessary.

In contrast, poisoning due to methanol, ethylene glycol, and isopropanol are much less common and typically result in death if treatment is delayed. Table 66-1 summarizes the most relevant characteristics of the presentation, diagnosis, and treatment of poisoning due to these agents.

Poisoning with methanol, usually resulting from the consumption of methanol-contaminated whiskey, and ethylene glycol, found in antifreeze, share many clinical similarities. First, they characteristically produce a high anion gap metabolic acidosis with rapid production of acid. Next, patients present as apparently drunk without the odor of ethanol or the presence of ethanol in the blood. Third, analysis of plasma electrolytes and osmolality aids in the diagnosis. The measured plasma osmolality exceeds the calculated osmolality, resulting in an osmolal gap. Osmolality is calculated by the formula:

TABLE 66-1 Acute Toxicity of the Alcohols

	Ethanol	Methanol	Ethylene Glycol	Isopropanol
CNS depressant	+	+	+	+
Convulsion	+	+	+	+
Odor	+	−	−	+(acetone)
Blood Gases	Respiratory acidosis ketoacidosis	severe metabolic acidosis	severe metabolic acidosis	mild metabolic acidosis
Anion gap	+	+ + +	+ + +	+
Osmolar gap	+	+	+	+
Oxalate crystaluria	−	−	+ +	−
Symptom onset	30 min	12–48 h	30 min–12 h	rapid
Lethal dose	5–8 g/kg	1–5 g/kg	1.5 g/kg	3–4 g/kg
Lethal blood level (mg/dL)	350–500	80	200	400
Special Rx treatment	HD	ETOH; HD	ETOH; HCO_3.HD	HD; HCO_3

HD = hemodialysis
(Reprinted with permission from Ellenhorn MJ: The Alcohols, in Hall JB, Schmidt GA, Wood LDH: Principles of Critical Care, McGraw-Hill, New York, 1992.)

2 Na + BUN/2.8 + glucose/18. The normal osmolal gap is 10 or less. Methanol and ethylene glycol uniquely produce both a severe metabolic acidosis and a discrepancy between measured and calculated serum osmolality. Furthermore, both are treated by ethanol infusion and hemodialysis. An intravenous solution of 10% ethanol is infused to maintain a serum level of 100 to 150 mg/dL to completely inhibit toxic metabolite formation. Folate (50 mg IV q 4 h) and pyridoxine (100 mg q 6 h) may aid in promoting the degradation of the toxic metabolites of methanol and ethylene glycol, respectively.

Isopropyl alcohol, isopropanol, is a potent central nervous system (CNS) and cardiovascular depressant. The principal metabolite of isopropanol, acetone, is not associated with severe metabolic acidosis, although an elevated osmolal gap is typical. As with ingestion of other alcohols, the usefulness of emesis, lavage, activated charcoal, and cathartics is minimal. Hemodialysis should be considered in patients with hypotension resistant to volume resuscitation or deep coma.

BARBITURATES AND OTHER SEDATIVE HYPNOTIC DRUGS

Barbiturates and other sedative-hypnotic drugs abolish central respiratory drive. Respiratory depression is the usual cause of death in patients without ventilatory support. At higher drug concentrations, skeletal, smooth, and cardiac muscle function is depressed, leading to decreased myocardial contractility, vasodilation, and hypotension. Despite depression of myocardial contractility by barbiturates, the low output and hypotension are frequently responsive to fluid challenges, without the need for inotropic support. There are no antidotes for these drugs. With only a few exceptions, the treatment of poisoning with sedative-hypnotic drugs requires support of the patient on a ventilator with adequate replacement of circulating volume for hypotension and careful attention to details of preventing complications until the coma resolves. Blood levels confirm drug ingestion but rarely impact upon patient management; because of tolerance, coingested drugs, large tissue stores, underlying medical disease, and active metabolites, clinical evaluation correlates better than blood levels with outcome. Gut decontamination and enhanced elimination, through gastric lavage and administration of charcoal, may be useful up to 6 to 8 h postingestion. Urinary alkalinization may increase phenobarbital excretion but is not useful for most other members of this class of drugs. Hemodialysis is effective for long-acting barbiturates.

BENZODIAZEPINES

Serious intoxication in adults following oral overdose with a benzodiazepine (BZD) alone is unusual. Indeed, the presence of coma following ingestion of a BZD should prompt a careful search for coingested drugs, trauma, or underlying medical disease. As with barbiturates, severe toxicity is related to respiratory and cardiovascular depression. When present, respiratory depression is treated with assisted ventilation and hypotension with volume expansion. Gastric lavage and administration of charcoal are useful when administered soon after ingestion. Forced diuresis, alkalinization, and hemodialysis are not effective. Flumazenil, a BZD antagonist, has been shown to reverse the respiratory and sedative effects of some BZDs.

NARCOTICS

The triad of decreased level of consciousness, constricted pupils, and respiratory depression suggests opioid intoxication and naloxone (Narcan®), an opiate antagonist, should be administered even before laboratory investigation confirms the diagnosis. Doses of 0.4 to 10 mg are given intravenously and titrated to patient response. Large doses may be required, especially in the setting of fentanyl overdose, and continuous infusion (4 mg in 1000 mL administered at 100 mL/h = 0.4 mg/h) may be required for ingestions of opioids with long half-lives. The majority of fatalities from opioid ingestion relate to respiratory depression and early institution of ventilatory assistance should be considered. Hypotension is usually due to a combination of venous vasodilation and hypoxemia and should be treated with supplemental oxygen and volume expansion. Hypoxemia due to noncardiogenic pulmonary edema, which may be severe, is not uncommon, responds to supplemental oxygen and positive end-expiratory pressure (PEEP), and resolves rapidly. Gastric lavage and charcoal administration may be useful after oral ingestion of opioids. Forced diuresis, alkalinization, and hemodialysis have no role in the management of opioid intoxication.

For further reading in *Principles of Critical Care,* see Chap 168 "General Management of Poisoning" Uri Taitelman/Matthew J Ellenhorn, Chap 170 "The Alcohols" Matthew J Ellenhorn, Chap 171 "Barbiturates and Other Sedative-Hypnotic Drugs" Matthew J Ellenhorn, Chap 172 "The Benzodiazepines" Matthew J Ellenhorn, Chap 174 "Narcotics" R Steven Thapratt/Timothy E Albertson

Stephen R. Amesbury

Cyclic antidepressants are commonly involved in suicide attempts and accidental overdoses. Because cardiovascular and neurologic complications of these drugs are life-threatening, the physician must be particularly alert to their occurrence.

In therapeutic doses, the cyclic antidepressants are well absorbed from the gastrointestinal tract. With overdose, however, the anticholinergic effects can dramatically impair gut motility and delay absorption. Therefore, measures to evacuate the stomach and to bind gut stores are important aspects of management. The fraction of free tricyclic antidepressant (TCA) in the serum is significantly affected by serum pH which may explain why acidosis potentiates toxicity. Metabolism of TCAs takes place primarily in the liver, and renal excretion is minimal, so forced diuresis and hemodialysis do not substantially enhance clearance. Drugs or diseases which impair hepatic metabolism can lead to protracted toxicity.

The usual therapeutic dose of the TCAs is 2 to 4 mg/kg/day and toxicity is increasingly prominent when more than 10 to 15 mg/kg/day is taken. Lower doses have been fatal in children. More than 2g is typically taken before life-threatening complications of ventilatory failure, arrhythmia, or seizure occur. The physician must always consider and exclude the possibility of multiple intoxicants.

MANIFESTATIONS OF ACUTE OVERDOSE

Central Nervous System (CNS) Abnormalities

The most common manifestation of overdose is depression of the level of consciousness, but agitation, confusion, extrapyramidal signs, and hallucinations have been described (Table 67-1). Progression from lethargy to coma and ventilatory failure can be extraordinarily rapid. Likewise, coma from uncomplicated TCA overdose tends to resolve rapidly, usually within 12 to 24 h. Protracted obtundation should prompt consideration of other causes, such as coingested drugs, anoxic encephalopathy related to shock, or occult trauma. Some of the newer non TCAs (e.g., maprotiline) have longer half-lives which may prolong coma.

Seizures are relatively common and are associated with increased mortality. Tonic-clonic seizure activity may potentiate cardiac toxicity by producing metabolic acidosis which increases free drug concentration.

TABLE 67-1 Major Toxicities in Acute Overdose

Central Nervous System Abnormalities
Hallucinations
Seizures
Coma
Anticholinergic Crisis
Mydriasis and blurred vision
Urinary retention
Dry mucous membranes
Constipation and ileus
Sinus tachycardia
Hyperthermia or hypothermia
Confusion, agitation, hallucination
Hypotension and Hypoperfusion
Cardiac Arrythmias
Supraventricular tachycardias
Ventricular tachycardia
Torsade de pointes
Ventricular fibrillation
Advanced heart block
Bradycardia and asystole

Anticholinergic Crisis

Sinus tachycardia is the most common rhythm abnormality and is due to an anticholinergic effect. Blurred vision, urinary retention, and dry mucous membranes are relatively common findings. Diminished peristalsis and delayed gastric emptying are anticholinergic effects and make drug recovery from the gut possible. The possibility of ileus must be considered when giving repeated doses of activated charcoal, since gastric overdistention may lead to aspiration.

Hypotension and Hypoperfusion

Peripheral alpha receptor blockade is the likely cause of hypotension in overdose, which may result in hypoperfusion and lactic acidosis. Hypotension can be followed shortly by cardiac arrest.

Cardiac Arrhythmias

Mortality in TCA overdose is most often related to severe hypotension or cardiac arrhythmia. The arrhythmias seen include tachyarrhythmias as well as advanced heart block and asystole (Table 67-1). Sinus tachycardia commonly precedes unstable rhythms, but malignant ventricular arrhythmias can interrupt normal sinus rhythm. The electrocardiographic signs of overdose include sinus tachycardia, QRS prolongation, rightward axis or right bundle branch block, PR and QT interval prolongation, and ST-T wave abnormalities. Limb lead QRS prolongation of greater than 100 msec identifies a subpopulation of patients at greater risk for both seizures and arrhythmias.

MANAGEMENT

Requirements for Admission and Monitoring

In any suspected cyclic antidepressant overdose, prolongation of the maximal initial limb lead QRS duration beyond 100 msec mandates continuous ECG monitoring and observation for CNS or circulatory deterioration. If the initial QRS duration is less than 100 msec and no anticholinergic manifestations or CNS abnormalities are present, the patient can be observed in the emergency department for 6 h. If no abnormalities develop, the likelihood of significant toxicity is very low and referral for psychiatric evaluation may be made. If any abnormalities develop during this period of observation, however, admission to the closely monitored environment of the ICU is warranted.

Modification of General Management

Because life-threatening arrhythmias may occur without warning, intravenous access should be established early (Table 67-2). Dextrose, naloxone hydrochloride, and thiamine should be given to address potentially correctable contributors to lethargy. Activated charcoal should be given, and syrup of ipecac should be avoided. Adequacy of ventilation should be monitored, and any degree of respiratory acidosis should be treated with prompt intubation and mechanical ventilation. Intubation may also be necessary for airway protection prior to gastric lavage with a large bore tube, followed by activated charcoal and a cathartic. Absence of bowel sounds, development of abdominal distention, or large gastric residuals should prompt discontinuation of charcoal and institution of gastric suction. If bowel peristalsis is present, repeat doses of charcoal can be given every 6 h. Forced diuresis, hemodialysis, and peritoneal dialysis have no role in the management of overdose, and hemoperfusion is not recommended.

TABLE 67-2 General Management Principles

Early IV access and activated charcoal
Avoid ipecac syrup and Type I antiarrhythmic drugs
Admit and monitor based on QRS duration, symptoms, and signs
Gastric lavage if airway is protected
Early intubation and mechanical ventilation
No role for diuresis, or dialysis
Maintain serum pH 7.45–7.55

Therapeutic Alkalemia

Acidemia increases the concentration of free drug in the serum, and overdose victims may develop acidemia from lactic acidosis following seizures and respiratory acidosis resulting from coma. Therefore, it is important to reverse respiratory acidosis with mechanical ventilation and to control seizures promptly. Either bicarbonate infusion (2 ampules sodium bicarbonate/L 5% dextrose solution) or hyperventilation (P_{CO_2} of 25 to 30) should be used to maintain serum pH between 7.45 and 7.55.

Physostigmine

We do not advise physostigmine use in tricyclic antidepressant overdose, since it has been associated with worsened seizures, bradycardia, vomiting, and asystole.

MANAGEMENT OF SPECIFIC COMPLICATIONS (TABLE 67-3)

Hypotension

Development of arterial hypotension should prompt rapid determination of serum pH and alkalinization. In the mechanically ventilated patient, hyperventilation should be achieved within minutes. Volume infusion should also be given, with repeated 500 ml boluses of crystalloid. If hypotension is not corrected with 2 or 3 L of fluid, particularly if other evidence of hypoperfusion exists, consideration should be given to right heart catheterization as a useful guide to resuscitation. Management should then follow the general princi-

TABLE 67-3 Treatment of Specific Complications

Hypotension
  Alkalinization
  Volume infusion
  Right heart catheterization in persistent hypotension
Seizures
  Alkalinization
  Diazepam (.15mg/kg IV, repeat as necessary)
  Phenytoin (15 mg/kg IV, over 30 min)
Arrhythmias (avoid class I agents)
  QRS widening
    Alkalinization
    Phenytoin (15 mg/kg IV, over 30 min)
  Ventricular arrhythmias
    Alkalinization
    Lidocaine (or over-drive pacing)
  Bradyarrhythmias/Asystole
    Isoproterenol (atropine usually ineffective)
    Pacemaker

ples of management of shock. Since malignant ventricular arrhythmias are the leading cause of death in cyclic antidepressant overdose, it seems particularly wise to avoid vasoactive drugs and their arrhythmogenic potential.

Seizures

Prophylactic antiepileptics do not have a clear role in TCA overdose. When seizures begin, alkalinization should be initiated and, except in rare circumstances, an endotracheal tube placed. Diazepam, 0.15 mg/kg, should be given intravenously and repeated at 15 to 20 min intervals until seizures are controlled or to a total of 30 to 40 mg. Phenytoin should also be given at the onset of seizures (15 mg/kg given intravenously over 30 min). Serum levels should dictate further doses to achieve a concentration of 20 μg/mL. Seizures that fail to respond to this regimen should be treated as other forms of status epilepticus (see Chap. 49).

Arrhythmias

Sinus tachycardia does not require treatment. Class Ia antiarrhythmic drugs (procainamide, diisopyramide, and quinidine) are contraindicated because their membrane effects amplify antidepressant toxicity. QRS widening, ventricular arrhythmia, and bradyarrhythmias should all prompt alkalinization of the blood. "Prophylactic" phenytoin for patients with QRS widening is recommended. Arrhythmias should be managed routinely, with the caution that class Ia antiarrhythmics be avoided. Also, atropine is unlikely to be effective in bradyarrhythmias. Beta blocking agents and bretylium have been reported to cause worsened hypotension. Patients may be successfully resuscitated from malignant arrhythmia after prolonged cardiopulmonary resuscitation.

Continuous ECG Monitoring

Patients should be monitored until they are fully awake, arrhythmia free, and with normal conduction for 24 h. In many patients this can be accomplished in a telemetry unit and may not require the ICU. At the earliest possible time, coordination of long-term care with psychiatric staff should be initiated.

For further reading in *Principles of Critical Care,* see Chap 173 "Cyclic Antidepressant Overdose" Jesse Hall/Gregory A Schmidt

Stephen R. Amesbury

INTRODUCTION

The toxicity of cyanide-liberating compounds is directly proportional to the amount and rate of hydrogen cyanide (HCN) formation. At body temperature and the pH of body fluids, it is in the form of nonionized HCN gas that diffuses rapidly through all body compartments. Inhibition of cytochrome aa_3 and interruption of aerobic respiration is the major mechanism of cyanide toxicity. Acute human intoxication occurs mainly during chemical and industrial procedures. HCN is a combustion product of fiber polymers, and many plants contain cyanogenic glycosides that may cause acute or chronic cyanide poisoning. Hospitalized patients receiving sodium nitroprusside may also develop cyanide poisoning.

TOXICOKINETICS

The rapidity of HCN formation in the stomach after ingestion of cyanide-containing compounds depends on gastric pH and the stability of the cyanide-liberating molecule. Ingestion when the stomach is full of alkaline food or buffered fluids may lead to a slowly developing clinical syndrome (delayed up to 1 h), since HCN is formed rapidly at an acid pH. The effects of inhalation of HCN is immediate with large exposures (above 280 ppm) being immediately fatal. HCN can be absorbed through human skin, but acute poisoning due to percutaneous absorption is not common.

The major route of biological cyanide detoxification in humans is by hepatic conversion to relatively nontoxic thiocyanate (SCN^-), which is rapidly excreted by normal kidneys. The most important enzyme for thiocyanate formation is rhodanese which is present in high intracellular concentrations in the liver and kidneys. The brain contains relatively small concentrations of rhodanese.

CLINICAL MANIFESTATIONS

The severity of clinical manifestations depends on the amount and rate of cyanide absorption. If exposure is by inhalation, absorption is immediate. Thus, a patient that is asymptomatic despite an inhalation exposure needs only a short period of observation and no antidotal therapy. Up to one-third of patients with smoke inhalation who are rescued from domestic fires will have high blood levels of cyanide.

If exposure is by ingestion, symptoms may develop slowly in three successive phases (Table 68–1). Following massive ingestion, the

TABLE 68-1 Manifestations of Progressive Acute Cyanide Poisoning by Ingestion

1. Excitement or stimulation phase	Anxiety, dyspnea, sensation of chest constriction, headache, hyperpnea, giddiness, confusion, hypertension, tachycardia
2. Depression phase	Auditory and visual disturbances, coma, fixed dilated pupils, convulsions, hypoventilation, apnea, hypotension, bradycardia, ventricular arrhythmias
3. Adynamic phase (*État de mort apparent*)	Deep coma, loss of muscular tone, loss of spontaneous activity and all reflexes, absence of blood pressure and pulse

patient may rapidly develop coma, seizures, apnea, and circulatory collapse, skipping the first phase.

The typical clinical syndrome is notable for the coexistence of rapidly developing coma, cardiac dysfunction, and severe lactic acidosis in the setting of a high mixed venous oxygen saturation due to the inability of tissues to consume delivered oxygen. The funduscopic examination may reveal bright red retinal veins, correlating with the elevated venous oxyhemoglobin saturation. When such findings are present in a setting consistent with cyanide exposure, empiric therapy should be given pending confirmation of the diagnosis.

DIAGNOSIS

A diagnosis of cyanide poisoning is typically made based upon the coincidence of exposure and a consistent clinical syndrome. It should be considered in comatose smoke inhalation victims who may have combined carbon monoxide and cyanide poisoning. Most suicide attempts are by chemists who have access to cyanides.

Whole blood cyanide levels should always be performed since they are valuable for confirmation of the diagnosis and for evaluation of the effects of treatment.

TREATMENT

Prompt cardiopulmonary resuscitation (CPR) and oxygen administration is the major determinant of survival from acute cyanide poisoning (Table 68–2). Several antidotes are available. Oxygen and thiosulfate are efficacious, and their use in cyanide poisoning is universally accepted. Ventilation with pure oxygen is a major

TABLE 68-2 Treatment of Cyanide Poisoning
_____
Widely agreed upon strategies
  Prompt cardiopulmonary resuscitation
  Ventilation with 100% oxygen
  Sodium thiosulfate, 25% solution, 150mg/kg intravenously
  Gastric decontamination
Additional therapies, not universally available or agreed upon
  Hydroxocobalamin, 4 g intravenously
  Induction of methemoglobinemia
    Amylnitrite 0.2 mL perle, crushed and inhaled 30 sec of each min until
      sodium nitrite is given
    Sodium nitrite 10% solution, 5–10 mg/kg, intravenously
    Paradimethylaminophenol (4-DMAP), 1–3 mg/kg intravenously
  Dicobalt EDTA, 300–600 mg intravenously
_____

therapeutic intervention, and potentiates the effect of other antidotes.

Sodium thiosulfate acts as an excellent sulfur donor to rhodanese
and other sulfane sulfur transferases which detoxify cyanide. At a
dose of 150 mg/kg administered intravenously, sodium thiosulfate
has practically no toxicity. The major disadvantage of thiosulfate is
its slow penetration of the intracellular compartment. The only
relative contraindication to thiosulfate administration is renal failure. Thiocyanate is readily removed by hemodialysis.

Additional therapies are not universally available or agreed
upon, but may be considered in certain institutions (Table 68–2).
Hydroxocobalamin, 4 g intravenously, dicobalt ethylenediamine-
tetracetate (EDTA), 300 to 600 mg intravenously, and induction of
methemoglobinemia are examples of such additional therapies
which are technically more difficult to administer, and potentially
dangerous for the patient.

DECONTAMINATION

In acute cyanide poisoning by ingestion, the order of therapeutic
interventions is **1**. prompt CPR as needed, **2**. 100% oxygen and
intravenous antidotes, and **3**. gastric lavage and decontamination
following initial therapy. Though several methods have been described in the literature for stomach decontamination after ingestion of cyanide salts, the most readily available is activated charcoal.

_____

For further reading in *Principles of Critical Care,* see Chap 176
  "Acute Cyanide Poisoning" Uri Taitelman

Stephen R. Amesbury

INTRODUCTION

The most commonly used salicylates are aspirin (ASA), salicylic acid, and methylsalicylic acid. The stomach and blood rapidly hydrolyze ASA to salicylic acid and acetic acid. Most toxic effects appear to be mediated by salicylic acid. ASA is a weak acid with a pKa of 3. Half an oral dose appears in the stomach in nonionized form and is rapidly absorbed. Peak therapeutic levels occur within 2 h. Enteric-coated preparations delay peak concentrations markedly. The standard nomogram for using serum level to predict toxicity cannot be applied to ingestions of these forms of aspirin. ASA is poorly soluble and often precipitates in the stomach, particularly in massive ingestions. Despite the relatively high intraluminal pH of the small bowel, ASA absorption at this site is substantial due to the large surface area. Once in the blood, acidosis enhances tissue penetration.

Drug elimination is largely by conjugation in the liver, but with multiple or large single doses, hepatic elimination pathways are saturated, and renal excretion of unchanged drugs becomes increasingly important. Under such conditions, the plasma half-life of therapeutic doses (2 to 5 h) can increase tenfold. Also, salicylates cross the placenta and are contraindicated in pregnancy.

ACID-BASE AND METABOLIC DISTURBANCES

Salicylate intoxication causes increased alveolar ventilation and endogenous acid production, resulting in respiratory alkalosis and metabolic alkalosis respectively. The metabolic acidosis is more prominent in infants, and respiratory alkalosis tends to dominate the acid-base disturbance in the elderly. Most patients exhibit a complex mixed acid-base disturbance. Lactate levels are usually modestly elevated, but severe lactic acidosis is rare unless shock supervenes.

CLINICAL PRESENTATION

The incidence of overdose from single ingestions in the pediatric population is decreasing, but chronic toxicity is still seen and is often unusual in presentation. Diagnosis is frequently delayed.

In general, acute ingestions of 150 to 300 mg/kg correlate to mild toxicity, 300 to 500 mg/kg to moderate toxicity, and >500 mg/kg to severe toxicity, with the potential for death (Table 69-1). The Done

TABLE 69-1 Toxicity Related to Ingested Dose and Serum Levels

Dose (mg/kg)	Level of Toxicity	Serum Level (mg/dL)
<150	None expected	<50
150–300	Mild to moderate	50–80
300–500	Severe	>80
>500	Potentially lethal	>160

nomogram may be used to predict severity of intoxication for single ingestions (Fig. 69-1). This predictor is not to be used for chronic ingestions, when enteric preparations are involved, or if coexisting disease or ingestion will complicate outcome. It is recommended that a level 6 h or longer after ingestions be used, to ensure that levels have reached their peak. Any serum level over 25 mg/dL in an adult with chronic ingestion and consistent findings should be considered to potentially indicate toxicity.

In the elderly, salicylism should be considered if obvious alternative explanations do not exist: 1. for any mixed respiratory alkalosis and metabolic acidosis; 2. in every patient with decreased level of consciousness, particularly when accompanied by typical acid-base disturbances; and 3. in every patient with respiratory distress due to low pressure pulmonary edema.

Neurologic signs tend to dominate the presentation and are a good gauge to the severity of the overdose. Symptoms begin with tinnitus and lethargy, progress to irritability or disorientation, and may culminate in hallucinations, seizures, and coma. Gastrointestinal symptoms of nausea and vomiting may represent central nervous system (CNS) disturbance or direct upper tract irritation. Hyperthermia is seen in as many as 20 percent of patients. Adult respiratory distress syndrome (ARDS) is most likely with chronic intoxication, in patients with significant metabolic acidosis, and with marked CNS abnormalities.

DIAGNOSIS

A high index of suspicion is necessary to make the diagnosis of salicylate toxicity because of its cryptic presentation in adults with chronic ingestion. When suspicion exists, plasma levels should be measured. Once a diagnosis is made, laboratory tests including complete blood count with platelet count, electrolytes, blood urea nitrogen (BUN), creatinine, glucose, urinalysis including pH, and arterial blood-gas levels should be obtained. A repeat salicylate level after 2 to 3 h will identify those patients with rising levels and potential for worsening toxicity. For more severe intoxications, prothrombin time (PT), serum calcium, chest radiograph, and liver function profile should be obtained.

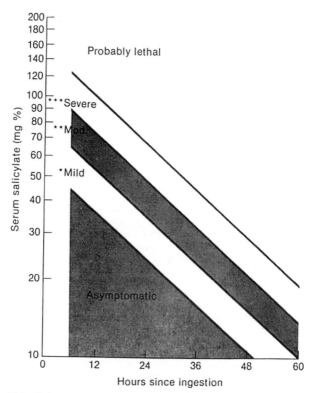

FIG. 69-1 Nomogram relating serum salicylate level to general severity of intoxication. This nomogram should not be applied to chronic intoxication or ingestion of enteric-coated preparations. Note that the nomogram begins 6 h after ingestion to provide that serum levels have peaked. (Reprinted with permission from Done AK: Aspirin overdose: Incidence, diagnosis and management. Pediatrics 62(Suppl):895, 1978.)

SUPPORTIVE THERAPY

Emesis or gastric lavage may be useful up to 12 h after massive ingestions. Once the airway is felt secure, activated charcoal should be given at a dose of 1.0 g/kg and repeated every 4 h for a total of three to four doses. Development of an ileus in critically ill patients often makes this impossible. Cathartics such as magnesium sulfate may also enhance elimination.

All patients presenting with coma should have glucose and naloxone administered immediately. Naloxone does not reverse the CNS effects of salicylates, but since profound CNS depression is an indication for dialysis, other sources of altered mental status should be considered and treated. Seizures should raise the possibility of a new electrolyte disturbance or hypoglycemia. Aside from correcting these metabolic abnormalities, seizures should be treated in the usual fashion.

Temperature in excess of 40°C (104°F) should be treated with passive cooling. Dehydration is common with severe intoxications, therefore fluid resuscitation should be vigorous and directed at achieving a urine output of 200 to 300 mL/h in the adult. During fluid resuscitation arterial oxygenation should be followed continuously with pulse oximetry, since low pressure pulmonary edema may necessitate more aggressive supportive measures. If hypocalcemia is associated with symptoms or electrocardiographic (ECG) changes, replacement therapy should be given intravenously with 10 mL calcium gluconate in the adult. An elevated PT can often be corrected with vitamin K therapy.

MANEUVERS TO ENHANCE ELIMINATION

Since metabolic acidosis promotes penetration of salicylate into tissues, pH correction should be undertaken immediately. It is usually possible to correct pH initially from 7.25 to 7.30 with boluses of bicarbonate (1 meq/kg each) while following serial arterial blood-gas levels. Serum electrolytes should be followed carefully since this bicarbonate preparation is extremely hypertonic and can induce hypernatremia. Critically ill patients require early intubation, muscle relaxation, mechanical ventilation, and correction of hypovolemia or ventricular dysfunction.

Alkalinization of the urine will markedly enhance renal excretion. At a urine pH of 7.5, renal clearance of free salicylate begins to increase dramatically. If possible, urine pH of 8.0 to 8.5 should ultimately be attained. Once the blood pH is corrected to approximately 7.30 and hypovolemia is treated, an infusion of 2 ampules bicarbonate in 1 L 5% dextrose solution should begin at a rate of 200 to 300 mL/h.

It is important that *hypokalemia* be rapidly corrected to avoid preferential tubular excretion of hydrogen ion, acidification of urine, and diminished salicylate excretion. In the presence of hypokalemia, alkalinization of the urine is impossible. If alkalinization of the urine continues to be difficult despite bicarbonate infusions over several hours, persistent or new hypokalemia should be considered and treated, if present, while bicarbonate infusion is continued at a higher rate. Hypocalcemia and pulmonary edema are always possible complications of this intervention. Drugs such as acetazolamide should not be used in salicylate overdose since they result in metabolic acidosis.

Hemodialysis is an effective means of removing drug while simultaneously correcting fluid and electrolyte abnormalities. This should be considered in single ingestions with levels above 120 mg/dL. It may be appropriate for chronic ingestions with lower levels of 50 to 100 mg/dL if complicating factors such as renal and cardiac failure make urine alkalinization difficult, if metabolic acidosis does not respond to standard measures, or if seizures and deep coma are present. Charcoal hemoperfusion is more effective in removing drug, but since hemodialysis also corrects the profound electrolyte and acid-base disturbances, it is the preferred therapy. Peritoneal dialysis should not be performed.

For further reading in *Principles of Critical Care,* see Chap 177 "Salicylates" Bianca Raikhlin-Eisenkraft/Jesse Hall

Ikeadi Maurice Ndukwu

Acetaminophen (APAP) is a widely used, effective antipyretic and analgesic agent which is safe when ingested in appropriate dosage. Hepatic and renal injuries may result from an overdose.

PATHOPHYSIOLOGY OF ACETAMINOPHEN POISONING

The liver is the site of APAP metabolism. Of an ingested APAP dose, 95 percent is metabolized by hepatocytes into nonhepatotoxic APAP-sulfate and APAP-glucuronide conjugates in equal parts.

The hepatic P-450 mixed function oxidase system oxidizes the remaining 5 percent of ingested APAP to an electrophilic compound, N-acetyl-p-benzoquinomine (NAPQI). NAPQI has very high avidity for sulfhydryl groups. Cysteine groups on cellular proteins and soluble thiols are the most significant sulfhydryl groups available. NAPQI combines with glutathione to form a conjugate; NAPQI-glutathione conjugate is excreted as a nonhepatotoxic mercapturic acid compound. When liver glutathione stores are reduced to approximately 70 percent, a protein-cysteine-APAP conjugate forms in greater quantity. This NAPQI pathway is thought to be solely responsible for necrotic hepatocellular damage seen in APAP poisoning.

THE CLINICAL PICTURE OF APAP TOXICITY

A patient presenting with APAP poisoning in the early phase ($\sim$20 h postingestion) may be totally asymptomatic, or only complain of mild to moderate abdominal discomfort. Nausea and vomiting may be present. In cases of extremely large ingestion, lethargy or coma may occur, although this is very rare. Measured circulating APAP levels are significantly elevated concomitant with high NAPQI synthesis.

The late phase (> 20 h) of APAP overdose is clinically manifested by evidence of chemical hepatitis and hepatocellular necrosis. Serum analysis reveals extremely elevated alanine aminotransferase (ALT), aspartate aminotransferase (AST) (10,000 to 20,000 IU/mL), bilirubin, and prothrombin time (PT).

The diagnosis of APAP poisoning in both the early and late clinical phases depends greatly on a high index of suspicion for drug overdose. Therefore, any patient suspected of having substance overdose should have an immediate circulating APAP level performed. Every attempt should be made to determine the time of APAP ingestion (Fig. 70-1). If historical and clinical evidence sup-

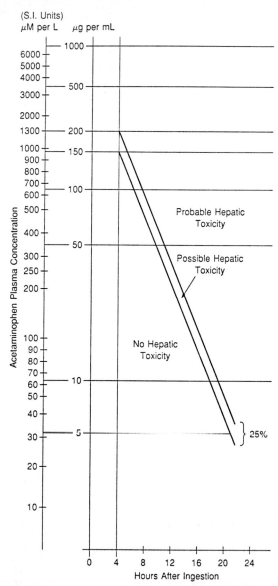

FIG. 70-1 Rumack-Matthew nomogram for predicting APAP hepatotoxicity. (From Rumack BH: Pediatr Clin North Am 33:698, 1986. Used with permission.)

port APAP poisoning despite unmeasurable APAP levels, then the diagnosis may be pursued with liver function tests, liver biopsy (if not contraindicated) looking for centrilobular necrosis pattern, and immunoassay for circulating NAPQI–cysteinyl adduct (an experimental assay at present).

THERAPY OF APAP POISONING

The best outcome in a patient with APAP poisoning is obtained when the diagnosis is made and specific therapy initiated within 8 h of ingestion.

The therapeutic strategy for a patient with APAP and multiple substance poisoning (see Chap. 66) should be induction of emesis, administration of oral activated charcoal, and administration of an oral loading dose of N-acetylcysteine (NAC), an antidote to APAP. This is followed every 4 h by administration of activated charcoal and NAC (NAC may be administered 2 h before charcoal). When APAP is the only agent ingested, then the best therapeutic approach may be induction of emesis, a single dose of activated charcoal, and then a loading dose of NAC followed by NAC every 4 h × 17 doses (Table 70-1). Maneuvers which improve tolerance of oral NAC include:

1. Dilution of the 20% stock solution to 5 percent (3:1) in soda or juice,
2. Serving as an ice cold solution with a straw in a covered container,
3. Repeating any dose vomited within 1 h of administration,
4. Giving antiemetic (droperidol or metaclopramide) if repeated emesis occurs, and
5. Administering via nasogastric tube (NGT) or duodenal tube as a slow drip if unable to stop emesis.

NAC administration protocols II and III (see Table 70-1) are used in Europe and Canada. The advantage of the parenteral route for NAC administration is avoidance of emesis. However, anaphylactoid reactions may occur with intravenous NAC.

Prognosis in APAP poisoning in patients treated within 20 h of ingestion is excellent. Patients usually will not respond to NAC after 20 h post APAP ingestion because of advanced hepatotoxicity, although some reports have suggested benefit even after onset of fulminant hepatic failure. These patients should be managed with the standard supportive care. Poor prognosis is suggested by bilirubin value greater than 4 mg/dL and PT ratio greater than 2.2. Liver transplantation (see Chap. 61) may be the only therapeutic option if there is a steeply rising bilirubin level, progressively worsening

TABLE 70-1 Protocols for NAC Administration*

	Length (hours)	Administration	Loading Dose	Doses	FDA Approval
I	72	Oral	140 mg/kg	70 mg/kg every 4 h for 17 doses	Yes
II	20	Intravenous	150 mg/kg over 15 min	50 mg/kg over 4 h followed by 100 mg/kg over 16 h	No
III	20	Intravenous	300 mg/kg over 20 h		No

*From Brent J. Rumack BH: Acetamunophen poisoning, in Harwood-Nuss A/(ed): *Clinical Practice of Emergency Medicine,* Philadelphia, PA, Lippincott, 1991, p. 456. Used with permission.

PT, and falling transaminase levels (indicating inpending hepatic failure).

For further reading in *Principles of Critical Care,* see Chap 178 "Acetaminophen Poisoning" Barry H Rumack/Jeffrey Brent

---

Kevin Simpson

Substance abuse has become increasingly common and the list of abused substances continues to grow, presenting an ever greater challenge to the intensive care physician. Complications related to abuse of cocaine, narcotics, and hallucinogens, as well as their management, are briefly reviewed.

COCAINE

Cocaine toxicity should be suspected in any patient who presents with otherwise unexplained acute myocardial infarction, severe hypertension, new seizures, rhabdomyolysis, intracranial hemorrhage, or spontaneous pneumomediastinum. These dramatic medical complications of cocaine abuse can be induced in young, otherwise healthy normal individuals without underlying medical problems. Cocaine-related fatalities often do not occur in close temporal relationship to the cocaine ingestion itself and may present up to 24 h later. As with all illicit street drugs, it is important to remember that these substances are unpredictable in terms of concentration or the presence of adulterants such as strychnine, which can mimic the hyperexcitability effect of cocaine, but which is associated with extreme muscular rigidity. When the possibility of cocaine abuse is suspected, one must initiate appropriate toxicology testing and screen for occult complications such as subarachnoid hemorrhage, acute myocardial infarction, and rhabdomyolysis. While the presenting complications of cocaine abuse are numerous and there is no specific antidote to cocaine, the initial focus of pharmacologic therapy for both the hyperkinetic and hyperdynamic states is diazepam.

While the first reported cardiac manifestations of cocaine toxicity were arrhythmias, and marked hypertension is to be expected, the aspect of cocaine's toxicity which has engendered the most attention is myocardial infarction.

Postulated mechanisms include vasospasm, endothelial abnormalities, and induction of platelet aggregation. Management of cocaine-related myocardial infarction is similar to treatment of the usual form of myocardial ischemia and includes nitrates and morphine. Although it is attractive to postulate that coronary vasospasm plays a prominent role, calcium channel blockers have not proven helpful. Coronary thrombosis has been demonstrated in these patients and thrombolytic therapy has been used successfully. However, severe hypertension is common with cocaine abuse and subarachnoid hemorrhage is not uncommon. Therefore, thrombolytic therapy should be used with caution. A hyperadrenergic state with tachycardia and hypertension is commonly seen with cocaine toxicity. While propranolol was previously used in this setting, there is a theoretical risk that beta blockade will allow an unopposed alpha effect, resulting in increased hypertension and coronary artery vasoconstriction. Labetalol, a combined α- and β-adrenergic antagonist, is now the drug of choice when diazepam alone is not successful. The cocaine-related arrhythmias generally respond to aggressive treatment of the hyperadrenergic state. If significant dysrhythmias continue, bretylium is the antiarrhythmic of choice.

The common central nervous system manifestations of cocaine toxicity include hyperactivity, tremors, fasciculations, and headache. Cocaine also causes both ischemic and hemorrhagic strokes. More commonly, cocaine has been associated with subarachnoid hemorrhage and generalized seizures. The seizures are most often self-limited; recurrent or prolonged seizures should be treated acutely with diazepam. If specific antiepileptics are required, phenobarbital appears to be more effective than phenytoin. Hyperthermia may occur as a result of the direct effects of cocaine on the temperature-regulating areas of the hypothalamus.

Pulmonary toxicity related to cocaine abuse includes noncardiogenic pulmonary edema, pulmonary hemorrhage, and pneumomediastinum. Rhabdomyolysis, with serum creatine phosphokinase levels reaching several hundred thousand, is usually associated with hyperpyrexia and hyperkinesis, and the release of myoglobin can cause acute renal failure. Cocaine abuse during pregnancy is associated with abruptio placentae, spontaneous abortion, and preterm labor, in addition to myocardial and cerebral infarction in the fetus.

NARCOTICS

The triad of decreased level of consciousness, constricted pupils, and respiratory depression strongly suggests opioid ingestion. While blood and urine assays may confirm the diagnosis, they are not necessary for clinical management as response to the opioid antagonist naloxone is virtually pathognomonic of opioid exposure. Indeed, response to administration of naloxone is strong evidence of the presence of opioids even in the face of negative results on drug screening.

Respiratory depression is the major threat to life; hence, aggressive airway control and maintenance of ventilation are essential. Indeed, the majority of fatalities from opioid ingestion relate to respiratory failure with resulting hypoxemia or aspiration pneumonia or both. Hypoxemia is usually secondary to hypoventilation.

When an abnormal alveolar-arterial gradient is present, opioid-induced noncardiogenic pulmonary edema must be considered.

Hypotension is usually due to a combination of venous vasodilation and hypoxemia. If oxygen administration fails to improve hypotension, fluid resuscitation with crystalloid is usually successful. Once again, aggressive control of the airway with endotracheal intubation, mechanical ventilation, and supplemental oxygen is the cornerstone of management of severe opioid intoxications.

Naloxone is the specific antidote of choice. In critical overdoses with hemodynamic instability, 0.4 mg should be given initially and rapidly titrated to stabilization of the patient or a total dose of 10 mg. In less critical patients without hemodynamic instability, an initial naloxone dosage of 0.4 to 2.0 mg is titrated to effect, observing for increased respirations, improved level of consciousness, or belligerent behavior. Fentanyl derivatives may require extremely large (10 to 20 mg) amounts of naloxone because of their extreme potency relative to morphine. The half-life of naloxone is approximately 60 min, whereas the half-lives of most opioid agonists are longer. Patients thus must be closely monitored for return of symptoms. Naloxone can be administered and titrated via continuous infusion (e.g., 4 mg in 1000 mL fluid administered at 100 mL/h=0.4 mg/h). If intravenous access is not readily available, alternate routes of administration include intramuscular, subcutaneous, sublingual injection, and endotracheal instillation although absorption and onset of action may be variable. Naloxone administration may precipitate acute withdrawal which, while unpleasant to the patient, is usually not life-threatening.

Gastric lavage and activated charcoal-cathartic may be useful after oral ingestion of opioids, especially if the opioid was combined with anticholinergics. However, forced diuresis, pH alteration, extracorporeal removal, or partial antagonist antidotes have no role in the management of opioid intoxication.

Opioids are frequently used in combination with a variety of other drugs. Management of mixed ingestions involves reversal of the opioid component with naloxone followed by specific supportive treatment of any other substances. Street samples of heroin typically contain 2 to 6 percent of the opioid, with the remainder consisting of various adulterants. Though usually inert from a toxicologic standpoint, contaminants can occasionally produce life-threatening symptoms requiring specific treatment. As the list of possible adulterants is long, including quinine, strychnine, lidocaine, procaine, lactose, mannitol, and dextrose, management is usually supportive and directed by an understanding of the adulterants commonly present in opioids and currently in use in a particular geographic location. Cotton fever refers to the fever and diffuse pulmonary infiltrates that develop within minutes of an intravenous injection of the water extract of the cotton used to filter a dose of heroin. Cotton fever requires only supportive therapy.

Opioids are widely used in the intensive care unit for their analgesic, sedative, and anesthetic properties and the fear of inducing dependence should not hinder their use for clear indications. Nonetheless, opioid tolerance is a common result. Once stable, a patient should have all opioids converted to a long-acting opioid such as methadone which is then withdrawn incrementally over 7 to 14 days. The long-acting opioid should be administered on a time-contingent basis, not on a symptom-contingent basis and no other opioid should be administered during this time.

HALLUCINOGENS

Hallucinogens refers to the broad group of compounds used primarily to produce hallucinations including amphetamines, PCP, mushrooms, LSD, and cannabinoids, among others. The major direct risks to the patient exposed to hallucinogens include associated effects on the central nervous and cardiovascular systems. Complications indirectly associated with exposure to hallucinogens include gastric aspiration, respiratory insufficiency, rhabdomyolysis, and the trauma associated with failure of the patient to appropriately respond to the environment due to distortion of perception.

Initial evaluation of the patient presenting with hallucinations attempts to determine if the hallucinations are due to a psychiatric or organic cause. All patients presenting with hallucinations should be presumed to have an organic etiology until proven otherwise. It is unusual to see the new onset of hallucinations or psychosis from a primary psychiatric cause in a patient older than age 40 who has no previous history of a psychiatric disorder. If the hallucinations are felt to be nonpsychiatric, the distinction between organic toxicologic exposure and other underlying medical disorders must be made. Many systemic diseases including electrolyte imbalances, ethanol withdrawal, and central nervous system infections may present with hallucinations and require specific management.

Hallucinogens themselves rarely result in direct life-threatening conditions. Death often results from trauma sustained because of altered perception of the environment, sympathomimetic stimulation, and cardiovascular collapse. Associated serious consequences include rhabdomyolysis secondary to isotonic muscle activity, electrolyte imbalance, and injuries resulting from forcible restraint. It is rarely necessary to know the specific identity of the hallucinogen since the management of toxicity resulting from these agents tends to be primarily supportive. Gastric decontamination is not generally indicated. Forced diuresis, alteration of pH, and extracorporeal drug removal have no role in the management of these ingestions.

For further reading in *Principles of Critical Care,* see Chap 174 "Narcotics" R Steven Tharratt/Timothy E Albertson, Chap 179 "Hallucinogens" R Steven Tharratt/Timothy E Albertson, Chap 180 "Cocaine" Edward A Panacek

INTRODUCTION

Pregnancy results in profound changes in cardiovascular and respiratory physiology. These changes, along with the special needs of the fetus must be taken into account in the evaluation and therapy of the critically ill pregnant patient. In addition, it should be understood that pregnancy and delivery introduce or increase the risk for development of several life-threatening conditions, including hemorrhagic shock, eclampsia, cardiomyopathy, amniotic fluid embolus, and disseminated intravascular coagulation. Finally, it should be emphasized that successful management of critical illness in pregnancy requires continuous integration of the intensive care team with obstetric, neonatal, and anesthesia consultants.

CARDIOPULMONARY PHYSIOLOGY OF PREGNANCY

Adaptation of the Circulation

Maternal blood volume begins to increase early in pregnancy, reaching a level 40 percent above baseline by the thirtieth week. Plasma volume increases 40 to 50 percent during this period, while red blood cell number increases by 20 to 40 percent; this results in a mild dilutional anemia. Plasma albumin concentration decreases and plateaus at 26 weeks, then decreases further postpartum. Coincident with the change in blood volume, maternal cardiac output (CO) increases 30 to 45 percent, with most of this change occuring during the first trimester. The increase in CO is due an increase in both the heart rate and stroke volume.

Later in the course of pregnancy CO becomes more dependent on body position. Particularly during the third trimester, the enlarged uterus can obstruct the inferior vena cava to reduce venous return. This effect is maximal in the supine position and less pronounced in the left lateral decubitus position. During labor, increasing venous return from uterine contactions can increase CO 10 to 15 percent, though this effect may be tempered by blood loss.

Blood pressure decreases early in pregnancy with maximum decreases seen at 16 to 28 weeks. Blood pressure then increases gradually reaching prepregnancy levels shortly postpartum. As a rule, diastolic blood pressure of 75 mmHg in the second trimester and 85 mmHg in the third trimester should be considered the upper limits of normal.

Adaptation of the Respiratory System

Oxygen consumption ($\dot{V}O_2$) increases 20 to 30 percent in pregnancy, and further rises to 40 to 100 percent of nonpregnant baseline levels during labor. Increased $\dot{V}O_2$ is associated with increased carbon dioxide production, though increased alveolar ventilation seen normally in pregnancy causes a net fall in P_{CO_2} to a partial pressure of 27 to 32 mmHg. The augmented alveolar ventilation results from a substantial increase in tidal volume while respiratory rate remains unchanged. Renal compensation results in a slightly alkalemic pH (7.40 to 7.45), with serum bicarbonate levels of 18 to 21 meq/L. Functional residual capacity (FRC) and expiratory reserve volume decrease by about 20 percent during gestation because of increased abdominal pressure from the enlarged uterus.

Fetal Oxygen Delivery

Oxygen delivery to fetal tissues depends on the O_2 content of uterine artery blood, and uterine artery blood flow as determined by CO. The anemia of pregnancy reduces the oxygen content of maternal blood by 20 to 25 percent. Thus, oxygen delivery to the pregnant mother and fetus is highly dependent on CO.

The uterine vasculature may be near maximally dilated under normal conditions and, thus, unable to increase flow and oxygen delivery under conditions of stress. Fetal oxygen delivery can be decreased, however, by uterine artery vasoconstriction. Maternal alkalosis, exogenous or endogenous catecholamines, and maternal hypotension can all elicit uterine artery vasoconstriction.

Compensatory mechanisms exist to maintain fetal oxygen delivery. Fetal hemoglobin has a higher affinity for oxygen than maternal hemoglobin, allowing aerobic metabolism under relatively hypoxic conditions. In addition, protective mechanisms, such as redistribution of blood flow to vital organs, decreased oxygen consumption under stress, and anaerobic metabolism in certain tissue beds may also exist.

Implications for Management of Critical Illness

Several generalizations regarding the approach to the critically ill pregnant patient can be made based on the cardiopulmonary physiology characteristic of the maternal–fetal interaction:

1. Assessment of adequacy of perfusion must be made with the understanding that baseline flow is increased, and that oxygen delivery is critically dependent upon CO.
2. Diminished placental blood flow represents a threat to fetal

well-being, especially in the presence of coexistent anemia or hypoxemia.

3. In general, measurements of oxygen delivery and acid-base status in the mother (as opposed to fetal monitoring) are the best measures of adequacy of O_2 delivery for mother and fetus.

4. Labor represents a tremendous aerobic load to the mother; the clinician must decide if labor should be avoided or postponed when oxygen delivery is marginal.

5. One effective way to reduce oxygen demand is to assume the work of breathing; early elective intubation and mechanical ventilation should be considered in selected patients.

CIRCULATORY DISORDERS OF PREGNANCY

Hypoperfused States

The initial approach to the hypoperfused pregnant patient is differentiation of a low flow state, due to hypovolemia or cardiac dysfunction, from a high flow state, due to sepsis or sepsis syndrome. This determination can often be made on the basis of clinical or historical information, though pulmonary artery catheterization may be required. When necessary, this procedure should be performed through the internal jugular or subclavian approachs; femoral vein catheterization is relatively contraindicated. In the healthy pregnant woman, right ventricular, pulmonary artery, and pulmonary capillary wedge pressures (P_{pw}) are unchanged from prepartum values.

Hemorrhagic Shock

The common causes of hemorrhagic shock in pregnancy are listed in Table 72-1. When hemorrhage occurs in pregnancy it is often massive, requiring aggressive intervention. Disseminated intravascular coagulation (DIC) frequently causes or complicates pregnancy-associated hemorrhage.

Patients at increased risk for bleeding should be identified early, and appropriate intravenous access and blood product support

TABLE 72-1 Etiology of Hemorrhagic Shock in Pregnancy

Early	Late (3rd Trimester)
Trauma	Trauma
Ectopic or abdominal pregnancy	Placenta previa
Abortion	Placental abruption
DIC	DIC
Hydatidiform Mole	Uterine Rupture
	Marginal Sinus rupture

(Reprinted with permission from Strek ME, Hall JB: Critical Illness in Pregnancy, in Hall JB, Schmidt GA, Wood LDH: Principles of Critical Care, McGraw-Hill, New York, 1992.)

should be obtained. The initial management of hemorrhage, as in nonpregnant patients, includes placement of two or three large bore peripheral venous catheters (16 gauge or larger) and immediate volume resuscitation with crystalloid or colloid until blood is available. Blood replacement with packed red blood cells should begin immediately. Massive obstetric hemorrhage is one setting in which initial resuscitation with unmatched type-specific blood may be indicated (see Chap. 3). Evidence for coagulopathy, particularly DIC, should be sought in any case of massive bleeding (see Chap. 51). Thrombocytopenia may result secondary to bleeding and dilution. Platelet transfusion should be considered when counts fall below 50,000/mm³. Fresh frozen plasma should be used to correct measured clotting abnormalities.

It is useful to position the patient in the left lateral decubitus position to assure that vena caval obstruction does not worsen already diminished venous return. If shock is not immediately reversed by volume resuscitation, intubation and mechanical ventilation should be performed to assure adequate oxygenation. Military antishock trousers (MAST) can be used to maintain blood pressure in profusely bleeding patients until adequate volume has been infused. They should not be applied to patients in pulmonary edema, and the abdominal compartment should not be inflated in the pregnant patient. The MAST suit is strictly a temporizing measure, and should be in place only as long as necessary to initiate definitive therapy.

Surgical evaluation should be performed immediately. Once the patient is stabilized, a decision should be made as to whether surgical intervention, conservative management, or angiographic localization with embolization of bleeding sites is most appropriate.

Trauma

The gravid woman is at increased risk of hemorrhage after trauma. Some injuries are unique to pregnancy, and include amniotic membrane rupture, placental abruption, uterine rupture, premature labor, and fetal trauma. Placental abruption and uterine rupture are the most serious complications of blunt abdominal trauma and rapid deceleration injury. Vaginal bleeding will usually be present, though not invariably. Displacement of abdominal contents upward increases the risk of visceral injury from penetrating trauma, and the bladder also is a target for injury due to displacement by the uterus. Hypovolemia may be initially difficult to evaluate due to tachycardia and supine hypotension attributable to pregnancy itself. When hypovolemia is clinically evident in the pregnant patient, blood loss may already be enormous. DIC may occur and coagulation profiles should be monitored. Physical findings of peritoneal injury may be masked by pregnancy; peritoneal lavage may be positive in the absence of signs or symptoms of injury. Fetal injuries are uncommon in blunt trauma. Fetal mortality is most often secondary to maternal shock.

Initial management includes assessment and stabilization of cardiorespiratory function. Intubation, if required, should be performed by a skilled individual due to the increased risk of aspiration in pregnancy. If hemorrhage is present, resuscitation should be carried out as discussed above. Once the cervical spine is cleared, the patient should be placed in lateral recumbancy and uterine lift performed if shock is present. Pelvic examination should assess for bleeding, urine, and amniotic fluid. Nitrazine paper can identify amniotic fluid and confirm rupture of amniotic membranes. Open peritoneal lavage, rather than needle paracentesis, should be performed to assess for blunt abdominal trauma. Ultrasound or computed tomography may assist in the diagnosis of pelvic or abdominal bleeding. Once the mother is stabilized, cardiotocographic monitoring of fetal cardiac activity and uterine activity should be performed for 4 h after the injury. Fetomaternal hemorrhage may be assessed by the Kleihauer-Betke test. If maternal death occurs despite aggressive resuscitation and the fetus is alive and undelivered, a postmortem cesarean section should be considered. Fetal prognosis is good if delivery is performed within 10 to 15 min of maternal death.

Cardiac Dysfunction

Cardiac dysfunction is most often caused by preexisting myocardial or valvular heart disease or cardiomyopathy arising de novo. Prior subclinical heart disease may manifest for the first time due to the physiologic changes of pregnancy. Maternal mortality is 7 percent in patients with class III or IV heart failure. Patients with valvular heart disease, pulmonary hypertension, or Eisenmenger's or Marfan's syndromes have an even higher mortality rate (25 to 50 percent).

Volume status should be assessed initially, and hypovolemia excluded. Pulmonary artery catheterization and echocardiography may be helpful in diagnosis and further management. Reversible metabolic disturbances such as hypocalcemia, hypophosphatemia, acidosis and hypoxemia should be corrected and avoided. If cardiogenic shock persists despite adequate preload, inotropic support may be indicated, with dobutamine being the drug of choice. This intervention should be reserved for life-threatening circumstances as dobutamine and other vasoactive drugs may reduce placental blood flow. Low dose dopamine (2 to 3 μg/kg/min) may improve splanchnic and renal perfusion, but should be reserved for situations where renal function is compromised. Pulmonary edema should be treated with intravenous furosemide; pulmonary artery catheterization is necessary to titrate this therapy.

If cardiogenic shock persists despite inotropic drug support, afterload reduction with nitroprusside or nitroglycerine should be considered. *Because of the risk of fetal cyanide poisoning, nitroprusside should be used only when the circulation cannot be stabilized with the aforementioned measures.* The dose and duration of therapy should be minimized, and the patient converted to oral hydralazine as soon as possible. Converting enzyme inhibitors are contraindicated in pregnancy.

The optimal method of delivery is an assisted vaginal delivery in the left lateral decubitus position. Epidural anesthesia may ameliorate tachycardia in response to pain, and beneficially lower SVR. As decreased SVR may lead to decompensation in patients with aortic stenosis, hypertrophic cardiomyopathy, or pulmonary hypertension, general anesthesia may be preferred in these patients. In general, cesarean section should be reserved for obstetric complications and fetal distress.

Septic Shock

Patients are at the greatest risk of sepsis in the peripartum and postabortion periods. Urinary and genital tract infections from the uterus, vagina, and episiotomy site are the most common sources. Cesarean section, prolonged rupture of membranes, retained products of conception, poor progress in labor, and prior instrumentation of the genitourinary tract increase the risk of sepsis. Postpartum endometritis or chorioamnionitis often precede septic shock. Bacterial organisms to be considered include *Staphylococcus aureus* and *epidermidis*; groups A, B, and D streptococci; *Escherichia coli; Proteus mirabilis; Enterobacter; Klebsiella; Pseudomonas*; anaerobic streptococci and bacteriodes; and *Clostridium perfringens*.

Data from pulmonary artery catheterization must be interpreted with caution in the diagnosis of sepsis in the gravid patient. Tachycardia, hypotension, low SVR and increased cardiac output, all signs of sepsis, may be seen to some degree in normal pregnant patients. Extreme values and rapid changes in hemodynamic parameters, however, suggest infection. As in other patients with sepsis, the risk of adult respiratory distress syndrome (ARDS) and DIC is increased.

Thorough culturing and evaluation of pelvic sites should be performed. Empirical antibiotic therapy to cover what is typically a polymicrobial infection shoud be given until specific bacteriologic cultures are available (e.g., cefoxitin, ampicillin-sulbactam). It is best to avoid aminoglycosides due to their potential fetal oto- and nephrotoxicities. Surgical drainage of pelvic and abdominal sources may be required.

Mechanical ventilatory support should be instituted if needed. Evidence of hypoperfusion requires optimization of volume status; pulmonary artery catheterization should be performed to guide this therapy due to the risk of precipitating low pressure pulmonary edema. Inotropic agents such as dobutamine may be of use in patients with abnormal ventricular function. Inotropic and vasoactive drugs are of less clear benefit in patients with high cardiac output, and may decrease placental blood flow. Elevated temperature should be controlled with acetaminophen and a cooling blanket; shivering induced by external cooling increases O_2 consumption and CO_2 production and should be controlled with sedation and muscle relaxation. Monoclonal antibodies to bacterial toxins and endogenous cytokines will likely play a role in future management of septic shock (see Chap. 37).

Preeclampsia-Eclampsia

Preeclampsia occurs in 5 to 10 percent of all pregnancies and is characterized by hypertension, proteinuria, and generalized edema. Preeclampsia may lead to a convulsive and potentially lethal phase, termed eclampsia, without warning. The hypertension observed in preeclampsia is labile, and the condition is characterized by diffuse vascular and possibly vascular endothelial dysfunction. Hemoconcentration, in part due to increased vascular permeability, occurs along with decreased renal and placental perfusion. Occasional patients develop a life-threatening thrombotic microangiopathy with evidence of thrombocytopenia and microangiopathic hemolytic anemia. Some of these patients fall into the category of the HELLP syndrome (*h*ypertension, *e*levated *l*iver enzymes, *l*ow *p*latelets), and may present with significant liver tenderness suggesting an acute abdomen. This is important to recognize since surgical intervention can be catastrophic.

Risk factors for the development of eclampsia include systolic or diastolic pressures > 160 and 110 mmHg respectively, headache, visual disturbances, epigastric pain, pulmonary edema, cyanosis, marked hemoconcentration, heavy proteinuria or renal dysfunction, and evidence of thrombotic microangiopathy (i.e. HELLP syndrome). However, a significant proportion of eclamptics may have minimal symptoms and elevations of blood pressure prior to convulsing.

Delivery is the therapy of choice in preeclamptic patients beyond the 36th week of pregnancy who have evidence of advanced disease (e.g., thrombocytopenia, elevated liver function tests). Hypertension (diastolic > 100 mmHg) should be treated with methyldopa as a first line agent. Hydralazine is the drug of second choice and may also be added to methyldopa for control of more severe hypertension. Nifedipine, labetalol, and diazoxide should be used only in patients who do not respond to methyldopa or hydralazine. *Nitroprusside is relatively, and converting-enzyme inhibitors are absolutely contraindicated in pregnancy*. Diuretics should not be used as they may add to reduced intravascular volume. Magnesium sulfate should be instituted to treat and prevent eclamptic convulsions.

Cardiopulmonary Resuscitation

Pregnancy limits the ability to adequately perform CPR due to impedance of venous return and arterial perfusion, and increased intrathoracic pressure caused by the gravid uterus. These considerations have prompted the following modifications to the usual approach in administration of CPR to the pregnant patient: **1.** the pregnant patient should receive standard CPR while being placed in the left lateral decubitus position to decrease aortocaval compression by the uterus, and **2.** if standard closed chest compression cannot generate a pulse, especially in late pregnancy, open-chest massage and emergency cesarean section should be considered. To facilitate this plan, obstetric, medical, and anesthesia staff need to be notified quickly of any circulatory deterioration of a critically ill gravida.

RESPIRATORY DISORDERS OF PREGNANCY

Ventilatory Failure

Asthma remains the most common respiratory problem encountered in pregnancy, though improved medical care has allowed patients with other chronic lung diseases to successfully bear children. When these conditions necessitate the institution of mechanical ventilatory support, attention to the unique cardiopulmonary physiology of pregnancy must be observed.

Mechanical Ventilation

Pregnancy increases the risk of airway management complications. Upper airway edema is common, and the highly vascularized upper airway may bleed from minor trauma. An increased risk of aspiration may exist due to delayed gastric emptying, increased intraabdominal pressure, and diminished competence of the gastroesophageal sphincter. Accordingly, airway management should include early and elective intubation by a skilled individual whenever possible. Other potentially useful measures include use of a relatively small endotracheal tube (6 to 7 mm), and use of cricoid pressure to minimize pulmonary aspiration.

Ventilator settings should be aimed at achieving eucapnia, which in this population is a P_{CO_2} of 28 to 35 mmHg. Alkalosis should be avoided due to the potential for decreasing uteroplacental blood flow. Initial guidelines include tidal volumes of 10 mL/kg and rates of 15 to 18 breaths/min. In patients with asthma, smaller tidal volumes will minimize the adverse effect of intrinsic positive pressure ventilation (PEEP) (see Chap. 32). In patients with stiff lungs (e.g., pulmonary edema, ARDS), smaller tidal volumes should be used to lower high airway pressures and decrease the risk of barotrauma. When toxic levels of oxygen are required due to a diffuse lung lesion, sufficient PEEP should be added to correct arterial hypoxemia on a nontoxic fraction of inspired oxygen ($FI_{O_2} \leq 0.6$). The patients should be placed in a lateral position when possible to maximize venous return. The use of PEEP, sighs, and alternating lateral position may minimize atelectasis. In unstable patients with severe lung lesions, muscle relaxation and sedation will decrease oxygen consumption and assist in stabilization. Pancuronium bromide and morphine sulfate are without adverse fetal effects with short-term use. Benzodiazepines increase the risk of cleft palate when used in early pregnancy. These agents all cross the placenta and, if given near delivery, will necessitate immediate intubation of the neonate.

Asthma

Pregnancy does not appear to alter the course of asthma in most patients. Adverse effects on maternal or fetal well being are uncommon, unless the asthma is poorly controlled. Thus, control of asthma and prevention of acute exacerbations are the most important factors in preventing poor outcomes such as fetal prematurity, and perinatal and maternal mortality.

The management of the pregnant patient with status asthmaticus is similar to that of the nonpregnant patient with a few exceptions. Even mild hypoxemia should be avoided due to potential detrimental effects on the fetus. Evaluation for, and prompt treatment of hypoxemia should be routine. Since baseline P_{CO_2} is decreased in pregnancy, an arterial blood-gas determination which shows a P_{CO_2} > 35 mmHg during status asthmaticus should alert the physician to impending ventilatory failure.

Most drugs used to treat asthma are considered safe for use during pregnancy. Inhaled β-agonists have been demonstrated safe and are standard therapy. Parenteral epinephrine should be limited to situations where inhaled bronchodilators have been ineffective due to the potential for decreased uteroplacental perfusion. Parenteral terbutaline may inhibit labor and precipitate pulmonary edema if given near term. Theophylline is safe during pregnancy with the only risk being neonatal theophylline toxicity when given at the time of delivery. Theophylline clearance is decreased in the third trimester so doses may require adjustment. Patients who do not respond to inhaled bronchodilators and theophylline should receive parenteral steroids. Adverse fetal effects due to corticosteroids appear to be rare. There is no definitive evidence to suggest that termination of pregnancy improves maternal outcome in asthma.

Chronic Lung Disease

Most chronic pulmonary diseases that can result in ventilatory failure, such as cystic fibrosis, kyphoscoliosis, neuromuscular diseases, pulmonary fibrosis, and chronic obstructive pulmonary disease (COPD), are uncommon in pregnancy. Patients with severe reductions in lung volumes have, however, successfully completed pregnancy. Patients with severe restrictive lung disease and progressive ventilatory insufficiency during pregnancy may benefit from nocturnal positive-pressure ventilation and oxygen administration. Pulse oximetry should be used to screen patients with marginal ventilatory function for nocturnal hypoxemia.

Acute Hypoxemic Respiratory Failure

Pregnancy predisposes to acute hypoxemic respiratory failure from disorders resulting in pulmonary edema such as amniotic fluid embolism, β-adrenergic tocolytic therapy, aspiration, and ARDS (see Chap. 30). Other causes of hypoxemic respiratory failure include venous air embolism and respiratory infections.

Amniotic Fluid Embolism

While amniotic fluid embolism is a rare event, it is associated with an extremely high mortality rate, and is estimated to cause 11 to 13 percent of all maternal deaths. Risk factors include: **1.** advanced maternal age; **2.** multiparity; **3.** amniotomy; **4.** cesarean section; **5.** insertion of intrauterine fetal or pressure monitoring devices; and **6.** term pregnancy in the presence of an intrauterine device. Clinical findings include abrupt onset of severe dyspnea, tachypnea, and cyanosis during labor or soon after delivery in the majority of cases. Shock and bleeding each are the initial presentation in 10 to 15 percent of cases. Pulmonary edema occurs in as many as 70 percent of cases, and has been associated with both left heart failure and increased pulmonary capillary leak. Bleeding due to DIC occurs in up to 50 percent of patients who survive the first 30 to 60 min, and most patients have laboratory evidence of DIC (see Chap. 51). Pulmonary artery catheterization may reveal acute elevation of pulmonary artery and central venous pressure or isolated left ventricular failure.

Management includes immediate intubation, administration of 100% oxygen, and mechanical ventilation with a small tidal volume (8 mL/kg) and rapid rate (24 breaths/min). Early sedation and muscle relaxation may assist in decreasing oxygen demand and achieving hemodynamic stability. PEEP should be utilized early to achieve a $PaO_2 > 90$ mmHg on a $FIO_2 \leq 0.6$. Vasoactive drugs are frequently required to reverse hypotension. Pulmonary artery catheterization and measurement of CO, Ppw and mixed venous oxygen saturation should be used to adjust vasoactive drugs and fluid management to achieve the least Ppw providing an adequate CO. Once DIC is established, appropriate therapy should be undertaken in conjunction with a hematology consultant (see Chap. 51).

Tocolytic Therapy

Pulmonary edema has been associated with intravenous administration of β-adrenergic agonists such as ritodrine, terbutaline, isoxuprine, and salbutamol to inhibit preterm labor. Associated risk factors include twin gestation and concurrent evidence of infection. Pulmonary edema develops acutely, within 30 to 72 h of the initiation of therapy. The development of pulmonary edema more than 24 h after the discontinuation of therapy suggests another cause. Symptoms usually consist of chest discomfort and dyspnea, with physical findings of tachypnea, tachycardia, and crackles on lung auscultation. Positive fluid balance in the hours to days preceding the onset of symptoms is often noted. Treatment should consist of discontinuation of tocolytic therapy, oxygen administration, and diuresis. Response is usually rapid, with resolution of tachypnea and hypoxemia often occurring within hours.

Aspiration

Factors that increase risk for aspiration in the pregnant woman include increased intragastric pressure resulting from external compression by the uterus, relaxation of the lower esophageal sphincter, delayed gastric emptying, and depressed mental status and vocal cord closure from analgesia. Early aspiration injury results from a chemical pneumonitis, and a diffuse lung injury with the development of ARDS may quickly result. A late complication of aspiration is the evolution to bacterial pneumonia, which tends to be focal and polymicrobial and occurs 24 to 72 h after the event.

Prevention of this complication should be the goal of all physicians involved in assessment and management of the patient's airway. If aspiration occurs, treatment is supportive (see Chap. 30). Antibiotics should be given only if bacterial pneumonia develops.

Venous Air Embolism

Venous air embolism is a rare but potentially lethal occurence. It occurs during normal labor, delivery of women with placenta previa, criminal abortions using air, orogenital sex, and insufflation of the vagina during gynecologic procedures. Symptoms include cough, dyspnea, dizziness, tachypnea, tachycardia, and diaphoresis.

Sudden hypotension may occur, often followed by respiratory arrest. A "mill-wheel murmur" or bubbling sound is occasionally heard over the precordium. Right heart strain, ischemia, and arrhythmias have been noted on the electrocardiogram. Patients who survive the initial cardiopulmonary collapse may develop noncardiogenic pulmonary edema.

Treatment includes immediate placement of the patient in the left lateral decubitus position. Aspiration of air from the right heart or pulmonary outflow tract should be attempted with a pulmonary artery catheter. The patient should be ventilated with 100% oxygen to decrease the size of the embolism by removing nitrogen.

Respiratory Infections

Pneumonia occuring during pregnancy is associated with an increased risk for respiratory failure requiring mechanical ventilation, preterm labor, and fetal and maternal mortality. The spectrum of organisms that result in bacterial pneumonia is similar to that in the nonpregnant population. Viral pneumonias caused by influenza virus and varicella zoster are also seen in pregnant women, though it is unclear whether pregnancy increases the risk for these infections, or whether increased morbidity and mortality result when they occur during pregnancy. Coccidioidomycosis is the fungal infection most commonly associated with increased risk of dissemination during pregnancy, especially if contracted in the second or third trimester.

The choice of antibacterial agents to treat pneumonia during pregnancy should include consideration of potential fetal toxicity. The penicillins, cephalosporins, and erythromycin (except for the estolate which increases the risk of cholestatic jaundice in pregnancy) are felt to be safe. Tetracycline is contraindicated, and sulfa-containing drugs should be avoided near term. The risks of amantadine use are unknown in pregnant women. Acyclovir is effective in treating varicella pneumonia during pregnancy when initiated early, and has not been associated with adverse effects; it should be started at the first sign of respiratory system involvement in pregnant patients with cutaneous varicella infection. Amphotericin B has not been associated with adverse effects on the fetus, and should be used to treat disseminated coccidioidal infections in pregnancy. Ketoconozole has not been studied in pregnancy, and should be used only in cases of hypersensitivity to amphotericin.

For further reading in *Principles of Critical Care,* see Chap 88 "Critical Illness in Pregnancy" Strek ME/Hall J

AN APPROACH TO SKIN DISEASE IN THE ICU

Dermatologic disorders are commonplace in the intensive care unit, and a methodical approach must be undertaken to discover the etiology and develop a therapeutic agenda. The skin functions to control the distribution of important electrolytes, restrict the loss of fluids, protect the underlying structures, and insulate against the loss of body heat. Loss of this barrier can quickly lead to fluid and electrolyte imbalance, shock, sepsis, malnutrition, and hypothermia. The examining physician must incorporate visual data to arrive at a differential diagnosis and the final diagnosis is often determined by microscopic examination in conjunction with the history and pattern of injury. The site of the initial abnormality, appearance and pattern of individual lesions, evolution of disease, and definition of possible provocative factors should always be noted. An assessment of the patient's general health, known allergies, previously diagnosed skin disorders, and other significant items of the past medical history are relevant. The lesions in question should be examined for arrangement, configuration, color, consistency, and distribution. An assessment of the overall condition includes the appearance of the entire integument including hair, nails, and all mucous membranes. The diagnostic workup may include gram stain, culture, dark field examination, Tzank smear, and skin biopsy (as appropriate). Withdrawal of suspicious precipitating factors and nonessential drugs, appraisal of the volume status, and aggressive nutritional support are required for the patient with severe dermatologic disease.

LIFE-THREATENING DERMATOLOGIC CONDITIONS

Toxic Epidermal Necrolysis (TEN)

Toxic epidermal necrolysis is classically manifested by widespread erythema and epidermal sloughing that resembles scalding. It may resemble erythema multiforme, drug reaction, or staphylococcal scalded skin syndrome. The precise mechanism of injury is unknown but may be immune mediated. Certain drugs (sulfonamides, butazones, hydantoins) have been implicated. Skin tenderness, conjunctival burning, fever, malaise, and arthralgias are often experienced. The syndrome presents as a morbilliform rash which often becomes confluent and diffusely erythematous, and proceeds to form vesicles and bullae which rupture. This results in large denuded areas on the back, shoulders, and face. Mucous membranes are often severely involved and occasionally target-like lesions appear on the palms and soles of the feet. This disorder often includes a positive Nikolsky sign. Over 50 percent of the body surface area can become involved and complications such as septic/hypovolemic shock, pulmonary edema, renal failure, gastrointestinal bleeding and pneumonia are common. TEN is associated with 25 to 50 percent mortality. Treatment is largely supportive and transfer to a burn unit is often needed. Topical antimicrobials are usually employed until progression of the skin disease ceases. Tissue grafts are routinely used to replace dermis over denuded areas. Corticosteroid therapy has fallen out of favor.

Pemphigus Vulgaris

This disorder describes flaccid weeping bullae on erythematous or normal appearing skin which result in denuded areas of skin. The scalp, mucous membranes, umbilical, and intertriginous areas are commonly involved. The mucosal lesions are painful. A Nikolsky sign is often present at affected sites. On Tzank preparation acantholytic cells are seen, and accumulations of eosinophils in the epidermis as well as separation above the basal layer of epidermis is seen in biopsy material. Direct immunofluorescence shows intercellular IgG and C3. The course of the disease is variable but mortality is greater than 70 percent without proper treatment. Therapy is based upon immunosuppression, (typically prednisone 240 mg/day) and is used until new blister formation is suppressed. Other immunosuppressive agents may be substituted to protect the patient from high dose steroids.

Pustular Psoriasis

Pustular psoriasis is a potentially lethal skin disorder which occurs in the setting of psoriasis and is characterized by extensive generalized erythroderma and pustule formation in conjunction with systemic symptoms. Apprehension, nausea, and shivering may occur hours before existing psoriatic plaques become bright red, tender, and acutely inflamed. Pinhead sized pustules appear which enlarge and coalesce to form lakes of pus. Within a day, the area exfoliates and new pustules appear. Alternatively at some point the process may spontaneously subside. Biopsy of affected areas reveals intense inflammation superimposed on characteristic findings of psoriasis. Suspected etiologies are varied and include infection, pregnancy, sunlight, and drugs (salicylate, iodide, lithium, phenylbutazone, oxyphenbutazone, among others). The disease is associated with the HLA-B27 antigen. This form of psoriasis is treated with frequent application of wet dressings and low-potency steroids which may be used in conjunction with photochemotherapy (psoralen and ultraviolet light). Methotrexate has also proven beneficial; however, oral corticosteroids should be avoided.

Exfoliative Dermatitis (Erythroderma)

Exfoliative dermatitis is an inflammatory disorder in which generalized erythema and scaling occur either as a specific phase of processes (such as drug eruptions and T cell lymphomas) or in the absence of preexisting disease. It has been attributed to drugs (sulfonamides, penicillins, barbiturates, antimalarials, and others), preexisting skin disease, and malignancies with dermatologic manifestations. Many cases are idiopathic and typically begin over the head, trunk, or genitals and extend over the entire cutaneous surface within the next several days to weeks. The skin becomes thickened and dry with scaling and hair loss. Hepatomegaly in this setting is usually associated with drug reaction or preexisting dermatoses. Splenomegaly may suggest an underlying lymphoproliferative disorder. Findings on skin biopsy are nonspecific. Treatment consists of systemic corticosteroids (100 to 300 mg/day cortisone acetate initially and tapered to 50 mg/day) in idiopathic cases when conservative therapy fails. Difficult cases should raise the suspicion of an underlying malignancy.

Erythema Multiforme

Erythema multiforme (EM) is an acute episodic cutaneous or mucocutaneous disease with characteristic target lesions. Two different syndromes are well described. EM minor is a milder form of the disease which has a tendency to recur. EM major is a severe disease sometimes indistinguishable from toxic epidermal necrolysis with significant morbidity due to systemic and mucocutaneous involvement. It is believed to be a hypersensitivity reaction and is commonly referred to as Stevens-Johnson syndrome. Prodromal symptoms include malaise, fever, headache, pharyngitis, rhinorrhea, cough, chest pain, nausea, vomiting, diarrhea, and arthralgias, which may occur up to one week before the skin disease appears. Early signs of EM include red edematous papules surrounded by blanching which enlarge to small plaques and progress to form target lesions with central areas of necrosis with or without blister formation. The distribution is usually symmetrical over the extensor aspects of the extremities and advances to involve the flexor surfaces and torso. Confluent areas of erosion may quickly form over the oral mucosa, lips and bulbar conjunctiva, and the pain from these lesions may cause difficulty in eating and breathing. Severe complications include corneal opacification, synechiae, blindness,

pneumonia, and toxic epidermal necrolysis. Skin biopsy is needed
to establish the diagnosis and shows perivascular lymphohistiocytic
infiltrates in the upper dermis, endothelial cell swelling, widespread
necrosis, and subepidermal blister formation. Treatment with steroids is unproved but is often employed with EM major (50 to 80
mg/day prednisone for 4 to 6 weeks). EM minor usually responds
to conservative therapy with topical or systemic corticosteroids.

DERMATOLOGIC COMPLICATIONS OF CRITICALLY ILL PATIENTS

Cutaneous Reactions to Drugs

The skin responds to a wide variety of insults in similar and therefore nonspecific ways. The mechanism for most drug reactions is
unknown and can not be clinically identified. The literature suggests
an incidence of adverse skin reactions to drugs at three per one
thousand courses of drug therapy. Over two thirds are caused by
sulfonamides, penicillins, and blood products. The only useful predictor of adverse skin reactions is a known allergic response to a
similar medication. Typically these reactions involve urticaria, an-
gioedma, and morbilliform eruptions which begin on the trunk and
progress peripherally. Less common reactions include cutaneous
vasculitis and fixed drug eruptions. The key to treatment is to
identify and discontinue the offending drug. Symptomatic relief can
be obtained with bland emollients and oral antihistamines.

Decubitus Ulcer

Approximately five percent of newly admitted patients develop
pressure sores during hospitalization. Decubitus ulcers usually
occur over bony prominences and are typically the result of excessive pressure for an extended period of time. Anoxia of the local
tissue follows, leading to epidermal and superficial dermal necrosis.
Shearing forces, friction, and moisture contribute to the formation
of pressure sores. Physical examination is important as detection of
early lesions is critical to proper management. Palpation of the ulcer
usually reveals a larger defect than can be appreciated visually.
Classification of pressure sores is as follows: stage 1—reversible
epidermal involvement (irregular, ill-defined area of soft tissue
swelling, induration, and warmth); stage 2—reversible inflammatory and fibroblastic response (extending through the dermis to the
subcutaneous fat); stage 3—full-thickness skin defect (extension in
the subcutaneous fat with undermining); stage 4—penetration into
deep fascia (muscle and bone involvement). Decubitus ulcers carry
a high complication rate, including osteomyelitis and polymicrobial
sepsis. Early lesions can be treated conservatively with usual wound

care. It is critical to relieve the pressure over the area thus the patient requires careful nursing care and turning every two h. Friction and moisture can be minimized with devices such as fluidized beds and sheep skin pads. More severe lesions require surgical debridement in addition to these measures.

Cutaneous Complications of Dopamine Infusion

Extravasation of dopamine can lead to severe vasoconstriction, digital ischemic necrosis, and gangrene. Patients with pre-existing vascular disease are at particular risk. Minor cases may require only topical nitroglycerin; however, if sloughing, discoloration, or skin necrosis occur after local extravasation of dopamine, the infusion should be immediately stopped and affected areas should be infiltrated with phentolamine (5 to 10 mg dissolved in 15 mL NS). This should yield immediate obvious local hyperemia if given within 24 h of the extravasation.

SELECTED CONDITIONS WITH DISTINCTIVE CUTANEOUS FINDINGS

Acquired Immunodeficiency Syndrome

Most dermatologic manifestations of acquired immunodeficiency syndrome (AIDS) arise from severe T cell immunodeficiency complicated by opportunistic infections. Many commonplace skin diseases can present in florid, aggressive, or complicated forms. These include dermatophyte infections, molluscum contagiosum, candidiasis, warts, and huge condyloma acuminata. Persistent herpes zoster may be a reliable indicator of human immunodeficiency virus (HIV) infection. AIDS patients can contract unusual primary and disseminated cutaneous fungal infections as well as mycobacterial infections.

Several types of cutaneous malignancies are seen in patients with AIDS. Lesions of Kaposi's sarcomas are often seen, and there is an increased frequency of oral squamous cell carcinoma, rectal carcinoma, and lymphoma. Oral lesions seen in AIDS patients include the white plaques of oral candidiasis and are a marker of disease progression. Papilloma and herpes viruses may produce oral lesions. The entity of "oral hairy leukoplakia" is a mixed infection of Epstein-Barr virus, herpes, and other viruses that appears as a hairy plaque on the sides of the tongue.

Drug reactions are seen with increased frequency in AIDS patients. Diffuse maculopapular erythematous eruptions are a common complication of trimethoprim-sulfamethoxazole therapy. The combination of KOH and Tzank preparations of skin scrapings in conjunction with skin biopsy with special stains for light microscopy and culture can give a preliminary diagnosis in many of these conditions.

Sepsis

Patients with certain forms of sepsis present with distinctive cutaneous findings. The lesions of gonococcemia are usually few and distributed distally, often near the joints. They consist of a primary macule that rapidly evolves into a small, tender, hemorrhagic papule or umbilicated pustule with a red halo. The skin lesions rarely yield organisms on usual smears and cultures, but they may have positive immunofluorescence studies. Meningococcemia can present with a rapidly progressive hemorrhagic rash associated with palpable petechiae and urticaria or maculopapular eruptions. Bullous and hemorrhagic lesions with central necrosis can occur when disseminated intravascular coagulation supervenes. Skin lesions associated with *Pseudomonas septicemia* include vesicles and bullae, which may become hemorrhagic and progress to ecthyma gangrenosum (round, indurated, painless lesions with surrounding erythema and a central necrotic gray-black eschar). Gangrenous cellulitis may occur in non-pressure bearing areas. Similar cutaneous manifestations of sepsis from other sources including disseminated fungal infections can occur.

For further reading in *Principles of Critical Care,* see Chap 71 "Dermatologic Conditions in the Critically Ill" Karen Timpe Schmidt/Gregory A Schmidt

---

74 | Hypothermia

Edward T. Naureckas

The diagnosis of hypothermia is often obvious as in victims of outdoor winter exposure or cold water immersion. In other cases, however, a high index of suspicion is required (see Table 74–1). Examples include elderly or drug intoxicated patients presenting with depressed mental status during winter months and patients returning to the ICU following a prolonged operative procedure. A reliable measurement of body temperature should be made immediately in these patients.

EFFECTS OF HYPOTHERMIA

A diagram of the progression of clinical events in hypothermia is summarized in Fig. 74–1. Below 30 to 32°C (86°–90°F), shivering ceases, the level of consciousness progressively declines, and cardiac arrhythmias become more common. Other major effects by system are noted below. It is important to remember that most of these abnormalities are best corrected by rewarming.

Central Nervous System

Intellectual function begins to be impaired at 34°C (93°F), unconsciousness occurs around 28°C (82°F), and a loss of electroencephalogram (EEG) activity occurs below 26° to 28°C (79°–82°F). These

TABLE 74-1 Clinical Presentation of Hypothermia

Clear Instances of Exposure
Immersion
Winter outdoor exposure
Postoperative state
Extensive burns

Hypothermia Complicating Other Disorders
Elderly patients with diverse injuries
Prolonged immobility, even indoors
Drug use
  Alcohol
  Psychotropics
  Barbiturates
Endocrinopathies
  Hypoglycemia
  Hyperosmolar coma and diabetic ketoacidosis
  Myxedema coma
Spinal cord injuries
Sepsis

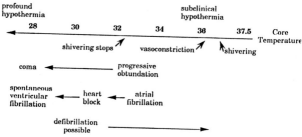

FIG. 74-1

changes to the central nervous system (CNS) are reversible with rewarming.

Respiration and Blood Gas Disturbances

Shivering increases oxygen consumption 400 to 600% above basal rate. Once shivering ceases oxygen consumption also falls markedly. Respiration becomes slow and shallow. Apnea may occur at temperatures below 24°C (75°F). It is thought as temperature decreases humans do not maintain a constant pH but rather allow an alkaline shift of 0.015 pH units/°C. This hypothesis is known as α-stat regulation. In order to maintain this regulation in the ICU, temperature correction nomograms should not be used with respect to pH and PCO_2. However, temperature correction should be used when measuring PO_2 and calculating hemoglobin saturation.

Cardiovascular Disorders

Cardiac output falls progressively below a body temperature of 30°C (86°F). However, blood pressure and systemic vascular resistance are usually preserved down to 25°C (77°F). Arrhythmias present a major cardiovascular problem and include atrial fibrillation, AV block and sinus bradycardia. These arrhythmias occur below 33°C (92°F) and are usually preceded by a characteristic J-junction elevation on the electrocardiogram (ECG), also known as the Osborne J wave. Prolongation of the PR and QT intervals may also be noted. Below 28°C (82°F) the heart becomes easily irritated and ventricular arrhythmias can occur spontaneously or in response to any mechanical, thermal or biochemical stimulus. Until the patient is warmed antiarrhythmic drugs tend to be ineffective with the possible exception of bretylium which may facilitate defibrillation.

Hypothermia also redistributes intravascular volume centrally, promotes diuresis, and causes peripheral vasoconstriction. Thus rewarming may require massive volume infusion as arterial and venous dilation occur. When hypotension persists despite adequate volume challenge, rewarming is the therapy of choice as inotropic drugs tend to be ineffective in hypothermia and are arrhythmogenic. In patients who do arrest, closed chest cardiac massage and intubation should, of course, be instituted and continued while the patient is rewarmed. A trial of electrical defibrillation may be indicated but has a low success rate at a temperature below 30°C (86°F).

Great caution should be applied when pronouncing death in patients who are hypothermic and have not yet been rewarmed. In patients presenting with the clinical scenarios outlined above, the patient should be rewarmed adequately before death is declared.

Other Disorders

Profound hypothermia (below 28°C (82°F)) results in granulocytopenia, hemoconcentration, and coagulation disorders which may or may not be evident on tests such as the prothrombin time or the partial thromboplastin time. Ileus is often seen in hypothermia and tends to resolve with rewarming.

MANAGEMENT

Instrumentation and Monitoring

It is important to measure temperature with a thermometer that can measure down to the severe hypothermia range. Many electronic devices are now available which fulfill this criterion. Measurement at multiple sites including rectal, sublingual, tympanic, pulmonary artery and esophageal, give the best perspective on the patient's overall thermal state. In profound hypothermia it is preferable to monitor at least two sites continuously if possible.

An arterial line should be placed to provide a continuous measurement of arterial blood pressure and to facilitate the measurement of arterial blood gases and other biochemical parameters. The ECG should be monitored due to the high risk of arrhythmias.

Endotracheal intubation should be performed for airway protection in any patient who is not readily responsive and is unable to follow commands. Nasal intubation is usually avoided due to the risk of epistaxis from hypothermia induced coagulopathy. An orogastric tube is also placed to reduce the risk of aspiration. A Foley catheter should be placed to monitor urine output.

Rewarming

The key therapy for hypothermia is effective rewarming. A summary of treatment options in hypothermia is shown in Figure 74–2.

TREATMENT OPTIONS IN HYPOTHERMIA

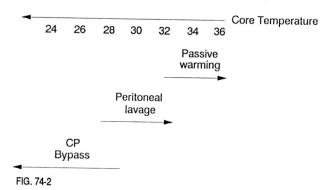

FIG. 74-2

Regardless of what technique is used to rewarm the patient steps must be taken to prevent further heat loss by keeping the patient dry and covered, humidifying inspired gases, and warming IV fluids.

Above 32°C (90°F) most patients will rewarm themselves and passive measures may be sufficient. Below 32°C (90°F) warming should be more aggressive especially in the elderly or in patients with intercurrent diseases. Peritoneal lavage is a practical means of invasive rewarming. Isotonic peritoneal dialysate can be warmed to 43°C (109°F). Gastric, bladder and pleural lavage have also been used. Other techniques such as administration of warm respiratory gases, radiant warmers and warm water immersion tend to be ineffective. In addition, shell rewarming may cause a fall in core temperature in these individuals by reversing peripheral vasoconstriction.

Below 25°C (77°F) or in patients with unstable hemodynamics the use of cardiopulmonary bypass should be considered. This technique can result in rewarming rates of up to 10°C/h (18°F/h).

For further reading in *Principles of Critical Care,* see Chap 72 "Hypothermia" Mitchell F Keamy/Jesse Hall

---

Manu Jain

Elevation of the core body temperature above 38.2°C (100.8°F) is known as hyperthermia. The differential diagnosis includes meningitis, sepsis, hypothalamic injury, thyroid storm, pheochromocytoma, cholinergic overdose, heat stroke, malignant hyperthermia and the neuroleptic malignant syndrome. Malignant hyperthermia and neuroleptic malignant syndrome occur in the presence of a normal anterior hypothalamic set point and they will be discussed in this chapter. Heat stroke will also be addressed.

MALIGNANT HYPERTHERMIA

Malignant hyperthermia (MH) is a true pharmacogenetic disease in that both an inherited predisposition and a triggering drug are necessary to induce the acute clinical manifestations. MH can be induced by inhalational anesthetics such as halothane, enflurane and others as well as the depolarizing muscle relaxants succinylcholine and decamethonium. The pathophysiology is a loss of calcium control which sets off a cascade of biochemical events which leads eventually to extreme metabolic activity, loss of adenosine triphosphate (ATP) production, and anaerobic metabolism.

The clinical presentation of MH varies in severity and all clinical features may not be present in every case. The classic features include muscle rigidity, hyperthermia, tachypnea, tachycardia, cyanosis, hypoxemia, and hypercapnia. One may also see skin mottling, rhabdomyolysis, hemolysis, disseminated intravascular coagulation (DIC), and arrhythmias (see Table 75-1). The onset of symptoms may be insidious or sudden, occurring intraoperatively or occasionally postoperatively.

Management of the acute MH crisis must be immediate and aggressive. The mainstay of treatment is discontinuation of the offending agent, supportive care, and dantrolene (see Table 75-2). Supportive care entails cooling the patient in almost any way to lower the patient's temperature. This could include cooling blankets, IV administration of cold saline, rectal, bladder, or nasogastric irrigation with sterile cold solutions. As a last resort cooling via cardiopulmonary bypass may be considered. Cooling should be halted at 38°C (100.4°F) to avoid inadvertent hypothermia. Other care includes maintaining an adequate volume status, ensuring adequate oxygenation and ventilation, and treating electrolyte abnormalities.

TABLE 75-1 Identification of Malignant Hyperthermia

Early Indicators
  Muscle Rigidity
  Sinus Tachycardia
  Skin Cyanosis with Mottling
  Increased End-Tidal CO_2
  Increased Mixed Venous CO_2
Late Indicators
  Marked Hyperthermia
  Hypotension
  Complex Arrhythmias
  Metabolic Acidosis
  Electrolyte Disturbances
  Rhabdomyolysis

(Reprinted with permission from Bristow G, Patel L: Hyperthermia, in Hall JB, Schmidt GA, Wood LDH, Principles of Critical Care, McGraw-Hill, New York, 1992.)

Dantrolene, which is a specific skeletal muscle relaxant, should be begun as soon as possible. The initial dose is 2.5 mg/kg IV. If no response is seen within 10 min the dose should be increased by 1 to 2 mg/kg until the maximum dose of 10 mg/kg is reached. However, the maximum dose can be exceeded if necessary. The half-life of dantrolene after intravenous administration is about 5 to 8 h. Cau-

TABLE 75-2 Treatment of Malignant Hyperthermia

1. Stop procedure, change anesthesia machine to a vapor free machine, increase minute ventilation to three times normal using 100% oxygen.
2. Give sodium bicarbonate, 1–2 mEq/kg.
3. Give dantrolene as soon as possible, 2.5 mg/kg, intravenously. If no response is evident within minutes, give further doses of 1–2 mg/kg at 10 min intervals. The maximum recommended dose is 10 mg/kg.
4. Cool the patient (surface cooling; intravenous cold saline; irrigation of wound, rectum, or stomach; cardiopulmonary bypass, if needed).
5. Maintain intravascular access. Monitor vital signs and rhythm. Consider invasive hemodynamic monitoring or esophageal echocardiography.
6. Initiate volume loading and osmotic diuretics.
7. Remain alert for coagulation disturbances and hyperkalemia (ECG signs may necessitate therapy before blood tests are available). Calcium should not be given.
8. Observe for 24–48 h, continue dantrolene 2.5 mg/kg intravenously every 5–8 h for three doses, followed by oral therapy 4 mg/kg/day for 2–3 days. Monitor for renal failure, DIC and temperature instability.

(Reprinted with permission from Bristow G, Patel L: Hyperthermia, in Hall JB, Schmidt GA, Wood LDH, Principles of Critical Care, McGraw-Hill, New York, 1992.)

tion must be exercised when using dantrolene with calcium antagonists since together they can cause profound myocardial depression.

The patient recovering from an episode of MH will need to be monitored closely since recrudescence of MH can occur up to 36 h after the first episode. They should also be monitored for DIC and renal failure as late complications.

NEUROLEPTIC MALIGNANT SYNDROME

Neuroleptic malignant syndrome (NMS) is likewise caused by trigger events in susceptible individuals. The major class of medications are the phenothiazines, thioxanthenes, and the butyrophenones. NMS is usually triggered in patients with psychiatric disorders within days of initiating treatment with one of the above mentioned medications. Occasionally, however, the onset of symptoms may be within hours or more rarely weeks.

There are four cardinal features of NMS and they manifest in the following order. There is a fluctuating level of consciousness which may range from random, nonpurposeful movements to coma. Second is autonomic instability which manifests in wide fluctuations in blood pressure and heart rate. Muscle stiffness, the third sign, is of the "lead pipe" variety. Lastly, hyperthermia develops. The most common complications are respiratory failure, rhabdomyolysis, DIC, hemolysis and arrhythmias.

Appropriate treatment consists of stopping the triggering agent, providing supportive care, controlling heat production and cooling the patient. Unlike the management of malignant hyperthermia however, non depolarizing muscle relaxants can be used to decrease muscle tone. Additional therapeutic agents include dantrolene and dopamine agonists such as bromocriptine and amantidine.

HEAT STROKE

Heat stroke is the most serious manifestation of the heat stress illnesses. It is usually related to high ambient temperature and humidity in the unacclimatized elderly. In the young, however, the onset is usually related to exercise and exertion in a hot environment. Certain drugs, notably alcohol and those with anticholinergic effects, can predispose to heat stroke. The clinical manifestations are related to severe volume and electrolyte depletion as well as a rise in core body temperature. Typical clinical features include mental status changes, cardiovascular collapse, muscle stiffness, rhabdomyolysis, DIC, and renal failure.

Treatment for heat stroke should be directed toward life-support and temperature-lowering efforts. Initially adequate oxygenation, ventilation, and volume repletion should be assured. Surface cooling is usually successful but may stimulate shivering. This can be controlled with non depolarizing muscle relaxants or a small dose of a phenothiazine.

For further reading in *Principles of Critical Care,* see Chap 73 "Hyperthermia" G Bristow/L Patel

---

BIOMEDICAL ETHICS

The bedrock of biomedical ethics was laid down thousands of years ago as part of the Hippocratic oath. Beneficence, nonmaleficence, autonomy, and justice are the four fundamental principles of biomedical ethics. Beneficence and nonmaleficence are best expressed as "I will use treatment to help the sick according to my ability and judgement but I will never use it to injure or wrong them." Autonomy means respecting the individuality and personhood of others which allow them to be self-determining agents. Consequently, if a critically ill, definitely salvageable patient who is legally competent and not clearly trying to commit suicide elects not to be admitted to an intensive care unit (ICU) where mechanical ventilation or other life support could save the patient's life and return the patient to a reasonable quality of life, it is the right of the patient through his or her ethical and legal autonomy to decide not to receive indicated critical care treatment. The decision-making capacity lies in the hands of the patient, not in the hands of health care providers. Justice supports the fair allocation of medical resources. At the present time in America, we do not have just allocation of medical resources. A high percentage of health care providers agree with the above and try to practice accordingly.

The American Hospital Association developed a code of patient's rights and this code has been enacted into law in many states. Some of the most important of these patient's rights are: **1.** to receive considerate and respectful care; **2.** to receive information about the illness, the course of treatment, and the prospects for recovery in terms the patient can understand; **3.** to receive as much information about any proposed treatment or procedure as the patient may need to give informed consent or to refuse this course of treatment; **4.** to participate actively in decisions regarding the medical care (to the extent permitted by law, this includes the right to refuse treatment); and **5.** to have patients' rights applied to the person who may have legal responsibility to make decisions about medical care on behalf of the patient.

INFORMED CONSENT

Informed consent is based on the ethical principles of autonomy and beneficence. In order to be considered legally effective, consent to medical treatment must meet three tests (in the absence of an exception such as an unforeseeable emergency). First, consent must be voluntary. The patient (or surrogate decision maker) must retain the ultimate power to accept or reject the available interventions. Second, consent must be adequately informed or knowing. A large minority of states, however, have adopted a more patient-oriented standard, requiring physicians to disclose all the information that the patient would want to know under the circumstances. Third, informed consent is sufficient only when it is given by an individual with adequate mental capacity and legal authority. An incapacitated patient needs a surrogate decision maker. A family member or someone designated by patient's advanced directive may serve as the patient's surrogate decision maker. A written consent form is not the equivalent of legally effective informed consent. Informed consent is the process of mutual communication and ultimate patient or surrogate choice. The written form is only tangible documentation or evidence that the communication process occurred. The legal issues become less dominating and intrusive, and ethical concerns become more central, when the critical care providers initiate and continue sensitive, complete, consistent, and honest communication with their patients and his or her family members.

LIFE SUPPORT AND DETERMINATION OF DEATH

The development of institutional protocols regarding critical care, especially do not resuscitate (DNR) orders, is now required by some states and by the Joint Commission on Accreditation of Healthcare Organizations (JCAHO). Critical care physicians must be completely familiar, and must assure familiarity on the part of nurses and other staff working as members of their team, with their own institutions' formal policies and procedures. The patient or surrogate of the patient may elect DNR that instructs caregivers to refrain from initiating cardiopulmonary resuscitation (CPR) for a patient who suffers an anticipated cardiac arrest.

Traditional standards of death based on cessation of cardiopulmonary functioning are no longer sufficient by themselves in light of modern medical technology that frequently can maintain the human organism almost indefinitely. A person is legally dead when there is irreversible cessation of all brain function (see Chap. 47).

DOCUMENTATION

The courts have held that creating and maintaining accurate records of patient care is an integral part of the duty that a health care provider owes to a patient. The watchwords of documentation are the same from the legal and medical perspectives: completeness, legibility (dictation is preferable, but dictated entries should be read and corrected before being signed), accuracy or truthfulness, timeliness, corrections made in a clear and unambiguous fashion, and objectivity.

The patient or surrogate has the right of access to the information contained in the medical record. A physician who is informed of a patient's or surrogate's request for access to records should offer to go through the record with the patient or surrogate, explain matters to them, and answer their questions.

Risk management programs should incorporate specific activities designed to address legal risks prevalent in the delivery of critical care. A critical care-sensitive risk management program should include the organization and administration of critical care units, the roles and responsibilities of the different professionals having contact with patients in those units, medical records, equipment maintenance, equipment modification, equipment records, analysis of equipment malfunctions, incident reporting, and trend analysis of unexpected incidents.

Perhaps the most influential aspect of effective risk management is the fostering of a positive relationship between the critical care team, led by the physician, and the patient and his or her family.

For further reading in *Principles of Critical Care,* see Chap 45 "Legal Issues in Critical Care" Marshall B Kapp, Chap 185 "Perspectives on Clinical Medical Ethics" Thomas A Raffin

---

INDEX

The letter *f* or *t* following a page number indicates that either a figure or a table is being referenced.